Pharmaceutical Perspectives of Nucleic Acid-Based Therapeutics

Pharmaceutical Perspectives of Nucleic Acid-Based Therapeutics

Edited by

Ram I. Mahato

University of Tennessee, Memphis, USA

and

Sung Wan Kim

University of Utah, USA

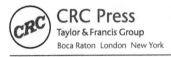
CRC Press
Taylor & Francis Group
Boca Raton London New York

CRC Press is an imprint of the
Taylor & Francis Group, an **informa** business
A TAYLOR & FRANCIS BOOK

CRC Press
Taylor & Francis Group
6000 Broken Sound Parkway NW, Suite 300
Boca Raton, FL 33487-2742

First issued in paperback 2020

© 2002 by Taylor & Francis Group, LLC
CRC Press is an imprint of Taylor & Francis Group, an Informa business

No claim to original U.S. Government works

ISBN-13: 978-0-367-45488-3 (pbk)
ISBN-13: 978-0-415-28385-4 (hbk)

Visit the Taylor & Francis Web site at
http://www.taylorandfrancis.com

and the CRC Press Web site at
http://www.crcpress.com

Typeset in Baskerville by
Integra Software Services Pvt. Ltd, Pondicherry, India

Every effort has been made to ensure that the advice and information in this book is true and accurate at the time of going to press. However, neither the publisher nor the authors can accept any legal responsibility or liability for any errors or omissions that may be made. In the case of drug administration, any medical procedure or the use of technical equipment mentioned within this book, you are strongly advised to consult the manufacturer's guidelines.

British Library Cataloguing in Publication Data
A catalogue record for this book is available
from the British Library

Library of Congress Cataloging in Publication Data
A catalog record for this book has been requested

We dedicate this book to the students from whom we continue to learn, to the patients who have had the courage to participate in early gene therapy clinical trials, and to the fellow colleagues who help keep up the pace.

Contents

Color plates

Figures

Tables

Contributors

Alessandra Poggi
Department of Molecular Biology
Beckman Research Institute
The City of Hope
Duarte, CA 91010-3011

Alessandro Michienzi
Department of Molecular Biology
Beckman Research Institute
The City of Hope
Duarte, CA 91010-3011

Alexander V. Kabanov
Department of Pharmaceutical Sciences
College of Pharmacy
Univeristy of Nebraska
Nebraska Medical Center
Omaha
NE 68198-6025

Alexander L. Rakhmilevich
Department of Human Oncology and
   UW Comprehensive Cancer Center
University of Wisconsin
600 Highland Avenue
Madison
WI 53792

Alison J. Lin
Departments of Materials, Physics and
   Biomolecular Science
University of California
Santa Barbara, CA 93106

Antonios G. Mikos
Departments of Chemical Engineering
   and Bioengineering
Rice University
6100 Main
MS 142, Houston
TX 77005-1892

Arthur M. Krieg
Coley Pharmaceutical Group
93 Worcester St.
Suite 101
Wellesley
MA 02481

Bernard Rayner
INSERM U386
Université Victor Segalen
Bordeaux, France

Chantal Pichon
Centre de Biophysique Moleculaire
CNRS UPR4301
rue Charles Sadron
45071 Orleans, Cedex 02
France

Cyrus R. Safinya
Departments of Materials and Physics
   and Biomolecular Science and
   Engineering Program
University of California
Santa Barbara
CA 93106

David G. Affleck
Division of Cardio-Thoracic Surgery
Department of Surgery
University of Utah Health Science
  Center
Salt Lake City, UT 84132

David A. Bull
Division of Cardio-Thoracic Surgery
Department of Surgery
University of Utah Health Science
  Center
Salt Lake City, UT 84132

David A. Dean
Division of Pulmonary and Critical
  Care Medicine
Northwestern University Medical School
Tarry 14-707
303 E. Chicago Ave.
Chicago, IL 60611

David Zaharoff
Department of Biomedical
  Engineering
Duke University, Box 90281
Durham, NC 27708

Delphine Lechardeur
Program in Cell and Lung Biology
Hospital for Sick Children and
  Department of Laboratory Medicine
  and Pathobiology
University of Toronto
555 University Av.
Toronto, Ontario, Canada, M5G 1X8

Dexi Liu
Department of Pharmaceutical Sciences
University of Pittsburgh School of
  Pharmacy
Pittsburgh, PA 15261

Eric Dausse
INSERM U386
Université Victor Segalen
Bordeaux, France

Eugene W. Gerner
The University of Arizona
Arizona Cancer Center
1515N. Campbell Avenue
P.O. Box 240524
Tucson
Arizona 85724

Fan Yuan
Department of Biomedical
  Engineering
Duke University
Durham
NC 27708

Fanny Santamaria
Institute of Human Virology
University of Maryland
Baltimore, MD

Fumiyoshi Yamashita
Department of Drug Delivery
  Research
Graduate School of Pharmaceutical
  Sciences
Kyoto University
Japan

Gan Wang
Institute of Environmental Health
  Sciences and Department
  of Pharmacology
Wayne State University School
  of Medicine
2727 Second Avenue
Detroit, MI 48201

Georg Widera
Genetronics, Inc.
San Diego, CA 92121

Gerardo Byk
Laboratory of Peptidomimetics and
  Genetic Chemistry
Department of Chemistry
Bar Ilan University
Ramat Gan 52900
Israel

Gergely L. Lukacs
Program in Cell and Lung Biology
  Hospital for Sick Children and
  Department of Laboratory Medicine
  and Pathobiology
University of Toronto
555 University Av.
Toronto
Ontario
Canada
M5G 1X8

Guisheng Zhang
Department of Pharmaceutical Sciences
University of Pittsburgh
Pittsburgh, PA 15261

Heather L. Davis
Coley Pharmaceutical Group
Wellesley, MA 02481

Holly M. Horton
Vical Inc. 9373 Towne Center Drive
Suite 100
San Diego
CA 92121

Heidi L. Holtorf
Departments of Chemical Engineering
  and Bioengineering
Rice University
6100 Main, MS 142
Houston, TX 77005-1892

Hui Wang
Department of Pharmacology and
  Toxicology
University of Alabama
Birmingham, AL 35294

Ileana Popa
Department of Microbiology and
  Immunology
University of Illinois
Chicago, IL 60612

Ilya Koltover
Materials Department
Northwestern University
Evanston, IL

Jean-Jacques Toulmé
INSERM U386, Université Victor
  Segalen Bordeaux 2
146, rue Léo-Saignat
33076 Bordeaux cédex
France

John J. Rossi
Department of Molecular Biology
Beckman Research Institute of the
  City of Hope
Duarte, CA 91010-3011

Kenichi Yoshikawa
Department of Physics
Graduate School of Science
Kyoto University
Kyoto 606-8502, Japan

Kimberly E. Fultz
The University of Arizona
Arizona Cancer Center
1515 N. Campbell Avenue
P.O. Box 240524
Tucson, Arizona 85724

Kyung Soo Ko
Center for Controlled Chemical
  Delivery
Department of Pharmaceutics and
  Pharmaceutical Chemistry
University of Utah
30 South 2000 East RM 201
Salt Lake City, UT 84112

Lei Yu
Center for Controlled Chemical
  Delivery
Department of Pharmaceutics and
  Pharmaceutical Chemistry
University of Utah
30 South 2000 East RM 201
Salt Lake City, UT 84112

Makiya Nishikawa
Department of Drug Delivery Research
Graduate School of Pharmaceutical
  Sciences
Kyoto University, Japan

Masahiko S. Satoh
DNA Repair Group
Health and Environment Unit
Laval University Medical Center
CHUQ
Faculty of Medicine
Laval University
2705 boul. Laurier
Ste-Foy
Quebec
G1V 4G2
Canada

Mikko O. Hiltunen
A.I. Virtanen Institute
University of Kuopio
Kuopio, P.O. Box 1627
Finland

Mikko P. Turunen
A.I. Virtanen Institute
University of Kuopio
Kuopio, P.O. Box 1627
Finland

Minhyung Lee
Center for Controlled Chemical
  Delivery
Department of Pharmaceutics and
  Pharmaceutical Chemistry
University of Utah
30 South 2000 East RM 201
Salt Lake City, UT 84112

Mitsuru Hashida
Department of Drug Delivery research
Graduate School of Pharmaceutical
Sciences
Kyoto University
Japan

Jun-ichi Miyazaki
Division of Stem Cell Regulation
  Research
Osaka University Medical School
2-2 Yamadaoka
Suita
Osaka 565-0871
Japan

Natalia A. Ignatenko
The University of Arizona
Arizona Cancer Center
1515 N. Campbell Avenue
P.O. Box 240524
Tucson, Arizona 85724

Nelle L. Slack
Departments of Physics, Materials and
  Biomolecular Sciences
University of California
Santa Barbara, CA 93106

Patrick Midoux
Centre de Biophysique Moléculaire
CNRS UPR4310
rue Charles Sadron
45071 Orléans cedex 02
France

Paul J. Payette
Coley Pharmaceutical Group
93 Worcester Street, Suite 101
Wellesley, MA 024841

Ruiwen Zhang
Dept. of Pharmacology and
  Toxicology
Division of Clinical
  Pharmacology
University of Alabama
Birmingham
AL 35294

Sarah McGuire
Department of Biomedical Engineering
Duke University
Durham, NC 27708

Seppo Ylä-Herttuala
Department of Molecular Medicine
A.I. Virtanen Institute
University of Kuopio
P.O. Box 1627
FIN-70211 Kuopio
Finland

Stephen H. Bailey
Division of Cardio-Thoracic Surgery
University of Utah
Salt Lake City, UT 84132

Suezanne E. Parker
Vical, Inc.
9373 Towne Center Drive, Suite 100
San Diego, CA 92121

Sung Wan Kim
Center for Controlled Chemical
  Delivery
University of Utah
Salt Lake City, UT 84112

Tatiana K. Bronich
Department of Pharmaceutical Sciences
University of Nebraska
Nebraska Medical Center
Omaha, NE 68198-6025

Tetsu M.C. Yung
DNA Repair Group
Health and Environment Unit

Laval University Medical Center
2705 boul, Laurier, Ste-Foy
Quebec, GIV 4G2
Canada

Thomas J. Hope
Department of Microbiology and
  Immunology
College of Medicine
University of Illinois at Chicago
Chicago, IL 60612

Xiaoxin Xu
Institute of Environmental Health
  Science
Wayne State University School of
  Medicine
Detroit, MI 48201

Yoshinobu Takakura
Department of Drug Delivery Research
Graduate School of Pharmaceutical
  Sciences
Kyoto University
Kyoto
Japan

Yuko Yoshikawa
Department of Food and Nutrition
Nagoya Bunri College
Nagoya 451-0077
Japan

Foreword

These are exciting times in the scientific world. There is, in fact, no other time in human history when the public all over the world is fascinated by the spectacular advances in gene therapy, tissue engineering, sequencing of the human genome, and stem cell research. That is all because of the hope these advances, when put into practice, promise to offer in the therapy of debilitating diseases. After the mission to the moon, the human genome project is perhaps the single largest project undertaken by the scientific community. With the entire blueprint of *homo sapiens* in hand, it is now possible to identify all of the genes and the mutations therein which underlie genetic disorders. The launching of the human proteome project has turned functional genomics and proteomics into powerful bullworks, which will give us an integrated scenario of turning nucleic acids into therapeutics. Perfecting the art of creating such nucleic acid-based therapeutics has been a tortuous path. It is only after backfires and misfires that we have reached a reasonable state of perfection in designing safe and effective molecular medicines. However, a long-standing impasse has been the lack of scientific breakthroughs in delivering these genetic medicines to the specific disease targets. The editors and authors of this book are in command of these issues, which have been richly illustrated in this book.

The development of effective gene medicines demands a multi-disciplinary approach. Its success hinges on selfless team work among scientists with expertise in molecular and cell biology, biochemistry, biophysics, polymer chemistry, colloid science, pharmaceutics, and medicine, just to name a few. In the last decade, significant progress has been made in the use of nucleic acids, such as plasmid DNA, antisense oligonucleotides, ribozymes, peptide nucleic acids (PNA) and aptamer nucleic acids for gene therapy. The spatial and temporal control of gene expression of therapeutic proteins plays an important role in determining the therapeutic index.

The editors have assembled a panel of international experts knowledgeable about the intricacies of molecular medicine. This book is an essential guide to aspiring entrants in the various aspects of nucleic acid based-therapeutics as well as a refresher to those scientists already in the gene therapy field.

Vincent H.L. Lee
Professor and Chair
Department of Pharmaceutical Sciences
University of Southern California
Los Angeles, CA

Preface

Progress in molecular biology and biotechnology has created many opportunities for the development of nucleic acid-based therapeutics for the treatment of genetic and acquired diseases. Gene therapy is a method for the prevention, correction or modulation of genetic and acquired diseases that uses genes to produce therapeutic proteins or inhibition of aberrant protein production. In the last decade, enormous progress has been made in various aspects of gene therapy. However, to realize its full potential to treat a variety of diseases, much basic science research and pre-clinical studies will be needed to establish efficacy and safety in relevant animal models of specific diseases. The lack of a comprehensive discussion on most of these inter-related fundamental science issues stimulated a grass root level work, the outcome of which is this book, entitled *Pharmaceutical Perspectives of Nucleic Acid-Based Therapeutics*.

The development of effective gene medicines demands a multi-disciplinary approach, which requires teamwork among scientists with different expertise, such as molecular and cell biology, biochemistry, biophysics, polymer chemistry, colloid science, pharmaceutics and medicine. In the last decade, significant progress has been made in the use of nucleic acids, such as plasmid DNA, antisense oligonucleotides, ribozymes, peptide nucleic acids (PNA) and aptamer nucleic acids for gene therapy. Plasmid-based gene expression systems contain cDNAs and several other elements, including intron, promoter/enhancer, polyadenylation sequences to control the protein production as well as the fidelity and duration of gene expression. The CpG motifs present in bacterial DNA have immense importance in cancer gene therapy and DNA vaccines. The spatial and temporal control of gene expression of therapeutic proteins plays an important role in the therapeutic index. Gene expression plasmids are used for the production of therapeutic proteins, whereas antisense oligonucleotides, ribozymes, peptide nucleic acid (PNA) and aptamers are used to decrease the level of abnormal proteins by specific interference with gene expression at transcription and translation levels. PNAs can also be linked to targeting ligands or nuclear localization signal (NLS) peptides for enhanced cell-targeting and intracellular trafficking. The use of DNA and RNA repair approaches, such as splicing and editing, which can correct a mutation by adding, deleting, or rewriting parts of mRNA transcripts will be of great interest.

Written by international experts knowledgeable about many aspects of nucleic acid-based therapeutics, this book will be an essential guide to aspiring scientists interested in the various aspects of nucleic acid-based therapeutics as well as established scientists in the gene therapy field and related disciplines. This book presents a comprehensive account of the structures and physicochemical properties of gene delivery and expression systems, with emphasis on their *in vivo* applications for the production of therapeutic proteins or the inhibition of aberrant protein production. The level of presentation assumes that the reader has basic knowledge of molecular and cell biology, physical chemistry, organic chemistry, pharmaceutical sciences and immunology. This book is broadly categorized into the following distinct arenas: (i) design of gene expression systems, (ii) modulation of gene expression, (iii) biophysical aspects of nucleic acids and carriers, (iv) intracellular trafficking, (v) nucleic acid delivery systems, (vi) biodistribution and pharmacokinetics, and (vii) clinical applications of gene therapy. Several key scientists consider the potential use of lipids, peptides, polymers, and micelles for the *in vivo* delivery of nucleic acids. The genesis of structure-synthesis-function interrelationships and the evolutionary approaches of these gene carriers are discussed at length. How the components of a viable gene expression system would influence the disease state by controlling gene regulation, transcription, translation and replication are also a central theme of this book. In addition, clinical applications of gene therapy are examined, with an emphasis on cardiovascular and autoimmune diseases, and cancer. Despite early setbacks, we need to reach equitable scientific resolutions and make every effort to reach our goal in treating diseases using gene medicines as pharmaceuticals. We hope that this book will provide stimulation for fundamental understanding of gene therapy and related sciences.

Ram I. Mahato
Sung Wan Kim

1 Basic components of gene expression plasmids

Jun-ichi Miyazaki

INTRODUCTION

Various plasmid vectors, including expression units for mammalian cells, have been developed for various purposes: to produce valuable proteins, to characterize gene products, to analyze the physiological consequences of overexpressing foreign genes, or to isolate genes of interest by screening recipient cells. Recently, plasmid vectors have also been used for nonviral gene therapy, owing to the development of novel gene delivery methods, such as naked DNA injection, *in vivo* electroporation, and lipofection. Various modifications have been added to optimize the preexisting plasmid vectors for such *in vivo* use, although the basic structure of the expression plasmid vectors remains unchanged. In this chapter, an overview of the essential elements of expression plasmid vectors from the viewpoint of their *in vivo* use will be given.

ESSENTIAL ELEMENTS OF EXPRESSION PLASMID VECTORS

In general, expression plasmid vectors are based on prokaryotic episomal plasmids, which are combined with eukaryotic gene transcription elements (Figure 1.1). Plasmid vectors always contain an origin of replication (*ori*) and a selection marker. These constituents are required for the selection and amplification of plasmid-containing bacterial cells, usually *Escherichia coli*. The selection marker is commonly a gene that confers resistance to some antibiotic, such as ampicillin, kanamycin, or tetracycline; of these, the ampicillin resistance gene is the most widely used. The eukaryotic part contains a single or multiple expression unit consisting of a transcriptional initiation element (enhancer/promoter), a multiple cloning site (MCS), and a sequence allowing for transcription termination. In most cases, the DNA inserted into the MCS for expression is not a genomic gene from the original exon/intron configuration, but a cDNA lacking introns. However, most expression plasmids contain an intron with splice consensus sequences 5' or 3' from the multiple cloning site. Apart from these basic elements, some expression plasmids contain additional elements that facilitate replication in mammalian cells. Expression plasmids for *in vitro* use may include a separate expression unit that confers resistance to selectable markers, permitting the isolation of stable transfectants.

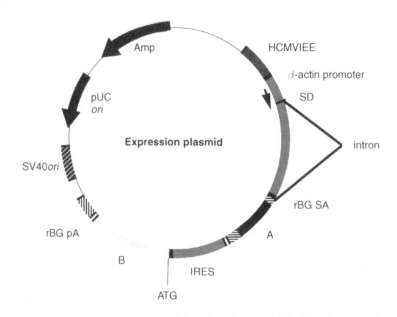

Figure 1.1 The basic constituents of an expression plasmid vector. The promoter and poly(A) addition site are the transcriptional control sequences supplied by the vector. A multiple cloning site for the insertion of the gene of interest is located in the empty vector between the transcriptional control elements. The intron may be located *3′* or preferably *5′* from the cloning site. The expression plasmid shown in this figure contains the CMV-IE enhancer, the chicken β-actin promoter, and a hybrid intron, the *5′* portion of a β-actin sequence and the *3′* portion of a β-globin sequence. This vector produces a bicistronic mRNA. In this case, the A coding sequence, placed in the *5′* portion of a bicistronic transcript, is translated in a cap-dependent manner, while the B coding sequence, placed downstream of the IRES, is translated in a cap-independent manner. Additional elements, e.g. to improve transcription, are integrated between the bacterial elements (resistance gene, origin of replication) and the basic transcriptional control elements. The abbreviations used in this figure are: HCMVIEE, human cytomegalovirus immediate early enhancer; SD, splice donor; rBG, rabbit β-globin, SA, splice acceptor; pA, poly(A) signal; IRES, internal ribosome entry site; *ori*, origin of replication.

TRANSCRIPTIONAL REGULATORY ELEMENTS

In eukaryotic cells, a gene consists of the transcribed portion, as well as the *5′* and *3′* flanking regulatory DNA sequences. Transcription initiation is usually regulated by the *5′* regulatory sequences, which include some common DNA elements. One of these elements, the TATA box (TATAAA), is located 25–35 base pairs upstream of the transcription start site for RNA polymerase II, and its function is to direct the transcription at the so-called cap site (Breathnach and Chambon, 1981). The CAAT box (GGCCAATCT) is known to be present upstream of the TATA box. Transcription is initiated by an interaction between these DNA elements and regulatory proteins.

Another important element is the enhancer sequence. This element was first identified in the SV40 and retrovirus genomes. Many cellular enhancer sequences have since been identified. The enhancers positively regulate transcription from the closest promoter and can act over several thousand base pairs in either orientation. They are usually found proximal to the promoter regions of genes, but are sometimes found within introns or even downstream of the transcribed region. They determine the strength, cell-type specificity, and developmental-stage specificity of the promoter. Enhancers can elevate transcription levels from several-fold to more than 1000-fold. Some enhancers are active in a wide variety of cell types, but others are active only in restricted cell types or at particular developmental stages. For example, the immunoglobulin gene enhancer is very active exclusively in B lymphocytes. The human cytomegalovirus (CMV) immediate early (IE) gene enhancer is extremely active in a wide range of cell types, although it shows some tissue preference (Boshart *et al.*, 1985).

Generally the rate of transcription initiation is the rate-limiting step in mRNA production, because the rate of transcriptional elongation is usually constant, except for some genes in which premature termination or pausing is seen. Therefore, the selection of an appropriate enhancer and promoter is crucial in the construction of expression plasmid vectors. In most experiments, both *in vitro* and *in vivo*, expression plasmids driven by a ubiquitously active enhancer and promoter are very useful. Examples of such promoters include the SV40 early promoter, RSV LTR promoter, CMV-IE promoter, β-actin promoter (Miyazaki *et al.*, 1989), and elongation factor-1α promoter (Mizushima and Nagata, 1990). The CMV-IE promoter has been shown to exhibit very high transcriptional activity in most tissues and cell types (Foecking and Hofstetter, 1986). However, when incorporated into retroviral vectors, which integrate into chromosomal DNA, the CMV-IE promoter is down-regulated, hampering long-term expression *in vivo* (Challita and Kohn, 1994). Furthermore, attenuation of the activity of the CMV and other viral promoters by cytokines, such as interferons (IFN-γ, IFN-β) and tumor necrosis factor (TNF-α), has been documented (Qin *et al.*, 1997). In contrast, attenuation of the activity of a cellular promoter (e.g., β-actin promoter) by cytokines has not been observed.

Heterologous enhancers can be combined with the promoter elements to achieve a desired expression level, or to increase expression. For example, the CMV-IE enhancer has been combined with the chicken β-actin promoter. As β-actin is the most abundant protein in most somatic cells, the β-actin promoter shows a broad expression pattern, independent of tissue or developmental stage (Miyazaki *et al.*, 1989). The CMV-IE enhancer is very active in a wide variety of cell lines. With the hope of combining the advantages of both the β-actin promoter and the CMV-IE enhancer, a composite promoter, designated the CAG promoter, was engineered by connecting the CMV-IE enhancer sequence to a modified chicken β-actin promoter (Niwa *et al.*, 1991). The strength of the resulting promoter was evaluated by a reporter assay after transient transfection into a number of cell lines derived from different cell types. This promoter showed higher transcriptional activity in the cell lines tested than did the CMV-IE promoter, chicken β-actin promoter, RSV-LTR, or SV40 early promoter.

The tissue specificity of an enhancer/promoter can best be characterized by making transgenic mice expressing a transgene under it. It may seem a reasonable assumption

Table 1.1 Structures of selected expression plasmids[a]

Plasmid	Promoter	Intron/location[b]	3'UTR/polyA	ori	Backbone	Reference
pSVT7	SV40	SV40/3'	SV40	SV40	pBR/amp	Bird et al., 1987
p91023(B)	SV40/AdV	AdV-Ig/5'	dhfr-SV40	SV40	pBR/Tc	Wong et al., 1985
pCDM8	CMV	SV40/3'	SV40	polyoma	ColE1/supF	Seed and Aruffo, 1987
pVR1012	CMV	CMV/5'	bGH		pUC/Km	Tripathy et al., 1996
pVR1255	CMV	CMV/5'	rBG		pUC/Km	Hartikka et al., 1996
pCAGGS	CAG	β-actin/5'	rBG	SV40	pUC/amp	Niwa et al., 1991

Notes

a Abbreviations used in this table: Adv, adenovirus; Ig, immunoglobulin; dhfr, dihydrofolate reductase; Tc, tetracycline; Km, kanamycin; bGH, bovine growth hormone; rBG, rabbit β-globin.

b 5' and 3' indicate the location of the intron relative to the cDNA insertion site on MCS.

that ubiquitous promoters can direct a broad specificity of expression when used in transgenic mice. However, this is not usually the case. For example, the RSV LTR promoter is very active in a variety of cell lines, but shows a rather restricted pattern of gene expression when used in transgenic mice. On the other hand, the CAG promoter shows ubiquitously high activity in transgenic mice (Kawamoto *et al.*, 2000).

CHROMOSOMAL ELEMENTS

Two other known factors that affect gene expression are the locus control region (LCR), and scaffold-associated region (SAR). However, when integrated into an expression plasmid, these elements do not affect the levels of expression in transiently transfected cells. Expression levels are affected only after the stable integration into the chromosomes, probably because these elements work specifically in the chromosomal context (Stief *et al.*, 1989; Klehr *et al.*, 1991). In fact, the LCR has been shown to confer copy number-dependent, position-independent, and tissue-specific expression of a transgene when integrated with the transgene, in a transgenic mouse study (Greaves *et al.*, 1989). However, it has been suggested that sequences associated with an origin of replication may increase nuclear retention, possibly by anchoring the plasmid to the nuclear matrix.

Another element, called the insulator, was identified as a chromosomal element that blocks the effects of an enhancer on the neighboring promoter when inserted between them (Muller, 2000). The insulator was also reported to protect some stably transfected genes from epigenetic silencing. The activity of the insulator is believed to be associated with the organization of a specialized chromatin structure. Insulator sequences have been found in the K14 gene, the chicken β-globin gene and others. This element may be used to disrupt the interference between two expression units that have been incorporated into a single plasmid or between an expression unit and viral enhancers in a viral vector (Inoue *et al.*, 1999; Steinwaerder and Lieber, 2000).

RNA PROCESSING

The conversion of the primary transcripts (heterogeneous nuclear RNA) to functional mRNA involves capping, splicing, polyadenylation (see below), and transport to the cytoplasm. These steps also strongly influence gene expression. Splicing refers to the elimination of intervening RNA sequences (introns) and requires consensus nucleotide sequences at the splice donor site, the splice acceptor site, and the branch point (Sharp, 1987). The exon/intron boundaries, as well as the sequences required for the correct recognition of these boundaries are conserved, and primary transcripts from heterologous species in the animal kingdom are usually recognized and processed in mammalian cells.

Most eukaryotic genes contain introns, although some intronless genes are known. When introduced into mammalian cells, some genes have been shown to depend on the presence of an intron for their efficient expression (Buchman and Berg, 1988; Ryu and Mertz, 1989; Yu *et al.*, 1991). Interestingly, the requirement for the presence of introns seems even stronger for DNA constructs introduced into transgenic mice (Brinster *et al.*, 1988). The construct in which the rat growth hormone gene is driven by the mouse metallothionein I promoter requires an intronic sequence for efficient expression in transgenic mice, but not for expression in stably transfected cultured cell lines. In this experiment, it was shown that introns from heterologous genes are about as effective for enhancing gene expression as endogenous introns. Although the molecular mechanisms underlying the dependency of genes on introns for efficient mRNA formation is not known, it is still recommended to include at least one intron in expression vectors. However, the use of introns can create artifacts resulting from aberrant splicing.

The SV40 small t-intron is one of the most commonly used introns in expression vectors and is also one of the shortest introns to produce a lariat branch site complex. During expression from vectors in which the SV40 small t-intron is present in the *3'* untranslated region (UTR), splice donor sites from the preceding cDNA genes may sometimes be preferentially used. Splicing from these sites to the splice acceptor site of the SV40 small t-intron may result in a deletion of mRNA within the protein coding region (Nordstrom and Westhafer, 1986). Splice donor sites in the cDNA could exist as a consequence of splice junctions from former introns. Furthermore, ordinarily inactive splice consensus sequences (cryptic splice donor or acceptor sites) are found in both the introns and exons of many genes. These may be utilized together with introns from expression vector sequences. Thus, introns should not be located in the *3'* UTR of cDNA expression vectors. If introns are included, they should be located in the *5'* UTR of the expression vector. Aberrant splicing between the splice donor site in the *5'* UTR and the cryptic splice acceptor site in the downstream cDNA is much less likely, because the splicing apparatus requires not only the splice acceptor site, but also the adjacent consensus sequence, including the branch point, for the splicing reaction to proceed.

The selection of appropriate introns is important for efficient RNA processing and to eliminate the utilization of the cryptic splice site in the coding region. Introns with splice sites and branch points that closely match the established consensus sequences are spliced more efficiently and accurately than ones that do not. Several introns have been used widely in mammalian expression vectors, including the second intron of the rabbit β-globin gene (O'Hare *et al.*, 1981), and intron A of CMV (Hartikka *et al.*, 1996). Some expression vectors include a hybrid intron, e.g., the *5'* portion of an adenovirus sequence and the *3'* portion of an immunoglobulin sequence (Choi *et al.*, 1991).

TRANSCRIPTIONAL TERMINATION SEQUENCES

Most mature mRNAs have a post-transcriptionally added poly(A) tract at their *3'* end (Wahle and Ruegsegger, 1999). Usually preceding the poly(A) addition site is a sequence transcribed from the sequence AATAAA on the DNA. This sequence, the so-called poly(A) signal, is the most conserved recognition element in eukaryotes. This sequence motif directs the cleavage of primary transcripts approximately 20 base pairs downstream. The cleavage process also requires another, less conserved, normally G/U-rich recognition sequence that is located downstream of the poly(A) signal (Zhao *et al.*, 1999). This sequence, in collaboration with the poly(A) signal, leads to the endonucleolytic attack. The poly(A) polymerase cleaves the transcripts after the U residue and adds 50–250 adenylate residues. Following poly(A) addition, the introns are cleaved and the mature mRNA is transported from the nucleus to the cytoplasm. This adenylation is believed to increase mRNA stability and is the convenient target for oligo(dT) primers in mRNA purification. Some poly(A) sites are promiscuous, which leads to a partial read-through and the production of mRNAs with different *3′* terminal ends. Therefore, in expression plasmid vectors it is important to include an effective poly(A) signal at the *3′* side of the cloning site. Poly(A) signals derived from the rabbit *β*-globin gene, bovine growth hormone gene, and SV40 T antigen gene are commonly used.

Note that termination of the transcription reaction takes place more than several hundred base pairs downstream of the poly(A) signal. The termination site is not known in most cases, and there is no well-defined consensus sequence. After the poly(A) signal-mediated cleavage, the *3′* part of the transcript is degraded in the nucleus. It is not well understood what contribution, if any, is made by the termination signal to efficient gene expression from an expression vector.

STABILITY OF TRANSCRIPTS

Translation of a specific mRNA is assumed to depend mainly on its concentration in the cytoplasm. Therefore, the mRNA turnover rate is believed to strongly affect specific protein production. The turnover rate of the mRNAs of several house-keeping genes is very low, with a half-life of more than 24 hours. In contrast, mRNAs for gene products that are required only for short periods, such as, cytokines, growth factors, and some proto-oncogenes (e.g., c-myc, c-fos), are short-lived, with half-lives of less than 30 minutes. These short-lived mRNAs are characterized by an A/U-rich region, and especially by the repeated occurrence of the sequence AUUUA in the *3′* UTR (Shaw and Kamen, 1986). The existence of these sequences in certain mRNA species has been shown to correlate with the enhanced degradation of the poly(A) tract, leading to a short mRNA half-life (Wilson and Treisman, 1988). However, the detailed mechanisms of mRNA turn-over are not fully understood (Ross, 1996; Wilusz *et al.*, 2001). The secondary structures of mRNAs are also involved in the regulation of the degradation rate.

In most cases, the DNA inserted into the MCS for expression is not a genomic gene with the original exon/intron configuration, but a cDNA. In exceptional cases, antisense RNA or ribozymes may be expressed. cDNA lacks intronic sequences, but still has the *5′* and *3′* UTR sequences. As discussed above, the presence of the *3′* UTR may reduce the stability of mRNA transcribed from the cDNA insert. Furthermore, the length and secondary structure of the *5′* UTR may influence the efficiency of translation. Therefore, it is generally recommended to use cDNA with only short *5′* and *3′* UTR sequences for expression with expression vectors.

TRANSLATION CONTROL

The process of translation can be divided into three stages: initiation, elongation, and termination. Usually, the AUG codon next to the mRNA cap is used to initiate translation. It is thought that a 43S preinitiation complex binds to the cap structure and moves along the 5′ untranslated region until an AUG codon in a favorable sequence context is reached (Kozak, 1989). This process is followed by the formation of a functional 80S complex by the association of the 60S subunit. The idea that a favorable context is involved comes from the results of compiling sequences from around the start codon of numerous vertebrate mRNAs. Two positions near the initiator AUG are most prominently conserved: position −3, which is often occupied by a purine residue, predominantly A, and position +4, which most often is a G residue. Experiments performed to test this model, using mutations at these positions, confirmed their importance for efficient translation, as mutations in −3 and +4 severely altered translational efficiency (Kozak, 1986). One of the most efficient sequence contexts for the start codon appears to be ACC<u>ATG</u>G, which includes the *NcoI* restriction enzyme recognition site (CCATGG).

Codon usage and termination codon context also influence the level of protein expression. For example, clusters of rare codons can severely retard ribosome movement, and scattered rare codons may also exert a negative effect. Rare codons are most likely to be encountered when genes from evolutionarily distant organisms, such as bacterial sources (e.g., the cytosine deaminase gene from *E. coli*), are expressed in mammalian cells, because each organism has a different pattern of codon usage. In these cases, a synthetic DNA sequence encoding the same peptide sequence using codons specific to the appropriate mammalian species will be translated more efficiently (Yang *et al.*, 1996; Andre *et al.*, 1998; Nagata *et al.*, 1999). In mammals, the UGA stop codon is preferred, and the adjacent bases can influence *in vivo* translation termination (Tate *et al.*, 1995). The stop codon may be duplicated or triplicated for efficient termination.

MULTIPLE GENE PRODUCTS FROM A SINGLE mRNA

Certain therapeutic proteins are heterodimers. For example, IL-12 is a heterodimer of p35 and p40 subunits that are joined by a single disulfide bond. Antibodies are heterodimers of heavy and light chain immunoglobulins that are joined by multiple disulfide bonds. Several strategies have been utilized to express multiple proteins from a single plasmid. One approach is to incorporate multiple transcription units, each with its own promoter and RNA processing signals, into a single plasmid. A second approach involves the utilization of internal ribosome entry sites (IRES), usually from picornaviruses, to construct multicistronic mRNAs. This approach utilizes a single transcription unit.

Picornaviruses are positive-strand RNA viruses. The single mRNA furnishes the codes for a long polyprotein, which is further processed to viral structural and non-structural proteins. Picornaviruses have unusually long 5′ untranslated leader regions, ranging from 600 to 1300 bp. In these leader sequences, up to 10 AUGs precede the AUG start codon. Analysis of the mechanism responsible for this unusual translation initiation showed that translation was performed by cap-independent, internal initiation and that the internal entry of ribosomes was mediated by an IRES. The contributing nucleotides of this cis-element in the leader, which is necessary for efficient internal initiation, has been determined. The potential for internal initiation in picornaviral 5′ UTRs has been exploited in eukaryotic expression vectors carrying polycistronic transcription units. This development provides a promising improvement in the expression of heterodimeric proteins.

The major histocompatibility (MHC) class 1 molecule is composed of a heavy chain, e.g., HLA-B7, and a light chain, β2-microglobulin. To express MHC class 1, both subunits must be expressed in the same cell. The inclusion of the IRES allows both polypeptide chains of a complete MHC class I molecule to be encoded by a single plasmid. In this case, the HLA-B7 heavy-chain coding sequence, placed in the 5' portion of a bicistronic transcript, is translated in a cap-dependent manner, while the β-microglobulin light-chain coding sequence, placed downstream of the IRES from encephalomyocarditis virus (EMCV) – a member of the picornavirus family – is translated in a cap-independent manner. Transfection of β2-microglobulin-deficient melanoma cells demonstrated that this bicistronic construct is capable of directing the synthesis of a complete MHC class I molecule (HLA-B7 heavy chain and β2-microglobulin light chain) on the cell surface (Parker *et al.*, 1995).

When the IRES is used, the coding sequence that is located downstream of the IRES seems to be expressed at several-fold levels lower than the upstream coding sequence. Equimolar expression of both cistrons seems difficult to achieve using the IRES, although stoichiometric expression is desirable for proteins built of similar or heterologous subunits. Fortunately, an increased tendency to integrate into oligomers is expected, as the close proximity of both subunits during coupled translation should favor their association. Nonetheless, the bicistronic approach may be best suited for applications where the protein translated in an IRES-dependent position is required at lower concentrations than the protein translated in the cap-dependent position. For example, bicistronic expression vectors have been used to screen high-level expression clones. The second, under-expressed cistron is used as an indicator for the expression of the first cistron.

Furthermore, genes can be designed with two IRES sequences, so as to permit three polypeptides to be encoded by a single transcript (Zitvogel *et al.*, 1994). However, such constructs result in long mRNAs, which may be more susceptible to degradation than are short mRNAs, and may thus result in low expression levels.

Recently, another method has been developed for the expression of multiple gene products, as fusion proteins, from a single cistron called a fusagene, in which linkers encoding cleavage sites for the Golgi-expressed endoprotease, furin, are incorporated between in-frame cDNA sequences encoding different secreted or membrane-bound proteins (Gaken *et al.*, 2000). The encoded proteins are post-synthetically cleaved and processed into each of their constituent proteins as individual, biologically active factors. Transfection of fusagene expression vectors into murine and human tumor cell lines demonstrates efficient expression and biological activity of each of the encoded proteins, such as IL-2 and B7.1, IL-4 and B7.1, IL-4 and IL-2, IL-12 p40 and p35, and IL-12 p40, p35 and IL-2. Thus, the fusagene vectors enable the coordinated expression of multiple gene products from a single monocistronic expression cassette.

MULTIPLE CLONING SITE OR POLYLINKER

The MCS is a stretch of unique restriction endonuclease cleavage sites between the promoter and the poly(A) signal in expression plasmid vectors, and is used as a common area to insert a cDNA or gene of interest. By using the MCS, the genes of interest can be inserted and assayed with ease. Sticky-end and blunt-end vector strands are available at different restriction sites. Although the MCS is very convenient, it should be noted that these sites usually remain in the mRNA transcribed from the expression unit of the vector and may reduce its stability or the efficiency of translation. Furthermore, one must be careful not to produce an ATG codon at the junctional sequence between the MCS and the insert, because it may work as a false start codon in the resulting mRNA and interfere with the production of the correct product.

In some expression plasmids, the MCS may be designed to connect the cDNA insert to specific DNA sequences to produce recombinant fusion proteins, which can be detected and purified without the use of an antibody or other protein-specific assay. Common fusion tags include the following: epitope tags (hemagglutinin, FLAG, and c-myc), reporter genes (green fluorescent protein [GFP], β-galactosidase [lacZ], chloramphenicol acetyltransferase [CAT], luciferase, and alkaline phosphatase), and affinity tags for purification (glutathione S-transferase [GST], calmodulin-binding protein [CBP], and FLAG). Some of these tags are designed to be removed by a cleavage enzyme, either enterokinase, factor Xa, or thrombin. Note that these tags usually have their own antigenicity. Therefore, *in vivo* expression of these fusion products may cause the production of antibodies against the tag portion, thus blocking the biological activity of the products.

PERSISTENCE OF GENE EXPRESSION

Delivery of expression plasmids to various tissues or solid tumors results in transient gene expression with a fast decline in expression levels (Doh *et al.*, 1997; Aihara and Miyazaki, 1998). Therefore, it is important to develop strategies to substantially increase the persistence of gene expression in transfected tissues.

Lack of persistence of gene expression is mainly due to DNA degradation and rapid clearance from the nucleus. The persistence of expression *in vivo* may be improved by using a replication plasmid, a strategy in which replication elements are included in the expression plasmid. In this technique, the ability to replicate may be provided by introducing an *ori* into the plasmid. The best-characterized origins are derived from viral sources, such as SV40, bovine papilloma virus (DiMaio *et al.*, 1982; DuBridge *et al.*, 1985), and Epstein-Barr virus (EBV) (Tsukamoto *et al.*, 1999; Mizuguchi *et al.*, 2000; Mucke *et al.*, 2000; Haan *et al.*, 2001). The function of these viral *ori* sequences requires the coexpression of specific viral proteins, such as SV40 T antigen or bovine papilloma E1 and E2 proteins (Ustav and Stenlund, 1991; Asselbergs and Grand, 1993). However, besides being potentially immunogenic, these viral replication proteins are known to have oncogenic properties, which restrict the use of these viral replication systems for expression plasmid vectors *in vivo*.

Plasmid vectors, including the replication system based on SV40, which is able to undergo a complete replication cycle in certain primate cells, have been developed for high-level expression *in vitro*. For SV40 replication, one of the early viral gene products, large T antigen and the SV40 *ori*, the latter of which is a fragment of less than 300 bp, are required. However, the T antigen has strong transforming activity *in vitro* and *in vivo*, as shown in transgenic mouse studies. In an attempt to overcome this limitation, an SV40 T antigen mutant that is deficient in its ability to bind to human tumor suppressor gene products, such as p53 and retinoblastoma, is being evaluated for its ability to facilitate the replication of plasmids in a safe manner *in vivo*.

Saeki *et al.* (1998) showed by Southern blot analysis that pEB, an EBV replicon-based plasmid containing the latent viral DNA replication origin (*oriP*) and EBV nuclear antigen-1 (EBNA-1), was maintained extrachromosomally in rodent cells (BHK-21) transfected with pEB. When pEB vector containing the luciferase gene was introduced into mouse liver, luciferase gene expression was observed for at least 35 days, whereas it was not detected on day 14 in the liver transfected with a luciferase expression plasmid lacking the EBV sequence. Prolonged transgene expression using the EBV replicon vector system was also shown in mouse kidney (Tsujie *et al.*, 2001). However, it is not known whether this EBV replicon system works in the other tissues or species.

In retrovirally transduced cells, promoters, like the CMV promoter, are known to be down-regulated. Chromatin structure, as well as DNA hypermethylation, is believed to play a significant role in this down-regulation. However, it is not clear whether the same mechanisms contribute to the decline of persistent expression with plasmid vectors.

CONCLUDING REMARKS

Transgene expression depends not only on the type of gene carriers, but also on the components of gene expression systems, which include a transcriptional initiation element (enhancer/promoter), an intron, a multiple cloning site, and a transcription termination sequence. Useful tools such as the IRES have been incorporated into these basic components. A thorough understanding of these components and their functions, together with further improvements of the methods of DNA delivery *in vivo*, is essential to manipulate transgene expression in the target tissues while minimizing unwanted side-effects accompanying the gene delivery and expression.

REFERENCES

Aihara, H. and Miyazaki, J. (1998) Gene transfer into muscle by electroporation *in vivo*. *Nat. Biotechnol.*, **16**, 867–870.

Andre, S., Seed, B., Eberle, J., Schraut, W., Bultmann, A. and Haas, J. (1998) Increased immune response elicited by DNA vaccination with a synthetic gp120 sequence with optimized codon usage. *J. Virol.*, **72**, 1497–1503.

Asselbergs, F.A. and Grand, P. (1993) A two-plasmid system for transient expression of cDNAs in primate cells. *Anal. Biochem.*, **209**, 327–331.

Bird, P., Gething, M.J. and Sambrook, J. (1987) Translocation in yeast and mammalian cells: not all signal sequences are functionally equivalent. *J. Cell Biol.*, **105**, 2905–2914.

Boshart, M., Weber, F., Jahn, G., Dorsch-Hasler, K., Fleckenstein, B. and Schaffner, W. (1985) A very strong enhancer is located upstream of an immediate early gene of human cytomegalovirus. *Cell*, **41**, 521–530.

Breathnach, R. and Chambon, P. (1981) Organisation and expression of eukaryotic split genes coding for proteins. *Annu. Rev. Biochem.*, **50**, 349–383.

Brinster, R.L., Allen, J.M., Behringer, R.R., Gelinas, R.E. and Palmiter, R.D. (1988) Introns increase transcriptional efficiency in transgenic mice. *Proc. Natl. Acad. Sci. USA*, **85**, 836–840.

Buchman, A.R. and Berg, P. (1988) Comparison of intron-dependent and intron-independent gene expression. *Mol. Cell. Biol.*, **8**, 4395–4405.

Challita, P.M. and Kohn, D.B. (1994) Lack of expression from a retroviral vector after transduction of murine hematopoietic stem cells is associated with methylation *in vivo*. *Proc. Natl. Acad. Sci. USA*, **91**, 2567–2571.

Choi, T., Huang, M., Gorman, C. and Jaenisch, R. (1991) A generic intron increases gene expression in transgenic mice. *Mol. Cell. Biol.*, **11**, 3070–3074.

DiMaio, D., Treisman, R. and Maniatis, T. (1982) Bovine papillomavirus vector that propagates as a plasmid in both mouse and bacterial cells. *Proc. Natl. Acad. Sci. USA*, **79**, 4030–4034.

Doh, S.G., Vahlsing, H.L., Hartikka, J., Liang, X. and Manthorpe, M. (1997) Spatial-temporal patterns of gene expression in mouse skeletal muscle after injection of lacZ plasmid DNA. *Gene Ther.*, **4**, 648–663.

DuBridge, R.B., Lusky, M., Botchan, M.R. and Calos, M.P. (1985) Amplification of a bovine papillomavirus-simian virus 40 chimera. *J. Virol.*, **56**, 625–627.

Foecking, M.K. and Hofstetter, H. (1986) Powerful and versatile enhancer-promoter unit for mammalian expression vectors. *Gene*, **45**, 101–105.

Gaken, J., Jiang, J., Daniel, K., van Berkel, E., Hughes, C., Kuiper, M. *et al.* (2000) Fusagene vectors: a novel strategy for the expression of multiple genes from a single cistron. *Gene Ther.*, **7**, 1979–1985.

Greaves, D.R., Wilson, F.D., Lang, G. and Kioussis, D. (1989), Human CD2 3' flanking sequence confer high-level, T cell-specific position-independent gene expression in transgenic mice. *Cell*, **56**, 979–986.

Haan, K.M., Aiyar, A. and Longnecker, R. (2001) Establishment of latent Epstein-Barr virus infection and stable episomal maintenance in murine B-cell lines. *J. Virol.*, **75**, 3016–3020.

Hartikka, J., Sawdey, M., Cornefert-Jensen, F., Margalith, M., Barnhart, K., Nolasco, M. *et al.* (1996) An improved plasmid DNA expression vector for direct injection into skeletal muscle. *Hum. Gene Ther.*, **7**, 1205–1217.

Inoue, T., Yamaza, H., Sakai, Y., Mizuno, S., Ohno, M., Hamasaki, N. *et al.* (1999) Position-independent human beta-globin gene expression mediated by a recombinant adeno-associated virus vector carrying the chicken beta-globin insulator. *J. Hum. Genet.*, **44**, 152–162.

Kawamoto, S., Niwa, H., Tashiro, F., Sano, S., Kondoh, G., Takeda, J. *et al.* (2000) A novel reporter mouse strain that expresses enhanced green fluorescent protein upon Cre-mediated recombination. *FEBS Lett.*, **470**, 263–268.

Klehr, D., Maass, K. and Bode, J. (1991) Scaffold-attached regions from the human interferon-beta domain can be used to enhance the stable expression of genes under the control of various promoters. *Biochemistry*, **30**, 1264–1270.

Kozak, M. (1986) Point mutations define a sequence flanking the AUG initiator codon that modulates translation by eukaryotic ribosomes. *Cell*, **44**, 283–292.

Kozak, M. (1989) The scanning model for translation: an update. *J. Cell Biol.*, **108**, 229–241.

Miyazaki, J., Takaki, S., Araki, K., Tashiro, F., Tominaga, A., Takatsu, K. *et al.* (1989) Expression vector system based on the chicken beta-actin promoter directs efficient production of interleukin-5. *Gene*, **15**, 269–277.

Mizuguchi, H., Hosono, T. and Hayakawa, T. (2000) Long-term replication of Epstein-Barr virus-derived episomal vectors in the rodent cells. *FEBS Lett.*, **472**, 173–178.

Mizushima, S. and Nagata, S. (1990) pEF-BOS, a powerful mammalian expression vector. *Nucleic Acids Res.*, **18**, 5322.

Mucke, S., Draube, A., Polack, A., Pawlita, M., Massoud, N., Staratschek-Jox, A. *et al.* (2000) Suppression of the tumorigenic growth of Burkitt's lymphoma cells in immunodeficient mice by cytokine gene transfer using EBV-derived episomal expression vectors. *Int. J. Cancer*, **86**, 301–306.

Muller, J. (2000) Transcriptional control: The benefits of selective insulation. *Curr. Biol.*, **10**, R241–R244.

Nagata, T., Uchijima, M., Yoshida, A., Kawashima, M. and Koide, Y. (1999) Codon optimization effect on translational efficiency of DNA vaccine in mammalian cells: analysis of plasmid DNA encoding a CTL epitope derived from microorganisms. *Biochem. Biophys. Res. Commun.*, **261**, 445–451.

Niwa, H., Yamamura, K. and Miyazaki, J. (1991) Efficient selection for high-expression transfectants with a novel eukaryotic vector. *Gene*, **108**, 193–199.

Nordstrom, J.L. and Westhafer, M.A. (1986) Splicing and polyadenylation at cryptic sites in RNA transcribed from pSV2-neo. *Biochim. Biophys. Acta.*, **867**, 152–162.

O'Hare, K., Benoist, C. and Breathnach, R. (1981) Transformation of mouse fibroblasts to methotrexate resistance by a recombinant plasmid expressing a prokaryotic dihydrofolate reductase. *Proc. Natl. Acad. Sci. USA*, **78**, 1527–1531.

Parker, S.E., Vahlsing, H.L., Serfilippi, L.M., Franklin, C.L., Doh, S.G., Gromkowski, S.H. *et al.* (1995) Cancer gene therapy using plasmid DNA: safety evaluation in rodents and non-human primates. *Hum. Gene Ther.*, **6**, 575–590.

Qin, L., Ding, Y., Pahud, D.R., Chang, E., Imperiale, M.J. and Bromberg, J.S. (1997) Promoter attenuation in gene therapy: interferon-gamma and tumor necrosis factor-alpha inhibit transgene expression. *Hum. Gene Ther.*, **8**, 2019–2029.

Ross, J. (1996) Control of messenger RNA stability in higher eukaryotes. *Trends Genet.*, **12**, 171–175.

Ryu, W.S. and Mertz, J.E. (1989) Simian virus 40 late transcripts lacking excisable intervening sequences are defective in both stability in the nucleus and transport to the cytoplasm. *J. Virol.*, **63**, 4386–4394.

Saeki, Y., Wataya-Kaneda, M., Tanaka, K. and Kaneda, Y. (1998) Sustained transgene expression *in vitro* and *in vivo* using an Epstein-Barr virus replicon vector system combined with HVJ liposomes. *Gene Ther.*, **5**, 1031–1037.

Seed, B. and Aruffo, A. (1987) Molecular cloning of the CD2 antigen, the T-cell erythrocyte receptor, by a rapid immunoselection procedure. *Proc. Natl. Acad. Sci. USA*, **84**, 3365–3369.

Sharp, P.A. (1987) Splicing of messenger RNA precursors. *Science*, **235**, 766–771.

Shaw, G. and Kamen, R. (1986) A conserved AU sequence from the 3' untranslated region of GM-CSF mRNA mediates selective mRNA degradation. *Cell*, **46**, 659–667.

Steinwaerder, D.S. and Lieber, A. (2000) Insulation from viral transcriptional regulatory elements improves inducible transgene expression from adenovirus vectors *in vitro* and *in vivo*. *Gene Ther.*, **7**, 556–567.

Stief, A., Winter, D.M., Stratling, W.H. and Sippel, A.E. (1989) A nuclear DNA attachment element mediates elevated and position-independent gene activity. *Nature*, **341**, 343–345.

Tate, W.P., Poole, E.S., Horsfield, J.A., Mannering, S.A., Brown, C.M., Moffat, J.G. *et al.* (1995) Translational termination efficiency in both bacteria and mammals is regulated by the base following the stop codon. *Biochem. Cell. Biol.*, **73**, 1095–1103.

Tripathy, S.K., Svensson, E.C., Black, H.B., Goldwasser, E., Margalith, M., Hobart, P.M. *et al.* (1996) Long-term expression of erythropoietin in the systemic circulation of mice after intramuscular injection of a plasmid DNA vector. *Proc. Natl. Acad. Sci. USA*, **93**, 10876–10880.

Tsujie, M., Isaka, Y., Nakamura, H., Kaneda, Y., Imai, E. and Hori, M. (2001) Prolonged transgene expression in glomeruli using an EBV replicon vector system combined with HVJ liposomes. *Kidney Int.*, **59**, 1390–1396.

Tsukamoto, H., Wells, D., Brown, S., Serpente, P., Strong, P., Drew, J. *et al.* (1999) Enhanced expression of recombinant dystrophin following intramuscular injection of Epstein-Barr virus (EBV)-based mini-chromosome vectors in mdx mice. *Gene Ther.*, **6**, 1331–1335.

Ustav, M. and Stenlund, A. (1991) Transient replication of BPV-1 requires two viral polypeptides encoded by the E1 and E2 open reading frames. *EMBO J.*, **10**, 449–457.

Wahle, E. and Ruegsegger, U. (1999) 3'-End processing of pre-mRNA in eukaryotes. *FEMS Microbiol. Rev.*, **23**, 277–295.

Wilson, T. and Treisman, R. (1988) Removal of poly(A) and consequent degradation of c-fos mRNA facilitated by AU-rich sequences. *Nature*, **336**, 396–399.

Wilusz, C.J., Wormington, M. and Peltz, S.W. (2001) The cap-to-tail guide to mRNA turnover. *Nat. Rev. Mol. Cell. Biol.*, **2**, 237–246.

Wong, G.G., Witek, J.S., Temple, P.A., Wilkens, K.M., Leary, A.C., Luxenberg, D.P. *et al.* (1985) Human GM-CSF: molecular cloning of the complementary DNA and purification of the natural and recombinant proteins. *Science*, **228**, 810–815.

Yang, T.T., Cheng, L. and Kain, S.R. (1996) Optimized codon usage and chromophore mutations provide enhanced sensitivity with the green fluorescent protein. *Nucleic Acids Res.*, **24**, 4592–4593.

Yu, X.M., Gelembiuk, G.W., Wang, C.Y., Ryu, W.S. and Mertz, J.E. (1991) Expression from herpesvirus promoters does not relieve the intron requirement for cytoplasmic accumulation of human beta-globin mRNA. *Nucleic Acids Res.*, **19**, 7231–7234.

Zhao, J., Hyman, L. and Moore, C. (1999) Formation of mRNA 3' ends in eukaryotes: mechanism, regulation, and interrelationships with other steps in mRNA synthesis. *Microbiol. Mol. Biol. Rev.*, **63**, 405–445.

Zitvogel, L., Tahara, H., Cai, Q., Storkus, W.J., Muller, G., Wolf, S.F. *et al.* (1994) Construction and characterization of retroviral vectors expressing biologically active human interleukin-12. *Hum. Gene Ther.*, **5**, 1493–1506.

2 Inducible gene expression strategies in gene therapy

*Eugene W. Gerner, Natalia A. Ignatenko
and Kimberly E. Fultz*

INTRODUCTION

Inducible expression of therapeutic gene products may be advantageous in certain applications of gene therapies (Castro *et al.*, 2000). For example, systemic treatment with antitumor cytokines like tumor necrosis factor (TNF) can be extremely toxic, making alternate methods of delivery of this cytokine necessary (Curnis *et al.*, 2000). Inducible, or conditional, expression of TNF in the regions surrounding tumors has the advantage of reducing systemic toxicity while retaining the anticancer effect (Weichselbaum *et al.*, 1994). Local delivery strategies, such as therapeutics encapsulated in liposomes, can reduce some systemic toxicity. However, locally delivered gene therapies using constitutive promoters still face the problem of the diffusion of potentially toxic gene products over time, and consequent regional or systemic toxicity (Crystal, 1999). Inducible gene expression strategies offer additional modes of regulation to optimize the delivery of gene products to target sites, while minimizing regional and systemic toxicities associated with the same gene products.

GENERAL APPROACHES

Conditional expression of therapeutic genes can be accomplished by a number of strategies. As depicted in Figure 2.1, multiple processes regulate gene expression. These processes affect gene transcription, RNA processing, translation and protein stability. Conceptually, any of these processes can be manipulated in therapeutic gene induction strategies. Combinations of strategies influencing more than one process may be beneficial.

Strategies for inducible gene transcription may affect any one of the general processes influencing levels of functional RNA. These processes include transcriptional preinitiation, initiation, promoter clearance, elongation, and termination (Shilatifard, 1998). Methods to modulate transcriptional initiation generally involve placing therapeutic genes under the control of promoters, which respond to specific physiological (e.g., hormones, growth factors) or environmental (e.g., physical stresses) stimuli (Green, 2000). These promoters contain specific DNA sequences, which respond to unique transacting factors (Leppa and Sistonen, 1997). Transcription elongation can be regulated to facilitate inducible gene expression. For example, the *Tat* gene of the human immunodeficiency virus (HIV)

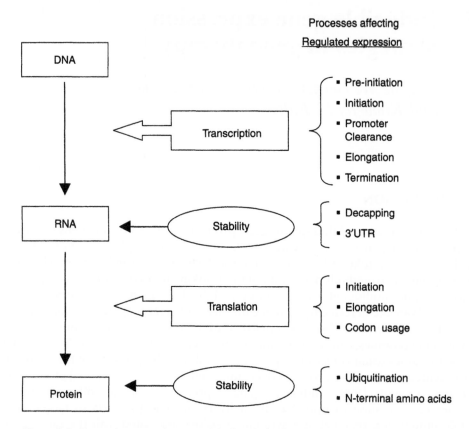

Figure 2.1 General approaches to achieving inducible gene expression in nucleic acid-based therapeutic strategies.

recognizes a stem loop RNA structure in the 5′ region of HIV transcripts. This recognition recruits other proteins, which promote transcription elongation of HIV messages (Roebuck and Saifuddin, 1999). Transcriptional attenuation or termination of gene expression are important regulatory processes in bacteria and animal cells (Spencer and Groudine, 1990; Yanofsky *et al.*, 1996). Strategies that artificially attenuate or terminate specific gene expression are being developed for applications in gene therapies (Morishita *et al.*, 1998; Ohi *et al.*, 1990; Rivera *et al.*, 1996).

An alternate approach to modification of therapeutic gene transcription is to modulate the stability of transcribed RNA. Examples of approaches to degrade RNAs have utilized DNA–RNA chimeric ribozymes (Teng *et al.*, 2000). Recent studies have identified unique regions in *3′* untranslated regions of natural genes (Guhaniyogi and Brewer, 2001). Therapeutic genes could be engineered to manipulate RNA regions required for degradation that would influence the stability of messenger RNAs transcribed from the therapeutic gene. An example of such a region would be AU-like response elements (AREs), which have been shown to regulate the stability of a number of messenger RNAs in mammalian tissues (Tierney and Medcalf, 2001).

Strategies for conditionally inducing gene expression could target other cellular processes, including translation or mechanisms affecting the stability of protein products translated from therapeutic genes. Recent studies describe the use of multiple internal ribosome entry sites (IRES) to enhance the expression of genes at the translational level (Owens *et al.*, 2001). Codon usage can also be altered to enhance, or suppress, gene expression in species specific manners (Zolotukhin *et al.*, 1996). Regulated degradation can drastically alter levels of certain proteins. Ubiquitin-dependent degradation can be influenced by amino-terminal amino acids and is one mode of regulated protein degradation in eukaryotic cells (Varshavsky *et al.*, 2000).

This chapter will focus on the application of inducible gene promoters to achieve inducible gene expression, although it is recognized that other strategies offer specific advantages for particular applications. At the end of the chapter, several approaches combining inducible promoters with other processes affecting gene expression will be discussed.

INDUCIBLE GENE EXPRESSION SYSTEMS

Designs of promoters to drive inducible gene expression systems could involve well understood mechanisms of induction by hormones, growth factors, metabolites and physiological or environmental stresses. Promoters can include several unique elements to achieve optimal application results. For example, in gene therapy applications targeted at specific tissues, promoters can be designed to include both tissue-specific and other regulated elements (Walther and Stein, 1996). Multiple promoter elements can have the advantage of high promoter activities. In some cases, this can lead to the disadvantage of 'leakiness,' or significant promoter activity in the absence of inducer (or presence of repressor). Advantages and disadvantages of 'leaky' versus tightly regulated promoter designs will be discussed at the end of this chapter, after consideration of specific types of inducible promoters.

STRESS INDUCIBLE PROMOTERS

Physical (e.g., heat shock, ionizing radiation) and physiological (e.g., hypoxia) stresses, along with metabolic factors (e.g., glucose), induce specific gene expression by mechanisms involving DNA sequence specific transcription factors (Table 2.1).

Table 2.1 Examples of DNA sequence specific transcription factors that regulate stress inducible promoters now being used in therapeutic applications. Shown are the stress inducers, transcriptional activating proteins and consensus response elements recognized by the transacting proteins

Transacting protein	Inducer	Consensus response element
Heat shock factor (HSF)	Heat shock	GAANNTTC
Oct-1	Ionizing radiation	ATGCAAAT
p53	Ionizing radiation	PuPuPuC(A/T)(T/A)GPyPy
Hypoxia inducible factor (HIF)	Hypoxia	(G/A)CGTG
Upstream stimulatory factor (USF)	Glucose	CACGTG

The regulated expression of inducible promoters offers advantages for selective activation of promoter activity in desired tissues. Activation can be achieved by either external factors (ionizing or non-ionizing radiations in the case of heat shock or radiation-inducible promoters), physiological characteristics unique to certain disease states, such as hypoxia in cancer, or the administration of non-toxic agents, such as glucose.

HEAT SHOCK PROMOTERS

Heat shock promoters regulate the response of cells to alterations in temperature and certain other stresses. The heat shock response is a ubiquitous cellular response to stresses (Gerner and Schneider, 1975; Carper *et al.*, 1987) and results in the induction of a family of proteins termed heat shock proteins (HSPs) (Lindquist, 1986; Lindquist and Craig, 1988). The mechanism of this induction, depicted in Figure 2.2, involves stress-induced denaturation of cellular proteins, which then recruit HSPs from protein complexes containing inactive heat shock factors (HSFs) (Zou *et al.*, 1998). HSFs are the proteins that recognize unique sequences (heat shock elements [HSEs]) in the promoter regions of heat inducible genes. The recruitment of HSPs from HSP-HSF complexes is part of the mechanism of HSF activation and, subsequently, HSP gene transcription.

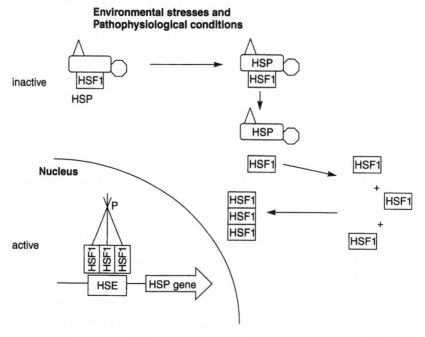

Figure 2.2 Proposed mechanism of inducible gene expression mediated by heat shock and certain other pathophysiological conditions. Adapted from Zou *et al.* (1998). Terminology: HSF1 (heat shock factor 1); HSP (heat shock proteins); HSE (heat shock element in DNA); P (phosphorylation).

HSPs are highly conserved in prokaryotes and eukaryotes, including organelles (mitochondria, chloroplasts), and a number of studies have indicated that HSPs play a significant role in cell survival responses to environmental stresses. The HSPs protect cells from damage, in part, by binding to partially denatured proteins or by dissociating protein aggregates, by regulating the correct protein folding and by functioning as a molecular chaperone for newly synthesized polypeptides (Beckman *et al.*, 1990; Craig, 1993).

The cellular heat shock response can be initiated by physical or pathophysiological stresses, as depicted in Figure 2.2. In most organisms, HSPs are activated in response to sublethal heat shock and other stresses, including UV light and different chemicals. Several HSPs are normally and/or differentially expressed during the cell cycle, and at specific stages of development and differentiation (Carper *et al.*, 1987). In pathophysiological states, HSPs inhibit genetic expression of pro-inflammatory cytokines (Yoo *et al.*, 2000). Induction of HSPs can contribute to cellular responses to tissue damage by oxygen and nutrient deprivation during the ischemic response (Marber *et al.*, 1993). The major stress-inducible heat shock protein is HSP70 (also known as HSP72 or HSP70i). Most cells constitutively express a 70-kD heat shock cognate protein (HSC70, also known as HSP73), which is highly homologous to HSP70 (Craig, 1993). Under normal conditions, HSP70 proteins function as ATP-dependent molecular chaperones by assisting in the folding of newly synthesized polypeptides, the assembly of multiprotein complexes, and the transport of proteins across cellular membranes (Craig, 1993; Marber *et al.*, 1993; Sarto *et al.*, 2000). Under various stress conditions, the accumulation of the inducible HSP70 enhances the ability of stressed cells to overcome high levels of unfolded/denatured proteins. The HSP70 protein can also function as an antiapoptotic chaperone protein that effectively inhibits apoptosis induced by a wide range of stimuli (Nylandsted *et al.*, 2000). Since HSP70 is abundant in malignant human tumors of various origins, it has been assumed that the high expression of HSP70 is a prerequisite for the survival of human cancer cells (breast, colon, prostate, liver, and glioblastoma). HSP70 neutralization by adenovirus expression of antisense HSP70 technology resulted in massive death of tumorigenic cancer cells (Nylandsted *et al.*, 2000).

In mammalian cells, the activation of HSPs in response to different stimuli is regulated at the transcriptional level via a stress-induced activation of specific transcriptional factors, termed heat shock factors (HSFs). The HSFs have been cloned from a variety of organisms. The single gene coding for HSF has been characterized in Drosophila and yeast (Saccharomyces cerevisiae and Schizosaccharomyces pombe), whereas multiple HSF genes are present in higher eukaryotes (Craig, 1993; Sarto *et al.*, 2000). HSF1 has been shown to activate transcription of various heat shock proteins in human and mouse cells in response to heat shock as well as other environmental stresses (Sarge *et al.*, 1991; Schuetz *et al.*, 1991; Mivechi *et al.*, 1992). HSF2 is not stress-responsive, but induces target gene expression during early embryogenesis, spermatogenesis and erythroid differentiation (Sistonen *et al.*, 1992; Mivechi *et al.*, 1994; Sarge *et al.*, 1994).

HSF3, identified in chicken, is induced by c-Myb in the absence of cellular stress (Nakai and Morimoto, 1993; Kanei-Ishii *et al.*, 1997). Another isoform of HSF found in human cells, HSF4, possesses transcription repressor properties *in vivo* (Frejtag *et al.*, 2001). Comparisons of HSF protein structure in these organisms indicate the presence of conserved DNA binding domain and three hydrophobic heptad repeats that constitute the trimerization domain. These domains are located within the amino-terminal region of the protein. The stress-responsive transcriptional activation domain is located in the carboxyl-terminal region of the molecule.

In the eukaryotic heat shock response, HSF1 binds to the conserved regulatory sequences in the HSP gene promoter known as heat shock elements. The heat shock elements (HSEs) consist of three inverted repeats of the sequence NGAAN located upstream of the heat shock genes (Amin *et al.*, 1988; Xiao and Lis, 1988). The molecular mechanism of HSPs activation by HSF involves HSF trimerization upon stress. Hyperphosphorylation and translocation to the nucleus follow trimerization. There, HSF cooperatively binds to the three DNA-binding domains followed by increased HSP transcription (Baler *et al.*, 1993; Sarge *et al.*, 1993). A mutant human HSF1 (HSF*), with the ability to activate a HSP promoter at non-heat shock temperatures, has been reported functional due to the deletions in carboxy-terminal residues 202–315 (Zuo *et al.*, 1995). HSF* provides a useful tool for the activation of HSP promoter in the absence of heat shock.

Heat inducible gene expression systems can be activated by a variety of technologies, all via the production of hyperthermia. Technologies used in clinical applications of hyperthermia include simple approaches, such as water baths, or more sophisticated methods, such as microwave or radiofrequency radiations and ultrasound (Gerner and Cetas, 1993). The magnitude of heat shock promoter activity induction is dependent on both the time of exposure to hyperthermia and the hyperthermic temperature (Gerner *et al.*, 2000). HSP promoter activity is activated by temperature in a species-specific manner. In flies, HSP promoter activity is activated by temperatures over $30\,°C$ (Lindquist, 1986). In human cells, temperatures of $40\,°C$ and above are required to activate HSP promoters (Gerner *et al.*, 2000).

HSP promoters are potent activators of gene expression. The human HSP70 promoter can be induced to activities similar to strong viral promoters, such as the cytomegalovirus (CMV) promoter. This induction requires that the HSP promoter be activated with temperatures of $42\,°C$ and above. However, HSP promoter activation is transient, persisting for periods up to 24 hours after heat shock before returning to the uninduced state (Gerner *et al.*, 2000). Thus, gene expression resulting from HSP promoter activation will be less than CMV, for example, unless repeated heat shock inductions are administered.

HSP promoters are under evaluation using a number of delivery vehicles for therapeutic applications. The adenoviral delivery of therapeutic genes under HSP promoter regulation can achieve high levels of expression in cells and tissues (Brade *et al.*, 2000; Borrelli *et al.*, 2001).

IONIZING RADIATION INDUCIBLE PROMOTERS

Radiotherapy for cancer generally utilizes ionizing forms of radiation. These radiations induce a variety of genes (Woloschak *et al.*, 1995), by mechanisms that are both oxygen dependent and independent. Some of these reported radiation-inducible genes require extremely toxic doses (greater than 10 Gy) for induction.

Promoters, which require extremely high radiotherapy doses (greater than 10 Gy) may not be exploitable in clinical applications.

One ionizing radiation-inducible gene is TNF alpha (Hallahan *et al.*, 1989). TNF alpha is weakly inducible by ionizing radiation via a mechanism involving protein kinase C signaling (Hallahan *et al.*, 1991). Seung *et al.* (1995) attempted to place TNF alpha expression under a more stringent control of ionizing radiation, by transfecting cells with a transgene containing TNF alpha cDNA downstream of a portion of the early response gene EGR-1 promoter. The DNA comprising this promoter, and promoters for several other genes, contains a radiation responsive DNA element. TNF alpha affects the expression of EGR-1 in some cell types, but the nature of the relationship between these two molecules is complex (Mechtcheriakova *et al.*, 2001).

The EGR-TNF transgene was inducible by ionizing radiation (Hallahan *et al.*, 1995). Radioisotopes have also been used to induce EGR-1 regulated gene expression in human pancreatic cancer cells (Takahashi *et al.*, 1997). A difficulty with this strategy is the rather limited level of radiation inducible gene expression using EGR-1 promoter elements. Manome *et al.* (1998) found that promoter activity was increased only three-fold after clinically relevant radiation doses of 2 Gy. There is evidence to suggest that this level of radiation inducible gene expression may be sufficient for certain therapeutic applications. Staba *et al.* (1998) found that the radiation-inducible EGR-TNF transgene enhanced the effectiveness of radiotherapy to control tumor growth in rodent models. The mechanism of this enhanced tumor control involved damage to tumor vasculature. It remains unclear if sufficient radiation-inducible gene products can be produced in human clinical applications to achieve the enhancements found in cell culture and animal models.

Radiation inducible promoters are also found in bacteria and these promoters are now being adapted for use in gene therapy applications in humans. Recent studies indicate that some of these bacterial promoters may be inducible by radiation doses used in clinical cancer therapy (2 Gy per day) (Nuyts *et al.*, 2001), and thus may find applications of gene therapy in clinical cancer management. Like many other promoters being considered for gene therapy applications, these promoters present challenging trade-offs between tightly regulated expression and inducibility. Bacterial promoters that showed the greatest sensitivity to induction by radiation also had the highest basal levels of activity. The promoter with lowest basal activity also was the least sensitive to induction.

HYPOXIA INDUCIBLE PROMOTERS

Many human cancers have regions that are hypoxic, or low in oxygen tension (Blancer and Harris, 1998). Hypoxia can influence a number of cellular parameters, including cell turnover and responses to cancer therapies. Tumor responses to radiotherapy are especially oxygen-dependent (Brown and Giaccia, 1998).

Hypoxia is a pathophysiological stress that causes the induction of specific genes (Blancer and Harris, 1998). Hypoxia-dependent gene expression is mediated by a hypoxia inducible factor (HIF). One member of this gene family, HIF-1, is a heterodimeric transcription factor that consists of α and β-subunits. The β-subunit is expressed independently of oxygen tension in the cell. The α-subunit becomes stabilized under hypoxia and is thus able to bind to the β-subunit and subsequently exert its effect on hypoxia regulated gene expression. When activated, HIF-1 mediates the differential expression of genes such as erythropoietin (Epo) and vascular endothelial growth factor (VEGF) (Shibata *et al.*, 1998).

Strategies are now being developed to use hypoxia-inducible promoters for applications in gene therapy (Rinsch *et al.*, 1997; Shibata *et al.*, 2000). Hypoxia provides not only a means of inducing HIF-dependent promoters, but also a means of selective expression in a pathophysiological state.

REGULATED EXPRESSION PROMOTERS

Metabolic genes

Organisms have evolved complex regulatory mechanisms for metabolic pathways. Gene therapy strategies are now being evaluated in inborn metabolic diseases, in which specific metabolic regulatory processes are altered (Lewin and Hauswirth, 2001). Metabolic genes, such as glucose-regulated genes, respond to a number of stimuli, including glucose and oxygen concentrations. A class of glucose regulated genes, the glucose-regulated proteins (GRPs) encode a family of molecular chaperones involved in protein folding and protein complex assembly (Little *et al.*, 1994). These genes are constitutively expressed in many cell types, but are further induced under stressful conditions. The stress-inducible features of promoters of GRPs, or other metabolically regulated genes, may provide targets for inducible gene therapies (Lewin and Hauswirth, 2001).

Insulin-dependent diabetes mellitus (IDDM) is an example of a metabolic disease under active consideration for inducible gene therapy strategies. In this disorder, inflammatory cytokines have been shown to activate apoptosis in pancreatic beta cells. Experimental studies indicate that expression of insulin-like growth factor-1 (IGF-1) can prevent the cytokine-mediated destruction of beta cells of the pancreas (Giannoukakis *et al.*, 2001). Regulated expression of IGF-1 in human pancreatic islets, to preserve beta cell function, may be a useful approach in the treatment of certain types of diabetes (Demeterco and Levine, 2001).

Metallothionein

Metallothionein proteins are the most abundant intracellular, metal-binding proteins (Andrews, 2000). Four metallothionein isoforms have been identified in the mouse (MT-I–MT-IV) and are clustered within 50 kilobases of each other. In humans, there is one MT II gene and a cluster of MT I genes on chromosome 16 (Searl *et al.*, 1984; West *et al.*, 1990; Heuchel *et al.*, 1995). The mammalian metallothioneins generally consist of 61 amino acids and 20 of these are cysteines (Heuchel *et al.*, 1995). These cysteines are important for the binding of such bivalent metal ions, such as zinc, copper and cadmium.

Metallothionein expression is mainly regulated at the transcriptional level and is induced by various heavy metals, such as zinc. There are seven short sequence motifs located in a region within 200 base pairs upstream of the transcription start site. These *cis*-acting DNA elements are responsible for heavy metal induction and are thus termed metal responsive elements (MREs) (Stuart *et al.*, 1984). Several regulatory proteins have been cloned which interact with these MREs. One of these, MRE-binding transcription factor-1 (MTF-1), is essential for the transcriptional activation of metallothionein genes by heavy metals like zinc and cadmium (Radtke *et al.*, 1993; Palmiter, 1994; Heuchel *et al.*, 1994; Koiszumi *et al.*, 1999).

The mechanism by which MTF-1 facilitates zinc-induction of metallothionein promoter through the MREs is not known, but several models have been proposed. First, zinc may act as a coinducer by binding to MTF-1 and creating an allosteric change, allowing MTF-1 to bind to the MREs. The model proposed for mammalian MTF-1/MRE interaction has already been proven for yeast copper metallothionein systems (Furst *et al.*, 1988). Another possibility may be that, under normal conditions, an inhibitor binds MTF-1. When an influx of zinc occurs, MTF-1 binds the zinc, undergoes a conformational change and is released from the inhibitor. The protein would then have the ability to bind to the MREs. Finally, upon an increase in intracellular zinc concentration, a specific coactivator may bind zinc and interact with MTF-1 to maximally induce transcription.

Since this promoter can be induced by the addition of zinc, it allows for the conditional expression of genes. This induction is especially important if the expression of a particular gene is deleterious to the cell. For example, the adenomatous polyposis coli (APC) tumor suppressor gene was inserted into a vector downstream of the MT II promoter (Morin *et al.*, 1996). Since continuous expression of APC is inhibitory to cell growth, an inducible expression system was necessary to examine the effects of APC expression on cells. This promoter was specifically chosen due to its low basal activity in the absence of zinc. The drawbacks to this system are the potential effects that increased zinc concentrations may have in the cell. These effects may include toxicity to the cell or altered gene expression due simply to the presence of zinc.

Tetracycline/Doxycycline 'gene switches'

Several systems have been established which can regulate gene expression. For instance, there are systems which rely on the addition of steroid hormones or heavy metal ions. However, certain physiologic or toxic effects may result and high basal-transcriptional activity may limit their usefulness (Furth *et al.*, 1994). Another approach has been developed which is based on the tetracycline-resistance operon *tet* from *E. coli* transposon Tn*10*.

This system utilizes a novel tetracycline-regulated trans-activator (tTA) protein. This novel chimera was constructed by fusing the *tet* repressor and the C-terminal activating domain of viral protein VP16 of herpes simplex virus (Furth *et al.*, 1994). The *tet* repressor binds to the *tet* operator sequences to sterically block the progression of RNA polymerase and inhibits transcription. When tetracycline is added, it binds to the repressor and causes a conformational change so that it can no longer bind to the operator sequences. The activating domain of VP16 is known to be essential for immediate early viral gene transcription (Triezenberg *et al.*, 1988). It strongly stimulates transcription from a minimal promoter from the human cytomegalovirus (hCMV) which is fused to *tet* operator sequences.

The fusion protein, or tTA, binds to the *tet* operator sequences in the absence of tetracycline and stimulates transcription. When tetracycline is added, it binds to the

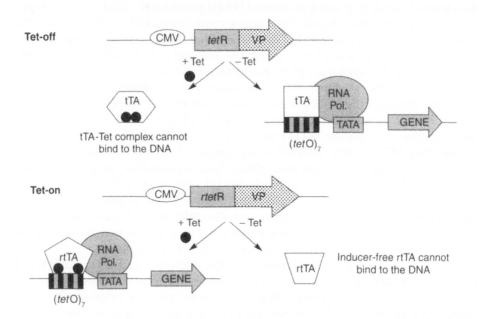

Figure 2.3 Tetracycline regulated gene expression (Adapted from: Applied Molecular Genetics, R. Miesfeld, Wiley publishing, New York, 1999, p. 190). Terminology: CMV (cytomegalovirus); VP (activating domain of viral protein VP16); *tet*R (Tet repressor); tTA (tetracycline-regulated trans-activator protein); rtTA (reverse *tet* transactivator protein); (*tet*O)$_7$ (repeat of 7 *tet* operator sequences); TATA (transcription initiation consensus sequence).

tTA and prevents it from binding to the *tet* operator sequences. Thus, transcription is repressed in the presence of tetracycline, as depicted in Figure 2.3. The gene of interest can be turned off and on simply by the administration of tetracycline, which is nontoxic to mammalian cells and mice (Shin, 2000).

This system is advantageous since *tet*R has high specificity for both its operator sequences and tetracycline (Hillen and Wissmann, 1989; Takahashi *et al.*, 1986). This allows the system to function at tetracycline concentrations well below toxic levels in mammalian cells (Gossen *et al.*, 1995). Tetracycline-derivatives, such as doxycycline, have been shown to be even better inducers than tetracycline. This is due to their increased affinity for *tet*R and high functional stability (Gossen *et al.*, 1995; Gossen and Bujard, 1993). This system is commonly referred to as 'Tet-off' since the gene is turned off in the presence of tetracycline.

A second, analogous system can be used in which the DNA binding domain of the *tet* repressor contains mutations that convert it from a repressor that only binds DNA in the absence of a ligand/inducer into a ligand-dependent DNA binding protein. In this system, the reverse *tet* transactivator (rtTA) has four amino acid changes in the *tet*R region. This mutation allows the transactivator to interact with the *tet*O sequences only when tetracycline is present (Shin, 2000). This system is therefore known as 'Tet-on' since the gene is turned on in the presence of tetracycline. The 'Tet-on' system was developed to rapidly induce tetracycline-dependent transcription because the 'Tet-off' system has a slow transcription reactivation time. This reactivation time is due to the biological half-life of tetracycline and its clearance from animals.

Recent efforts have focused on using these highly regulated gene expression systems in gene therapies for disease. Applications include modification of stem cells (Moutsatsos *et al.*, 2001), treatment of retinal diseases (Dejneka *et al.*, 2001) and immunotherapy for cancer (Nakagawa *et al.*, 2001).

COMBINATION STRATEGIES

Previous sections have discussed a number of inducible promoters and their applications in nucleic acid-based therapeutics. Enhanced regulated gene expression can be achieved by combining several strategies.

We have developed a multiple promoter vector, depicted in Figure 2.4, which utilizes a minimal heat shock promoter to drive the HIV *Tat* gene and a region of the HIV1 long terminal repeat (LTR), containing the TAR element, to drive expression of therapeutic genes. Thus, we are combining strategies affecting transcription initiation (the heat shock promoter elements) and transcription elongation (the HIV1 TAR elements) (Gerner *et al.*, 2000).

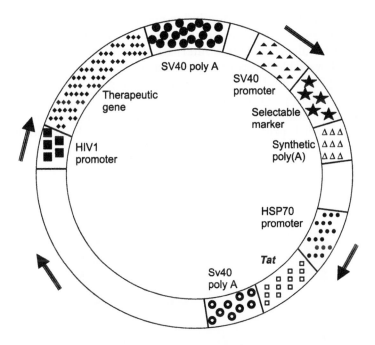

Figure 2.4 Three promoter vector for high level regulated gene expression. Experimental results are described in Gerner *et al.* (2000). Features shown include the minimal HSP70 promoter driving HIV *Tat* expression in the same vector with the HIV1 LTR up stream of a therapeutic gene. A marker gene under SV40 promoter control is included. All expressed genes contain poly(A) sequences to enhance protein expression.

This novel approach has several advantages over single promoter strategies. The major advantage is that it is capable of achieving levels of therapeutic gene production that are greater than by using either of these promoters alone. Second, the levels of achievable promoter activity exceed the activity of the CMV promoter, which is widely used in gene therapy applications, by a factor of five. Finally, the multiple promoter strategy retains heat shock inducibility. The threshold temperature (~40 °C) for heat inducibility in human tumor cells is unaffected and the transient nature of the response is retained.

The major disadvantage of this multiple promoter strategy is that the combination promoter activity is leaky. Positive and negative aspects of leaky versus tightly controlled promoters will be discussed in the next section.

Other research groups are combining stress inducible promoters with the Cre-LoxP site specific recombination system of P1 bacteriophage. Scott *et al.* (2000) have combined the ionizing radiation inducible EGR-1 promoter with this recombination system to express herpes simplex virus thymidine kinase (HSV-tk). With this combination system, radiation doses relevant for cancer treatment can be used to amplify expression of HSV-tk, hopefully, at higher levels and in a more regulated manner than in single promoter systems.

LEAKY VERSUS TIGHTLY CONTROLLED EXPRESSION

Strategies to conditionally induce gene transcription may be tightly regulated, with essentially no gene expression in the absence of inducer (Donovan *et al.*, 1996) or presence of inhibitor (Chevalet *et al.*, 2000). Alternatively, inducible gene expression may be leaky, with variable levels of expression, in the absence of specific inducers/presence of specific inhibitors (see Lieu and Wagner, [2000] for an example). The utility of tightly controlled or leaky promoters in gene therapy depends on the specific application. Figure 2.5 depicts two examples, one in which a tightly regulated promoter is preferable and another in which a leaky inducible

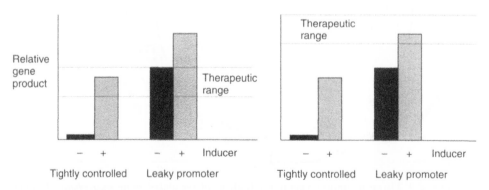

Figure 2.5 Conceptual examples of benefits and limitations of tightly regulated and leaky promoters. Therapeutic ranges for expressed genes are depicted by dotted lines. The left panel describes a situation in which the tightly-controlled promoter achieves regulated expression of therapeutic levels of gene product. The right panel illustrates an example where the leaky promoter is optional.

promoter is beneficial. The common factor in deciding efficacious promoter design is the level of required therapeutic gene product. As recognized by Felgner (1997), efficacy of nucleic acid based therapies often depends on expression of 'adequate' gene product (either RNA or protein products).

A tightly regulated inducible gene expression is advantageous if low levels of gene product are sufficient for the application. For example, certain toxins produced by gene therapy may be required in only a few molecules per cell to induce cell death (Martin *et al.*, 2000). As depicted in Figure 2.5, tight control of gene expression would be critical in these applications.

For many applications in gene therapy, however, a major problem is insufficient therapeutic gene production to achieve the desired physiological response. An example is the attempt to synthesize adequate levels of certain cytokines to stimulate local immune responses in cancer gene therapy (Clark *et al.*, 2000). A leaky, but strong, promoter, as discussed earlier for glucose-regulated promoters (Little *et al.*, 1994) and our combination vectors containing both HSP and HIV promoters (Figure 2.4 and Gerner *et al.*, 2000), may be useful in situations conceptualized in Figure 2.5 (right panel).

The classification of a promoter as tightly regulated or leaky sometimes depends on the context. A promoter containing several response elements may be tightly regulated in tissues where only proteins recognizing the regulated response element are present, while this same promoter could be leaky in tissues making proteins that recognize other response elements.

CONCLUDING REMARKS

Inducible, or regulated, gene expression can be achieved by a number of strategies affecting gene transcription, translation and protein stability. These strategies can be used alone or in combination to achieve the desired levels of regulated gene expression. This review focused on strategies manipulating transcriptional processes, including transcriptional initiation and, for the example of the HIV TAR element, transcriptional elongation.

Stress inducible promoters are under active consideration and investigation in gene therapy applications, and include heat shock, radiation, hypoxia and metabolite inducible promoters. Each has advantages and disadvantages to be considered when addressing specific applications.

Tightly regulated gene expression is attainable in therapeutic applications, but achieving adequate levels of therapeutic gene products remains an important problem in gene therapy. Consequently, leaky but highly active regulated systems may be useful, compared to more tightly regulated, but less active, systems.

ACKNOWLEDGMENT

Varian Biosynergy, Inc. and the Arizona Disease Control Research Commission (#9829) supported some of the work reviewed in this chapter.

REFERENCES

Amin, J., Ananthan, J. and Voellmy, R. (1988) Key features of heat shock regulatory elements. *Mol. Cell. Biol.*, **8**, 3761–3769.

Andrews, G.K. (2000) Regulation of metallothionein gene expression by oxidative stress and metal ions. *Biochem. Pharmacol.*, **59**, 95–104.

Baler, R., Dahl, G. and Voellmy, R. (1993) Activation of human heat shock genes is accompanied by oligomerization, modification, and rapid translocation of heat shock transcription factor HSF1. *Mol. Cell. Biol.*, **13**, 2486–2496.

Beckmann, R.P., Mizzen, L.E. and Welch, W.J. (1990) Interaction of Hsp70 with newly synthesized proteins: implication for protein folding and assembly. *Science*, **238**, 850–854.

Blancher, C. and Harris, A.L. (1998) The molecular basis of the hypoxia response pathway: tumour hypoxia as a therapy target. *Cancer Metastasis Rev.*, **17**, 187–194.

Borrelli, M.J., Schoenherr, D.M., Wong, A., Bernock, L.J. and Corry, P.M. (2001) Heat-activated transgene expression from adenovirus vectors infected into human prostate cancer cells. *Cancer Res.*, **61**, 1113–1121.

Brade, A.M., Ngo, D., Szmitko, P., Li, P.X., Liu, F.F. and Klamut, H.J. (2000) Heat-directed gene targeting of adenoviral vectors to tumor cells. *Cancer Gene Ther.*, **7**, 1566–1574.

Brown, J.M. and Giaccia, A.J. (1998) The unique physiology of solid tumors: opportunities (and problems) for cancer therapy. *Cancer Res.*, **58**, 1408–1416.

Carper, S.W., Duffy, J.J. and Gerner, E.W. (1987) Heat shock proteins in thermotolerance and other cellular processes. *Cancer Res.*, **47**, 5249–5255.

Castro, M.G., Cowen, R., Smith-Arica, J., Williams, J., Ali, S., Windeatt, S. *et al.* (2000) Gene therapy strategies for intracranial tumours: glioma and pituitary adenomas. *Histol. Histopathol.*, **15**, 1233–1252.

Chevalet, L., Robert, A., Gueneau, F., Bonnefoy, J.Y. and Nguyen, T. (2000) Recombinant protein production driven by the tryptophan promoter is tightly controlled in ICONE 200, a new genetically engineered *E. coli* mutant. *Biotechnol. Bioeng.*, **69**, 351–358.

Clark, P.R., Stopeck, A.T., Ferrari, M., Parker, S.E. and Hersh, E.M. (2000) Studies of direct intratumoral gene transfer using cationic lipid-complexed plasmid DNA. *Cancer Gene Ther.*, **7**, 853–860.

Craig, E. (1993) Chaperones: helpers along the pathways to protein folding. *Science*, **60**, 1902–1903.

Crystal, R.G. (1999) *In vivo* and *ex vivo* gene therapy strategies to treat tumors using adenovirus gene transfer vectors. *Cancer Chemother. Pharmacol.*, **43**, S90–S99.

Curnis, F., Sacchi, A., Borgna, L., Magni, F., Gasparri, A. and Corti, A. (2000) Enhancement of tumor necrosis factor alpha antitumor immunotherapeutic properties by targeted delivery to aminopeptidase N (CD13). *Nature Biotech.*, **18**, 1185–1190.

Dejneka, N.S., Auricchio, A., Maguire, A.M., Ye, X., Gao, G.P., Wilson, J.M. *et al.* (2001) Pharmacologically regulated gene expression in the retina following transduction with viral vectors. *Gene Ther.*, **8**, 442–446.

Demeterco, C. and Levine, F. (2001) Gene therapy for diabetes. *Front. Biosci.*, **6**, D175–D191.

Donovan, R.S., Robinson, C.W. and Glick, B.R. (1996) Review: optimizing inducer and culture conditions for expression of foreign proteins under the control of the Lac promoter. *J. Indust. Microbiol.*, **16**, 145–154.

Felgner, P.L. (1997) Nonviral strategies for gene therapy. *Scientific Am.*, **276**, 102–106.

Frejtag, W., Zhang, Y., Dai, R., Anderson, M.G. and Mivechi, N.F. (2001) Heat shock –4 (HSF4a) represses basal transcription through interaction with TFIIF. *J. Biol. Chem.*, **276**, 14685–14694.

Furst, P., Hu, S., Hackett, R. and Hamer, D. (1988) Copper activates metallothionein gene transcription by altering the conformation of a specific DNA binding protein. *Cell*, **55**, 705–717.

Furth, P.A., St. Onge, L., Böger, H., Gruss, P., Gossen, M., Kistner, A. *et al.* (1994) Temporal control of gene expression in transgenic mice by a tetracycline-responsive promoter. *Proc. Natl. Acad. Sci. USA*, **91**, 9302–9306.

Gerner, E.W. and Schneider, M.J. (1975) Induced thermal resistance in HeLa cells. *Nature*, **256**, 500–502.

Gerner, E.W. and Cetas, T.C. (1993) *Hyperthermic Oncology 1992*, Volume 2, Plenary and Symposia Lectures, University of Arizona Press, Tucson AZ.

Gerner, E.W., Hersh, E.M., Pennington, M., Tsang, T.C., Harris, D., Vasanwala, F. *et al.* (2000) Heat-inducible vectors for use in gene therapy. *Int. J. Hyperthermia*, **16**, 171–181.

Giannoukakis, N., Mi, Z., Rudert, W.A., Gambotto, A., Trucco, M. and Robbins, P. (2001) Prevention of beta cell dysfunction and apoptosis activation in human islets by adenoviral gene transfer of the insulin-like growth factor I. *Gene Ther.*, **7**, 2015–2022.

Gossen, M., and Bujard, H. (1993) Anhydrotetracycline, a novel effector for tetracycline controlled gene expression systems in eukaryotic cells. *Nucleic Acids Res.*, **21**, 4411–4412.

Gossen, M., Freundlieb, S., Bender, G., Muller, G., Hillen, W. and Bujard, H. (1995) Transcriptional activation by tetracyclines in mammalian cells. *Science*, **268**, 1766–1769.

Green, M.R. (2000) TBP-associated factors (TAFIIs): multiple, selective transcriptional mediators in common complexes. *Trends Biochem. Sci.*, **25**, 59–63.

Guhaniyogi, J. and Brewer, G. (2001) Regulation of mRNA stability in mammalian cells. *Gene*, **265**, 11–23.

Hallahan, D.E., Mauceri, H.J., Seung, L.P., Dunphy, E.J., Wayne, J.D., Hanna, N.N. *et al.* (1995) Spatial and temporal control of gene therapy using ionizing radiation. *Nature Med.*, **1**, 786–791.

Hallahan, D.E., Spriggs, D.R., Beckett, M.A., Kufe, D.W. and Weichselbaum, R.R. (1989) Increased tumor necrosis factor alpha mRNA after cellular exposure to ionizing radiation. *Proc. Natl. Acad. Sci. USA*, **86**, 10104–10107.

Hallahan, D.E., Virudachalam, S., Sherman, M.L., Huberman, E., Kufe, D.W. and Weichselbaum, R.R. (1991) Tumor necrosis factor gene expression is mediated by protein kinase C following activation by ionizing radiation. *Cancer Res.*, **51**, 4565–4569.

Heuchel, R., Radtke, F., Georgiev, O., Stark, G., Aguet, M. and Schaffner, W. (1994) The transcription factor MTF-1 is essential for basal and heavy metal-induced metallothionein gene expression. *EMBO J.*, **13**, 2870–2875.

Heuchel, R., Radtke, F. and Schaffner, W. (1995) Transcriptional regulation by heavy metals, exemplified at the metallothionein genes. In: P.A. Baeuerle (ed.) *Inducible Gene Expression, Vol. I*, Birkhäuser, Boston.

Hillen, W. and Wissmann, A. (1989) Protein-nucleic acid interaction. In: W. Saenger and U. Heinemann (eds.) *Topics in Molecular and Structural Biology, Vol. 10.*, Macmillan, London, pp. 143–162.

Kanei-Ishii, C., Tanikawa, J., Nakai, A., Morimoto, R.I. and Ishii, S. (1997) Activation of heat shock transcription factor 3 by c-myb in the absence of cellular stress. *Science*, **277**, 246–248.

Koizumi, S., Suzuki, K., Ogra, Y., Yamada, H. and Otsuka, F. (1999) Transcriptional activity and regulatory protein binding of metal-responsive elements of the human metallothionein-IIA gene. *Eur. J. Biochem.*, **259**, 635–642.

Leppa, S. and Sistonen, L. (1997) Heat shock response-pathophysiological implications. *Ann. Med.*, **29**, 73–78.

Lewin, A.S. and Hauswirth, W.W. (2001) Ribozyme gene therapy: applications for molecular medicine. *Trends Mol. Med.*, **7**, 221–228.

Lieu, P.T. and Wagner, E.K. (2000) Two leaky-late HSV-1 promoters differ significantly in structural architecture. *Virology*, **272**, 191–203.

Lindquist, S. (1986) The heat shock response. *Annu. Rev. Biochem.*, **55**, 1151–1191.

Lindquist, S. and Craig, E.A. (1988) The heat shock proteins. *Annu. Rev. Genet.*, **22**, 631–677.

Little, E., Ramakrishnan, M., Roy, B., Gazit, G. and Lee, A.S. (1994) The glucose-regulated proteins (GRP78 and GRP94): functions, gene regulation, and applications. *Crit. Rev. Eukaryotic Gene Expression*, **4**, 1–18.

Manome, Y., Kunieda, T., Wen, P.Y., Koga, T., Kufe, D.W. and Ohno, T. (1998) Transgene expression in malignant glioma using a replication-defective adenoviral vector containing the Egr-1 promoter: activation by ionizing radiation or uptake of radioactive iododeoxy-uridine. *Hum. Gene Ther.*, **9**, 1409–1417.

Marber, M.S., Latchman, D.S., Walker, J.M. and Yellon, D.M. (1993) Cardiac stress protein elevation 24 hours after brief ischemia or heat stress is associated with resistance to myocardial infraction. *Circulation*, **88**, 1264–1272.

Martin, V., Cortes, M.L., de Felipe, P., Farsetti, A., Calcaterra, N.B. and Izquierdo, M. (2000) Cancer gene therapy by thyroid hormone-mediated expression of toxin genes. *Cancer Res.*, **60**, 3218–3224.

Mechtcheriakova, D., Schabbauer, G., Lucerna, M., Clauss, M., De Martin, R., Binder, B.R. *et al.* (2001) Specificity, diversity, and convergence in VEGF and TNF-alpha signaling events leading to tissue factor up-regulation via EGR-1 in endothelial cells. *FASEB J.*, **15**, 230–242.

Mivechi, N.F., Ouyang, H. and Hahn, G.M. (1992) Lower heat shock factor activation and binding and faster rate of HSP-70A messenger RNA in heat sensitive human leukemias. *Cancer Res.*, **52**, 6815–6822.

Mivechi, N.F., Park, Y.M., Ouyang, H., Shi, X.Y. and Hahn, G.M. (1994) Selective expression of heat shock during differentiation of human myeloid leukemic cells. *Leukemia Res.*, **18**, 597–608.

Morin, P.J., Vogelstein, B. and Kinzler, K. (1996) Apoptosis and APC in colorectal tumor-igenesis. *Proc. Natl. Acad. Sci. USA*, **93**, 7950–7954.

Morishita, R., Higaki, J., Tomita, N. and Ogihara, T. (1998) Application of transcription factor 'decoy' strategy as means of gene therapy and study of gene expression in cardio-vascular disease. *Circulation Res.*, **82**, 1023–1028.

Moutsatsos, I.K., Turgeman, G., Zhou, S., Kurkalli, B.G., Pelled, G., Tzur, L. *et al.* (2001) Exogenously regulated stem cell-mediated gene therapy for bone regeneration. *Mol. Ther.*, **3**, 449–461.

Nakagawa, S., Massie, B. and Hawley, R.G. (2001) Tetracycline-regulatable adenovirus vectors: pharmacologic properties and clinical potential. *Eur. J. Pharm. Sci.*, **13**, 53–60.

Nakai, A. and Morimoto, R.I. (1993) Characterization of a novel chicken heat shock transcription factor, HSF3, suggests a new regulatory pathway. *Mol. Cell. Biol.*, **13**, 1983–1997.

Nuyts, S., Landuyt, W., Lambin, P. and Anne, J. (2001) The use of radiation-induced bacterial promoters in anaerobic conditions: a means to control gene expression in clostridium-mediated therapy for cancer. *Radiation Res.*, **155**, 716–723.

Nylandsted, J., Rohde, M., Brand, K., Bastholm, L., Elling, F. and Jaattela, M. (2000) Selective depletion of heat shock protein 70 (HSP70) activates a tumor-specific death program that is independent of caspases and bypasses Bcl-2. *Proc. Natl. Acad. Sci. USA*, **97**, 7871–7876.

Ohi, S., Dixit, M., Tillery, M.K. and Plonk, S.G. (1990) Construction and replication of an adeno-associated virus expression vector that contains human beta-globin cDNA. *Gene*, **89**, 279–282.

Owens, G.C., Chappell, S.A., Mauro, V.P. and Edelman, G.M. (2001) Identification of two short internal ribosome entry sites selected from libraries of random oligonucleotides. *Proc. Natl. Acad. Sci. USA*, **98**, 1471–1476.

Palmiter, R.D. (1994) Regulation of metallothionein genes by heavy metals appears to be mediated by a zinc-sensitive inhibitor that interacts with a constitutively active transcrip-tion factor, MTF-1. *Proc. Nat. Acad. Sci. USA*, **91**, 1219–1223.

Radtke, F., Heuchel, R., Georgiev, O., Hergersberg, M., Gariglio, M., Dembic, Z. and Schaffner, W. (1993) Cloned transcription factor MTF-1 activates the mouse metallothionein I promoter. *EMBO J.*, **12**, 1355–1362.

Rinsch, C., Regulier, E., Deglon, N., Dalle, B., Beuzard, Y. and Aebischer, P. (1997) A gene therapy approach to regulated delivery of erythropoietin as a function of oxygen tension. *Hum. Gene Ther.*, **8**, 1881–1889.

Rivera, V.M., Clackson, T., Natesan, S., Pollock, R., Amara, J.F., Keenan, T. *et al.* (1996) A humanized system for pharmacologic control of gene expression. *Nature Med.*, **2**, 1028–1032.

Roebuck, K.A. and Saifuddin, M. (1999) Regulation of HIV-1 transcription. *Gene Expression*, **8**, 67–84.

Sarge, K.D., Murphy, S.P. and Morimoto, R.I. (1993) Activation of heat shock gene transcription by heat shock factor 1 involves oligomerization, acquisition of DNA-binding activity, and nuclear localization and can occur in the absence of stress. *Mol. Cell. Biol.*, **13**, 1392–1407.

Sarge, K.D., Park-Sarge, O.Y., Kirby, J.D., Mayo, K.E. and Morimoto, R.I. (1994) Regulated expression of heat shock factor 2 in mouse testis: potential role as a regulator of HSP gene expression during spermatogenesis. *Biol. Reproduct.*, **50**, 1334–1343.

Sarge, K.D., Zimarino, V., Holm, K., Wu, C. and Morimoto, R.I. (1991) Cloning and characterization of two mouse heat shock factors with distinct inducible and constitutive DNA-binding ability. *Genes Develop.*, **5**, 1902–1911.

Sarto, C., Binz, P.A. and Mocarelli, P. (2000) Heat shock proteins in human cancer. *Electrophoresis*, **6**, 1218–1226.

Schuetz, T.J., Gallo, G.J., Sheldon, L., Tempst, P. and Kingston, R.E. (1991) Isolation of cDNA for HSF2: evidence of two heat shock factor genes in humans. *Proc. Natl. Acad. Sci. USA*, **88**, 6910–6915.

Scott, S.D., Marples, B., Hendry, J.H., Lashford, L.S., Embleton, M.J., Hunter, R.D. *et al.* (2000) A radiation-controlled molecular switch for use in gene therapy of cancer. *Gene Ther.*, **7**, 1121–1125.

Searl, P.F., Davison, B.L., Stuart, G.W., Wilkie, T.M., Norstedt, G. and Palmiter, R.D. (1984) Regulation, linkage and sequence of mouse metallothionein I and II genes. *Mol. Cell. Biol.*, **4**, 1221–1230.

Seung, L.P., Mauceri, H.J., Beckett, M.A., Hallahan, D.E., Hellman, S. and Weichselbaum, R.R. (1995) Genetic radiotherapy overcomes tumor resistance to cytotoxic agents. *Cancer Res.*, **55**, 5561–5565.

Shibata, T., Akiyama, N., Noda, M., Sasai, K. and Hiraoka, M. (1998) Enhancement of gene expression under hypoxic conditions using fragments of the human vascular endothelial growth factor and the erythropoietin genes. *Int. J. Radiat. Oncol. Biol. Phys.*, **42**, 913–916.

Shibata, T., Giaccia, A.J. and Brown, J.M. (2000) Development of a hypoxia-responsive vector for tumor-specific gene therapy. *Gene Ther.*, **7**, 493–498.

Shilatifard, A. (1998) Factors regulating the transcriptional elongation activity of RNA polymerase II. *FASEB J.*, **12**, 1437–1446.

Shin, M.K. (2000) Controlling gene expression in mice with tetracycline: Application in pigment cell research. *Pigment Cell Res.*, **13**, 326–331.

Sistonen, L., Sarge, K.D., Phillips, B., Abravaya, K. and Morimoto, R. (1992) Activation of heat shock factor 2 during hemin-induced differentiation of human erythroleukemia cells. *Mol. Cell. Biol.*, **12**, 4104–4111.

Spencer, C.A. and Groudine, M. (1990) Transcription elongation and eukaryotic gene regulation. *Oncogene*, **5**, 777–785.

Staba, M.J., Mauceri, H.J., Kufe, D.W., Hallahan, D.E. and Weichselbaum, R.R. (1998) Adenoviral TNF-alpha gene therapy and radiation damage tumor vasculature in a human malignant glioma xenograft. *Gene Ther.*, **5**, 293–300.

Stuart, G.W., Searl, P.F., Chen, H.Y., Brinster, R.L. and Palmiter, R.D. (1984) A 12-base-pair DNA motif that is repeated several times in metallothionein gene promoters confers metal regulation to a heterologous gene. *Proc. Natl. Acad. Sci. USA*, **81**, 7318–7322.

Takahashi, M., Altschmied, L. and Hillen, W. (1986) Kinetic and equilibrium characterization of the Tet repressor-tetracycline complex by fluorescence measurements. Evidence for divalent metal ion requirement and energy transfer. *J. Mol. Biol.*, **187**, 341–348.

Takahashi, T., Namiki, Y. and Ohno, T. (1997) Induction of the suicide HSV-TK gene by activation of the Egr-1 promoter with radioisotopes. *Hum. Gene Ther.*, **8**, 827–833.

Teng, J., Fukuda, N., Hu, W.Y., Nakayama, M., Kishioka, H. and Kanmatsuse, K. (2000) DNA-RNA chimeric hammerhead ribozyme to transforming growth factor-beta (1) mRNA inhibits the exaggerated growth of vascular smooth muscle cells from spontaneously hypertensive rats. *Cardiovasc. Res.*, **48**, 138–147.

Tierney, M.J. and Medcalf, R.L. (2001) Plasminogen Activator Inhibitor Type 2 Contains mRNA Instability Elements within Exon 4 of the Coding Region. *J. Biol. Chem.*, **276**, 13675–13684.

Triezenberg, S.J., Kingsbury, R.C. and McKnight, S.L. (1988) Functional dissection of VP16, the trans-activator of herpes simplex virus immediate early gene expression. *Genes Develop.*, **2**, 718–729.

Varshavsky, A., Turner, G., Du, F. and Xie, Y. (2000) The ubiquitin system and the N-end rule pathway. *Biol. Chem.*, **381**, 779–789.

Walther, W. and Stein, U. (1996) Cell type specific and inducible promoters for vectors in gene therapy as an approach for cell targeting. *J. Mol. Med.*, **74**, 379–392.

Weichselbaum, R.R., Hallahan, D.E., Beckett, M.A., Mauceri, H.J., Lee, H., Sukhatme, V.P. *et al.* (1994) Gene therapy targeted by radiation preferentially radiosensitizes tumor cells. *Cancer Res.*, **54**, 4266–4269.

West, A.K., Hildebrand, C.E., Karin, M. and Richards, R.I. (1990) Human metallothionein genes: Structure of the functional locus at 16q13. *Genomics*, **8**, 513–518.

Woloschak, G.E., Felcher, P. and Chang-Liu, C.M. (1995) Combined effects of ionizing radiation and cycloheximide on gene expression. *Mol. Carcinogenesis*, **13**, 44–49.

Xiao, H. and Lis, J.T. (1988) Germline transformation used to define key features of heat shock response elements. *Science*, **239**, 1139–1142.

Yanofsky, C., Konan, K.V. and Sarsero, J.P. (1996) Some novel transcription attenuation mechanisms used by bacteria. *Biochimie*, **78**, 1017–1024.

Yoo, C.G., Lee, S., Lee, C.T., Kim, Y.W., Han, S.K. and Shim, Y.S. (2000) Anti-inflammatory effect of heat shock protein induction is related to stabilization of IkappaB alpha through preventing IkappaB kinase activation in respiratory epithelial cells. *J. Immunol.*, **164**, 5416–5423.

Zolotukhin, S., Potter, M., Hauswirth, W.W., Guy, J. and Muzyczka, N. (1996) A 'humanized' green fluorescent protein cDNA adapted for high-level expression in mammalian cells. *J. Virol.*, **70**, 4646–4654.

Zou, J., Guo, Y., Guettouche, T., Smith, D.F. and Voellmy, R. (1998) Repression of heat shock transcription factor HSF1 activation by HSP90 (HSP90 complex) that forms a stress-sensitive complex with HSF1. *Cell*, **94**, 471–480.

Zuo, J., Rungger, D. and Voellmy R. (1995) Multiple layers of regulation of human heat shock transcription factor 1. *Mol. Cell. Biol.*, **15**, 4319–4330.

3 Modulation of gene expression by antisense oligonucleotides

Ruiwen Zhang and Hui Wang

INTRODUCTION

One of the major developments in modern biomedical research is genetic therapy, which is based on progress made in molecular biology and genetics, especially the identification, cloning, sequencing and characterization of pathogenic genes. Major efforts in the development of genetic therapy can be summarized in two general approaches. The first is the introduction of a vector that is capable of inserting into the genetic code a gene of interest that may restore a normal function or correct an abnormal function. This approach is termed gene therapy. The second, termed antisense therapy, delivers to the target cells antisense molecules that target RNA or DNA with which they hybridize and specifically inhibit the expression of pathogenic genes. In the past, the term **antisense** has been used to include four distinct approaches, including classical antisense or anticode, ribozyme or catalytic RNA, triplex or antigene, and aptamer technologies. These antisense technologies are compared in Table 3.1.

Antisense nucleic acids are single-strand oligonucleotides that are complementary to the sequence of target RNA or DNA. Since the idea of antisense therapy was first introduced over 20 years ago (Zamecnik, 1996), antisense oligonucleotides have been developed into a vigorously investigated area of research. In the mid-1970s, the laboratory of Zamecnik and Stephenson demonstrated that a synthetic oligonucleotide disrupted protein synthesis in Rous sarcoma virus 35S RNA in a cell-free system and also prevented the viral replication in mammalian cells (Zamecnik and Stephenson, 1978; Stephenson and Zamecnik, 1978). In the same period, the laboratory of Ts'o and Miller demonstrated that chemically modified oligonucleotides could be utilized as a probe to determine the structure and function of nucleic acids in living cells (Miller *et al.*, 1977, 1988). However, this pioneering work did not generate a significant research interest, with very few scientific papers being published in the field from the late 1970s to the mid-1980s. The contributions of the forementioned researchers to the antisense field were recognized after the discovery of natural regulation of gene expression by antisense RNA (Simons, 1988). In the 1980s, major effort was devoted to establish useful techniques for automated total oligonucleotide synthesis, yielding sufficient amount of oligonucleotides. In the last 15 years, antisense RNA and DNA techniques have been rapidly developed and widely used for investigating gene function, gene expression regulation and modulation of gene expression, as well as validation of new therapeutic targets. Antisense oligonucleotides are being investigated for the

Table 3.1 A brief comparison of antisense technologies

Approach	Active molecule	Molecular target	Cellular site of action[1]	Suggested mechanisms of action	Stage of drug development
Antisense	DNA or RNA	RNA[2]	Cytoplasm	Translation arrest, RNase H activation, inhibition of splicing, disruption of RNA structure	Clinical use[3] clinical trials
Ribozyme	RNA	RNA	Cytoplasm	Translation arrest, Destruction of RNA	Clinical trials
Triplex	DNA	DNA	Nucleus	Blockage of transcription	Preclinical
Aptamer	DNA or RNA	Protein	Nucleus, cytoplasm, or extracellular	Interference with protein function	Clinical phase I trial

Notes
1 Site of action is referred to the initial site of interaction of antisense molecule with its target molecule and may be not the same as biological activity occurs.
2 Any kind of RNA can be targeted: pre-RNA, mRNA or viral RNA.
3 The first antisense drug Vitravene has now been approved for the treatment of patients with cytomegalovirus-induced retinitis. Several other antisense oligonucleotides have entered clinical phase I–III trials.

treatment of various human diseases such as hypertension, cardiovascular diseases, cancer, genetic disorders, and viral infections, including those caused by HIV, hepatitis virus B, and herpes simplex virus (HSV).

Over the years, however, there have been many concerns that have limited enthusiasm for the development of antisense drugs from the preclinical to the clinical pharmacologic level (Stein and Cheng, 1993; Diasio and Zhang, 1997). Until recently, these major concerns have included: (1) ability to synthesize sufficient quantities of oligonucleotides for use as a drug that meets GMP (Good Manufacturing Practice) requirements; (2) biostability of synthetic oligonucleotides *in vivo*; (3) capability and efficiency of oligonucleotides to enter the target cell that contains the gene of interest; (4) retention of oligonucleotides within the target cells to maintain sufficient inhibitory effects on the expression of target genes; (5) extent of metabolism of oligonucleotides *in vivo* and the effect of the metabolites on both pharmacology and toxicology of oligonucleotides; (6) interaction of the antisense oligonucleotides with their specific mRNA targets and the efficiency of such an interaction; (7) significance of non-sequence specific interactions with other macromolecules *in vivo*, including proteins and nucleic acids; (8) *in vivo* biological efficacy of oligonucleotides particularly in clinical setting; (9) safety and side effects of both intact and metabolic derivatives of oligonucleotides particularly in clinical setting, and; (10) regulatory issues in the development of antisense oligonucleotides as drugs. Perhaps the most significant advances in responding to these concerns have been: (1) the development of improved synthetic methods yielding sufficient quantities of antisense oligonucleotides to permit extensive preclinical pharmacologic and toxicologic studies and, more importantly clinical studies; (2) advanced antisense chemistry providing various modifications of oligonucleotides, resulting in improved pharmacokinetic, pharmacodynamic and toxicologic profiles of antisense oligonucleotides; (3) better understanding of biological effects of antisense oligonucleotides including both antisense and non-antisense mechanisms and both sequence-dependent and -independent effects, and; (4) the evaluation of several antisense oligonucleotides in clinical trials addressing the areas of concern listed above by either demonstrating that the concerns were unfounded or by developing alternative approaches to overcome the concerns. The first antisense drug Vitravene has now been approved for the treatment of patients with cytomegalovirus-induced retinitis (Crooke, 1998b). Several other antisense oligonucleotides have entered clinical phase I-III trials (Agrawal, 1996, 1999; Crooke, 1998a; Wickstrom, 1998; Kushner and Silverman, 2000; Monia *et al.*, 2000; Gewirtz, 2000; Zhang and Wang, 2000a).

MECHANISMS OF ACTION OF ANTISENSE OLIGONUCLEOTIDES

Although rapid progress has been made in the development of antisense therapy, the technology remains in its infancy and many questions remain unanswered. In the beginning of antisense investigation, the principle of gene function by antisense oligonucleotides was thought to be simple and straightforward. Antisense oligonucleotides were thought to bind to and interact with their complimentary target RNA or DNA in a sequence-specific manner and block gene translation or transcription. This process was named hybrid-arrest, and resulted in therapeutic effects in a sequence-dependent manner. Now it has been revealed that antisense oligonucleotides distribute their inhibiting effects on target genes through several distinct mechanisms. It is also true that antisense molecules may exert their biological activity through both antisense and non-antisense mechanisms. Readers are directed to several recently published reviews (Crooke, 1998a,b, 1999, 2000a,b; Gewirtz, 2000; Agrawal, 1999; Agrawal and Kandimalla, 2000; Lebedeva and Stein, 2001). Amongst many proposed mechanisms, hybrid-arrest and RNase H activation are generally accepted and are briefly reviewed below.

Hybrid-arrest

Early studies suggest that antisense oligonucleotides bind to and interact with code region, cause blockage of ribosomal read-through mRNA and stop translation. Later it was demonstrated that antisense can also be targeted to the initiation code region and can inhibit downstream gene expression more efficiently. Now it is known that oligonucleotides may produce antisense effects through binding to 5' cap region, 3' poly(A), and/or to the splicing site of the pre-RNA, the latter interfering with RNA splicing, maturation and transport (Crooke, 1999).

Cleavage of target sequences

Several types of antisense oligonucleotides, such as oligonucleotide phospho-thioates (PS-oligos), may bind with their target RNA to form a RNA:DNA duplex, whilst simultaneously activating enzyme RNase H, resulting in RNA degradation.

Other types of oligonucleotides, such as methylphosphonate oligonucleotides and α-oligonucleotides, however, do not possess this property (Boiziau *et al.*, 1992a,b). Ribozymes also possess the capacity to degrade target RNA more efficiently.

ANTISENSE CHEMISTRY

According to the chemical composition, physicochemical and/or biochemical properties, antisense oligonucleotides can be divided into antisense RNA and antisense DNA (Table 3.1).

Antisense RNA

Natural antisense RNA is known to be involved in gene regulation in normal organisms (Simons, 1988). Manmade antisense RNAs have also been used in antisense studies. There are two major approaches used to apply antisense RNA into living cells; nuclear expression of RNA by engineered antisense genes and microinjection of artificial antisense RNA. Thus far, antisense RNA has shown limited application in the development of therapeutic agents. Interested readers are directed to recent published reviews and books (Obertstra and Nellen, 1997; Bunnell and Morgan, 1997; Zhang *et al.*, 1997).

Nuclear expression of RNA by engineered antisense genes

The concept of gene regulation by antisense RNA is straight forward: after RNA that is complementary to the target mRNA is introduced to target cells, a specific RNA:RNA duplex is formed by base pairing between antisense RNA and the target RNA, resulting in a blockage of gene expression. This result can be achieved by the introduction and expression of an antisense gene. Using this approach, a part or full length of the normal gene sequences are placed under a promoter in an inverted orientation. The complementary strand, therefore, is transcribed into a noncoding antisense RNA that hybridizes with the target mRNA and specifically interferes with its expression. These antisense expression vectors can be constructed and introduced into living cells using standard procedures and have been found to be useful in studies of gene function and regulation. However, as seen with other gene therapy vectors, antisense expression vectors have shown limited efficacy *in vivo*. Other problems include the availability of suitable promoters or vectors and levels of antisense RNA expression to meet the needs for regulation of the target mRNA expression.

Microinjection of in vitro transcribed RNA

This approach includes the production and purification of antisense transcripts *in vitro* and then the introduction of the antisense RNA into cells by microinjection. Compared to the antisense gene approach described above, a major advantage of this method is that a much larger amount of antisense RNA can be introduced into cells. Also, antisense RNA can be injected at a specific time and can therefore result in the transient inhibition of gene expression, which can be used in studies of gene expression at a specific time within a particular window of development. However, as RNAs are extremely sensitive to nuclease degradation, the potential pharmacological uses of antisense RNA are limited.

Liposomal encapsulation of RNA

Alternatively, anitsense RNA can be delivered both *in vitro* and *in vivo* by the use of liposomes. Certain protection against nuclease may be achieved by liposomal encapsulation. In addition, liposomes may be targeted to certain cells by coupled antibodies that specifically interact with cells that carry corresponding surface antigens.

Antisense DNA

In contrast to antisense RNA, antisense oligodeoxynucleotides are short sequences of single stranded DNA and can be produced in large quantities using automated synthetic organic chemistry with various modified linkages or terminal groups. Thus, antisense DNA are now being used much more frequently in antisense investigations than antisense RNA and ribozymes. Almost all of the clinically tested antisense oligonucleotides are modified antisense DNA.

Unmodified phosphodiester oligodeoxynucleotides

In general, phosphodiester oligonucleotides (PO-oligos), and their methylphosphonate and phosphorothioate analogs, are considered as the first generation of antisense DNA. With high affinity to their targets, PO-oligos bind to the target mRNA stably and the melting temperature (Tm) of PO-oligos:RNA duplex is high. PO-oligos also possess the ability to activate RNase H. The major disadvantage of PO-oligos is that they are sensitive to nucleases and degrade rapidly in plasma and/or cytoplasm. Another problem is that the cellular uptake of PO-oligos is poor. Even after the uptake, PO-oligos are still subject to attack by the nucleases, although this process is much slower than in plasma. Therefore, PO-oligos are merely used in early antisense investigation and limited to *in vitro* cell-free, serum-free systems.

Oligonucleotide analogs with backbone modifications

For over a decade, great efforts have been given to synthesize nucleases-resistant antisense oligos. Different backbone modifications have been made to improve the cellular uptake and resistance to nucleases of antisense oligos. Among them, phosphorothioate (PS-oligos) and methylphosphonate (MP-oligos) oiligonucleotides have been extensively investigated.

Substitution of sulfur for oxygen on the phosphorus residue of DNA generates phosphorothioate analogs, PS-oligos. As unmodified oligos, PS-oligos retain the negative charge and thus are more aqueous soluble than MP-oligos. PS-oligos are much more resistant to nucleases than PO-oligos. The duplex of PS-oligos:RNA is a good substrate for RNase H. The problems are that PS-oligos are less well taken up by the cells and appear to produce non-specific toxicities in some systems. Thus far, most clinically tested antisense oligonucleotides are PS-oligos.

MP-oligos, where -CH$_3$ replaces -O, were first synthesized in the late 1970s by Miller and his colleagues (Miller *et al.*, 1981). It has been confirmed that MP-oligos are much more resistant to extra- and intra-cellular nucleases. The Tm of a MP-oligos:RNA duplex is also higher than that of PO-oligos. MP-oligos are uncharged oligos and thus pass through plasma membrane much better than PO-oligos. The major disadvantage of this class of analogue is its relatively poor hybridization efficiency and inability to activate RNase H (Carter and Lemoine, 1993).

Several other types of backbone modification have also been proposed, which produce nuclease-resistant oligos. Of these, α-oligos have been extensively studied. In α-oligos the base is transposed from the natural β-orientation to the unnatural α-orientation to form a parallel duplex with target sequence. This parallel duplex is nuclease-resistant, but does not elicit RNase H activity (Cazenave *et al.*, 1989). These modifications have generated limited interest and application in antisense research.

Oligonucleotides with terminal modification

To enhance the cellular uptake and nuclease resistance of oligonucleotides, different terminal modifications at the *5'* or *3'* terminus of oligonucleotides have been attempted. Polylysine, avidin (such as acridine), and cholesterol have been used to improve cellular uptake and antisense effects of oligos (Nechers, 1989, 1993). However, the value of these approaches remains uncertain and needs to be further determined, especially in *in vivo* settings.

Mixed-backbone oligonucleotides (MBOs)

In the development of second generation antisense oligonucleotides, major efforts have been devoted to stabilizing PS-oligonucleotides by various modifications to their structures (Agrawal and Iyer, 1995; Agrawal *et al.*, 1997; Agrawal and Zhang, 1998; Wang *et al.*, 1999a). More stable oligonucleotides have at least two advantages: an intact antisense oligonucleotide provides a longer duration of action; and the generation of fewer degradation products would avoid potential unwanted side-effects from these metabolites. One of the novel structures is mixed-backbone oligonucleotides (MBOs). These novel oligonucleotides have segments of 2'-O-methyl oligoribonucleotide phosphorothioates at both the *3'-* and *5'-*ends. Modified oligonucleotides have been shown to increase *in vivo* stability and, therefore, increase cellular uptake and decrease total elimination (Agrawal *et al.*, 1997; Agrawal and Zhang, 1998; Wang *et al.*, 1999a).

Uptake of antisense oligonucleotides

It is generally agreed that oligonucleotides enter cells by some form of endocytosis. It is also believed that the extent of oligonucleotide uptake is associated with cell type, type of oligonucleotides, nuclease activity, and the intra- and inter-cellular stability of oligonucleotoides. Although the exact mechanisms for cellular uptake and tissue distribution and retention/accumulation are not clear, PS-oligonucleotides are distributed to all major tissues after *in vivo* administration by various means of dosing (Agrawal *et al.*, 1997; Agrawal and Zhang, 1997, 1998). Although there are no significant difference in uptake and distribution amongst oligonucleotides with backbone modifications, remarkable differences in biostability may count for improved pharmacokinetics and safety profiles. MBOs have a similar tissue distribution pattern as PS-oligonucleotides, but they have greater stability, as shown in several studies (Agrawal *et al.*, 1997; Zhang *et al.*, 1995a,b,c).

TARGET VALIDATION OF ANTISENSE OLIGONUCLEOTIDES

Like any other kinds of new drugs, antisense drugs need to undergo intense, systemic, and thorough evaluation before they can be used in the clinics. Table 3.2 summarizes the major elements in the research and development of antisense drugs. Perhaps the most important aspect of pharmacologic studies of antisense oligonucleotides is the target effectiveness of these agents. There are now numerous published studies that have demonstrated the effectiveness of antisense oligonucleotides directed against mRNA targets in a variety of preclinical and clinical settings, including cancer, various infectious diseases, as well as other conditions (Crooke, 1998a,b, 2000a; Agrawal, 1996; Wickstrom, 1998; Kushner and Silverman, 2000; Monia *et al.*, 2000; Gewirtz, 2000; Zhang and Wang, 2000a; Agrawal and Iyer, 1995). For example, more than 100 gene targets have been tested for cancer therapy (Agrawal, 1996; Wickstrom, 1998; Kushner and Silverman, 2000; Monia *et al.*, 2000; Gewirtz, 2000; Zhang and Wang, 2000a; Wang *et al.*, 1999a; Stein and Cheng, 1997).

Design of antisense oligonucleotides

Although the design of antisense oligos is theoretically straightforward (to identify a complementary oligonucleotide on the basis of the nucleotide sequence of the mRNA), the selection of an effective and specific antisense oligo has so far been largely based on investigators' experience and trial-based experiments. Since certain oligo sequences, such as CpG and GGGG, have been shown to have non-antisense effects, these sequences should be avoided to demonstrate sequence-specific antisense effects. In addition, since PS-oligos have certain side-effects and undergo extensive metabolism *in vivo*, advanced antisense chemistry may be needed for *in vivo* studies. Some general features of optimal antisense oligos will be described below, with an emphasis on the selection of appropriate target sites.

Random 'sequence-walking' approach

Based on Watson-Crick base pairing rules and a known sequence of the target gene, a linear, sequence-walking method has been used to design and select antisense oligos. Usually, a relatively large number of 15 ~ 30 mer 'random' oligos (10–100 depending on the length of the gene of interest), targeted to various region of the target mRNA, are synthesized individually and their antisense activity assessed using a defined cell free or *in vitro* screening assay. This conventional method has been used in many antisense experiments and yielded good results, although it is expensive, time and labor-consuming. Only less than 5% of the oligos

Table 3.2 Key components in antisense drug development

Stage and goals	Test system	Approaches and requirements
I. Design of oligonucleotides		Following Watson-Crick pairing rules, design the sequence of the oligo to interact with target gene. Synthesize and purify the oligo in high quality and sufficient quantity
II. Target validation: specificity and efficiency	Cell-free system Cell culture	Demonstrate specific down regulation of target gene by western and northern blot, RT-PCR or bioassay
III. *In vitro* biological activity specificity and efficiency	Cell culture	Demonstrate specific antisense effect by various bioassays such as anti-viral and anti-proliferation effect, induction of apoptosis
IV. *In vivo* biological activity specificity and efficiency	Animal	Using animal disease models, demonstrate specific antisense effect by various bioassays such as anti-viral and anti-tumor effect, induction of apoptosis, improving survival
V. *In vivo* pharmacology pharmacokinetics pharmacology screening	Animal	Determine pharmacokinetic profile of oligos, i.e., absorption, distribution, metabolism, and elimination Determine pharmacological effects of oligos on host tissues other than desired effects
VI. *In vivo* toxicology toxicokinetics toxicity testing	Animal	Determine toxicokinetic profile of oligos Determine toxicological effects of oligos in a GLP (Good Laboratory Practice) setting
VII. Large-scale oligo synthesis		Produce sufficient oligo that meet GMP (Good Manufacture Practice) regulation
VIII. Clinical evaluation	Humans	Phase I: Safety and pharmacokinetics Phase II: Initial clinical efficacy Phase III: Clinical efficacy Phase IV: Post-marketing trials
IV. Regulatory issues		Meet regulatory body such as FDA requirements on investigational new drug and new drug applications.

are generally found to be effective antisense reagents. For example, in a study of HSV-1 antisense screening, only one out of 100 tested oligos showed antisense activity in cell culture (Peyman *et al.*, 1995). One out of 34 oligos targeted to C-*raf* kinase mRNA had significant effect on the reduction of C-*raf* kinase mRNA in cultured lung cancer A549 cells (Monia *et al.*, 1996).

Computer-aided target selection: computer folding of mRNA

Lack of antisense efficacy of oligos may be largely due to the selection of inaccessible sites of the target RNA. It is often seen that a single or a few bases shift has no significant change in oligo:RNA binding, but may have large differences in antisense activity. It is now accepted that the binding of complementary oligos is mainly determined by the secondary and tertiary structures of the target RNAs (Milner *et al.*, 1997). Therefore, major effort has been devoted in this area to make possible the prediction of accessible sites in mRNAs through various approaches, such as the use of computer programs to predict the secondary structure of RNA (Zuker, 1989). Using a RNA folding program such as MFOLD (Genetics Computer Group, Madison, WI), antisense oligos are designed to target against the regions of mRNA that are predicted by the computer program to be free from intramolecular base pairing. However, this approach has not yet yielded much success in correctly predicting RNA structure and guiding antisense design (Milner *et al.*, 1997).

Oligonucleotide scanning arrays

Recent advances in DNA array technologies have led to the development of oligonucleotide scanning arrays as a novel approach to identify active antisense reagents (Milner *et al.*, 1997; Elder *et al.*, 1999). This method allows combinatorial synthesis of a large number of oligonucleotides and parallel measurement of the binding strength of all oligonucleotides to the target mRNA. It appears that there is a correlation between the binding strength and the antisense activity of test oligonucleotides (Milner *et al.*, 1997; Elder *et al.*, 1999). However, the potential of this method in selecting optimal antisense oligonucleotides has yet to be demonstrated.

Oligonucleotide library/RNase H digestion-based screening

As mentioned above, there is convincing evidence that RNase H is involved in antisense activity. This involvement has led to the use of RNase H screening assays to identify effective antisense reagents (Ho *et al.*, 1998; Lima *et al.*, 1997). In this method, RNase H is used in combination with a random or semi-random oligonucleotide library. The target mRNA is transcribed *in vitro*, end-labeled, and mixed with the oligo library. The RNase H cleavage sites are then identified by gel electrophoresis. However, RNase H mapping method may not precisely define the accessible sites of target mRNA since RNase H cleavage can occur at more than one location, and it will therefore be difficult to predict the antisense activity.

Other methods of selecting antisense oligonucleotides

Several other methods have been proposed to select optimal antisense oligonucleotides. They include DNA enzymes (deoxyribozymes) that cleave RNA in a way similar to ribozymes (Santon and Joyce, 1997) and RNase T1 foot-printing that identifies single stranded regions of target RNA (Gewirtz, 1997). However, the potential of these methods in selecting optimal antisense oligonucleotides has yet to be demonstrated.

Pharmacological evaluation of antisense oligonucleotides

As illustrated in Table 3.2, the pharmacological effects of antisense oligos can be evaluated both *in vitro* and *in vivo*. Antisense effects are usually first examined in cell-free systems, confirming that antisense oligos selectively hybridize with the specific mRNA targets, resulting in decreased expression of target proteins. Those antisense oligos that have been found effective are then further examined at cellular and molecular levels. While there is some variability on cellular uptake, depending on the chemistry of antisense oligos, many oligos can apparently cross the plasma membrane into the cytosol in sufficient quantities to cause the desired antisense effect. Cellular pharmacokinetic studies have also examined various approaches to increase cellular uptake of antisense oligos by using liposomes, phospholipids, and other means to increase membrane penetrability of these oligos.

The *in vivo* preclinical pharmacologic evaluation of antisense oligos has employed animal studies, predominantly in murine species. Pharmacokinetic studies examining the fate of antisense oligos *in vivo*, i.e., absorption, distribution, metabolism and excretion, have mainly been undertaken after administration of PS-oligos, representing the first generation antisense oligos. PS-oligos have a short distribution half-life and a longer elimination half-life in plasma, and are distributed widely into and retained in all major tissues following intravenous, intraperitoneal, or subcutaneous administration (Zhang *et al.*, 1995a,b,c, 1996; Agrawal and Zhang, 1997a,b, 1998). Extensive metabolism of antisense oligos has been observed, although the mechanisms are not fully understood. PS-oligos are degraded primarily from the *3'*-end, but degradation from the *5'*-end or both the *3'*- and *5'*-ends has been observed, as well (Agrawal and Zhang, 1997a,b). Pharmacokinetic profiles of PS-oligo are, in general, not associated with the length or primary sequence of oligo, but associated with the modification of the backbone and specific segments at the *3'* and/or *5'* end (Zhang *et al.*, 1995a,b,c, 1996; Agrawal and Zhang, 1997a,b, 1998; Agrawal *et al.*, 1995, 1997).

Compared with pre-clinical studies, far fewer clinical studies of oligos have been reported. Most clinical studies so far have used PS-oligos (Crooke, 1998a, 2000a; Wickstrom, 1998; Kushner and Silverman, 2000; Zhang and Wang, 2000a). Examples of clinical trials currently underway with antisense oligos as anticancer agents include those targeted to mutant p53, *bcl-2*, protein kinase C, protein kinase A, *c-raf* kinase, and Ha-*ras* (Crooke, 1998a, 2000a; Wickstrom, 1998; Kushner and Silverman, 2000; Zhang and Wang, 2000a). Clinical trials of oligos with advanced antisense chemistry have also begun (Chen *et al.*, 2000). In this chapter, we are presenting the antisense anti-MDM2 oligo with advanced antisense chemistry as an example to illustrate the protocol for *in vitro* and *in vivo* evaluation of antisense oligo therapeutics in pre-clinical settings.

ANTI-MDM2 ANTISENSE OLIGONUCLEOTIDES AS ANTITUMOR AGENTS

MDM2 as a target for cancer therapy

Oncogene and tumor suppressor genes have been shown to play a major role in formation, growth and progression of human cancers. Perhaps the most important and studied tumor suppressor gene is p53 (Prives, 1999). Abnormalities of p53 tumor suppressor gene are among the most frequent molecular events in human and animal neoplasia. Studies have also shown that the tumor suppressor function of p53 can be inhibited without mutation. A major advancement in the under-standing of p53 pathway is the discovery of mouse double minute 2 (MDM2) and its role in controlling p53 levels (Cahilly-Snyder *et al.*, 1987; Piette *et al.*, 1997). There is an MDM2-p53 autoregulatory feedback loop that regulates intracellular functions of p53: the MDM2 gene is a target for the direct transcriptional activation of p53 and MDM2 protein is a negative regulator of p53 (Zhang and Wang, 2000b). In addition, MDM2 protein interacts with other cellular proteins that involve in cell cycle regulation, including pRb, E2F1/DP1 and p19ARF. Therefore, MDM2 plays a crucial role in cell cycle control and tumor transformation and growth. Like p53, MDM2 has become a target for the rational drug design for cancer therapy (Cahilly-Snyder *et al.*, 1987; Zhang and Wang, 2000b). Several recent reviews provide comprehensive discussion of MDM2 oncogene and its functions, as well as its interaction with various cellular proteins (Momand and Zambetti, 1997; Prives, 1998; Lozano and Montes de Oca Luna, 1998; Juven-Gershon and Oren, 1999; Freedman *et al.*, 1999; Freedman and Levine, 1999).

MDM2 has also been shown to play a role in DNA damaging treatment. MDM2 is transcriptionally induced by p53 following DNA damage (Barak *et al.*, 1993; Perry *et al.*, 1993). The MDM2 gene product MDM2 oncoprotein, in turn, binds to p53 and directly blocks p53 function as a transcription factor and tumor suppressor and induces p53 degradation. This p53-MDM2 loop may play a role in p53-mediated response to DNA damaging treatment in tumor cells and, there-fore, can be modulated to improve the therapeutic effectiveness of DNA damaging agents or radiation therapy.

The connection between MDM2 and cancer has been shown in many studies of human cancers. Over-expression of MDM2 is shown in a variety of human tumors and may be due to one or more of the three mechanisms: (1) gene amplification (Momand *et al.*, 1998; Watanabe *et al.*, 1994); (2) increased transcription (Landers *et al.*, 1994), or; (3) enhanced translation (Landers *et al.*, 1997). Over-expression of the MDM2 gene has been shown to be associated with many human tumors, including soft tissue tumors, osteosarcomas, esophageal carcinomas, brain tumor, breast cancer, ovarian carcinoma, cervical cancer, lung cancer, colon cancer, bronchogenic carcinoma, nasopharyngeal carcinoma, neuroblastomas, testicular germ-cell tumor, urothelial cancers, bladder cancer, leukemia, large B-cell lymphoma as well as to pediatric solid tumors (Momand *et al.*, 1998; Zhang and Wang, 2000b). In general, human cancer cell lines or tumor tissues with MDM2 gene amplifications or overexpression often have wild-type p53 (Momand *et al.*, 1998), presumably inactivated by MDM2.

Many cancer therapeutic agents exert their cytotoxic effects through activation of wild-type p53, and the restoration of wild-type p53 can increase the sensitivity of tumors to DNA-damaging agents (Dorigo *et al.*, 1998; Nielsen and Maneval, 1998). However, the activation of p53 by DNA damage, such as cancer chemotherapy and radiation treatment, may be limited in cancers with MDM2 expression, especially those with MDM2 over-expression. Therefore, inactivation of the MDM2 negative feedback loop may increase the magnitude of p53 activation following DNA damage, thus enhancing the therapeutic effectiveness of DNA damaging drugs and radiation therapy. In the past, several strategies have been used to test the hypothesis that, by disrupting p53-MDM2 interaction, the negative regulation of p53 by MDM2 will be diminished and the cellular functional level of p53 will increase, especially after DNA damaging treatment, resulting in tumor growth arrest and/or apoptosis. These strategies included polypeptides that bind to MDM2 protein (Bottger *et al.*, 1997), antibody against MDM2 protein (Midgley and Lane, 1997), as well as small molecular MDM2 inhibitors (Arriola *et al.*, 1999).

In our laboratories, an antisense approach has been tested to inhibit MDM2 expression that can be used in both gene function study and the development of therapeutic agents (Figure 3.1; Zhang and Wang, 2000b). We have successfully identified anti-MDM2 antisense oligos that effectively inhibit MDM2 expression in tumor cells containing MDM2 gene amplifications (Chen *et al.*, 1998, 1999; Wang *et al.*, 1999b). We are now using the specific anti-MDM2 oligos as a research tool to investigate the role of MDM2 oncogene in the development and treatment of

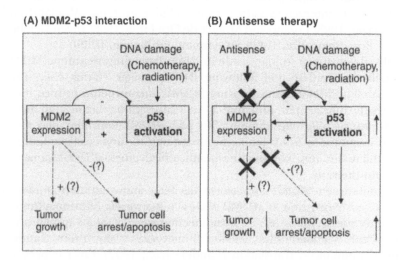

Figure 3.1 MDM2 as an antisense target for cancer therapy. Panel (A) MDM2-p53 Interaction. In normal and cancer cells, there is a MDM2-p53 feedback autoregulatory loop. The MDM2 expression is induced by p53 and MDM2 inhibits p53 activity by forming a MDM2-p53 complex and promoting p53 degradation. Therefore, both p53 and MDM2 expression and their activity in normal circumstances are under control and remain in basal levels. Following DNA damaging treatment such as cytotoxic agent chemotherapy and radiation therapy, p53 is activated and then MDM2 induced, which in turn inhibits p53 function and induces p53 degradation, resulting in limitation on p53 activation by DNA damaging treatment. In addition, MDM2 may have p53-independent activity that promotes tumor growth. Panel (B) The antisense approach to inhibit MDM2 function. Antisense anti-MDM2 oligonucleotide will specifically inhibit MDM2 expression, resulting in inactivation of MDM2-p53 feed back loop. The levels and function of p53 will be increased, resulting in increased cell growth arrest, apoptosis, and tumor growth inhibition. Antisense inhibition of MDM2 expression will diminish other MDM2 activities that are p53-independent. Following DNA damaging treatment in combination with antisense anti-MDM2 therapy, the activation of p53 will be significantly increased, resulting in greater response to therapy.

human cancers by systematically evaluating these antisense oligos as therapeutic agents alone or in combination with other therapeutics. These studies will not only provide the proof of principle for anti-MDM2 oligonucleotides but also evaluate the usefulness of antisense therapy in general.

The selected antisense anti-MDM2 oligo has been shown to specifically inhibit the MDM2 expression *in vitro* (Chen *et al.*, 1998). Inhibition of MDM2 expression in cultured human cancer cell lines results in the activation of p53 and induces apoptosis or cell arrest. The p53 activation activity of the antisense oligo has been shown in all tested cell lines containing wild-type p53 with various levels of MDM2 expression (Chen *et al.*, 1999). This oligo has no effect on the levels of mutant p53, while MDM2 expression is inhibited in cells with mutant p53. In a recent study using mixed-backbone oligos, we demonstrated that the new anti-MDM2 antisense oligo specifically inhibited MDM2 expression in cultured cells and in tumor tissues. The oligo had significant *in vivo* anti-tumor activity when administered alone and had synergistic effects when used in combination with DNA damaging agents (Wang *et al.*, 1999b).

PS-oligonucleotides targeted to MDM2

Design of anti-MDM2 oligonucleotides

Recently, we have successfully identified an anti-MDM2 antisense PS-oligonucleotide that effectively inhibits MDM2 expression in tumor cells containing MDM2 gene amplifications (Chen *et al.*, 1998). Effective anti-human-MDM2 antisense PS-oligonucleotides were initially screened in two cell lines, JAR (choriocarcinoma) and SJSA (osteosarcoma), that contained wild type p53, amplified MDM2 genes, and an overexpression of MDM2 oncoprotein. The cells were treated with PS-oligonucleotides in the presence of cationic lipids to facilitate their cellular uptake. Steady state levels of MDM2 were determined by Western blot analysis. Of nine PS-oligonucleotides screened, Oligo AS5 (5'-GATCACTCCCACCTTCAAGG-3'), which can hybridize to a position ~360 bp downstream of the translation start codon, was found to reproducibly decrease MDM2 protein levels in both cell lines by three- to five-fold at concentrations of 100–400 nM (Chen *et al.*, 1998). In contrast, the mismatched control Oligo M4 (5'-GATGACTCACACCATC AAGG-3') had no effect on MDM2 expression (Chen *et al.*, 1998).

Anti-MDM2 oligos activate RNase H

Oligo AS5 has been shown to induce RNase H cleavage of the target MDM2 mRNA, resulting in truncation and degradation of the target. Following Northern blot hybridization, AS5 was shown to cause a slight decrease in the molecular weight of MDM2 mRNA (Chen *et al.*, 1998). This is consistent with RNase H cleavage at the target of AS5 (~700 nt from the 5' end), which would reduce the molecular weight of the mRNA (~5500 nt) by ~12%.

Anti-MDM2 oligos activate p53 and induce apoptosis

Further studies demonstrated that, following AS5 treatment, the p53 protein level was elevated and its activity was increased (Chen *et al.*, 1998). A dose-dependent induction of p21 expression by AS5 was observed up to 6.6-fold at the optimal concentration of 200 nM (Chen *et al.*, 1998), suggesting that p53 transcriptional activity be increased following inhibition of MDM2 expression.

JAR cells treated with AS5 showed a significant increase in the levels of apoptosis (Chen *et al.*, 1998). Cells exhibiting a blebbing of the cellular membrane began to appear after incubation with the antisense oligo for eight hours. Incubation with oligo AS5 for 24 hours or longer resulted in a ~80% loss of attached cells (Chen *et al.*, 1998). Control oligos caused significantly less cell death. AS5 did not cause visible apoptosis in H1299 cells that lacked p53 (Chen *et al.*, 1998). These results suggest that apoptosis induced by AS5 is due to activation of p53 following MDM2 inhibition by the oligonucleotides.

Optimization of anti-MDM2 oligos

After publishing these encouraging observations with PS-oligo AS5 (Chen *et al.*, 1998), we continued the screening project with the following primary goals: (1) to obtain new oligos with better *in vivo* stability that could be used in future *in vivo* studies; (2) to determine the effects of anti-MDM2 oligos on human tumor cells with varying status of p53 and/or MDM2 expression, and; (3) to identify the candidate cell lines that could be used in future *in vivo* studies. In this study, PS-oligo AS5-2 (5′-TGACACCTGTTCTCACTCAC-3′) was shown to have the highest activity in tested cell lines and was used in further studies. Thus, 26 cell lines (16 types of human cancers) have so far been tested with AS5-2 in comparison with control oligonucleotides. Oligo AS5-2 significantly activated p53 activity in all cells with low levels of wild-type p53, even in those with a very low level of MDM2 expression (Chen *et al.*, 1999). AS5-2 has no effect on cells with null p53, H1299 and SK-N-MC, or those with mutant p53 (Chen *et al.*, 1999). Based on these results, AS5-2 and its mixed-backbone analogs were chosen as candidate oligonucleotides to be used in further *in vitro* and *in vivo* studies.

Mixed-backbone antisense oligonucleotides targeted to MDM2

Design of anti-MDM2 MBO

Based on the above screening, a modified analog of AS5-2 with advanced antisense chemistry was designed (Wang *et al.*, 1999b). The structures of Oligo AS and its mismatched control ASM are as follows:

AS: 5′-**UGA**CACCTGTTCTCAC**UCAC**-3′
ASM: 5′-**UGA**G̲ACC̲AGTTG̲TCAG̲**UCAC**-3′

Two nucleosides at the 5′-end and four nucleosides at the 3′-end are 2′-*O*-methyl ribonucleosides (bold letters); the remaining are deoxynucleosides. The underlined nucleosides of Oligo ASM are those of mismatched controls compared to Oligo AS. For both modified oligonucleotides, all internucleotide linkages are phosphorothioate.

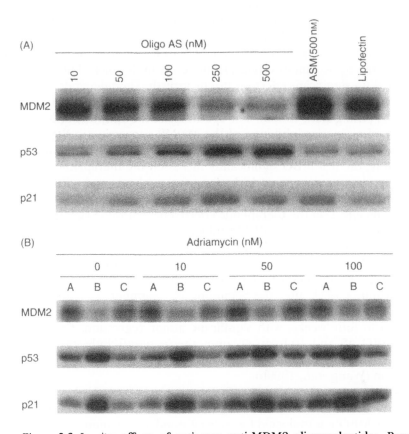

Figure 3.2 In vitro effects of antisense anti-MDM2 oligonucleotides. Panel (A) Dose-dependent, sequence specific MDM2 inhibition, p53 activation and p21 induction. AS; Anti-MDM2 MBO; ASM: mismatched control MBO. Human colon cancer LS174T cells were exposed to MBOs at various concentrations in presence of Lipofectin (7 μL/ml). Protein levels of MDM2, p53 and p21 were analyzed by Western blotting. Equal amounts (20 μg) of protein were used in each lane. Panel (B) Antisense anti-MDM2 MBO increases chemotherapy-associated p53 activation. Human colon cancer LS174T cells were exposed to MBOs for 18 hours at various concentrations in presence of Lipofectin (7 μL/ml) prior to incubation with chemotherapeutic agent adriamycin for 24 hours. Protein levels of MDM2, p53 and p21 were analyzed by Western blotting. Equal amount (20 μg) of protein were used in each lane. Following DNA damaging treatment in combination with antisense anti-MDM2 therapy, the activation of p53 will be significantly increased. Lanes A: Lipofectin + Adriamycin; Lanes B: MBO AS + Adriamycin; and Lanes C; Control MBO ASM + Adriamycin.

In vitro and in vivo activities

The novel anti-MDM2 MBO AS specifically inhibited MDM2 expression in SJSA cells and p53 levels were elevated accordingly. The mismatched control ASM had no effect. The test MBO AS also inhibited the growth of tumor cell lines *in vitro* in a dose-dependent manner (Wang *et al.*, 1999b). Figure 3.2 illustrates the dose-dependent effects of the anti-MDM2 MBO in human colon cancer LS174T cells when the cells were treated with antisense MBOs alone or in combination with anticancer agent adriamycin.

The *in vivo* anti-tumor effects of the test MBO on tumor growth were first evaluated using the SJSA tumor xenograft model in nude mice. The mismatch control ASM had no significant effect on tumor growth. Dose-dependent growth inhibition on SJSA tumor xenografts was found following the treatment of anti-MDM2 MBO AS (Wang *et al.*, 1999b). The specificity of the anti-MDM2 MBO was further confirmed by *in vivo* inhibition of the MDM2 expression in SJSA tumor tissues in a dose-dependent manner. The mismatch control ASM showed no effect. More importantly, the test MBO significantly increased the therapeutic effects of the cancer chemotherapeutic agents 10-hydroxycamptothecin and adriamycin in SJSA xenografts in a dose-dependent manner (Wang *et al.*, 1999b). The mismatch control showed no effect on the therapeutic effectiveness of these agents.

The synergistic effects between MDM2 inhibition and cancer cytotoxic agents were further demonstrated in the JAR xenograft model (Wang *et al.*, 1999b). In this case, we directly injected the MBO AS or 10-hydroxycamptothecin into large tumors (average 2,000 mg), mimicking the clinical late stage of tumors. All control animals died within a week after the beginning of treatment. 10-hydroxycamptothecin alone had no effect on animal survival. 25% of animals treated with MBO AS survived up to four weeks, with significant tumor regression. Combination treatment of MBO AS and 10-hydroxycamptothecin significantly improved the survival rate: 50% of the animals survived over six weeks with almost complete tumor regression (Wang *et al.*, 1999b).

The novel MBO targeted at MDM2 oncogene has now been further evaluated in other types of human cancers, including colon, lung, breast and prostate. The selected antisense MBO was evaluated for its *in vitro* and *in vivo* antitumor activity in human cancer models: those containing wild type p53 and those containing mutant p53. In cancer cells with wild type p53, the p53 and p21 levels were elevated, resulting from specific inhibition of MDM2 expression by the antisense MBO. In cancer cells with mutant p53, following the inhibition of MDM2 expression, p21 levels were elevated, although the p53 levels remained unchanged. *In vivo* antitumor activity of antisense MBO occurred in a dose-dependent manner in nude mice bearing human cancer xenografts. In both models (p53 wild-type or mutant), *in vivo* synergistic or additive therapeutic effects of MDM2 inhibition and the cancer chemotherapeutic agents Irinotecan, 5-fluorouracil, and Taxol were observed. These results suggest that MDM2 has a role in tumor growth through both p53-dependent and p53-independent mechanisms. We speculate that MDM2 inhibitors such as antisense oligonucleotides have a broad spectrum of anti-tumor activities in human breast cancers; regardless of p53 status. These studies should provide a basis for the future development of anti-MDM2 antisense oligonucleotides as cancer therapeutic agents used alone or in combination with conventional chemotherapeutics.

CONCLUDING REMARKS

Over the years, there have been many concerns that have limited enthusiasm for the development of antisense oligonucleotides as therapeutic agents. The recent advances in antisense technology have made this approach to the treatment of human disease a reality. Perhaps the most important aspect of therapeutic oligonucleotides is the target effectiveness of these agents. With the progress made in the last decade, it is believed that antisense oligos will have a promising future as therapeutic agents, alone or in combination with other therapeutic agents, if the specific disease or gene targets are carefully identified. Future studies are needed not only to provide the proof of principle for antisense effects *in vitro* and *in vivo*, but also to meet the full requirement for antisense therapy as a widely accepted therapeutic approach. To that end, more rational selection of both targets and antisense drugs, more and well-designed clinical studies, as well as new concept and approaches to resolve regulatory issues related to antisense drugs are urgently needed.

ACKNOWLEDGMENT

Experimental studies in our laboratory were supported by a grant from the National Institute of Health, National Cancer Institute to R. Zhang (R01 CA 80698).

REFERENCES

Agrawal, S. (1996) Antisense oligonucleotides: towards clinical trial. *Trends Biotech.*, **14**, 376–387.

Agrawal, S. (1999) Importance of nucleotide sequence and chemical modifications of antisense oligocnucleotides. *Biochim. Biophys. Acta.*, **1489**, 53–68.

Agrawal, S. and Iyer, R.P. (1995) Modified oligonucleotides as therapeutic and diagnostic agents. *Curr. Opinion Biotechnol.*, **6**, 112–119.

Agrawal, S. and Kandimalla, E.R. (2000) Antisense therapeutics: Is it simple as complementary base recognition? *Mol. Med. Today*, **6**, 72–81.

Agrawal, S. and Zhang, R. (1997a) Pharmacokinetics of phosphorothioate oligonucleotide and its novel analogs. In: B. Weiss (ed.) *Antisense Oligodeoxynucleotides and Antisense RNA as Novel Pharmacological and Therapeutic Agents*, CRC Press, Boca Raton, FL, pp. 58–78.

Agrawal, S. and Zhang, R. (1997b) Pharmacokinetics of Oligonucleotides. In: *Oligonucleotides as Therapeutic agents. Ciba Foundation Symposium 209*, Wiley, Chichester, pp. 60–78.

Agrawal, S. and Zhang, R. (1998) Pharmacokinetics and bioavailability of oligonucleotides following oral and colorectal administrations in experimental animals. In: S. Crooke (ed.) *Antisense Research and Applications*, Springer-Verlag, Heidelberg, pp. 525–543.

Agrawal, S., Jiang, Z., Zhao, Q., Shaw, D., Cai, Q., Roskey, A. *et al.* (1997) Mixed-backbone oligonucleotides as second generation antisense oligonucleotides: *In vitro* and *in vivo* studies. *Proc. Natl. Acad. Sci. USA*, **94**, 2620–2625.

Agrawal, S., Zhang, X., Zhao, H., Lu, Z., Yan, J., Cai, H. *et al.* (1995) Absorption, tissue distribution and *in vivo* stability in rats of a hybrid antisense oligonucleotide following oral administration. *Biochem. Pharm.*, **50**, 571–576.

Arriola, E.L., Lopez, A.R. and Chresta, C.M. (1999) Differential regulation of p21/waf-1/cip-1 and mdm2 by etoposide: etoposide inhibits the p53-mdm2 autoregulatory feedback loop. *Oncogene*, **18**, 1081–1091.

Barak, Y., Juven, T., Haffner, R. and Oren, M. (1993) MDM2 expression is induced by wild type p53 activity. *EMBO J.*, **12**, 461–468.

Boiziau, C., Larrouy, B., Moreau, S., Cazenave, C., Shire, D. and Toulme, J.-J. (1992a) Ribonuclease H-mediated inhibition of translation and reverse transcription by antisense oligodeoxynucleotides. *Biochem. Soc. Transactions*, **20**, 764–767.

Boiziau, C., Thuong, N.T. and Toulmé, J.-J. (1992b) Mechanisms of the inhibition of reverse transcription by antisense oligonucleotides. *Proc. Natl. Acad. Sci. USA*, **89**, 768–772.

Bottger, A., Bottger, V., Sparks, A., Liu, W.L., Howard, S.F. and Lane, D.P. (1997) Design of a synthetic MDM2-binding mini protein that activates the p53 response *in vivo*. *Curr. Biol.*, **7**, 860–869.

Bunnell, B.A. and Morgan, R.A. (1997) Development of retroviral vectors expressing antisense RNA to inhibit replication of the human immunodeficiency virus. In: B. Weiss (ed.) *Antisense Oligodeoxynucleotides and Antisense RNA, Novel Pharmacological and Therapeutic Agent*, CRC Press, Inc., Boca Raton, FL, pp. 197–212.

Cahilly-Snyder, L., Yang, F.T., Francke, U. and George, D.L. (1987) Molecular anlaysis and chromosomal mapping of amplified genes isolated from a transformed mouse 3T3 cell line. *Somat. Cell Mol. Gene.*, **13**, 235–244.

Carter, G. and Lemoine, N.R. (1993) Antisense technology for cancer therapy: Dose it make sense? *Br. J. Cancer*, **67**, 869–876.

Cazenave, C., Stein, C.A., Loreau, N. *et al.* (1989) Comparative inhibition of rabbit globin mRNA translation by mordified antisense oligodeoxynucleotides. *Nucleic Acids Res.*, **17**, 4255–4273.

Chen, H.X., Marchall, J.L., Ness, E., Martin, R.R., Dvorchik, B., Rizi, N. *et al.* (2000) A safety and pharmacokinetic study of a mixed-backbone oligonucleotide (GEM231) targeting the type I protein kinase A by two-hour infusion in patients with refractory solid tumors. *Clin. Cancer Res.*, **6**, 1259–1266.

Chen, L., Agrawal, S., Zhou, W., Zhang, R. and Chen, J. (1998) Synergistic activation of p53 by inhibition of MDM2 expression and DNA damage. *Proc. Natl. Acad. Sci. USA*, **95**, 195–200.

Chen, L., Lu, W., Agrawal, S., Zhou, W. Zhang, R. and Chen, J. (1999) Ubiquitous induction of p53 in tumor cells by antisense inhibition of MDM2 expression. *Mol. Med.*, **5**, 21–34.

Crooke, S.T. (1998a) *Antisense Research and Applications*. Springer-Verlag, Berlin.

Crooke, S.T. (1998b) Vitravene – another piece in the mosaic. *Antisense Nucleic Acid Drug Dev.*, **8**, vii–viii.

Crooke, S.T. (1999) Molecular mechanisms of action of antisense drugs. *Antisense Biochim. Biophys. Acta.*, **1489**, 31–44.

Crooke, S.T. (2000a) Comments on evaluation of antisense drugs in the clinic. *Antisense Nucleic Acid Drug Dev.*, **10**, 225–227.

Crooke, S.T. (2000b) Progress in antisense technology: the end of beginning. *Methods Enzymol.*, **313**, 3–45.

Diasio, R.B. and Zhang, R. (1997) Pharmacology of therapeutic oligonucleotides. *Antisense Nucleic Acid Drug Dev.*, **7**, 239–243.

Dorigo, O., Turla, S.T., Lebedeva, S. and Gjerset, R.A. (1998) Sensitization of rat glioblastoma multiforme to cisplatin *in vivo* following restoration of wild-type p53 function. *J. Neurosurg.*, **88**, 535–540.

Elder, J.K., Johnson, M., Milner, N., Mir, K.U., Sohail, M. and Southern, E.M. (1999) Antisense oligonucleotide scanning arrays. In: M. Schena (ed.) *DNA Microarrays: a Practical Approach*, IRL Press, Oxford, pp. 77–99.

Freedman, D.A., and Levine, A.J. (1999) Regulation of p53 protein by MDM2 oncoprotein-Thirty eighth G.H.A. Clowes memorial award lecture. *Cancer Res.*, **59**, 1–7.

Freedman, D.A., Wu, L. and Levine, A.J. (1999) Functions of the MDM2 oncoprotein. *Cell Mol. Life Sci.*, **55**, 96–107.

Gewirtz, A.M. (1997) Oligonucleotide therapeutics for human leukaemia. In: D.J. Chadwick and G. Cardew (eds) *Oligonucleotides as Therapeutic Agents. Ciba Foundation Symposium 209*, Wiley, Chichester, pp. 169–194.

Gewirtz, A.M. (2000) Oligonucleotide therapeutics: a step forward. *J. Clin. Oncol.*, **18**, 1809–1811.

Ho, S.P., Bao, Y., Lesher, T., Malhotra, R., Ma, L.Y., Fluharty, S.J. *et al.* (1998) Mapping of RNA accessible sites for antisense experiments with oligonucleotide libraries. *Nat. Biotechnol.*, **16**, 59–63.

Juven-Gershon, T. and Oren, M. (1999) MDM2: the ups and downs. *Mol. Med.*, **5**, 71–83.

Kushner, D.M. and Silverman, R.H. (2000) Antisense cancer therapy: the state of the science. *Curr. Oncol. Rep.*, **2**, 23–30.

Landers, J.E., Cassel, S.L. and George, D.L. (1997) Translational enhancement of MDM2 oncogene expression in human tumor cells containing a stablized wild-type p53 protein. *Cancer Res.*, **57**, 3562–3568.

Landers, J.E., Haines, D.S., Strauss, J.F. and George, D.L. (1994) Enhanced translation: a novel mechanism of MDM2 oncogene overexpression identified in human tumor cells. *Oncogene*, **9**, 2745–2750.

Lebedeva, I. and Stein, C. (2001) Antisense oligonucleotides: promise and reality. *Ann. Rev. Pharmacol. Toxicol.*, **41**, 403–419.

Lima, W.F., Brown-Driver, V., Fox, M., Hanecak, R. and Bruice, T. (1997) Combinatorial screening and rational optimization for hybridisation to folded Hepatitis C virus RNA of oligonucleotides with biological antisense activity. *J. Biol. Chem.*, **272**, 626–638.

Lozano, G. and Montes de Oca Luna, R. (1998) MDM2 function. *Biochim. Biophys. Acta.*, **1377**, M55–M59.

Midgley, C.A. and Lane, D.P. (1997) P53 protein stability in tumor cells is not determined by mutation but is dependent on MDM2 binding. *Oncogene*, **15**, 1179–1189.

Miller, P.S. and Ts'o, P.O.P. (1988) Oligonucleotide inhibitors of gene expression in living cells: new opportunities in drug design. *Ann. Reports Med. Chem.*, **23**, 295–304.

Miller, P.S., Braiterman, L.T. and Ts'o, P.O.P. (1977) Effects of a trinucleotide ethyl phosphotriester, Gmp(Et)Gmp(Et)U on mammalian cells in culture. *Biochemistry*, **16**, 1988–1996.

Miller, P.S., McParland, K.B., Jayaraman, K. and Ts'o, P.O.P. (1981) Biochemical and biological effects of nonionic nucleic acid methylphosphonates. *Biochemisty*, **20**, 1874–1880.

Milner, N., Mir, K.U. and Southern, E.M. (1997) Selecting effective antisense reagents on combinatorial oligonucleotide arrays. *Nat. Biotechnol.*, **15**, 537–541.

Momand, J. and Zambetti, G.P. (1997) Mdm-2: 'big brother' of p53. *J. Cell Biochem.*, **64**, 343–352.

Momand, J., Jung, D., Wilczynski, S. and Niland, J. (1998) The MDM2 gene amplification database. *Nucleic Acids Res.*, **26**, 3453–3459.

Monia, B.P., Holmlund, J. and Dorr, F.A. (2000) Antisense approaches for the treatment of cancer. *Cancer Invest.*, **18**, 635–650.

Monia, B.P., Johnson, J.F., Geiger, T., Muller, M. and Fabbro, D. (1996) Antitumor activity of a phosphorothioate antisense oligodeoxynucleotide targeted against C-*raf* kinase. *Nat. Med.*, **2**, 668–675.

Nechers, L.M. (1989) Antisense oligonucleotides as a tool for studying cell regulation: mechanism of uptake and application to the study of oncogene function. In: J.S. Cohen (ed.) *Oligodeoxyribonucleotides: Antisense Inhibitors of Gene Expression*. Macmillan Press, London.

Nechers, L.M. (1993): Cellular internalization of oligodeoxynucleotides. In: S.T. Crooke and B. Lebleu (eds) *Antisense Research and Applications*, CRC Press, Inc., Boca Raton, FL, pp. 451–460.

Nielsen, L.L. and Maneval, D.C. (1998) p53 tumor suppressor gene therapy for cancer. *Cancer Gene Ther.*, **5**, 52–63.

Obertstra, J. and Nellen, W. (1997) Regulation genes with antisense RNA. In: B. Weiss (ed.) *Antisense Oligodeoxynucleotides and Antisense RNA, Novel Pharmacological and Therapeutic Agents*, CRC Press, Inc., Boca Raton, FL, pp. 171–195.

Perry, M.E., Piette, J., Zawadzki, J.A., Harvey, D. and Levine, A.J. (1993) The MDM-2 gene is induced in response to UV light in a p53-dependent manner. *Proc. Natl. Acad. Sci. USA*, **90**, 11623–11627.

Peyman, A., Helsberg, M., Kretzschmar, G., Mag, M., Grabley, S. and Uhlmann, E. (1995) Inhibition of viral growth by antisense oligonucleotides directed against the IE110 and the UL30 mRNA of Herpes Simplex Virus Type-1. *Biol. Chem. Hoope-Seyler*, **376**, 195–198.

Piette, J., Neel, H. and Marechal, V. (1997) MDM2: keeping p53 under control. *Oncogene*, **15**, 1001–1010.

Prives, C. (1998) Signaling to p53: breaking the MDM2-p53 circuit. *Cell*, **95**, 5–8.

Prives, C. and Hall, P.A. (1999) The p53 pathway. *J. Pathol.*, **187**, 112–126.

Santon, S.W. and Joyce, G.F. (1997) A general purpose of RNA-cleaving DNA enzyme. *Proc. Natl. Acad. Sci. USA*, **94**, 4262–4266.

Simons, R.W. (1988) Naturally occurring antisense RNA control – a brief review. *Gene*, **72**, 35–44.

Stein, C.A. and Cheng, Y.C. (1993) Antisense oligonucleotides as therapeutic agents – Is the bullet really magical? *Science*, **261**, 1004–1012.

Stein, C.A. and Cheng, Y.C. (1997) Antisense inhibition of gene expression. In: V.T. DeVita, S. Hellman and S.A. Rosenberg (eds) *Cancer: Principles and Practice of Oncology*, Lippincott-Raven, Philadelphia, pp. 3059–3074.

Stephenson, M.L. and Zamecnik, P.C. (1978) Inhibition of Rous sarcoma virus RNA translation by a specific oligodeoxyribonucleotide. *Proc. Natl. Acad. Sci. USA*, **75**, 285–288.

Wang, H., Cai, Q., Zeng, X., Yu, D., Agrawal, S. and Zhang, R. (1999a) Anti-tumor activity and pharmacokinetics of a mixed-backbone antisense oligonucleotide targeted to RIα subunit of protein kinase A after oral administration. *Proc. Natl. Acad. Sci. USA*, **96**, 13989–13994.

Wang, H., Oliver, P., Zeng, X., Le, L.P., Chen, J., Chen, L. *et al.* (1999b) MDM2 oncogene as a target for cancer therapy: an antisense approach. *Intl. J. Oncol.*, **15**, 653–660.

Watanabe, T., Hotta, T., Ichikawa, A., Kinoshita, T., Nagai, H. and Uchida, T. (1994) The MDM2 oncogene overexpression in chronic lymphocytic leukemia and low-grade lymphoma of B-cell origin. *Blood*, **84**, 3158–3165.

Wickstrom, E. (1998) *Clinical Trials of Genetic Therapy with Antisense DNA and DNA Vectors*. Marcel Dekker, New York.

Zamecnik, P.C. (1996) History of antisense oligonucleotides. In: S. Agrawal (ed.) *Antisense Therapeutics*, Humana Press, Totowa, pp. 1–12.

Zamecnik, P.C. and Stephenson, M.L. (1978) Inhibition of Rous sarcoma virus replication and cell transformation by a specific oligodeoxynucleotide. *Proc. Natl. Acad. Sci. USA*, **75**, 280–284.

Zhang, R. and Wang, H. (2000a) Antisense oligonucleotides as anti-tumor therapeutics. *Recent Res. Dev. Cancer*, **2**, 61–76.

Zhang, R. and Wang, H. (2000b) MDM2 oncogene as a novel target for human cancer therapy. *Curr. Pharm. Design*, **6**, 393–416.

Zhang, R., Diasio, R.B., Lu, Z., Liu, T., Jiang, Z., Galbraith, W.M. and Agrawal, S. (1995a) Pharmacokinetics and tissue disposition in rats of an oligodeoxynucleotide phosphorothioate (GEM 91) developed as a therapeutic agent for human immunodeficiency virus type-1. *Biochem. Pharm.*, **49**, 929–939.

Zhang, R., Lu, Z., Zhao, H., Zhang, X., Diasio, R.B., Habus, I. *et al.* (1995b) *In vivo* stability, disposition, and metabolism of a 'hybrid' oligonucleotide phosphorothioate in rats. *Biochem. Pharmacol.*, **50**, 545–556.

Zhang, R., Yan, J., Shahinian, H., Amin, G., Lu, Z., Liu, T. *et al.* (1995c) Pharmacokinetics of an oligodeoxynucleotide phosphorothioate (GEM 91) in HIV-infected subjects. *Clin. Pharmacol. Ther.*, **58**, 44–53.

Zhang, R., Iyer, P., Yu, D., Zhang, X., Lu, Z., Zhao, H. and Agrawal, S. (1996) Pharmacokinetics and tissue disposition of a chimeric oligodeoxynucleotide phosphorothioate in rats following intravenous administration. *J. Pharm. Exp. Ther.*, **278**, 971–979.

Zhang, S.-P., Zhou, L.-W., Nichols, R.A. and Weiss, B. (1997) Use of plasmid antisense RNA expression vectors in neurobiology. In: B. Weiss (ed.) *Antisense Oligodeoxynucleotides and Antisense RNA, Novel Pharmacological and Therapeutic Agents*, CRC Press, Inc., Boca Raton, FL, pp. 213–241.

Zuker, M. (1989) On finding all suboptimal folding of an RNA molecule. *Science*, **244**, 48–52.

4 Ribozymes as therapeutic agents and genetic tools

Alessandra Poggi, Alessandro Michienzi and John J. Rossi

INTRODUCTION

Ribozymes are RNA molecules capable of acting as enzymes even in the complete absence of proteins. They have the catalytic activity of breaking and/or forming covalent bonds with extraordinary specificity, accelerating the rate of these catalytic reactions. The ability of RNA to serve as a catalyst was first shown for the self-splicing Group I intron of *Tetrahymena* and the RNA moiety of RNAse P (Cech, 1990; Guerrier-Takada *et al.*, 1983; Kruger *et al.*, 1982). Group I introns, which range in size from 200 to 1500 nucleotides, are classified by phylogenetically conserved secondary structures, as well as by certain functional characteristics. These introns possess many of the attributes of protein enzymes, including substrate and co-factor binding domains. The well studied *Tetrahymena* intron has been shown to harbor important tertiary interactions with the substrate molecule and to undergo conformational shifts. It can also be engineered to bind, cleave and release multiple substrates. RNAse P is a ubiquitous enzyme that cleaves the $5'$ precursor segment from pre-transfer RNA molecules. The holoenzyme is comprised of at least one protein and one RNA subunit (ranging in size from 140 to 490 nucleotides, depending on the organism) (Kurz and Fierke, 2000). The RNA of the bacterial enzyme alone, under the appropriate salt and ionic conditions, can site specifically cleave the $5'$ leader segment from precursor t-RNAs (Guerrier-Takada *et al.*, 1983).

Subsequent to the discovery of these two RNA enzymes, RNA mediated catalysis has been associated with the self-splicing group II introns of yeast, fungal and plant mitochondria (as well as chloroplasts) (Michel and Ferat, 1995), single-stranded plant viroid and virusoid RNAs (Buzayan *et al.*, 1986, 1987; Hutchins *et al.*, 1986), hepatitis delta virus (Nishikawa *et al.*, 1992) and a satellite RNA from *Neurospora* mitochondria (Saville and Collins, 1990). Recently proposed ribozyme functions are the possibilities of ribosomal RNA functioning as a peptidyltransferase (Cech, 2000) and the spliceosomal snRNAs functioning as a ribozyme in complex with the pre-mRNA to catalyze pre-messenger RNA splicing (Steitz and Steitz, 1993). It is highly likely that additional RNA catalytic motifs and new roles for RNA mediated catalysis will also be found as we learn more about the genomes of a variety of organisms.

Ribozymes occur naturally, but can also be artificially engineered and synthesized to target specific sequences in *cis* or *trans*. New biochemical activities are being developed using *in vitro* selection protocols as well (Wilson and Szostak, 1999). Ribozymes can easily be manipulated to act on novel substrates. These custom-designed RNAs have great potential as therapeutic agents and are becoming a powerful tool for molecular biologists.

The discovery of catalytic RNA molecules has revolutionized views on the origins of life. RNA molecules, once thought to be primarily passive carriers of genetic information, can carry out some functions previously thought to be catalyzed only by proteins, indicating that RNA can confer not only a genotype (as in many RNA viruses), but also a phenotype. The RNA catalyzed reactions include self-cleavage, or *trans* cleavage reactions, ligation, and *trans*-splicing. These observations have led to speculation that RNA might have been an early self-replicating molecule in the pre-biotic world. Evidence supporting this notion comes from the fact that group I introns can exhibit RNA polymerase-like activities under certain conditions (Doudna *et al.*, 1991). In addition, the catalytic core of group I introns shares homology with several small satellite RNAs associated with plant viruses, which are also homologous to the human hepatitis delta virus (HDV), suggesting a common and ancient origin.

CATALYTIC MOTIFS

There are six ribozymes that have been successfully modified and/or adapted for use in therapeutic and functional genomic applications. These are the group I introns, RNAse P, the hammerhead and hairpin motifs, the hepatitis delta ribozyme and the reverse splicing reaction of group II introns. Each of these ribozymes requires a divalent metal cation for activity (usually $Mg++$), which may participate in the chemistry of the cleavage/ligation reaction and/or may be important for maintaining the structure of the ribozyme.

The group I intron of *Tetrahymena* was the first ribozyme for which the *cis*-cleaving (on a portion of the same RNA strand) reaction was converted into a *trans*-(on an exogenous RNA molecule) reaction (Cech, 1990). An altered form of the ribozyme lacking the 5' and 3' exons, but with a guanosine covalently attached to the 3' end of the intron, was shown to be capable of binding RNA substrates with complementarity to an internal guide sequence, cleaving the bound RNA, releasing the cleavage products and recycling the ribozyme itself. These elegant *in vitro* experiments demonstrated that self-cleaving RNAs could be engineered to carry out *trans*-cleavage reactions. A more recent application of the group I intron is that of correcting defective mRNAs in what has been termed 'trans-splicing' (Sullenger and Cech, 1994). In its *trans*-splicing configuration, the group I intron is not attached to a 5' exon, but has appended to the intron a 3' exon which is to be *trans*-spliced onto a target RNA. Figure 4.1 shows the Group I intron structure and model for *trans*-splicing. *Trans*-splicing may be of clinical importance in the future for repairing defective messages such as mutant forms of globin or the tumor suppressor p53 mRNAs. *Trans*-splicing ribozymes have been shown to simultaneously reduce mutant p53 expression and restore wt p53 activity in various human cancers. The corrected transcripts were translated to produce functional p53 that could *trans*activate p53-responsive promoters and down-modulate expression of the multi-drug resistance (MDR1) gene promoter. There was a 23-fold induction of a p53-responsive promoter and a three-fold reduction in MDR1 promoter expression in *trans*fected cancer cells (Watanabe and Sullenger, 2000).

Group I Intron

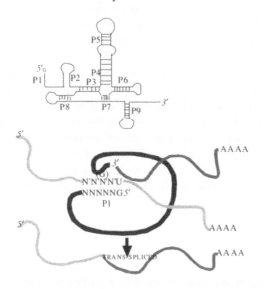

Figure 4.1 Group I intron structure and model for *trans*-splicing. The upper diagram
depicts the generalized secondary structure of the Group I intron. P1-P9
depict the various conserved helices. P1 is the internal guide sequence that
pairs with the 5′ exon in *cis*-splicing, and with the target mRNA in *trans*-
splicing. The bottom part of this figure depicts a *trans*-splicing reaction. The
(G) is the guanosine co-factor that acts as the nucleophile in the splicing
reaction. (*See Color plate 1*)

The group II intron was first identified as a self-splicing ribozyme in fungal
mitochondrial transcripts. Since the initial discovery, these introns have been
found in chloroplasts as well as in some bacteria (Michel and Ferat, 1995). The
intron has two sequences called 'exon binding sites' (EBS), which pair with
sequences in the exons during self-splicing. The released intron can reinsert itself
into spliced RNA as well as DNA by a reversal of the splicing mechanism. The
sequence requirements for binding of the EBS elements to a target DNA have been
elucidated, allowing engineering of the EBS for targeted integration of the group
II introns into a variety of gene sequences (Guo *et al.*, 2000). The implications of
this work are that group II introns can be engineered for targeted gene disruption,
or for insertion of therapeutic genes in a site-specific fashion into a host genome.

The endoribonuclease RNAse P is found in organisms throughout nature. As
stated above, this enzyme has RNA and one or more protein components. The
RNA component from the *E. coli* and *B. subtilis* enzymes can act as a site specific
cleavage agent in the absence of the protein under certain salt and ionic conditions
(Kurz and Fierke, 2000). Studies of the substrate requirements for this enzyme-
isolated from either bacteria or humans – have been carried out. The minimal substrates for either the bacterial or human enzymes resemble a segment of a transfer
RNA molecule (Forster and Altman, 1990; Kawa *et al.*, 1998). This structure can be
mimicked by uniquely designed antisense RNAs, which pair to the target RNA, and
serve as substrates for RNAse P mediated site-specific cleavage. Several investigators

have taken advantage of this property in the design of antisense RNAs which pair with target mRNAs of interest to stimulate both the site-specific cleavage of the target and the recycling of the antisense. It has also been shown that the antisense component can be covalently joined to the RNAse P RNA, thereby directing the enzyme only to the target RNA of interest (Liu and Altman, 1996).

One category of intramolecular RNA catalysis produces a $2'$, $3'$-cyclic phosphate and $5'$-OH terminus on the reaction products. A number of small plant pathogenic RNAs (viroids, satellite RNAs, and virusoids), a transcript from a *Neurospora* mitochondrial DNA plasmid, and the animal virus hepatitis delta virus (HDV) undergo a self-cleavage reaction *in vitro* in the absence of protein. The reactions require neutral pH and Mg^{2+}. It is thought that the self-cleavage reaction is an integral part of their *in vivo* rolling circle mechanism of replication. These self-cleaving RNAs can be subdivided into groups depending on the sequence and secondary structure formed about the cleavage site. Small ribozymes have been derived from a motif found in single stranded plant viroid and virusoid RNAs that replicate via a rolling circle mechanism. Based upon a shared secondary structure and a conserved set of nucleotides, the term 'hammerhead' has been given to one group of this self-cleavage domain (Forster and Symons, 1987; Haseloff and Gerlach, 1988). The hammerhead ribozyme is composed of approximately 30 nucleotides. The simplicity of the hammerhead catalytic domain (Figures 4.2 and 4.3) has made it a popular choice in the design of *trans*-acting ribozymes. Utilizing Watson-Crick base

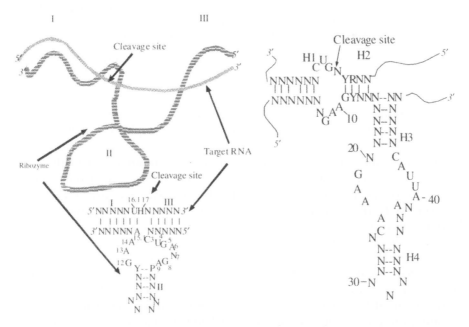

Figure 4.2 The hammerhead and hairpin ribozymes. Secondary structures for both the hammerhead and hairpin ribozymes are depicted. N = any nucleotide, R = Purine and Y = Pyrimidine. A diagram of the tertiary structure of the hammerhead ribozyme is depicted above the secondary structure model. The corresponding stems I, II and III in both structures are shown. In the hammerhead ribozyme H = A, C or U at the cleavage site. In the hairpin ribozymes H1, H2, etc. refer to the helical regions of the RNA structure.

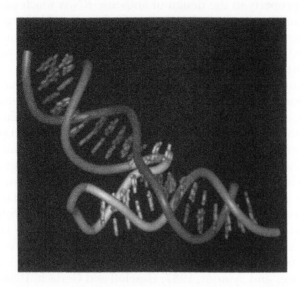

Figure 4.3 Chimeric hammerhead ribozyme structure. The ribozyme structure was computer modeled after the work of Pley *et al.* (1994). The yellow ribbon (backbone) and bases depict the catalytic core of the ribozyme, while the green ribbon (backbone) and bases depict the binding arms, which in this case are DNA from the work of Taylor *et al.* (1992). The magenta bases and ribbon (backbone) are the target RNA. The orange ribbon depicts the backbone of stem II, which can be minimally reduced to four propane diols and one G:C base pair (J. Rossi and P. Swiderski, unpublished data). The blue ribbon represents the target backbone at the site of ribozyme-mediated cleavage. (*see Color Plate 2*)

pairing, the hammerhead ribozyme can be designed to cleave any target RNA. The requirements at the cleavage site are relatively simple, and virtually any UH (where H is U, C or A) can be targeted.

A second plant derived self-cleavage motif, initially identified in the negative strand of the tobacco ringspot satellite RNA, has been termed the 'hairpin' or 'paperclip' (Buzayan *et al.*, 1986). The hairpin ribozymes cleave RNA substrates in a reversible reaction that generates 2', 3'-cyclic phosphate and 5'-hydroxyl termini. Engineered versions of this catalytic motif have also been shown to be capable of cleaving and turning over multiple copies of a variety of targets in *trans* (Figure 4.2) (Hampel *et al.*, 1990). Substrate requirements for the hairpin include a GUC, with cleavage occurring immediately upstream of the G. The hairpin ribozyme is also capable of catalyzing a ligation reaction, although it is more frequently used for cleavage reactions. Hairpin ribozyme-mediated cleavage and ligation proceed through a catalytic mechanism that does not require direct coordination of metal cations to phosphate or water oxygens.

Hepatitis delta virus (HDV) genomic and antigenomic RNAs contain a self-cleavage site hypothesized to function during rolling circle replication of this satellite virus. Like the plant pathogens, the sites in HDV are postulated to have a related secondary structure, three models of which have been proposed: *cloverleaf; pseudoknot* and *axehead* (Perrotta and Been, 1993), none of which is similar to the catalytic domains previously described. Like the other ribozyme motifs, the HDV ribozymes require a divalent cation and cleavage results in products with $2'$, $3'$-cyclic phosphate and $5'$-OH termini. Investigations of *trans*-cleavage with the HDV ribozyme have not advanced as far as those of the hammerhead or hairpin ribozymes.

The *Neurospora* mitochondrial VS RNA (Saville and Collins, 1990), a single-stranded circular RNA of 881 nt, shares some features of the self-catalytic RNAs of HDV, group I introns, and some plant viral satellite RNAs. Although VS RNA can be drawn to have a secondary structure like group I introns, it is missing essential base-pairing regions, the cleavage site is in a different position, and the termini produced are $2'$, $3'$-cyclic phosphate and $5'$-OH. Like the hammerhead ribozymes, the VS RNA requires divalent cations for cleavage *in vitro*. The catalytic core of *Neurospora* VS RNA has been shown to consist of 154 nt.

RIBOZYME APPLICATIONS

Ribozymes have been applied as anti-viral agents, for the treatment of cancer and genetic disorders, and as tools for pathway elucidation and target validation. Initial uses of ribozymes focused on anti-viral, primarily for the treatment of HIV (Rossi, 1999). Viruses that go through a genomic RNA intermediate in their replication cycle, such as HIV, hepatitis B virus and hepatitis C virus are attractive targets because a single species of ribozyme can target both viral genomic RNA and mRNAs. Ribozymes have also been widely used to target cellular genes, including those aberrantly expressed in cancers. One early ribozyme target was the *bcr-abl* fusion transcript created from the Philadelphia chromosome associated with chronic myelogenous leukemia (Kuwabara *et al.*, 1998; Lange, 1995; Snyder *et al.*, 1993, 1997). This chromosome is characterized by a translocation that results in the expression of a *trans*forming *bcr-abl* fusion protein. In this case, ribozymes have been designed to specifically target the fusion mRNA and not the normal *bcr* or *abl* mRNAs, preventing the function of *bcr-abl* oncogenes. The mutation at codon 12 in c-H-*ras* from GGU to GUU creates a site for hammerhead ribozyme mediated cleavage. An endogenously expressed ribozyme targeted to this site was effective in preventing focus formation in about 50% of NIH3T3 cells *trans*fected with this activated *ras* gene. In contrast, cells expressing this same ribozyme, but *trans*fected with an activated *ras* in which the codon change was at position 61 instead of 12, were not protected from foci formation by the ribozyme (Koizumi and Ohtsuka, 1992; Tsuchida *et al.*, 1998). Ribozymes targeting over-expressed *HER-2/neu* in breast carcinoma cells effectively reduced the tumorigenicity of these cells in mice (Czubayko *et al.*, 1997; Lui *et al.*, 2001).

In addition to directly targeting oncogenes, ribozymes have also been applied more indirectly as anti-cancer therapies. For example, ribozymes targeting the multiple drug resistance-1 (MDR1) (Kobayashi *et al.*, 1994; Scanlon *et al.*, 1994; Wang *et al.*, 1999) or fos mRNAs (Funato *et al.*, 1997; Scanlon *et al.*, 1994) in cancer cell lines effectively made the cells more sensitive to chemotherapeutic agents. Alternatively, a ribozyme targeting *bcl-2* triggered apoptosis in oral cancer cells (Gibson *et al.*, 2000). Factors required for metastasis are also attractive targets for ribozymes. Ribozymes targeted against *CAPL/mts* (Maelandsmo *et al.*, 1996) matrix metalloproteinase-9 (Sehgal *et al.*, 1998), pleiotrophin (Czubayko *et al.*, 1994) and VLA-6 integrin (Feng *et al.*, 1995; Yamamoto *et al.*, 1996) all reduced the metastatic potential of the respective tumor cells. Angiogenesis is also an important target for cancer therapy, and has been blocked in mice by ribozymes targeting fibroblast growth factor binding protein and pleiotrophin (Czubayko *et al.*, 1994). Ribozyme-based therapies have also been tested in animals to inhibit other proliferative disorders, such as coronary artery restenosis (Frimerman *et al.*, 1999; Gu *et al.*, 2001; Jarvis *et al.*, 1996a).

Heritable and spontaneous genetic disorders represent additional applications for therapeutic ribozymes targeting cellular genes. These include the beta-amyloid peptide precursor mRNA involved in Alzheimer's disease (Currie *et al.*, 1997; Dolzhanskaya *et al.*, 2000), and an autosomal-dominant point mutation in the rhodopsin mRNA that gives rise to photoreceptor degeneration and *retinitis pigmentosa* (Hauswirth and Lewin, 2000; LaVail *et al.*, 2000).

OPTIMIZING INTRACELLULAR FUNCTION OF RIBOZYMES

In contrast to the rather extensive knowledge of the rules governing ribozyme function *in vitro*, where free diffusion of ribozyme and target in solution is unrestricted, there are only a limited set of rules for predicting ribozyme efficacy in a complex intracellular environment. The parameters that affect ribozyme function in cells are: intracellular stability, expression levels of the ribozyme RNA, intracellular co-localization with the target RNA, stability of the ribozyme transcripts, and interactions of proteins with the ribozymes. The most effective strategies for achieving ribozyme function *in vivo* involve mechanisms for maximizing the ability of the ribozyme to pair with its target RNA. Since the *trans*-cleaving and *trans*-ligation applications of ribozymes involve Watson-Crick base pairing of the ribozyme, or the guide sequence (for RNAse P) to the target RNA, this interaction is the rate-limiting step *in vivo*. Various strategies have been used to identify accessible pairing sites on target RNAs. Not all target sites for these ribozymes are accessible for cleavage; secondary structures, binding of proteins and nucleic acids, and other factors influence intracellular ribozyme efficacy. Computer- assisted RNA folding predictions and *in vitro* cleavage analyses are not necessarily predictive for intracellular or *in vivo* activity, and the best ribozyme target sites must often be determined empirically *in vivo*. Strategies utilizing cell extracts with native mRNAs have proven useful for determining accessible ribozyme binding sites (Castanotto *et al.*, 2000; Scherr *et al.*, 2000; Scherr and Rossi, 1998).

Expression levels and intracellular localization of the ribozyme *trans*cripts are critical for the successful application of the ribozymes in gene therapy. For transcripts, various promoters can be used to obtain either constitutive or regulated expression (Bertrand *et al.*, 1997; Good *et al.*, 1997). The transcripts themselves can be engineered to localize within the same cellular or sub-cellular compartment as the target RNA. In order for *trans*-cleaving ribozymes to be effective in down-regulating mRNAs, the efficiency of cleavage must be greater than the steady state rates of synthesis and decay of the target.

For ribozyme down-regulation to be effective, the decay mediated by the ribozyme at a given ribozyme concentration must exceed the steady state level of target turnover in the absence of ribozyme. This condition can be best achieved by identifying highly accessible target sites combined with high levels of ribozyme expression in the appropriate cellular compartment. Using these parameters, down-regulation can exceed 90%. A combination of the above elements has been applied to an anti-HIV-1 ribozyme. A ribozyme targeted to a highly accessible and highly conserved site in the HIV genomic and mRNAs was inserted within a small RNA element that directs localization of the *trans*cripts into the nucleolus (Figure 4.4) (Michienzi *et al.*, 2000). Since HIV encoded regulatory proteins Tat and Rev have nucleolar localization signals, and both bind HIV RNA, it was reasoned that these proteins could direct trafficking of HIV RNAs into this organelle. The chimeric ribozyme transcripts were made from a strong Pol III promoter element, producing high levels of the transcript, which localized primarily in the nucleolus. These nucleolar localized ribozymes were positioned to bind and cleave HIV-1

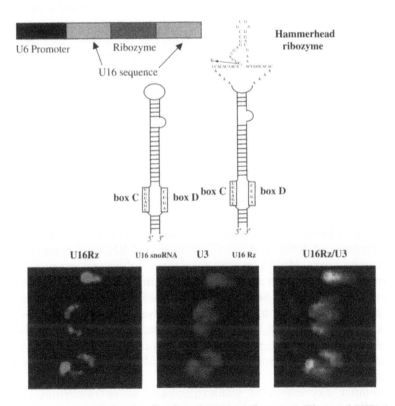

Figure 4.4 Nucleolar localized anti-HIV-1 ribozyme. The anti-HIV-1 ribozyme was inserted within the apical loop of the small nucleolar RNA U16. The chimeric U16-ribozyme was placed behind the Pol III U6 snRNA promoter. Transcripts of the chimeric RNA localize to the nucleolus, as shown by the *in situ* hybridization and co-localization with the small nucleolar RNA U3. The *in situ* hybrids were performed in transfected 293 cells. The ribozyme probe was fluorescein labeled (green), whereas the U3 probe was labeled with Cy3 (red). Reproduced with permission from Michienzi *et al.* (2000). (*see Color Plate 3*)

RNAs as they trafficked through the nucleolus, and in fact provided nearly complete inhibition of HIV replication in cell culture (Michienzi *et al.*, 2000). Other strategies for co-localizing ribozymes and substrates to enhance ribozyme function include: the use of viral dimerization/packaging domains on ribozyme and target, nuclear versus cytoplasmic localization, and the use of localized mRNA 3′ UTRs on ribozyme and target (Bertrand *et al.*, 1997; Sullenger and Cech, 1993). To achieve maximal ribozyme efficacy, it is important to have some knowledge of the intracellular trafficking of the target RNA. In many instances the RNAs will not have unique intracellular partitioning, and therefore it becomes necessary to test high levels of ribozyme expression in either the cytoplasm or nucleus to determine which is the best compartment for obtaining optimal ribozyme function.

As the use of ribozymes progresses from cell culture systems into animal models, additional control over ribozyme expression will be required. Ribozyme expression can be restricted to specific organs or cell types through the use of tissue-specific promoters. This specificity has been successfully achieved in tissue culture using the tyrosinase promoter, which is exclusively expressed in melanocytes (Ohta *et al.*, 1996). In another example, *trans*genic mice were created that carried a ribozyme gene driven by the insulin promoter, and were only expressed in the pancreatic beta-cell islets (Efrat *et al.*, 1994). Alternatively, inducible promoters, such as those regulated by tetracycline, have shown utility in both cell culture and in animals, allowing ribozyme expression to be turned on and off at will (Benedict *et al.*, 1998; Thomas *et al.*, 2001).

RIBOZYME DELIVERY

Whatever type of ribozyme is chosen, it must be introduced into its target cells. Two general mechanisms exist for introducing catalytic RNA molecules into cells: exogenous delivery of the preformed ribozyme and endogenous expression from a *trans*criptional unit. Preformed ribozymes can be delivered into cells using liposomes, electroporation, or microinjection. Many exciting developments in the chemical synthesis of RNA and modified forms of RNA have taken place over the past several years. Molecules with long-term stability in serum or intra-cellular environments have been synthesized (Burgin *et al.*, 1996; Heidenreich *et al.*, 1994; Jarvis *et al.*, 1996b). Several of these backbone-modified ribozymes still maintain the site specificity and catalytic turnover features of unmodified RNAs, and some have enhanced catalytic properties, making them candidates for *ex vivo* delivery. Chemically modified ribozymes have been shown to be capable of being delivered without encapsulation and can be taken up by cells (Flory *et al.*, 1996).

Stable intracellular expression of transcriptionally active ribozymes can be achieved by viral vector-mediated delivery. Currently, retroviral vectors are the most commonly used in cell culture, primary cells and in transgenic animals (Morgan and Anderson, 1993). Retroviral vectors have the advantage of stable integration into a dividing host cell genome, and the absence of any viral gene expression reduces the chance of an immune response in animals. In addition, retroviruses can be easily pseudo-typed with a variety of envelope proteins to broaden or restrict host cell tropism, thus adding an additional level of cellular targeting for ribozyme gene delivery. Adenoviral vectors can be produced at high titers and provide very efficient transduction, but they do not integrate into the host genome and, consequently, expression of the transgenes is only *transient* in actively dividing cells (Perlman *et al.*, 2000; Suzuki *et al.*, 2000; Tsuchida *et al.*, 2000). Other viral delivery systems are actively being pursued, such as the adeno-associated virus, alpha viruses and lentiviruses (Giordano *et al.*, 2000; Horster *et al.*, 1999; Kunke *et al.*, 2000; L'Huillier *et al.*, 1992; Lipkowitz *et al.*, 1996; Sczakiel *et al.*, 1997; Welch *et al.*, 1998). Adeno-associated virus is attractive as a small, non-pathogenic virus that can stably integrate into the host genome. An alpha virus system, using recombinant Semliki Forest virus, provides high transduction efficiencies of mammalian cells along with cytoplasmic ribozyme expression (Smith *et al.*, 1997).

Another vehicle for the *ex vivo* delivery of ribozyme genes is cationic lipids (Hope *et al.*, 1998). Since there are a variety of formulations for these lipids, it is usually best to test a panel of lipids for those that provide the highest efficiency of gene transfer with the least toxicity.

FUNCTIONAL GENOMICS AND TARGET VALIDATION

Ribozymes can be used to inactivate specific gene expression, and can thereby be used to help identify the function of a protein or the role of a gene in a functional biochemical pathway. Target validation is an increasingly important tool in basic biological research and drug development. With the recent completion of the human genome sequencing initiative, there are tens of thousands of transcriptomes that have no assigned function. Ribozymes provide a facile and highly specific tool for interfering with the expression of these transcripts to monitor their biological function.

Ribozyme-mediated target validation can also be used to identify specific member(s) of a protein family involved in a specific phenotype. Carefully designed ribozymes can selectively knock down expression of each protein in a gene family.

TRANSGENIC ANIMALS EXPRESSING RIBOZYMES

Therapeutics and target validation studies will certainly be tested in animals. Ribozymes have been used in transgenic mice to create disease models such as diabetes by selectively down-regulating the hexokinase mRNA in pancreatic islets (Efrat *et al.*, 1994). In this case the ribozyme expression was under the control of the insulin promoter, and was therefore only expressed in the pancreatic beta cells. Retroviral delivery of ribozymes targeted against neuregulin-1 in a chick blastoderm resulted in the same embryonic lethal phenotype as a gene knockout. Localized retroviral delivery of the same ribozyme later in the development allowed dissection of the neuregulin biochemical pathway (Zhao and Lemke, 1998). The use of a heat inducible ribozyme against *Fushi tarzu* in *Drosophila* allowed the developmentally timed disruption of this gene function in *Drosophila* embryos (Zhao and Pick, 1993).

RIBOZYME-MEDIATED RNA REPAIR

A novel therapeutic application of ribozymes exploits the *trans*-splicing activity of the *Tetrahymena* ribozyme. This ribozyme has been used to repair defective mRNAs by *trans*-splicing onto these RNAs a functional sequence (Sullenger and Cech, 1994; Watanabe and Sullenger, 2000). These ribozymes are designed to bind and cleave the target RNAs 5' of the undesired mutation. Since the ribozyme in this case is an intron, it is engineered to carry with it the correct RNA sequence as the 3' exon. Following cleavage of the mutant target RNA, the ribozyme catalyzes ligation of wild-type sequence onto the cleaved transcript. This process was first successfully demonstrated with the correction of a mutant *lac*Z transcript (Sullenger and Cech, 1994) in bacteria, and subsequently with the correction of a sickle cell message in erythroid cells (Lan *et al.*, 1998).

RIBOZYME-BASED GENE DISCOVERY

The necessity of ribozymes to selectively base-pair with the target RNAs prior to catalysis has been exploited to discover new gene functions involved in a particular phenotype. This protocol has been termed 'inverse genomics' (Beger *et al.*, 2001). A combinatorial ribozyme library has been introduced into cultured cells, and selection or scoring for a particular phenotype has led to the identification of several new gene functions (Kruger *et al.*, 2000; Li *et al.*, 2000; Welch *et al.*, 2000). A hairpin ribozyme library containing roughly 2×10^7 different ribozymes was stably transduced into tumor cells in culture and cells able to grow in soft agar were identified. Ribozymes isolated from these cells were sequenced, and the complement to the ribozyme pairing arms was determined. This approach has potential applications in many systems (therapeutic or otherwise) where a phenotype is of interest but the genes involved are unknown.

RIBOZYME EVOLUTION

The discovery of the ribozyme sparked new debate on the 'RNA world' hypothesis, where all biological processes were carried out by RNA-based enzymes. Since then, RNA evolution has been forced *in vitro* to come up with RNA enzymes capable of carrying out a wide variety of biochemical reactions, as far-reaching as carbon–carbon bond and peptide bond formation. *In vitro* RNA evolution has been used to create RNA-cleaving ribozymes with smaller catalytic domains, DNA cleaving ribozymes and new catalytic motifs (Szostak, 1997). Even RNA cleaving DNAzymes have been generated through *in vitro* evolution (Santoro and Joyce, 1997). These 'evolved' enzymes exemplify the power of *in vitro* evolution and will no doubt find many applications.

It is reasonable to conclude that achieving effective ribozyme-substrate interactions and ribozyme function in an intracellular environment is not a straightforward task, and that new strategies for expression and localization of ribozymes in the intracellular mileu will be required to permit the general utility of ribozymes as therapeutic agents.

OTHER CONSIDERATIONS

Although base-pairing specificity confers target selectivity, minimizing the potential for general toxicity, the question of toxicity must be rigorously tested since mispairing by a ribozyme to a non-targeted substrate could elicit undesired antisense inhibitory effects. Since every ribozyme sequence has different potential base-pairing interactions, an accumulation of data from many different ribozyme experiments will be required to assess this potential problem. Some of the potential sources of toxicity are non-specific interactions of ribozymes with cellullar proteins, the generation of high intracellular concentrations of the cleavage products, and the inhibitory effects on cellular metabolism of various chemically generated backbone modifications used to stabilize pre-synthesized ribozymes.

A different problem is loss of ribozyme activity due to base-pairing mismatches or mutations at the site of cleavage. This is an especially significant problem in designing ribozymes against genetically variable targets such as HIV. By choosing targets in highly conserved sequences and simultaneously using multiple ribozymes to a number of targets, loss of ribozyme activity can be minimized. Such strategies are already being tested by a number of laboratories.

One of the potential advantages of ribozymes versus antisense RNAs is their catalytic activity, which could theoretically lead to inactivation of multiple targeted substrates. It has yet to be demonstrated that this type of catalytic activity can occur intracellularly. The recently described protein facilitation of hammerhead ribozyme mediated cleavage (Bertrand and Rossi, 1994; Herschlag *et al.*, 1994) suggests that intracellular ribozyme mediated substrate turnover may be possible. Experiments designed to exploit the intracellular protein facilitation of ribozyme turnover are currently underway in several laboratories. The inclusion of RNA binding proteins in *in vitro* evolution strategies to enrich ribozyme-protein combinations with enhanced catalytical activities should also be exploited. Finally, the design and chemical synthesis of ribozymes capable of high catalytic turnover as a consequence of specific base and backbone modifications is a distinct possibility.

FUTURE PROSPECTS

The notion that ribozymes could be used as therapeutic agents has only existed for a few years, yet there is a great deal of interest in deploying clinically useful ribozymes in the very near future. At this time it is premature to conclude that ribozymes will have a place in the repertoire of therapeutic agents available to modern medicine. We must learn a great deal more about the movement of RNA inside the cells as well as the cellular factors that can impede or enhance ribozyme utilization. These are not simple problems, but they are not confined to those studying the application of ribozymes. As techniques in cell biology become more refined, answers to some of these problems will be forthcoming.

Basic studies of ribozyme structure and mechanisms of catalysis are flourishing in the midst of commercial interests. Based upon the research and development taking place in both academic and commercial settings, we can expect to see many new developments in ribozyme design and applications in the near future.

Table 4.1 Partial list of successful ribozyme mediated target mRNA down-regulation

Target	Effect	Reference
HIV-1	Block viral replication *in vitro*	(Sarver *et al.*, 1990; Yu *et al.*, 1993)
CCR5	Block HIV-1 cell entry *in vitro*	(Bai *et al.*, 2000; Cagnon and Rossi, 2000; Feng *et al.*, 2000)
Chronic myelogenous leukemia bcr/abl mRNA	Block cell proliferation *in vitro*	(Kuwabara *et al.*, 1998; Lange, 1995; Snyder *et al.*, 1993, 1997)
Ras	Block tumor foci formation *in vitro* and *in vivo*	(Koizumi and Ohtsuka, 1992; Tsuchida *et al.*, 1998)
Her2/neu	Block tumorigenicity *in vivo*	(Czubayko *et al.*, 1997a; Lui *et al.*, 2001)
MDR1 Cfos	Make cells more sensitive to chemotherapeutic agents *in vitro*	(Kobayashi *et al.*, 1994; Scanlon *et al.*, 1994; Wang *et al.*, 1999; Funato *et al.*, 1997)
Bcl2	Trigger apoptosis *in vitro*	(Gibson *et al.*, 2000)
CAPL/mts MMP9 Pleiotrophin VLA-6 integrin	Reduce or eliminate metastatic potential of cells *in vivo*	(Maelandsmo *et al.*, 1996; Sehgal *et al.*, 1998; Czubayko *et al.*, 1994; Feng *et al.*, 1995; Yamamoto *et al.*, 1996)
FGFBP VegF Receptor	Block angiogenesis *in vitro* and *in vivo*	(Czubayko *et al.*, 1997; Pavco *et al.*, 2000)
PNA1 c-Myb Lipoxygenase	Block restenosis *in vivo*	(Frimerman *et al.*, 1999; Gu *et al.*, 2001; Jarvis *et al.*, 1996a,b)
Beta-amyloid peptide mRNA	Block amyloid plaque formation *in vitro*	Currie *et al.*, 1997; Dolzhanskaya *et al.*, 2000)
Rhodopsin	Block photoreceptor degeneration *in vivo*	(Hauswirth and Lewin, 2000)
Ftz	Block pattern formation *in vivo*	(Zhao and Pick, 1993)
Hexokinase	Generate type II diabetes model *in vivo*	(Efrat *et al.*, 1994)

The transformation of ribozyme sequences from naturally-occurring, *cis*-cleaving (and ligating) molecules to target-specific, *trans*-cleaving (and ligating) reagents has stimulated a great deal of interest in their potential applications. Ribozymes targeting viral genes are now in clinical evaluation, ribozymes targeting cellular genes are moving into transgenic animals and the use of ribozymes is expanding into RNA evolution, mRNA repair and gene discovery. Table 4.1 shows the partial list of successful ribozyme-mediated target mRNA down-regulation.

For ribozymes to become generally useful surrogate genetic tools and realistic therapeutic agents, several obstacles first need to be overcome. These obstacles are the efficient delivery to a high percentage of the cell population, efficient expression of the ribozyme from a vector or intracellular ribozyme concentration, colocalization of the ribozyme with the target, specificity of ribozyme for the desired mRNA, and an enhancement of ribozyme-mediated substrate turnover. As our knowledge of RNA structure, secondary and tertiary, increases, we will be able to target RNAs more rationally, which may help with the problems of specificity. At the same time, the understanding of the physical localization of RNA in cells and its tracking as it moves from the nucleus to the cytoplasm will also help in ensuring co-localization of the ribozyme and target. Modifications of the ribozymes, e.g., the $2'$ ribose with various agents such as methyl, allyl, fluoro and amino groups, increase the stability to nucleases quite dramatically. Similarly, chimeric DNA-RNA ribozymes increase the stability. The efficiency of delivery to cells with viral vectors or liposomes is also continually improving. These molecules must retain their catalytic potential, reach an accessible site on the substrate, and effectively impact on the steady state levels of target molecules to be useful as either surrogate genetic tools or as therapeutic agents. Great progress has been made in all of these areas and should allow extensive use of the highly specific reagents for down-regulating expression of target RNAs.

ACKNOWLEDGMENTS

JJR was supported by NIH grants AI 29329 and AI 42552.

REFERENCES

Bai, J., Gorantla, S., Banda, N., Cagnon, L., Rossi, J. and Akkina, R. (2000) Characterization of anti-CCR5 ribozyme-transduced CD34+ hematopoietic progenitor cells *in vitro* a SCID-hu mouse model *in vivo*. *Mol. Ther.*, **1**, 244–254.

Beger, C., Pierce, L.N., Kruger, M., Marcusson, E.G., Robbins, J.M., Welsh, P. *et al.* (2001) Identification of Id4 as a regulator of BRCA1 expression by using a ribozyme-library-based inverse genomics approach. *Proc. Natl. Acad. Sci. USA*, **98**, 130–135.

Benedict, C.M., Pan, W., Loy, S.E. and Clawson, G.A. (1998) Triple ribozyme-mediated down-regulation of the retinoblastoma gene. *Carcinogenesis*, **19**, 1223–1230.

Bertrand, E., Castanotto, D., Zhou, C., Carbonnelle, C., Lee, N.S., Good, P. *et al.* (1997) The expression cassette determines the functional activity of ribozymes in mammalian cells by controlling their intracellular localization. *RNA*, **3**, 75–88.

Bertrand, E.L. and Rossi, J.J. (1994) Facilitation of hammerhead ribozyme catalysis by the nucleocapsid protein of HIV-1 and the heterogeneous nuclear ribonucleoprotein A1. *EMBO J.*, **13**, 2904–2912.

Burgin, Jr., A.B., Gonzalez, C., Matulic-Adamic, J., Karpeisky, A.M., Usman, N., McSwiggen, J.A. and Beigelman, L. (1996) Chemically modified hammerhead ribozymes with improved catalytic rates. *Biochemistry*, **35**, 14090–14097.

Buzayan, J.M., Hampel, A. and Bruening, G. (1986) Nucleotide sequence and newly formed phosphodiester bond of spontaneously ligated satellite tobacco ringspot virus RNA. *Nucleic Acids Res.*, **14**, 9729–9743.

Buzayan, J.M., McNinch, J.S., Schneider, I.R. and Bruening, G. (1987) A nucleotide sequence rearrangement distinguishes two isolates of satellite tobacco ringspot virus RNA. *Virology*, **160**, 95–99.

Cagnon, L. and Rossi, J.J. (2000) Downregulation of the CCR5 beta-chemokine receptor and inhibition of HIV-1 infection by stable VA1-ribozyme chimeric transcripts. *Antisense Nucleic Acid Drug Dev.*, **10**, 251–261.

Castanotto, D., Scherr, M. and Rossi, J.J. (2000) Intracellular expression and function of antisense catalytic RNAs. *Methods Enzymol.*, **313**, 401–420.

Cech, T.R. (1990) Self-splicing of group I introns. *Annu. Rev. Biochem.*, **59**, 543–568.

Cech, T.R. (2000) Structural biology. The ribosome is a ribozyme. *Science*, **289**, 878–879.

Currie, J.R., Chen-Hwang, M.C., Denman, R., Smedman, M., Potempska, A., Ramakrishna, N. *et al.* (1997) Reduction of histone cytotoxicity by the Alzheimer beta-amyloid peptide precursor. *Biochim. Biophys. Acta.*, **1355**, 248–258.

Czubayko, F., Downing, S.G., Hsieh, S.S., Goldstein, D.J., Lu, P.Y., Trapnell, B.C. and Wellstein, A. (1997a) Adenovirus-mediated *trans*duction of ribozymes abrogates HER-2/neu and pleiotrophin expression and inhibits tumor cell proliferation. *Gene Ther.*, **4**, 943–949.

Czubayko, F., Liaudet-Coopman, E.D., Aigner, A., Tuveson, A.T., Berchem, G.J. and Wellstein, A. (1997b) A secreted FGF-binding protein can serve as the angiogenic switch in human cancer. *Nat. Med.*, **3**, 1137–1140.

Czubayko, F., Riegel, A.T. and Wellstein, A. (1994) Ribozyme-targeting elucidates a direct role of pleiotrophin in tumor growth. *J. Biol. Chem.*, **269**, 21358–21363.

Dolzhanskaya, N., Conti, J., Merz, G. and Denman, R.B. (2000) *In vivo* ribozyme targeting of beta APP(+) mRNAs. *Mol. Cell Biol. Res. Commun.*, **4**, 239–247.

Doudna, J.A., Couture, S. and Szostak, J.W. (1991) A multisubunit ribozyme that is a catalyst of and template for complementary strand RNA synthesis. *Science*, **251**, 1605–1608.

Efrat, S., Leiser, M., Wu, Y.J., Fusco-DeMane, D., Emran, O.A., Surana, M. *et al.* (1994) Ribozyme-mediated attenuation of pancreatic beta-cell glucokinase expression in transgenic mice results in impaired glucose-induced insulin secretion. *Proc. Natl. Acad. Sci. USA*, **91**, 2051–2055.

Feng, B., Rollo, E.E. and Denhardt, D.T. (1995) Osteopontin (OPN) may facilitate metastasis by protecting cells from macrophage NO-mediated cytotoxicity: evidence from cell lines down-regulated for OPN expression by a targeted ribozyme. *Clin. Exp. Metastasis*, **13**, 453–462.

Feng, Y., Leavitt, M., Tritz, R., Duarte, E., Kang, D., Mamounas, M. *et al.* (2000) Inhibition of CCR5-dependent HIV-1 infection by hairpin ribozyme gene therapy against CC-chemokine receptor 5. *Virology*, **276**, 271–278.

Flory, C.M., Pavco, P.A., Jarvis, T.C., Lesch, M.E., Wincott, F.E., Beigelman, L. *et al.* (1996) Nuclease-resistant ribozymes decrease stromelysin mRNA levels in rabbit synovium following exogenous delivery to the knee joint. *Proc. Natl. Acad. Sci. USA*, **93**, 754–758.

Forster, A.C. and Altman, S. (1990) External guide sequences for an RNA enzyme. *Science*, **249**, 783–786.

Forster, A.C. and Symons, R.H. (1987) Self-cleavage of plus and minus RNAs of a virusoid and a structural model for the active sites. *Cell*, **49**, 211–220.

Frimerman, A., Welch, P.J., Jin, X., Eigler, N., Yei, S., Forrester, J. *et al.* (1999) Chimeric DNA-RNA hammerhead ribozyme to proliferating cell nuclear antigen reduces stent-induced stenosis in a porcine coronary model. *Circulation*, **99**, 697–703.

Funato, T., Ishii, T., Kanbe, M., Scanlon, K.J. and Sasaki, T. (1997) Reversal of cisplatin resistance *in vivo* by an anti-fos ribozyme. *In Vivo*, **11**, 217–220.

Gibson, S.A., Pellenz, C., Hutchison, R.E., Davey, F.R. and Shillitoe, E.J. (2000) Induction of apoptosis in oral cancer cells by an anti-bcl-2 ribozyme delivered by an adenovirus vector. *Clin. Cancer Res.*, **6**, 213–222.

Giordano, V., Jin, D.Y., Rekosh, D. and Jeang, K.T. (2000) Intravirion targeting of a functional anti-human immunodeficiency virus ribozyme directed to pol. *Virology*, **267**, 174–184.

Good, P.D., Krikos, A.J., Li, S.X., Bertrand, E., Lee, N.S., Giver, L. *et al.* (1997) Expression of small, therapeutic RNAs in human cell nuclei. *Gene Ther.*, **4**, 45–54.

Gu, J.L., Pei, H., Thomas, L., Nadler, J.L., Rossi, J.J., Lanting, L. and Natarajan, R. (2001) Ribozyme-mediated inhibition of rat leukocyte-type 12-lipoxygenase prevents intimal hyperplasia in balloon-injured rat carotid arteries. *Circulation*, **103**, 1446–1452.

Guerrier-Takada, C., Gardiner, K., Marsh, T., Pace, N. and Altman, S. (1983) The RNA moiety of ribonuclease P is the catalytic subunit of the enzyme. *Cell*, **35**, 849–857.

Guo, H., Karberg, M., Long, M., Jones III, J.P., Sullenger, B. and Lambowitz, A.M. (2000) Group II introns designed to insert into therapeutically relevant DNA target sites in human cells. *Science*, **289**, 452–457.

Hampel, A., Tritz, R., Hicks, M. and Cruz, P. (1990) 'Hairpin' catalytic RNA model: evidence for helices and sequence requirement for substrate RNA. *Nucleic Acids Res.*, **18**, 299–304.

Haseloff, J. and Gerlach, W.L. (1988) Simple RNA enzymes with new and highly specific endoribonuclease activities. *Nature*, **334**, 585–591.

Hauswirth, W.W. and Lewin, A.S. (2000) Ribozyme uses in retinal gene therapy. *Prog. Retin. Eye Res.*, **19**, 689–710.

Heidenreich, O., Benseler, F., Fahrenholz, A. and Eckstein, F. (1994) High activity and stability of hammerhead ribozymes containing 2'-modified pyrimidine nucleosides and phosphorothioates. *J. Biol. Chem.*, **269**, 2131–2138.

Herschlag, D., Khosla, M., Tsuchihashi, Z. and Karpel, R.L. (1994) An RNA chaperone activity of non-specific RNA binding proteins in hammerhead ribozyme catalysis. *EMBO J.*, **13**, 2913–2924.

Hope, M.J., Mui, B., Ansell, S. and Ahkong, Q.F. (1998) Cationic lipids, phosphatidylethanolamine and the intracellular delivery of polymeric, nucleic acid-based drugs. *Mol. Membr. Biol.*, **15**, 1–14.

Horster, A., Teichmann, B., Hormes, R., Grimm, D., Kleinschmidt, J. and Sczakiel, G. (1999) Recombinant AAV-2 harboring gfp-antisense/ribozyme fusion sequences monitor transduction, gene expression, and show anti-HIV-1 efficacy. *Gene Ther.*, **6**, 1231–1238.

Hutchins, C.J., Rathjen, P.D., Forster, A.C. and Symons, R.H. (1986) Self-cleavage of plus and minus RNA *trans*cripts of avocado sunblotch viroid. *Nucleic Acids Res.*, **14**, 3627–3640.

Jarvis, T.C., Alby, L.J., Beaudry, A.A., Wincott, F.E., Beigelman, L., McSwiggen, J.A., Usman, N. and Stinchcomb, D.T. (1996a) Inhibition of vascular smooth muscle cell proliferation by ribozymes that cleave c-myb mRNA. *RNA*, **2**, 419–428.

Jarvis, T.C., Wincott, F.E., Alby, L.J., McSwiggen, J.A., Beigelman, L., Gustofson, J. *et al.* (1996b) Optimizing the cell efficacy of synthetic ribozymes. Site selection and chemical modifications of ribozymes targeting the proto-oncogene c-myb. *J. Biol. Chem.*, **271**, 29107–29112.

Kawa, D., Wang, J., Yuan, Y. and Liu, F. (1998) Inhibition of viral gene expression by human ribonuclease P. *RNA*, **4**, 1397–1406.

Kobayashi, H., Dorai, T., Holland, J.F. and Ohnuma, T. (1994) Reversal of drug sensitivity in multidrug-resistant tumor cells by an MDR1 (PGY1) ribozyme. *Cancer Res.*, **54**, 1271–1275.

Koizumi, M. and Ohtsuka, E. (1992) Design of RNAs that inhibit the activated c-Ha-ras gene in mammalian cells. *Ann. N. Y. Acad. Sci.*, **660**, 276.

Kruger, K., Grabowski, P.J., Zaug, A.J., Sands, J., Gottschling, D.E. and Cech, T.R. (1982) Self-splicing RNA: autoexcision and autocyclization of the ribosomal RNA intervening sequence of Tetrahymena. *Cell*, **31**, 147–157.

Kruger, M., Beger, C., Li, Q.X., Welch, P.J., Tritz, R., Leavitt, M., Barber, J.R. and Wong-Staal, F. (2000) Identification of eIF2Bgamma and eIF2gamma as cofactors of hepatitis C virus internal ribosome entry site-mediated *trans*lation using a functional genomics approach. *Proc. Natl. Acad. Sci. USA*, **97**, 8566–8571.

Kunke, D., Grimm, D., Denger, S., Kreuzer, J., Delius, H., Komitowski, D. and Kleinschmidt, J.A. (2000) Preclinical study on gene therapy of cervical carcinoma using adeno-associated virus vectors. *Cancer Gene Ther.*, **7**, 766–777.

Kurz, J.C. and Fierke, C.A. (2000) Ribonuclease P: a ribonucleoprotein enzyme. *Curr. Opin. Chem. Biol.*, **4**, 553–558.

Kuwabara, T., Warashina, M., Tanabe, T., Tani, K., Asano, S. and Taira, K. (1998) A novel allosterically *trans*-activated ribozyme, the maxizyme, with exceptional specificity *in vitro* and *in vivo*. *Mol. Cell*, **2**, 617–627.

Lan, N., Howrey, R.P., Lee, S.W., Smith, C.A. and Sullenger, B.A. (1998) Ribozyme-mediated repair of sickle beta-globin mRNAs in erythrocyte precursors. *Science*, **280**, 1593–1596.

Lange, W. (1995) Cleavage of BCR/ABL mRNA by synthetic ribozymes-effects on the proliferation rate of K562 cells. *Clin. Padiatr.*, **207**, 222–224.

LaVail, M.M., Yasumura, D., Matthes, M.T., Drenser, K.A., Flannery, J.G., Lewin, A.S. and Hauswirth, W.W. (2000) Ribozyme rescue of photoreceptor cells in P23H *trans*genic rats: long-term survival and late-stage therapy. *Proc. Natl. Acad. Sci. USA*, **97**, 11488–11493.

L'Huillier, P.J., Davis, S.R. and Bellamy, A.R. (1992) Cytoplasmic delivery of ribozymes leads to efficient reduction in alpha-lactalbumin mRNA levels in C127I mouse cells. *EMBO J.*, **11**, 4411–4418.

Li, Q.X., Robbins, J.M., Welch, P.J., Wong-Staal, F. and Barber, J.R. (2000) A novel functional genomics approach identifies mTERT as a suppressor of fibroblast *trans*formation. *Nucleic Acids Res.*, **28**, 2605–2612.

Lipkowitz, M.S., Klotman, M.E., Bruggeman, L.A., Nicklin, P., Hanss, B., Rappaport, J. and Klotman, P.E. (1996) Molecular therapy for renal diseases. *Am. J. Kidney Dis.*, **28**, 475–492.

Liu, F. and Altman, S. (1996) Requirements for cleavage by a modified RNase P of a small model substrate. *Nucleic Acids Res.*, **24**, 2690–2696.

Lui, V.W., He, Y. and Huang, L. (2001) Specific down-regulation of HER-2/neu mediated by a chimeric U6 hammerhead ribozyme results in growth inhibition of human ovarian carcinoma. *Mol. Ther.*, **3**, 169–177.

Maelandsmo, G.M., Hovig, E., Skrede, M., Engebraaten, O., Florenes, V.A., Myklebost, O. *et al.* (1996) Reversal of the *in vivo* metastatic phenotype of human tumor cells by an anti-CAPL (mts1) ribozyme. *Cancer Res.*, **56**, 5490–5498.

Michel, F. and Ferat, J.L. (1995) Structure and activities of group II introns. *Annu. Rev. Biochem.*, **64**, 435–461.

Michienzi, A., Cagnon, L., Bahner, I. and Rossi, J.J. (2000) Ribozyme-mediated inhibition of HIV 1 suggests nucleolar trafficking of HIV-1 RNA. *Proc. Natl. Acad. Sci. USA*, **97**, 8955–8960.

Morgan, R.A. and Anderson, W.F. (1993) Human gene therapy. *Annu. Rev. Biochem.*, **62**, 191–217.

Nishikawa, S., Suh, Y.A., Kumar, P.K., Kawakami, J., Nishikawa, F. and Taira, K. (1992) Identification of important bases for the self-cleavage activity at two single-stranded regions of genomic HDV ribozyme. *Nucleic Acids Symp. Ser.*, **27**, 41–42.

Ohta, Y., Kijima, H., Ohkawa, T., Kashani-Sabet, M. and Scanlon, K.J. (1996) Tissue-specific expression of an anti-ras ribozyme inhibits proliferation of human malignant melanoma cells. *Nucleic Acids Res.*, **24**, 938–942.

Pavco, P.A., Bouhana, K.S., Gallegos, A.M., Agrawal, A., Blanchard, K.S., Grimm, S.L. *et al.* (2000) Anticancer and anti-metastatic activity of ribozymes targeting the messenger RNA of vascular endothelial growth factor receptors. *Clin. Cancer Res.*, **6**, 2094–2103.

Perlman, H., Sata, M., Krasinski, K., Dorai, T., Buttyan, R. and Walsh, K. (2000) Adeno-virus-encoded hammerhead ribozyme to Bcl-2 inhibits neointimal hyperplasia and induces vascular smooth muscle cell apoptosis. *Cardiovasc. Res.*, **45**, 570–578.

Perrotta, A.T. and Been, M.D. (1993) Assessment of disparate structural features in three models of the hepatitis delta virus ribozyme. *Nucleic Acids Res.*, **21**, 3959–3965.

Pley, H.W., Flaherty, K.M. and McKay, D.B. (1994) Three-dimentional structure of a hammerhead ribozyme. *Nature*, **372(6501)**, 68–74.

Rossi, J.J. (1999) Ribozymes, genomics and therapeutics. *Chem. Biol.*, **6**, R33–R37.

Santoro, S.W. and Joyce, G.F. (1997) A general purpose RNA-cleaving DNA enzyme. *Proc. Natl. Acad. Sci. USA*, **94**, 4262–4266.

Sarver, N., Cantin, E.M., Chang, P.S., Zaia, J.A., Ladne, P.A., Stephens, D. *et al.* (1990) Ribozymes as potential anti-HIV-1 therapeutic agents. *Science*, **247**, 1222–1225.

Saville, B.J. and Collins, R.A. (1990) A site-specific self-cleavage reaction performed by a novel RNA in Neurospora mitochondria. *Cell*, **61**, 685–696.

Scanlon, K.J., Ishida, H. and Kashani-Sabet, M. (1994) Ribozyme-mediated reversal of the multidrug-resistant phenotype. *Proc. Natl. Acad. Sci. USA*, **91**, 11123–11127.

Scherr, M., Reed, M., Huang, C.F., Riggs, A.D. and Rossi, J.J. (2000) Oligonucleotide scanning of native mRNAs in extracts predicts intracellular ribozyme efficiency: ribozyme-mediated reduction of the murine DNA methyl*trans*ferase. *Mol. Ther.*, **2**, 26–38.

Scherr, M. and Rossi, J.J. (1998) Rapid determination and quantitation of the accessibility to native RNAs by antisense oligodeoxynucleotides in murine cell extracts. *Nucleic Acids Res.*, **26**, 5079–5085.

Sczakiel, G., Palu, G. and James, W. (1997) Delivery of recombinant HIV-1-directed antisense and ribozyme genes. *Methods Mol. Biol.*, **63**, 389–400.

Sehgal, G., Hua, J., Bernhard, E.J., Sehgal, I., Thompson, T.C. and Muschel, R.J. (1998) Requirement for matrix metalloproteinase-9 (gelatinase B) expression in metastasis by murine prostate carcinoma. *Am. J. Pathol.*, **152**, 591–596.

Smith, S.M., Maldarelli, F. and Jeang, K.T. (1997) Efficient expression by an alphavirus replicon of a functional ribozyme targeted to human immunodeficiency virus type 1. *J. Virol.*, **71**, 9713–9721.

Snyder, D.S., Wu, Y., McMahon, R., Yu, L., Rossi, J.J. and Forman, S.J. (1997) Ribozyme-mediated inhibition of a Philadelphia chromosome-positive acute lymphoblastic leukemia cell line expressing the p190 bcr-abl oncogene. *Biol. Blood Marrow Transplant.*, **3**, 179–186.

Snyder, D.S., Wu, Y., Wang, J.L., Rossi, J.J., Swiderski, P., Kaplan, B.E. and Forman, S.J. (1993) Ribozyme-mediated inhibition of bcr-abl gene expression in a Philadelphia chromosome-positive cell line. *Blood*, **82**, 600–605.

Steitz, T.A. and Steitz, J.A. (1993) A general two-metal-ion mechanism for catalytic RNA. *Proc. Natl. Acad. Sci. USA*, **90**, 6498–6502.

Sullenger, B.A. and Cech, T.R. (1994) Ribozyme-mediated repair of defective mRNA by targeted, *trans*-splicing. *Nature*, **371**, 619–622.

Sullenger, B.A. and Cech, T.R. (1993) Tethering ribozymes to a retroviral packaging signal for destruction of viral RNA. *Science*, **262**, 1566–1569.

Suzuki, T., Anderegg, B., Ohkawa, T., Irie, A., Engebraaten, O., Halks-Miller, M. *et al.* (2000) Adenovirus-mediated ribozyme targeting of HER-2/neu inhibits *in vivo* growth of breast cancer cells. *Gene Ther.*, **7**, 241–248.

Szostak, J.W. (1997) *In vitro* selection and directed evolution. *Harvey Lect.*, **93**, 95–118.

Taylor, N.R., Kaplan, B.E., Swiderski, P., Li, H. and Rossi, J.J. (1992) Chimeric DNA-RNA hammerhead ribozymes have enhanced *in vitro* catalytic efficiency and increased stability *in vivo*. *Nucleic Acids Res.*, **20**, 4559–4565.

Thomas, M.K., Devon, O.N., Lee, J.H., Peter, A., Schlosser, D.A., Tenser, M.S. and Habener, J.F. (2001) Development of diabetes mellitus in aging *trans*genic mice following suppression of pancreatic homeoprotein IDX-1. *J. Clin. Invest.*, **108**, 319–329.

Tsuchida, T., Kijima, H., Hori, S., Oshika, Y., Tokunaga, T., Kawai, K. *et al.* (2000) Adenovirus-mediated anti-K-ras ribozyme induces apoptosis and growth suppression of human pancreatic carcinoma. *Cancer Gene Ther.*, **7**, 373–383.

Tsuchida, T., Kijima, H., Oshika, Y., Tokunaga, T., Abe, Y., Yamazaki, H. *et al.* (1998). Hammerhead ribozyme specifically inhibits mutant K-ras mRNA of human pancreatic cancer cells. *Biochem. Biophys. Res. Commun.*, **253**, 368–373.

Wang, F.S., Kobayashi, H., Liang, K.W., Holland, J.F. and Ohnuma, T. (1999) Retrovirus-mediated transfer of anti-MDR1 ribozymes fully restores chemosensitivity of P-glycoprotein-expressing human lymphoma cells. *Hum. Gene Ther.*, **10**, 1185–1195.

Watanabe, T. and Sullenger, B.A. (2000) Induction of wild-type p53 activity in human cancer cells by ribozymes that repair mutant p53 *transcripts. Proc. Natl. Acad. Sci. USA,* **97**, 8490–8494.

Welch, P.J., Marcusson, E.G., Li, Q.X., Beger, C., Kruger, M., Zhou, C. *et al.* (2000) Identification and validation of a gene involved in anchorage-independent cell growth control using a library of randomized hairpin ribozymes. *Genomics,* **66**, 274–283.

Welch, P.J., Yei, S. and Barber, J.R. (1998) Ribozyme gene therapy for hepatitis C virus infection. *Clin. Diagn. Virol.,* **10**, 163–171.

Wilson, D.S. and Szostak, J.W. (1999) *In vitro* selection of functional nucleic acids. *Annu. Rev. Biochem.,* **68**, 611–647.

Yamamoto, H., Irie, A., Fukushima, Y., Ohnishi, T., Arita, N., Hayakawa, T. and Sekiguchi, K. (1996) Abrogation of lung metastasis of human fibrosarcoma cells by ribozyme-mediated suppression of integrin alpha6 subunit expression. *Int. J. Cancer,* **65**, 519–524.

Yu, M., Ojwang, J., Yamada, O., Hampel, A., Rapapport, J., Looney, D. *et al.* (1993) A hairpin ribozyme inhibits expression of diverse strains of human immunodeficiency virus type 1. *Proc. Natl. Acad. Sci. USA,* **90**, 6340–6344.

Zhao, J.J. and Lemke, G. (1998) Selective disruption of neuregulin-1 function in vertebrate embryos using ribozyme-tRNA transgenes. *Development,* **125**, 1899–1907.

Zhao, J.J. and Pick, L. (1993) Generating loss-of-function phenotypes of the fushi tarazu gene with a targeted ribozyme in Drosophila. *Nature,* **365**, 448–451.

5 Peptide nucleic acids (PNA) binding-mediated target gene transcription

Gan Wang and Xiaoxin Xu

INTRODUCTION

Peptide nucleic acids (PNAs) are synthetic oligonucleotides with modified backbones (Figure 5.1) (Nielsen *et al.*, 1991). In PNAs, the deoxyribose phosphate backbones are replaced with polyamide backbones. PNAs can bind to DNA and RNA targets in a sequence-specific manner to form PNA/DNA and PNA/RNA Watson-Crick double helical structures. When binding to double-stranded DNA targets, the PNA molecule replaces one DNA strand in the target duplex by strand displacement, while the displaced DNA strand exists as a single-stranded D-loop at the PNA binding site (Kurakin *et al.*, 1998; Lohse *et al.*, 1999; Nielsen *et al.*, 1991). A [PNA]$_2$/DNA triple helix structure can form when PNAs bind to a homopurine/homopyrimidine sequence (Figure 5.2). In this case, a second molecule of PNA binds to the DNA strand of the PNA/DNA duplex by Hoogsteen hydrogen bonds to form a triplex structure at the target site and the displaced DNA strand remains as a single stranded D-loop (Hanvey *et al.*, 1992; Nielsen *et al.*, 1991). Studies have shown that the triplexes formed with PNAs are pyrimidine-motif in that the pyrimidine PNA strand binds parallel to the purine strand in DNA targets

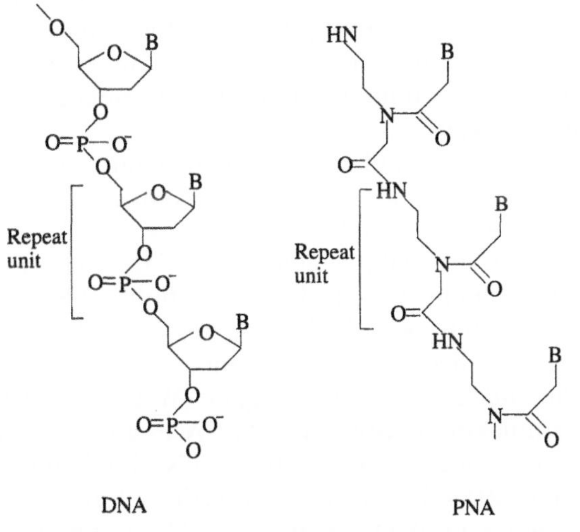

Figure 5.1 Structures of DNA and PNA oligonucleotides.

(A)

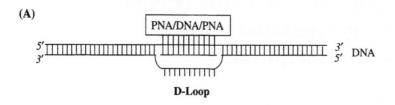

D-Loop

(B)

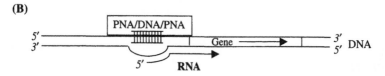

Figure 5.2 PNA binding to duplex DNA target generated [PNA]$_2$/DNA triplex and single-stranded D-loop structure.

(Demidov *et al.*, 1994; Hanvey *et al.*, 1992; Knudsen and Nielsen, 1996; Nielsen *et al.*, 1991). The [PNA]$_2$/DNA triplex structure stabilizes both the bound PNAs and the single stranded D-loop at the PNA binding site (Nielsen *et al.*, 1991; Lohse and Nielsen, 1999).

PNAs have been used in a variety of applications. For antisense therapy, PNAs designed to bind to mRNA sequences of target genes have been used to block expression of many target genes both *in vitro* and *in vivo* (Aldrian-Herrada *et al.*, 1998; Cutrona *et al.*, 2000; Efferth *et al.*, 2000; Penichet *et al.*, 1999; Pooga *et al.*, 1998; Scarfi *et al.*, 1999; Tyler *et al.*, 1999). For mutation detection, PNAs have been used to detect low levels of single base mutations from large populations because of their very high binding affinity and specificity (Orum *et al.*, 1993; Tyler *et al.*, 1999). In targeted mutagenesis studies, PNAs also have been used to introduce mutations into target genes (Faruqi *et al.*, 1998). However, one of the most important potentials of PNAs that has not been well studied is their ability to induce transcription and expression of target genes. The strategy of using PNA to induce expression of specific target gene attracts very little attention because of the lack in understanding of the molecular mechanism of PNAs binding-induced transcription and its effect on gene re-modulating in living cells.

Binding of PNAs to duplex DNA targets could generate single-stranded D-loops and these D-loops were demonstrated to initiate transcription from *in vitro* systems (Mollegaard *et al.*, 1994). We have been interested to find out whether PNA binding-generated D-loops can be used as artificial promoters to initiate transcription and lead to expression of target genes in living cells. For these studies, PNAs were designed to bind to the human γ-globin gene 5′ flanking region and the PNA binding-induced transcription was studied both *in vitro* and *in vivo* using both reporter gene constructs and the endogenous γ-globin gene (Wang *et al.*, 1999). The results obtained from these studies demonstrated that PNA binding generated D-loops could initiate transcription in HeLa nuclear extracts. PNA binding generated D-loops have also been demonstrated to lead to expression of green fluorescent protein (GFP) reporter gene in mammalian cells. More importantly, treatment of cultured human cells with the PNAs also resulted in transcription of the endogenous γ-globin gene from the PNA binding sites. These results suggest that PNA binding-mediated target gene expression strategy may provide a very useful tool in inducing transcription of specific target genes. This strategy may provide a novel approach to remodeling the gene expression that will have great implication in clinical treatment and other industrial applications, such as pharmaceutical and agricultural industrial application. PNA binding-induced transcription strategy will be important in scientific research as it will provide a powerful tool to study gene transcription remodeling and regulation. However, due to the lack of the molecular mechanism of PNA binding-induced transcription, several issues need to be addressed before this technology can be used in general application.

PNA BINDING AFFINITY

PNAs can bind to both DNA and RNA targets with very high affinity. The binding of PNAs to DNA and RNA is much higher than the DNA/DNA or DNA/RNA bindings. For example, the melting temperature (T_m) of a normal dA_{10}-dT_{10} DNA hybrid is 23 °C; however, the T_m of a similar dA_{10}-dT_{10} DNA/PNA hybrid is 86 °C (Nielsen *et al.*, 1991). This high binding affinity is attributed to the lack of electrostatic repulsion between the PNA strand and the DNA or RNA strand in the duplex hybrid. The higher binding affinity can also result from the [PNA]$_2$/DNA triplex formation at the PNA binding site since the [PNA]$_2$/DNA triplex structure formed at the homopurine/homopyrimidine sequences can stabilize the bound PNAs. In our previous studies, the Kd of a 12 mer PNA was found to be at 7×10^{-8} M (Figure 5.3), which was more than 200-fold higher than that of the regular 12 mer triplex forming oligonucleotides (TFO).

PNA BINDING SPECIFICITY

Because of the high binding affinity of PNA to DNA and RNA targets, the binding specificity of PNA is much higher than that of DNA or RNA. For this reason, mismatches between PNA and the target DNA or RNA will greatly reduce the binding affinity of PNAs to the targets, resulting in a much higher binding specificity of the PNA to the targets (Doyle *et al.*, 2001; Nielsen *et al.*, 1991, 1993, 1994; Taylor *et al.*, 1997). In our recent studies using a series of PNAs with different lengths, high specific PNA binding was demonstrated. For example, a target sequence was well protected with PNAs as short as 10 mer in length in a plasmid construct (Wang, unpublished data); however, this specificity was not achieved with a 10 mer control PNA or regular 10 mer TFO at the same target site.

DETECTION OF PNA BINDING-INDUCED TRANSCRIPTION
IN VITRO

Binding of PNAs to homopurine/homopyrimidine sequence of double-stranded DNA targets generates a [PNA]$_2$/DNA triplex and single stranded D-loop structure

(A) Structure of pUSAG3

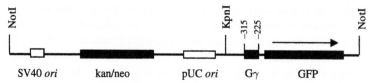

(B) Sequence of the Gγ-globin gene −300 region.

```
   -324                                                        -265
5'-CTTCTATGGTGGGAGAAGAAAACTAGCTAAAGGGAAGAATAAATTAGAGAAAAATTGGAA-3'
3'-GAAGATACCACCCTCTTCTTTTGATCGATTTCCCTTCTTATTTAATCTCTTTTTAACCTT-5'
```

(C) Sequences of PNA oligonucleotides

PNA-1   NH2-T CTTCCCTTT-OOO-*TTTJJJTTJT*-COOH

PNA-2   NH2-TTTTCTTCTCCC-OOO-*JJJTJTTJTTTT*-COOH

CP-1   NH2-TTCCTTCCTT-OOO-*TTJJTTJJTT*-COOH

Figure 5.3 Structure of pUSAG3 and sequences of the human Gγ-globin gene −300 region and the PNAs. (A) Structure of pUSAG3. (B) DNA sequences around the Gγ-globin gene −300 region. The underlined nucleotide sequences show the PNA binding sites. (C) Sequences of PNA oligonucleotides used in the study. Cytosines were replaced by pseudoisocytosines (J) for third strand binding; three linkers (O) were incorporated to link the DNA binding domain and the triplex binding domain. The ltalic sequences in the PNA oligonucleotides were designed for triplex binding.

at the PNA binding sites. To investigate if PNA binding-generated D-loops can initiate transcription in HeLa nuclear extracts, an *in vitro* transcription assay was performed. The plasmid pUSAG3 was constructed to contain a promoterless GFP gene with a 60 bp human γ-globin gene 5′ UTR region sequence (−315 to −255) in front of the coding sequence of the GFP reporter gene (Figure 5.3A). This 60 bp DNA region contains 10 bp and a 12 bp homopurine/homopyrimidine sequences that are potential PNA binding targets (Figure 5.3B). Two PNAs, PNA-1 and PNA-2, were designed to bind to the 10 bp and 12 bp homopurine sequences to form [PNA]$_2$/DNA triplex and single-stranded D-loop structures (Figure 5.3C). A gel mobility shift assay was performed to confirm the specificity and affinity of these two PNAs (Figure 5.4). For transcription assay, the pUSAG3 plasmid DNA was linearized with *Eag*I restriction enzyme. The linearized pUSAG3 DNA was incubated with PNAs in 10 mM Tris (pH 7.5) at 37 °C for three hours for PNAs binding to the target sites and forming [PNA]$_2$/DNA triplex and single-stranded D-loop structures. The PNA/DNA complexes were incubated in HeLa nuclear extracts supplemented with ATP, CTP, UTP, and [α-^{32}P] GTP at 30 °C for 60 minutes for RNA synthesis. Nascent RNA was isolated from the reactants and analyzed by polyacrylamide gel electrophoresis using a 5% gel containing 7 M urea. The newly synthesized RNA was visualized by autoradiography and quantitated by phosphor-imaging analysis (Figure 5.5). No specific RNA transcripts were synthesized from

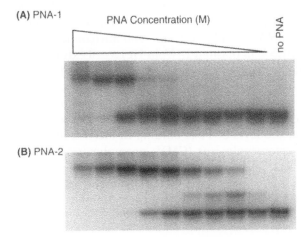

Figure 5.4 Determining the binding affinity of both PNA-1 and PNA-2 with gel mobility shift assay. A fixed concentration of the ^{32}P-labeled 60bp DNA fragment
$(5 \times 10^{-9} \text{ M})$ was incubated with increasing concentrations of PNA in TE
buffer (10 mM Tris, pH7.5, 1mM EDTA) at 37 °C for four hours. The
reactants were analyzed by polyacrylamide gel electrophoresis in a 20%
gel followed by autoradiography. (**A**) Binding of PNA-1 to DNA target.
(**B**) Binding of PNA-2 to DNA target.

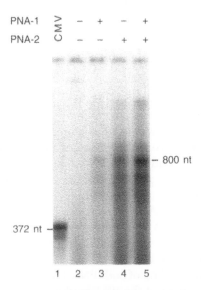

Figure 5.5 Detection of PNA binding-mediated GFP transcription in HeLa nuclear
extract. Plasmid DNA encoding green fluorescent protein (pUSAG3) was
linearized and used as a template for *in vitro* transcription in a HeLa
nuclear extract transcription system. Lane 1, CMV promoter-driven
372 nt RNA transcript as a positive control; lane 2, pUSAG3 plasmid DNA
alone; lane 3, pUSAG3 plasmid DNA in the presence of PNA-1; lane 4,
pUSAG3 plasmid DNA in the presence of PNA-2; lane 5, pUSAG3 plasmid
DNA in the presence of both PNA-1 and PNA-2.

these two homopurine/homopyrimidine sequence sites of the plasmid in the plasmid DNA alone due to the lack of a mammalian promoter (Figure 5.5 lane 2). However, in the presence of both PNA-1 and PNA-2, an $\sim$800 nucleotide (nt) RNA transcript was synthesized from pUSAG3 plasmid DNA in HeLa cell extract, which is in agreement with transcription initiating from the PNA binding site (Figure 5.5 lane 5). The $\sim$800 nt RNA transcript was also detected in the presence of either PNA-1 or PNA-2 (Figure 5.5 lanes 3 and 4); however, the amounts of RNA transcript in these reactions were much less than that observed in the reaction with both PNAs. In comparison, the level of PNA binding-induced transcription was comparable to the level of cytomegalovirus (CMV) promoter induced transcription in HeLa nuclear extracts, and the CMV promoter is a known strong mammalian promoter (Figure 5.5 lane 5 versus lane 1). This result suggests that PNA binding generated D-loops provide relatively strong promoter activity in HeLa nuclear extracts *in vitro*.

DETERMINATION OF TRANSCRIPTION INITIATION SITES OF PNA BINDING-INDUCED TRANSCRIPTION

To determine whether the RNA transcripts obtained from the PNA binding-induced transcription in HeLa nuclear extract were indeed initiated from the PNA binding sites, a reverse transcription-based primer extension assay was performed (Figure 5.6). Nascent RNA was isolated from the *in vitro* transcription assay in similar experiments. This RNA was used as a template for a reverse transcription assay and a $[\gamma\text{-}^{32}\text{P}]$-labeled primer that binds to the 5' coding sequence of the GFP gene was used as the extension primer. Plasmid pUSAG3 DNA alone or pUSAG3 DNA pre-incubated with a control PNA (CP-1) (which does not bind to the plasmid) did not induce any specific RNA transcripts from either PNA-1 or PNA-2 binding sites (Figure 5.6 lanes 1 and 2). In contrast, when PNA-bound pUSAG3 plasmid DNA was used as a template, specific RNA transcripts were synthesized from the PNA binding sites. When the PNA-1-bound pUSAG3 plasmid DNA was used as a template, two specific RNA transcripts were observed: one started from the 3' end of the PNA-1 binding site and the other one started from the 5' end of the PNA-1 binding site (Figure 5.6 lane 3). When the PNA-2-bound pUSAG3 plasmid was used as a template, one RNA transcript starting from the 3' end of the PNA-2 binding site was generated (Figure 5.6 lane 4). Interestingly, when pUSAG3 DNA treated with both PNA-1 and PNA-2 was used as a template, three RNA transcripts, corresponding to the two PNA-1 and one PNA-2-specific transcripts, were produced (Figure 5.6 lane 5). This result suggests that binding of either PNA-1 or PNA-2 to the target site was able to initiate RNA transcription; however, the binding of both PNA-1 and PNA-2 to the targets enhanced the D-loop transcription activity at the PNA binding targets.

PNA BINDING GENERATED D-LOOPS LEAD TO GFP GENE EXPRESSION IN MAMMALIAN CELLS

To study if binding of PNAs to their target sites can induce gene expression *in vivo*, we investigated whether binding of PNAs to pUSAG3 plasmid could induce GFP

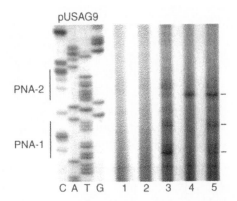

pUSAG9

PNA-2

PNA-1

C A T G   1   2   3   4   5

Figure 5.6 Determining the initiation sites of RNA transcripts synthesized from the PNA-bound pUSAG3 plasmid DNA in HeLa nuclear extracts. The pUSAG3 plasmid was constructed by inserting a 60bp DNA fragment containing the −315 to −255 region sequence of the human Gγ-globin gene into the Sma I site of the pEGFP-1 plasmid, a green fluorescent protein (GFP) promoter reporter vector (Clontech Laboratories; Palo Alto, CA) (Figure 5.3A). A DNA sequencing reaction of the pUSAG3 plasmid was performed using a primer binding to the 5′ coding region of the GFP gene. The same primer was used as a primer for the reverse transcription. Lane 1, pUSAG3 plasmid DNA alone; lane 2, pUSAG3 plasmid DNA treated with control PNA (CP-1); lane 3, pUSAG3 plasmid DNA treated with PNA-1; lane 4, pUSAG3 plasmid DNA treated with PNA-2; lane 5, pUSAG3 plasmid DNA treated with PNA-1 and PNA-2. The sequences show both the PNA-1 (lower) and the PNA-2 (upper) binding site in the plasmid pUSAG3.

expression in mammalian cells. The pUSAG3 plasmid DNA with or without *in vitro* bound PNAs was microinjected into the nuclei of CV1 monkey embryonic kidney fibroblast cells and GFP expression was monitored at various times by fluorescence microscopy (Figure 5.7). No GFP expression was observed in CV1 cells injected with pUSAG3 plasmid DNA alone (Figure 5.7C). In contrast, when PNA-bound pUSAG3 plasmid DNA was injected into CV1 cells, GFP expression was detected in the cells (Figure 5.7A and B). As a positive control for GFP expression, pGreen Lantern-1, a plasmid which carries a CMV promoter-driven GFP gene (Life Technologies, Inc., Gaithersburg, MD), was microinjected into CV1 cells in a parallel experiment and GFP expression was detected (data not shown). This result and the *in vitro* transcription result suggest that PNA binding generated D-loops cannot only be recognized as promoters *in vitro* to initiate transcription, but they can also be recognized as promoters in living cells to initiate transcription and eventually lead to expression of target genes.

PNA-INDUCED ENDOGENOUS γ-GLOBIN GENE EXPRESSION IN HUMAN CELLS

To investigate whether PNAs can be used to induce endogenous target gene expression, we explored the possibility of inducing endogenous human γ-globin gene

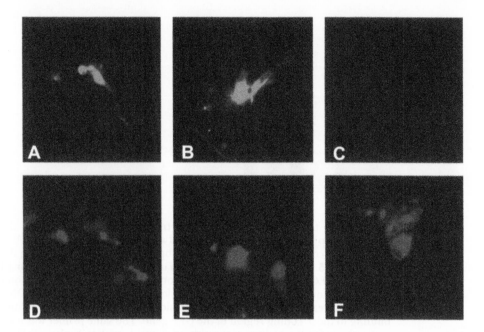

Figure 5.7 Detection of PNA binding-mediated GFP gene expression in CV1 cells.
Twenty hours post-injection of plasmid or plasmid-PNA complexes, GFP
expression was determined. GFP fluorescence is shown in the top panels
and the rhodamine-labeled BSA signal is shown in the bottom panels. (A)
and (D), CV1 cells injected with pUSAG3.PNA-1; (B) and (E), CV1 cells
injected with pUSAG3.PNA-2; (C) and (F), CV1 cells injected with pUSAG3
plasmid DNA alone. In all cases, rhodamine-labeled BSA was co-injected
with the DNAs to the cells. (*see Color Plate 4*)

expression with the PNAs. PNA-mediated γ-globin gene expression was studied in
K562 human erythroleukemia cells that have low levels of endogenous γ-globin gene
expression. K562 cells were treated with both PNA-1 and PNA-2 by a co-electro-
poration procedure. At various time points after the PNA treatment, total RNA was
isolated from the cells and a RNase protection assay was performed to determine the
amount of γ-globin gene mRNA (Figure 5.8). The γ-globin mRNA transcript was
increased 1.8-fold when K562 cells were treated with both PNAs for 48 hours compared with the untreated K562 cells (Figure 5.8 lane 2 versus lane 1). In a similar
experiment in which K562 cells were treated with 75 μM hemin, a γ-globin gene-
specific inducer, for three days the levels of γ-globin expression increased 4.6-fold
(Figure 5.8 lane 5). Expression of glyceraldehyde phosphate dehydrogenase (GAPD)
gene was used as an internal control and did not change in any of the experiments.
This result suggests that the PNAs designed to bind to 5′ UTR region of γ-globin
gene could induce endogenous γ-globin transcription in K562 cells.

To determine if the increased γ-globin transcripts in PNA-treated K562 cells
were synthesized from the PNA binding sites, a reverse transcription assay was
performed using total RNA isolated from PNA-treated K562 cells as a template
(Figure 5.9A). Treatment of K562 cells with PNAs induced a specific γ-globin

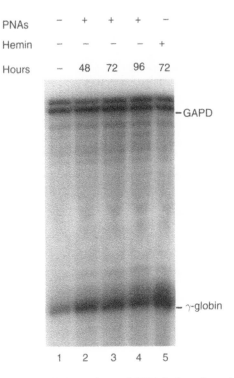

Figure 5.8 Detection of PNA-induced γ-globin gene expression in K562 cells with RNase Protection Assay. Lane 1, K562 cells; lane 2 to lane 4, K562 cells treated with PNAs for two, three, and four days, respectively; lane 5, K562 cells treated with hemin (75 µM) for three days.

transcript at the PNA binding sites; however, this RNA transcript was not synthesized in untreated K562 cells or the cells treated with PNA-1 alone. This result provides direct evidence that PNAs can bind to endogenous gene targets and initiate transcription at the PNA binding-generated D-loops.

CORRELATION BETWEEN PNA BINDING GENERATED D-LOOPS AND NATURAL PROMOTER IN TARGET GENE TRANSCRIPTION

PNA binding can initiate transcription from the PNA binding-generated D-loops. However, the normal promoters exist in most of the target genes. The correlation between PNA-binding generated D-loops and the gene's natural promoter in target gene transcription will be important to study. We have studied this correlation by determining the levels of transcription from both PNA binding-generated D-loop sites and γ-globin gene promoter in PNA-treated K562 cells using a reverse transcription assay (Figure 5.9B). Without PNA treatment or the cells treated with control PNA, low levels of RNA transcription initiated from γ-globin gene promoter were detected in K562 cells (Figure 5.9B lane 6). However, in PNA treated K562 cells, much higher

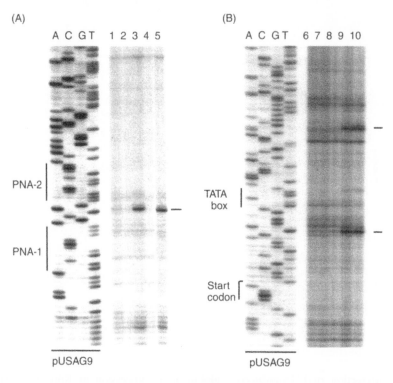

Figure 5.9 Determining PNA binding-induced endogenous γ-globin gene transcription
with reverse transcription primer extension. The plasmid pUSAG9 was used as
sequence templates in this experiment. The pUSAG9 plasmid was constructed
by inserting a DNA fragment containing the β-globin gene minimal locus
control region (mLCR) HS2 sequence, the Aγ-globin gene, and the β-globin
gene (the corresponding nucleotide positions of HS2, Aγ-, and β-globin genes
in EMBL GeneBank are 7759 to 9182, 38084 to 43975, and 60409 to 65475,
respectively; EMBL ID: HSHBB4R1; accession number: K01891) into the KpnI
restriction enzyme digestion site of pEGFP-1 plasmid. (A) Detection of γ-globin
transcripts initiated from the PNA binding sites. A primer that binds to the
γ-globin gene at the position −207 to −225 (5′CCAAGAGGATACTGCTGCT3′)
was used for both reverse transcription primer extension and DNA sequencing
reactions. (B) Detection of γ-globin transcripts initiated from the γ-globin
promoter. A primer that binds to the γ-globin gene coding region at the
position 80 to 61 (5′TCTCCTCCAGCATCTTCCAC3′) was used for both
reverse transcription primer extension and DNA sequencing reactions. Lane 1
and lane 6, total RNA isolated from K562 cells; lane 2 and lane 7, total RNA
isolated from control PNA-treated K562 cells; lane 3 and lane 9, total RNA
isolated from PNA-2 treated K562 cells; lane 4 and lane 8, total RNA isolated
from PNA-1 treated K562 cells; lane 5 and lane 10, total RNA isolated from
PNA-1 plus PNA-2 treated K562 cells.

levels of RNA transcription initiated from γ-globin gene promoter were detected
(Figure 5.9B lanes 9 and 10). Interestingly, additional transcripts initiated from different positions of γ-globin promoter also were detected (Figure 5.9B lanes 9 and 10
versus lanes 6 and 7). This result indicates that binding of PNA to an upstream
sequence of target gene promoter not only leads to transcription from the PNA

binding generated D-loops, but also results in enhanced transcription from the natural promoter of target genes. Therefore, PNA binding generated D-loops have a dual effect on transcription: they induce transcription from the D-loops and enhance transcription from the normal promoter of the target genes. The molecular mechanism of this enhanced transcription is unknown. It is possible that transcription of the target gene from an upstream sequence makes the natural promoter of the gene more accessible for the transcription components, leading to an increased transcription from its normal promoter.

PNA LENGTH REQUIREMENT FOR INDUCING TRANSCRIPTION FROM PNA BINDING SITES

The PNAs used in our studies were designed to bind to a 10 bp and a 12 bp target, respectively. Studies by others have used a 10 mer PNA (Mollegaard *et al.*, 1994). To determine the PNA length requirement for inducing transcription from the PNA binding sites, a new plasmid, pJK-1, was constructed to contain a promoterless luciferase reporter gene with a 20 bp homopurine/homopyrimidine sequence in front of the coding sequence of luciferase gene. A series of PNAs with different lengths were synthesized to bind to the PNA binding site to generate D-loops of various sizes. A gel mobility shift assay confirmed binding of these PNAs to the target site (Wang, unpublished data). To determine the level of transcription initiated from various D-loops generated by PNAs, an *in vitro* transcription experiment was performed to synthesize RNA from the plasmid DNA and then a reverse transcription-based primer extension assay was performed to determine the transcription levels (Figure 5.10). No specific RNA transcripts were synthesized from the PNA binding site when pJK-1 plasmid DNA alone or pJK-1 plasmid-DNA treated with control PNA were used as templates. Specific RNA transcripts initiated from the PNA binding site were also not detected when pJK-1 plasmid DNA treated with 10 mer PNA (which binds sequence-specifically to the target site, as demonstrated by PNA binding assay) was used as templates for the *in vitro* transcription assay. In contrast, specific RNA transcripts initiated from the PNA binding site were detected when pJK-1 plasmid DNA treated with the 12 mer, 14 mer, 16 mer, 18 mer, and 20 mer PNAs were used as templates for the *in vitro* transcription assay (Figure 5.10 lanes 2, 3, 4, 5, and 6 versus lanes 1 and 7). Phosphorimaging analysis indicated that the highest levels of transcription were detected when the 16 mer and 18 mer PNA-treated plasmid DNAs were used as templates. When the PNA-bound plasmid DNAs were transfected into COS-7 cells and GFP expression was monitored by fluorescent microscope, a similar result was obtained (Wang, unpublished data). These results suggest that PNAs with lengths of 16–18 mer were more effective in inducing transcription *in vitro* and inducing expression of the target genes in living cells than PNAs of other lengths.

TRANSCRIPTION COMPONENTS INVOLVED IN PNA BINDING-INDUCED TRANSCRIPTION

Although PNA binding generated D-loops have been demonstrated for their abilities in inducing transcription (Wang *et al.*, 1999), little is known about the

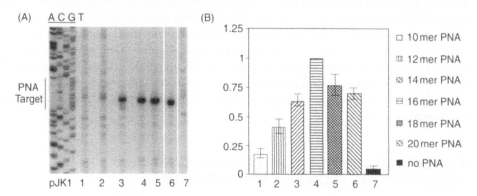

Figure 5.10 Determining the transcription activity of D-loops generated by individual PNAs bound to the pJK-1 plasmid DNA. Nascent RNA was generated from individual PNA bound pJK-1 plasmid DNA via HeLa nuclear extract *in vitro* transcription. The RNA was used as a template in a reverse transcription assay. The amount of RNA transcripts initiated from the PNA binding site region was quantified using phosphorimaging analysis. The initiation sites of the transcripts were determined by comparison with the DNA sequence ladder. (A) Reverse transcription assay to detect specific RNA transcripts initiated from the PNA binding site region. (B) Comparison of the transcription activity of the D-loops generated by individual PNA. The results are mean data from five individual experiments. The amount of RNA transcripts initiated from the PNA binding site versus PNA binding was counted as 100% and the amount of RNA transcripts synthesized from the pJK-1 versus other PNAs was calculated as percentage to that of PNA6. Lane1, pJK-1 plasmid DNA +10 mer PNA; lane 2, pJK-1 plasmid DNA +12 mer PNA; lane 3, pJK-1 plasmid DNA +14 mer PNA; lane 4, pJK-1 plasmid DNA +16 mer PNA; lane 5, pJK-1 plasmid DNA +18 mer PNA; lane 6, pJK-1 plasmid DNA +20 mer PNA; lane 7, pJK-1 plasmid DNA alone.

molecular mechanism of the PNA binding-induced transcription process. However, detection of PNA binding-mediated GFP expression in living cells suggests that the mechanism of normal protein-related transcription (class II nuclear gene transcription) may be applicable to PNA binding-induced transcription. Therefore, the transcription model for the class II nuclear gene transcription may be used for PNA binding-induced transcription. The well-established model of class II nuclear gene transcription in mammalian cells (Nikolov and Burley, 1997) suggests that during normal eukaryotic transcription initiation the TATA binding protein (TBP), a component of TFIID, recognizes and binds to the TATA sequence in the promoter region. This binding recruits RNA polymerase II and other basal transcription factors including TFIIB, TFIIE, TFIIF, and TFIIH to the promoter region resulting in the opening of the promoter region for approximately 17 bp (Holstege *et al.*, 1996). At the same time, the RNA polymerase undergoes a major conformational change, yielding a stable and highly processive elongation complex that completes synthesis of the nascent RNA transcripts. Although the general transcription process may be similar, the initiation process may still be different because of the distinguishable structures between PNA binding generated D-loops and the natural promoter organization. For example, in PNA binding-induced transcription single-stranded loops have already been generated into the DNA targets prior to the binding of the transcription machinery. Therefore, recognition of the TATA site with TBP seems unnecessary for PNA binding-induced transcription initiation. However, this binding is essential to the transcription initiation of class II nuclear genes. Therefore, the molecular mechanism of PNA binding-induced transcription, especially the transcription initiation process, needs to be studied to provide a better understanding of this process.

LIMITATION OF PNA BINDING-INDUCED TARGET GENE EXPRESSION

Although great potential exists for PNA binding-induced target gene expression, PNA binding-induced gene expression technology has its limitation in application in current time. One of the biggest challenges in applying PNAs to living cells is its poor delivery efficiency into cells (Hanvey *et al.*, 1992; Pardridge *et al.*, 1995). This is possibly due to the uncharged nature of PNAs since the uncharged PNAs may not bind to the charged cell membrane as effectively as those charged oligonucleotides used in the antisense studies and, therefore, may not effectively be taken up by the cell endocytosis process. Another obstacle that needs to be overcome in PNA technology is the fact that the binding of PNAs to duplex DNA targets can be inhibited in the presence of high concentrations of salts. The positively charged ions can bind to the negatively charged DNAs and, therefore, block the interaction of PNA with the DNA targets (Cherny *et al.*, 1993; Nielsen *et al.*, 1994; Peffer *et al.*, 1993). Unfortunately, most living cells maintain relatively high concentrations of salts inside the cells.

Several strategies can be used to overcome these difficulties. To increase PNA delivery efficiency, the incorporation of positively charged groups such as lysine into PNAs may enhance the attachment of PNAs to the cell membrane and hence increase the PNA uptake by the cells. Coupling PNAs with ligands has already been demonstrated to lead to increased PNA delivery efficiency (Aldrian-Herrada *et al.*, 1998; Basu and Wickstrom, 1997; Chinnery *et al.*, 1999; Cutrona *et al.*, 2000; Pooga *et al.*, 1998; Scarfi *et al.*, 1999; Simmons *et al.*, 1997). Both strategies may be used to improve PNA delivery efficiency. Several strategies may also be used to overcome the PNA binding inhibition in the presence of high concentrations of salts. Incorporation of positively charged groups into PNA molecules may help PNAs in competing with other positively charged ions for binding to negatively charged DNA targets and improve binding efficiency of PNA to duplex DNA targets in the presence of high concentrations of salts (Mollegaard *et al.*, 1994). Increasing target gene transcription also has been demonstrated to lead to increased PNA binding efficiency in the presence of high concentrations of salts (Larsen and Nielsen, 1996). The sequence context of the PNA binding targets may contribute to PNA binding inhibition in the presence of high concentrations of salts, as well. In our previous studies, binding of PNA-2 to the DNA target was more salt concentration-independent than that of PNA-1 (Wang *et al.*, 1999) and the target sequences of these two PNAs were slightly different and were separated by only six base pairs in human cells. Therefore, if the salt inhibition effect is observed in one chosen PNA target site, changing PNAs' binding target sites to other positions may overcome this inhibition effect.

CONCLUDING REMARKS

PNA binding-induced transcription and target gene expression provides an ideal strategy to induce expression of specific target genes. This strategy will have a broad range of applications, including treatment of many human diseases and inducing expression of therapeutic genes. PNA binding-induced transcription and target gene expression also provides a powerful method to study the molecular mechanism of transcription initiation and gene regulation. However, some difficulty exists in the technology that has limited its applications. The molecular mechanism of PNA binding induced transcription and target gene expression needs to be established to provide a better understanding of the molecular basis of this important approach. Once these issues are resolved, the great implication of this technology in the treatment of many human diseases and other applications will be predictable.

REFERENCES

Aldrian-Herrada, G., Desarmenien, M.G., Orcel, H., Boissin-Agasse, L., Mery, J., Brugidou, J. *et al.* (1998) A peptide nucleic acid (PNA) is more rapidly internalized in cultured neurons when coupled to a retro-inverso delivery peptide. The antisense activity depresses the target mRNA and protein in magnocellular oxytocin neurons. *Nucleic Acids Res.*, **26**, 4910–4916.

Basu, S. and Wickstrom, E. (1997) Synthesis and characterization of a peptide nucleic acid conjugated to a D-peptide analog of insulin-like growth factor 1 for increased cellular uptake. *Bioconj. Chem.*, **8**, 481–488.

Cherny, D.Y., Belotserkovskii, B.P., Frank-Kamenetskii, M.D., Egholm, M., Buchardt, O., Berg, R.H. *et al.* (1993) DNA unwinding upon strand-displacement binding of a thymine-substituted polyamide to double-stranded DNA. *Proc. Natl. Acad. Sci. USA*, **90**, 1667–1670.

Chinnery, P.F., Taylor, R.W., Diekert, K., Lill, R., Turnbull, D.M. and Lightowlers, R.N. (1999) Peptide nucleic acid delivery to human mitochondria. *Gene Ther.*, **6**, 1919–1928.

Cutrona, G., Carpaneto, E.M., Ulivi, M., Roncella, S., Landt, O., Ferrarini, M. *et al.* (2000) Effects in loive cells of a c-myc anti-gene PNA linked to a localization signal. *Nature Biotech.*, **18**, 300–303.

Demidov, V.V., Cherny, D.I., Kurakin, A.V., Yavnilovich, M.V., Malkov, V.A., Frank-Kamenetskii, M.D. *et al.* (1994) Electron microscopy mapping of oligopurine tracts in duplex DNA by peptide nucleic acid targeting. *Nucleic Acids Res.*, **22**, 5218–5222.

Doyle, D.F., Braasch, D.A., Simmons, C.G., Janowski, B.A. and Corey, D.R. (2001) Inhibition of gene expression inside cells by peptide nucleic acids: effect of mRNA target sequence, mismatched bases, and PNA length. *Biochemistry*, **40**, 53–64.

Efferth, T., Fabry, U. and Osieka, R. (2000) Leptin contributes to the protection of human leukemia cells from cisplatinum cytoxicity. *Anticancer Res.*, **20**, 2441–2546.

Faruqi, A.F., Egholm, M. and Glazer, P.M. (1998) Peptide nucleic acid-targeted mutagenesis of a chromosomal gene in mouse cells. *Proc. Natl. Acad. Sci. USA*, **95**, 1398–1403.

Goodrich, J.A. and Tjian, R. (1994) Transcription factors IIE and IIH Band ATP hydrolysis direct promoter clearance by RNA polymerase II. *Cell*, **77**, 145–156.

Hanvey, J.C., Peffer, N.J., Bisi, J.E., Thomson, S.A., Cadilla, R., Josey, J.A. *et al.* (1992) Antisense and Antigene Properties of Peptide Nucleic Acids. *Science*, **258**, 1481–1485.

Holstege, F.C.P., van der Vliet, P.C. and Timmers, H.T.M. (1996) Opening of an RNA polymerase II promoter occurs in two distinct steps and requires the basal transcription factors IIE and IIH. *EMBO J.*, **15**, 1666–1677.

Knudsen, H. and Nielsen, P.E. (1996) Antisense properties of duplex- and triplex-forming PNAs. *Nucleic Acids Res.*, **24**, 494–500.

Kurakin, A., Larsen, H.J. and Nielsen, P.E. (1998) Cooperative strand displacement by peptide nucleic acids (PNA). *Chem. & Biol.*, **5**, 81–89.

Larsen, H.J. and Nielsen, P.E. (1996) Transcription-mediated binding of peptide nuclei acid (PNA) to double-stranded DNA: sequence-specific suicide transcription. *Nucleic Acids Res.*, **24**, 458–463.

Lohse, J., Dahl, O. and Nielsen, P.E. (1999). Double duplex invasion by peptide nucleic acid: a general principle for sequence-specific targeting of double-stranded DNA. *Proc. Natl. Acad. Sci. USA*, **96**, 11804–11808.

Mollegaard, N.E., Buchardt, O., Egholm, M. and Nielsen, P.E. (1994) Peptide nucleic acid. DNA strand displacement loops as artificial transcription promoters. *Proc. Natl. Acad. Sci. USA*, **91**, 3892–3895.

Nielsen, P.E., Egholm, M., Berg, R.H. and Buchardt, O. (1993) Sequence specific inhibition of DNA restriction enzyme cleavage by PNA. *Nucleic Acids Res.*, **21**, 197–200.

Nielsen, P.E., Egholm, M., Berg, R.H. and Buchardt, O. (1991) Sequence-selective recognition of DNA by strand displacement with a thymine-substituted polyamide. *Science*, **254**, 1497–1500.

Nielsen, P.E., Egholm, M. and Buchardt, O. (1994) Sequence-specific transcription arrest by peptide nucleic acid bound to the DNA template strand. *Gene*, **149**, 139–145.

Nikolov, D.B. and Burley, S.K. (1997) RNA polymerase II transcription initiation: A structural view. *Proc. Natl. Acad. Sci. USA*, **94**, 15–22.

Orum, H., Nielsen, P.E., Egholm, M., Berg, R.H., Buchardt, O. *et al.* (1993) Single base pair mutation analysis by PNA directed PCR clamping. *Nucleic Acids Res.*, **21**, 5332–5336.

Pardridge, W.M., Boado, R.J. and Kang, Y.-S. (1995) Vector-mediated delivery of a polyamide ('peptide') nucleic acid analogue through the blood-brain barrier *in vivo*. *Proc. Natl. Acad. Sci. USA*, **92**, 5592–5596.

Peffer, N.J., Hanvey, J.C., Bisi, J.E., Thomson, S.A., Hassman, C.F., Noble, S.A. *et al.* (1993) Strand-invasion of duplex DNA by peptide nucleic acid oligomers. *Proc. Natl. Acad. Sci. USA*, **90**, 10648–10652.

Penichet, M.L., Kang, Y.S., Pardridge, W.M., Morrison, S.L. and Shin, S.U. (1999) An antibody-avidin fusion protein specific for the transferrin receptor serves as a delivery vehicle for effective brain targeting: initial applications in anti-HIV antisense drug delivery to the brain. *J. Immunol.*, **163**, 4421–4426.

Pooga, M., Soomets, U., Hallbrink, M., Valkna, A., Saar, K., Rezaei, K. *et al.* (1998) Cell penetrating PNA constructs regulate galanin receptor levels and modify pain transmission *in vivo*. *Nature Biotech.*, **16**, 857–861.

Scarfi, S., Giovine, M., Gasparini, A., Damonte, G., Millo, E., Pozzolini, M. *et al.* (1999) Modified peptide nucleic acids are internalized in mouse macrophages RAW 264.7 and inhibit inducible nitric oxide synthase. *FEBS Letters*, **451**, 264–268.

Simmons, C.G., Pitts, A.E., Mayfield, L.D., Shay, J.W. and Corey, D.R. (1997) Synthesis and permeability of PNA-peptide conjugates. *Bioorg. Med. Chem. Lett.*, **7**, 3001–3007.

Taylor, R.W., Chinnery, P.F., Turnbull, D.M. and Lightowlers, R.N. (1997) Selective inhibition of mutant human mitochondrial DNA replication *in vitro* by peptide nucleic acids. *Nature Genetics*, **15**, 212–215.

Tyler, B.M., Jansen, K., McCormick, D.J., Douglas, C.L., Boules, M., Stewart, J.A. *et al.* (1999) Peptide nucleic acids targeted to the neurotensin receptor and administered i.p. cross the blood-brain barrier and specifically reduce gene expression. *Proc. Natl. Acad. Sci. USA*, **96**, 7053–7058.

Wang, G., Xu, X., Pace, B., Dean, D.A., Glazer, P.M., Chan, P. *et al.* (1999) Peptide nucleic acid (PNA) binding-mediated induction of human g-globin gene expression. *Nucleic Acids Res.*, **27**, 2806–2813.

Zawel, L. and Reinberg, D. (1995) Common themes in assembly and function of eukaryotic transcription complexes. *Annu. Rev. Biochem.*, **64**, 533–561.

6 Aptamers for controlling gene expression

Jean-Jacques Toulmé, Eric Dausse,
Fanny Santamaria and Bernard Rayner

INTRODUCTION

Over the last twenty years a number of strategies making use of synthetic oligo-nucleotides for modulation of gene expression have been developed. These approaches share a working hypothesis according to which nucleic acids are not considered as the recipient of genetic information. They rather constitute ligands designed to specifically bind to a pre-determined target, thus interfering with its function. This target molecule is generally an RNA sequence but can occasionally be a DNA region or even a protein playing a major role in gene expression through the selective binding to a promotor region.

The idea of making use of nucleic acids to address modification to an RNA target in a sequence-dependent way dates back to 1967 when Belikova *et al.* (1967) described what would be, a few years later, recognized as the antisense strategy. Multiple examples of successful inhibition of gene expression by antisense RNA generated *in situ* or by chemically-modified oligonucleotides have been reported (Cohen, 1989; Couvreur and Malvy, 2000; Crooke and Lebleu, 1993; Weiss, 1997). The discovery that RNA can act as a catalyst for RNA cleavage offered new possibilities for artificially controlling gene expression (Cech and Bass, 1986). Ribozyme can be considered as active antisense RNAs, the specificity of the cleaving reaction being controlled by base-pairing between the flanking stretches and the target RNA. Interestingly, ribozymes are formally equivalent to the combination of an antisense oligodeoxynucleotide and of ribonuclease H (RNase H), a class of ubiquitous enzymes which specifically cleave the RNA strand of an RNA-DNA duplex and which have been demonstrated to play a key role in antisense effects (Toulmé and Tidd, 1998). A number of applications have been described with either chemically-modified ribozymes or catalytic transcripts generated within cells, thus offering a wide potential in gene therapy (Eckstein and Lilley, 1997). Recently, a phenomenon known as double-stranded RNA interference provided a rational for unexplained results obtained in the frame of antisense studies. It has been demonstrated in various organisms that double-stranded RNA delivered to a cell, or to a living organism by various means, triggered the selective degradation of the homologous mRNA sequence (Elbashir *et al.*, 2001; Montgomery *et al.*, 1998; Zamore *et al.*, 2000). The process which involves the recruitment of a specialized RNase is not fully understood. RNAi offers an alternative to the antisense strategy, at least in the tissues in which RNA interference has been shown to take place.

The approaches described above target RNA and most often induce its selective degradation. The so-called 'triplex' or 'antigene' strategy rests upon the binding of an oligopyrimidine or an oligopurine to a DNA double-strand exclusively containing purines on one strand and pyrimidines on the other strand (Thuong and Hélène, 1993). Even though the number of successful inhibitions of gene expression by triple-helix forming oligonucleotides is much lower than the available examples reported for antisense oligomers or ribozymes, this strategy has been demonstrated to be efficient in biological models (Giovannangeli and Hélène, 2000; Vasquez *et al.*, 2000).

The sense approach, in which a short nucleic acid sequence mimicking the natural binding site of a DNA- or RNA-binding protein, has been essentially used for functional analysis of a target gene. The competition between the decoy and the natural binding site abolishes the formation of the authentic nucleic acid/protein complexes and thus inhibits the process mediated by this complex (Clusel *et al.*, 1993).

All the above strategies depend upon the rational design of the oligonucleotide ligand. Knowledge of the target molecule as well as the rules allowing the binding of the oligonucleotide to this target are absolute pre-requisites for the conception of antisense, ribozymes, sense or triplex-forming sequences. In contrast, *in vitro* selection of RNA or DNA sequences displaying a property of interest can be undertaken without prior sequence or structure information on either partner, i.e., the target or the ligand. This strategy, known as Systematic Evolution of Ligands by EXponential enrichment (SELEX), is a combinatorial one: the sequences of interest of so-called aptamers are selected in a randomly synthesized pool of nucleic acids (Ellington and Szostak, 1990; Tuerk and Gold, 1990) (Figure 6.1). Moreover, in contrast to the rational design of antisense, ribozyme and triplex-forming oligomers, no hypothesis has to be made regarding the type of interaction engaged in by aptamer-target complexes: aptamers are selected on a functional basis. High affinity oligomers binding selectively to a wide range of molecular targets have been identified using this approach (Ellington and Conrad, 1995; Famulok and Mayer, 1999; Gold *et al.*, 1995). This approach includes molecular species involved in the control of gene expression, either protein or nucleic acid elements. The association of aptamers with the regulatory element may perturb these natural processes, making them artificial modulators of gene expression. Therefore, aptamers constitute an alternative to rationally designed oligonucleotides and *in vitro* selection expands the repertoire of strategies available for selectively interfering with several steps of gene expression. As for antisense oligonucleotides, unless RNA aptamers are produced *in situ*, it is necessary to stabilize them against nucleases and to deliver them to the appropriate cellular compartment. The requirement to maintain the shape of the selected oligomer, however, restricts the use of chemical modifications. This chapter will focus on *in vitro* selection for the identification of aptamers which may be used to regulate gene expression by targeting either proteins or RNA structures. Specific procedures to generate chemically-modified aptamers will be discussed.

SELECTING THE SHAPE

Very generally, the identification of a molecule of interest by a combinatorial strategy requires: (i) the random synthesis of a balanced library in which the different candidates are statistically equi-represented, (the over-representation of some compounds and the under-representation of others will bias the population and subsequently may affect the outcome of the selection); (ii) the efficient partitioning of candidates which display the desired property depends upon a carefully adjusted 'selection pressure' combined with an effective procedure allowing the physical separation of the winners, and; (iii) the identification of these winning molecules and their defined synthesis at high yield and low cost for further use. This means either a very sensitive analytical method to determine the chemical structure of the selected molecules must be used or the use of a procedure in which the identification step is coupled to the synthesis or to the selection (for instance, by position scanning or by omission).

Nucleic acid libraries make step 'iii' (identification) much more easy than for any other compound, allowing the simultaneous screening of up to 10^{15} different molecules, i.e., 10^6–10^{11}-fold more than with non-nucleic acid derivatives. This case of identification is essentially due to the fact that RNA or DNA sequences bear the necessary information to be replicated. Indeed, following selection, the selected sequences can be amplified by polymerase chain reaction (PCR), thus regenerating a new pool of sequences. This new pool can be further used for an additional step of selection (Figure 6.1). Therefore, SELEX is an iterative process, each selection/amplification round enriching the population of sequences with respect to the desired property. The process can be continued until the pool does not evolve anymore, typically after 5 to 15 cycles, depending on the complexity of the library, the relative number of sequences displaying the expected character in the starting pool and the stringency of the selection. Moreover, the selected oligomers can be cloned, propagated in bacteria and sequenced according to routine procedures. In addition, the random synthesis of the balanced starting pool (and the synthesis of the winning oligomer for specific studies and use) is well controlled using standard phosphoramidite chemistry. These advantages have led a wide number of researchers to use this powerful method for different purposes: identification of a consensus binding site for RNA or DNA binding proteins, selection of new catalytic activities, need of high affinity ligands for diagnostic or therapeutic applications (Ellington and Conrad, 1995; Jayasena, 1999; Toulmé, 2000).

The primary sequence dictates higher order structures. Therefore, a collection of sequences actually corresponds to a collection of shapes, each one displaying a unique three-dimensional distribution of elementary groups able to engage diverse types of interaction with any kind of target molecule. *In vitro* selection of an oligonucleotide sequence should, therefore, be viewed as the selection of an RNA or DNA structure 'complementary' to a portion of the target.

In vitro selection is now routinely used in a number of laboratories. We discuss below the major features for running a SELEX experiment which typically involves three major steps: (i) the synthesis of the library; (ii) the selection of the oligomers of interest, and; (iii) the amplification of the selected sequences (Figure 6.1). The use of RNA libraries makes it necessary to include a transcription step prior to selection and a reverse transcription step prior to amplification. More details can be found in recent reviews (Brody and Gold, 2000; Ellington, 1994; Famulok and Jenne, 1998; Famulok *et al.*, 2000; Toulmé, 2000).

The design of the library (chemistry and length of the random sequence) and the selection procedure must be decided first. Unless the process aims at identifying the natural motif recognized by nucleic acid binding proteins (in that case RNA libraries will be used for RNA-binding proteins and DNA libraries for DNA-binding proteins), there is no rule for guiding the choice of the chemistry. Both RNA and DNA aptamers displaying similar affinity and specificity have been selected against a given target. In general, however, different molecules have been sieved, e.g., for the reverse transcriptase of the Human Immunodeficiency Virus-1 (HIV-1) (Tuerk *et al.*, 1992) and for thrombin (Bock *et al.*, 1992; Kubik *et al.*, 1994). In other words, generally homologous DNA sequences derived from selected RNA aptamers will not bind and vice versa, illustrating the relationship between oligonucleotide chemistry and conformation.

The molecular diversity of the library is linked to the length of the random window and varies as 4^n (where n is the length in nucleotide of the randomized stretch; Figure 6.1a). The theoretical complexity of the pool may surpass the experimental limit which is equal to about 10^{14}–10^{15} different sequences. How-ever, aptamers have been identified even in cases where sequence coverage was incomplete, due to the use of pools of oligonucleotides longer than 25 nucleotides ($4^{25} \approx 10^{15}$). This identification is likely related to the fact that frequently selected aptamers display essential motifs containing less than 15–20 nucleotides. For instance, an anti-thrombin DNA aptamer has been selected from a library with 60 randomized positions (Bock *et al.*, 1992). The starting pool presented a com-plexity of about 10^{13} individual species, i.e., only $1/10^{23}$ of the possible candidates. A strong ligand (Kd $\approx$ 30 nM at 25 °C (Sumikura *et al.*, 1997)) 15 nucleotide long was identified, meaning that this sequence was present $> 10^4$ times in the initial pool. A limited number of scaffolds have been selected which display essential residues for binding; these include stem-loops, internal loops and bulges, pseudo-knots and four-stranded structures.

Extraction of candidates of interest from the pool can be carried out by any of the following methods, which allow the physical separation between free and target-bound oligonucleotides: affinity chromatography, filtration on cellulose filters, or polyacrylamide gel electrophoresis. For those techniques in which either one partner is immobilized or the complex is retained, the support is always in vast excess compared to the intended target. The enrichment of sequences which interact with the chromatographic support or with the filter can be minimized by passing the pool of random sequences on unliganded support or on the filter in the absence of the target prior to each selection step. Alternatively one can switch from one type of support to another or from one method to another.

The molecular evolution of the pool is driven by the competition between the various candidates for binding to the target. This can be controlled by adjusting the ionic concentration, the temperature, the target concentration, and the number of washes prior to eluting the bound sequences. These conditions can be varied from step to step during a SELEX procedure to get aptamers of the highest affinity. Alternatively, a known ligand of the target can be introduced as a competitor.

Numerous studies have taken advantage of *in vitro* selection for the identification of aptamers. Many of them are relevant to the control of gene expression. This includes the determination of consensus RNA (or DNA) motifs recognized by proteins which naturally bind to RNA (or DNA) regions and play a role in gene expression, and the identification of oligonucleotide ligands exhibiting high affin-ity and specificity for a protein involved in a regulatory process. In both cases,

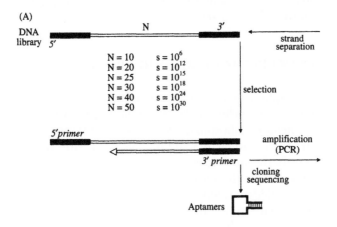

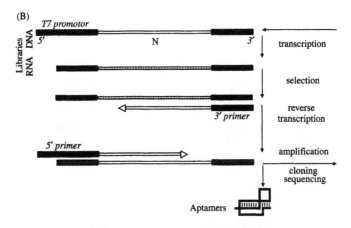

Figure 6.1 Scheme of the key steps for *in vitro* selection of DNA or RNA aptamers. The filled boxes correspond to the fixed portions of the candidates which are identical for every oligomer in the library. The open bars correspond to the random sequence whose length N dictates the complexity of the library. The number of theoretical sequences for N = 10–50 is given in panel A. Alternatively, partly randomized regions can be inserted between the fixed region for the optimization of aptamers through biazed libraries. (A) Scheme for the selection of DNA aptamers such as hairpins obtained against the TAR RNA element of HIV-1 (Boiziau *et al.*, 1999). (B) Scheme for the selection of RNA aptamers such as pseudoknots identified against the reverse transcriptase of HIV-1 (Tuerk *et al.*, 1992). RNA sequences obtained by *in vitro* transcription of the DNA library are indicated with dotted boxes.

selected aptamers will work as decoys, trapping the protein in a non-informative complex. *In vitro* selection has also been performed against RNA structures to identify sequences that take into account the folded RNA chain. Another application deals with the use of aptamers to small molecules (dyes, for instance) to generate dye-controlled expression cassettes. These various applications of SELEX will be reviewed in the following sections.

APTAMERS TO NUCLEIC ACID-BINDING PROTEINS

In vitro selection of aptamers has been carried out against a large number of proteins interacting with nucleic acids, from both prokaryotic and eukaryotic origins. Targets include ribosomal proteins, translational regulators and initiation factors, transcription factors and polymerases. Most of these studies were undertaken to identify the nucleic acid sequences or structures which guide the binding of these proteins. To this end RNA or DNA libraries containing either fully randomized or partly degenerated sequences were prepared. Due to the large number of variants which can be sampled in a single experiment such studies are much more informative than the tedious investigations carried out with a series of point-mutated sequences.

Polymerases

In vitro selection of RNA was performed against the yeast RNA polymerase II (Thomas *et al.*, 1997) to get information on its functional interactions with transcripts. Heparin was added to the medium after the ninth round of selection to increase the stringency and reduce the diversity of the selected sequences. After six additional rounds at high stringency, one class of ligand characterized by a GNXGAGG motif was identified. Aptamers which contact the largest Pol II subunit inhibit template DNA binding. One aptamer was shown to selectively inhibit yeast Pol II but not the Pol I or Pol III *in vitro* transcription activity. RNA aptamers characterized by a hairpin structure with a six base pair stem and a CAA loop preceded by a CCCCA consensus pentamer were shown to bind tightly to the *E. coli* rho factor, essential for the transcription termination (Schneider *et al.*, 1993). In agreement with the known preference of rho for C rich sequence, a large number of selected aptamers showed a high cytosine content. This study significantly increased the number of RNA sequences recognized by the rho factor but the size of the randomized region (30 nt) did not cover that of the natural hexamer binding site (70–80 nt), and therefore did not allow for the full characterization of the recognition motif responsible for transcription termination.

The Qβ replicase is the RNA-dependent RNA polymerase responsible for replicating the genome of the coliphage Qβ. It consists of four subunits, one of them being the host-encoded ribosomal protein S1. To elucidate the specific RNA features that make the coliphage genome preferentially replicated compared to the vast excess of host sequences, *in vitro* selection was carried out by filter binding within a pool of 10^{13} different sequences. One set of RNA was identified which folds as a pseudo-knot with conserved loop sequences (Brown and Gold, 1995). Similar aptamers were previously selected against S1 ribosomal protein and 30S ribosomal particles (Ringquist *et al.*, 1995). To get rid of the S1 binding RNAs, a second selection was carried out with a counter selection step against the 30S subunit of *E. coli* ribosomes. Most of the molecules selected at the end of eleven rounds showed no shared structural motif but a high pyrimidine content. This class of molecules bind poorly to the protein S1 compared to the Qβ replicase.

SELEX experiments were also performed with 2'-5' oligoadenylate synthase (Hartmann *et al.*, 1998) and the thermostable Taq polymerase (Dang and Jayasena, 1996) in different perspectives. In the first case, unstructured RNA oligomers were shown to activate 2'-5'A synthase, an enzyme which was previously believed to be activated only by double-stranded RNA. Dang and Jayasena (1996) screened a single-stranded DNA library to isolate sequences inhibiting the Taq Pol at room temperature but not above 40 °C, thus making 'hot start' PCR dispensable. The selection procedure, which included a binding step at room temperature and amplification at high temperature with the same enzyme, yielded reversibly inhibitory sequences, selective for the Taq polymerase. Two families of aptamers were identified displaying Kds in the low picomolar range. Heterodimeric aptamers resulting from the head to tail combination of two parent ligands showed a 75-fold increased affinity and a 10-fold decreased IC_{50} compared to the monomeric aptamers.

Reverse transcriptases are key enzymes for the development of retroviruses. Tuerk *et al.* (1992) have isolated high affinity RNA ligands from a pool of sequences randomized at 32 nucleotide positions against the reverse transcription of HIV-1. A fairly large number of the selected aptamers adopted a pseudo-knot fold (Figure 6.1b) with one helix specified at the primary sequence level, whereas the second one (stem 2) did not show sequence preference (Green *et al.*, 1995). These pseudo-knotted RNAs bind to the HIV-1 RT with a high affinity and inhibit the *in vitro* reverse transcriptase (DNA polymerase) activity with an IC_{50} of about 30 nM. Stopped flow experiments monitored by fluorescence energy transfer and filter binding assay showed that the extremely high affinity of the pseudo-knot for the enzyme ($K_d = 25$ pM) was essentially due to a very low dissociation rate constant compared to DNA–DNA or DNA–RNA complexes (Kensch *et al.*, 2000). A low resolution (4.8 Å) structure of an HIV-1 RT/RNA pseudo-knot crystal has shown that the kinked aptamer binds along the cleft lying between the polymerase and the RNase H catalytic sites, presumably overlapping the binding region of duplex DNA and that of the primer tRNA (Jaeger *et al.*, 1998). Other RNA ligands of the HIV-1 RT, adopting different structures, but displaying similar binding and inhibitory properties, have recently been identified (Burke *et al.*, 1996). All of them are selective for the HIV-1 RT and do not inhibit the avian or murine reverse transcriptases.

In vitro selection carried out against other reverse transcriptases led to the identification of high affinity RNA ligands: aptamers to the enzymes from avian, feline and murine retroviruses show stem-loop structures (Chen and Gold, 1994; Chen *et al.*, 1996). The different RNA ligands share very little properties, thus demonstrating that specific inhibitors can be selected against enzymes displaying identical catalytic properties.

A single-stranded DNA library was also screened against the HIV-1 RT. K_d values for the selected DNA sequences were in the nanomolar range and they inhibited the DNA polymerase activity of this enzyme with a K_i as low as 1 nM (Schneider *et al.*, 1995). The best DNA aptamer folds as a hairpin with an internal loop and competes with the RNA pseudo-knot for RT binding. These two ligands share very little structural similarity.

Nucleases

In vitro selection of aptamers can also be carried out against nucleases. Similar to the selection of artificial ribozymes, one should be able to regenerate a pool of sequences of interest from the products of the enzymatic reaction. Jayasena *et al.* (1996) were interested in the characterization of the recognition site of the Reg B endonuclease from the T4 bacteriophage. This enzyme was known to cleave at GGAG sequences. However, not every GGAG tetranucleotide is processed by Reg B. In addition, the endonucleolytic activity is strongly stimulated by the *E. coli* ribosomal protein S1. A library of 10^{14} circular sequences was prepared by the transcription of a DNA library bearing a 30 nucleotide randomized stretch followed by a ligation step. After incubation with Reg B in the presence of S1, the product of the reaction was run on a gel for partitioning cleaved products form unreacted circular substrates. The selected RNAs were religated to regenerate the randomized region and reverse-transcribed prior to PCR amplification. After 12 rounds of this procedure the library was enriched in sequences with a -GGAG- tetranucleotide cleavage site, but unfortunately no consensus was identified except that a family of selected sequences possessed fairly long stretches of As and Cs (Jayasena *et al.*, 1996). As expected, the cleavage rate of these sequences was increased in the presence of S1.

Ribonucleases H are ubiquitous enzymes which cleave the RNA strand of RNA–DNA duplex. They are crucial for the lifecycle of retroviruses, are involved in DNA replication and play a key role for antisense effects mediated by oligodeoxynucleotides (Crouch and Toulmé, 1998). Selection of DNA aptamers to the human ribonuclease H type has been carried out by nitrocellulose filter binding. A series of G-rich sequences were identified as high affinity ligands (Kd ≈ 100 nM) of this enzyme. One of the aptamers was suggested to generate a four-stranded guanine scaffold, which inhibited the *in vitro* RNase H activity of the human RNase H in a selective manner; in particular, the two best inhibitory aptamers did not inhibit the RNase H activity of HIV-1 RT (Pileur *et al.*, submitted). Interestingly, a selection of DNA oligonucleotides performed against this retroviral enzyme by alternatively binding to the natural heterodimer p66-p51, which carries the RNase H activity, and to the p51-p51 homodimer, devoid of the RNase H domain (counter-selection step), led to G-rich oligomers. The G-rich oligomers displayed a selective affinity for the p66-p51 reverse-transcriptase and did not bind to the homodimer, suggesting that the aptamer binding site involved the RNase H domain of the retroviral enzyme (Andréola *et al.*, 2001). In addition, these anti-RT aptamers inhibited the retroviral RNase H activity but not the human RNase H.

Transcription factors

More than ten years ago random selection of sequences were used to determine the DNA sequence recognized by transcription factors. Blackwell and Weintraub (1990) developed the selected and amplified binding site (SAAB) methodology to identify the preferred motif of a class of DNA-binding proteins containing a basic-helix-loop-helix (bHLH) motif. Using this technique they were able to select by electrophoretic mobility shift assay the double-stranded DNA sequence recognized by the proto-oncogene c-Myc, a protein containing a bHLH domain; a carboxy-terminal polypeptide of human c-Myc binds, in a sequence-dependent way, to the hexamer CACGTG (Blackwell *et al.*, 1990). Using a similar strategy Pollock and Treisman (1990) isolated by immuno precipitation-the DNA fragments associated to the transcription factor serum response factor (SRF) and to the oncoprotein c-Fos. They suggested that this method might be used for the identification of binding sites of proteins contained in cell-free extracts or produced by cell-free translation. The potential of *in vitro* selection has also been demonstrated for characterizing the binding site of *E. coli* regulatory proteins such as the Leucine-responsive protein (Lrp) (Cui *et al.*, 1995).

The Tax protein of the human T-cell lymphotropic virus (HTLV-1) is a transcription factor which *trans*-activates the expression of both viral and cellular genes, in part by interacting with DNA binding proteins such as the cyclic AMP-response element binding (CREB) protein. An RNA pool having a core of 120 nucleotide random sequence (roughly 10^{13} different candidates) was used for *in vitro* selection against Tax; after six rounds approximately 40% of the selected population bound to this protein (Tian and Kole, 1995). The analysis of eight clones revealed a single RNA species which selectively bound to Tax with a Kd of about 70 nM and blocked its association with CREB. This study provides an example of aptamers targeted to a protein not known for binding nucleic acids.

Translation and splicing factors

Translation and splicing machineries involve a fairly large number of RNA and RNA-binding proteins. Specific interactions between these multiple partners responsible for functional and regulatory complexes are far from being fully understood. Numerous selections have been carried out against ribosomal proteins (Moine *et al.*, 1997; Ringquist *et al.*, 1995), initiation and elongation factors (Hornung *et al.*, 1998; Klug *et al.*, 1999; Méthot *et al.*, 1996; Nazarenko and Uhlenbeck, 1995), and proteins involved in splicing (Burd and Dreyfuss, 1994; Shi *et al.*, 1997; Tsai *et al.*, 1991). These selections have been conducted to elucidate the RNA motif recognized by these proteins. A few representative examples will be described below which exemplify the interest of such studies.

Klug *et al.* (1999) selected RNA sequences that bind the Sel B protein of *E. coli*, an elongation factor which recognizes a stem-loop structure and drives the incorporation of selenocysteine in response to an opal (UGA) codon immediately upstream of the structure. The wild-type hairpin recognized by Sel B in the dehydrogenase G mRNA was used as a competitor for the selection allowing the RNA pool to evolve very quickly. In four cycles high affinity aptamers ($K_d \approx 1$ nM) were selected. Several aptamers bound 50-fold better than the natural RNA hairpin. This binding is not uncommon for *in vitro* selection and has been reported in several instances (Bartel *et al.*, 1991; Burd and Dreyfuss, 1994; Méthot *et al.*, 1996). Natural RNA (and DNA) binding sites have been 'selected' on functional criteria which are generally more demanding than high affinity, may involve optimal interactions with several partners and should ultimately be reversible under various conditions. Extremely high affinity is definitely not the best way to switch rapidly from an 'on' to 'off' (from expressed to repressed) status. Indeed, although it provided high affinity aptamers, the selection against the Sel B protein (Klug *et al.*, 1999) identified many different sequences which generally did not resemble tRNA or mRNA natural structures recognized by this elongation factor. This nonresemblance of tRNA or mRNA natural structures strongly suggests that the RNA motifs recognized by the selenocysteine-incorporating machinery have evolved in response to many different biological constraints. These aptamers have not been evaluated for their ability to drive the incorporation of selenocysteine.

In vitro selection has been used for the identification of RNA ligands which recognize the translation initiation factor eIF-4B. This 80 kDa phosphoprotein contains an RNA recognition motif (RRM) near the N-terminus, and stimulates the helicase activity of eIF-4A and eIF-4F. Sonenberg and co-workers (Méthot *et al.*, 1996) performed selection against intact or truncated eIF-4B in the absence or in the presence of eIF-4A and demonstrated that the RRM is responsible for the recognition of a stem-loop structure containing a GGAA/C motif. Moreover, eIF-4B can bind simultaneously to two different RNA molecules, supporting a model whereby this simultaneous binding could promote the recruitment of both the mRNA and the ribosome through interactions with the 18S rRNA.

A few examples of translational repressor/operator are known which involve the selective recognition of an RNA structure by a protein. Bacteriophages such as R17 are well documented model systems. The R17 coat protein represses the translation of the replicase gene by binding to a 19 nt hairpin whose stem sequesters the Shine/Dalgarno sequence and the AUG start codon. Selection of RNA ligands against the R17 coat protein identified a consensus stem-loop structure with a tetranucleotide loop and a single base-bulged stem (Schneider *et al.*, 1992) which confirmed the essential features established from the investigation of more than 100 variants of the R17 coat protein binding sites by Uhlenbeck and colleagues (Witherell *et al.*, 1991). Remarkably, had the natural binding site not have been previously known, the consensus derived from *in vitro* selection would have facilitated the location of the translational hairpin operator in the R17 bacteriophage genome. Similar experiments were carried out with the MS2 coat protein, which recognizes the same RNA hairpin as the R17 coat protein. Interactions between two A residues in the tetraloop (position -4) and in the bulge (position -10) with the protein are crucial for complex formation. Interestingly, crystallographic studies showed that an aptamer with a trinucleotide loop and an additional base-pair in the upper stem region restored the crucial A(-4)-A(-10) interactions with protein pockets through a concerted rearrangement of the $3'$ strand of the RNA hairpin, which does not interact with the R17 coat protein, showing that different RNA scaffolds present similar recognition surfaces (Convery *et al.*, 1998).

SELEX has also allowed the characterization of the RNA hairpin, which constitutes the iron responsive element (IRE) recognized by the iron regulatory factor (IRF) protein to post-transcriptionally regulate translatability and decay of mRNAs involved in iron import and storage in eukaryotic cells (Henderson *et al.*, 1994).

Control of gene expression by aptamer-protein complexes

Several examples demonstrate that aptamers selected against a purified protein in the test tube retain their binding activity in a cell context and may exert a regulatory function. Potentially, every aptamer targeted to a protein involved in the transmission of the genetic information can act as a decoy and, therefore, perturb the mechanisms in which the target protein is involved. Obviously, trapping a factor widely used in the cell is of limited interest as this will result in the inhibition of multiple or even every gene. For instance, RNA sequences selected against yeast RNA polymerase II induced a growth defect when expressed, under a Pol III-dependent promotor, in cells having an artificially reduced level of Pol II activity (Thomas *et al.*, 1997).

Aptamers can be used to dissect the involvement of a protein in gene expression. Translation of the Hepatitis C Virus (HCV) mRNA is initiated by the internal ribosome entry site (IRES), which constitutes a binding site for *trans*-acting cellular factors, such as the polypyrimidine tract-binding protein (PTB). To assess the function of PTB in IRES-mediated translation initiation, Anwar *et al.* (2000) used previously selected (Singh *et al.*, 1995) RNA aptamers. These sequences character-ized by a (U/G)C(A/Y)GCCUG(Y/G)UGCY$_4$CY$_4$(G/Y)G consensus bound specifi-cally PTB with a K$_d$ of 1–5 nM. Three anti-PTB aptamers inhibited *in vitro* translation in reticulocyte lysate of mono- or bicistronic constructs, in which the luciferase gene was under the control of the HCV IRES, in a selective manner: no inhibition of cap-dependent translation was detected. As expected for a decoy effect, adding back recombinant human PTB relieved the inhibition mediated by the aptamers. Interestingly, a selective inhibition was also detected following the co-transfection of a liver-derived cell line by an HCV IRES-Luciferase construct, along with an anti-PTB aptamer, thus demonstrating that PTB is required for efficient HCV IRES-dependent translation.

PTB, also known as hnRNP 1, was originally proposed as a splicing factor on the basis of its affinity for several pyrimidine tracts of adenoviral major late (Ad-ML) and α-tropomyosin pre-mRNAs. Singh *et al.* (1995), who identified the anti-PTB RNA aptamers, used it to unambiguously demonstrate that PTB actually regulates alternative splicing by selectively repressing the *3'* splice site of Ad-ML pre-mRNA in a concentration dependent-manner. A similar approach was used to investigate the properties of B52, a member of the *Drosophila* SR protein family, which was expected to play a role in splicing a subset of pre-mRNAs. Nine rounds of selec-tion allowed the identification of RNA sequences, displaying a specific affinity (Kd = 20–50 nM) for B52 (Shi *et al.*, 1997). These aptamers were characterized by a hairpin structure containing two absolutely conserved hexamers separated by a variable nucleotide. Deletion analysis led to a stem-loop structure about 20 nucleotide long, which constituted the minimal motif recognized by B52. This motif served as the basis for the design of a multivalent inhibitory RNA further used *in vivo*. As the presence of several binding sites in the same molecule increased the affinity for the target, a pentameric unit was built which contained five individually selected hairpins against B52. To make sure that each of the five aptamers folded properly, the stems were reorganized and/or elongated. In add-ition, a hairpin structure with a structurally stable UNCG tetraloop was engineered near the *3'* end of the construct. Such units were linked 'head-to-tail' with a hammerhead ribozyme incorporated at the *3'* end of each unit to yield the mature pentavalent aptamer. The multivalent aptamers were shown to bind B52 10-fold more efficiently than the monomer and to efficiently inhibit the splicing of the *ftz* pre-mRNA of *Drosophila* when provided *in trans*, in an *in vitro* assay.

The level of B52 was shown to be critical to fly development. Genes expressing such B52 multivalent binding aptamers were introduced in cultured *Drosophila* cells and in transgenic flies (Shi *et al.*, 1999). The expression of the aptamer construct caused up to 50% reduction in survival. Conversely, the over-expression of B52 is responsible for developmental abnormalities, such as undeveloped larval salivary glands. Interestingly, the salivary gland development is restored by the co-expression of inhibitory aptamers in a B52 overproducing strain, supporting the hypothesis that anti-B52 aptamers can inhibit the function of the protein *in vivo*.

When the target is a viral protein, the aptamer may interfere with the development of the virus. For human pathogens these sequences may be of therapeutic interest. Aptamers have been raised against almost all proteins from HIV-1. In several instances the aptamers isolated *in vitro* were shown to retain their binding properties in infected cells and prevented the multiplication of the virus. Two G-rich oligodeoxynucleotides selected against the RNase H domain of the HIV-1 reverse-transcriptase displayed inhibitory properties in a cell-free assay (Andréola *et al.*, 2001). The inhibitory mechanism is unknown. It might be related to the effect on RNase H but G-rich oligomers susceptible to give rise to four-stranded structures were shown to block the adsorption and penetration of the virus into the cell (Wyatt *et al.*, 1994).

The HIV-1 Tat is an 86 amino acid long protein which contains a cysteine-rich region and a highly basic domain. Both are essential for function, the arginine-rich portion being responsible for binding to the *trans*-activation response region (TAR) of the retroviral RNA. The Tat-TAR complex is crucial for the efficient transcription of the HIV-1 genome. In addition, the Tat protein influences the metabolism and growth of the host cell. Authentic TAR-RNA supplied as a decoy inhibits *in vitro* transcription, however the cytotoxicity associated to such oligomers, likely due to the specific interaction with cellular factors, is a major concern (Sullenger *et al.*, 1991). *In vitro* selection has been used by several teams to isolate high affinity RNA ligands of Tat which would not be recognized by host cell proteins. Marozzi *et al.* (1998) started from a library corresponding to the TAR sequence in which the central 21 nt encompassing the Tat and cell protein binding sites were randomized. TAR RNA which could not be amplified in the process was used as a competitor. The presomptive secondary structure of the selected candidates was characterized by a stem-loop interrupted by bulges. The two characterized aptamers showed a conserved sequence at a position crucial for Tat binding, but not located in a bulge in contrast to the authentic TAR sequence. These sequences bound to a Tat-derived peptide with an affinity similar to that of TAR (K_d = 20–30 nM) but did not support *in vitro* transcription when introduced in the promotor in place of the TAR sequence, indicating that the anti-Tat aptamers had likely lost the ability to bind essential cell factors (Marozzi *et al.*, 1998). HIV types 1 and 2 encode closely related Tat-1 and Tat-2 proteins. The above study was carried out with Tat-1. Aptamers to the 99 amino-acid protein Tat-2 were also characterized which looked alike the authentic TAR motif (Rhim and Rice, 1997).

Recently, a new selection (Yamamoto *et al.*, 2000) was carried out against Tat-1 using a pool of RNA with a large (120 nt) randomized sequence under similar conditions to the ones used previously (Marozzi *et al.*, 1998). This SELEX experiment led to aptamers called RNA^{Tat} able to bind Tat more than 100 times better than the authentic TAR RNA. This outcome was ascribed to the presence of two inverted repeats of TAR-like motifs characterized by a double two nucleotide bulge; deleting either bulge reduced the binding activity significantly. However, the stoichiometry of the Tat/aptamer complex was 1:1. Such aptamers could not have been identified in the selection carried out by Marozzi *et al.* (1998) due to the size of the randomized region placed in the context of a TAR-hairpin.

The high affinity of RNA^{Tat} was responsible for the efficient competition of binding to Tat compared to the authentic RNA. Interestingly, such RNA aptamers efficiently competed out the binding of a Tat-2-derived peptide, suggesting a similar type of binding to the Tat protein from HIV-1 or HIV-2 (Yamamoto *et al.*, 2000). In a cell-free transcription assay, the presence of RNA^{Tat} decreased two to three-fold the level of transcription of a luciferase reporter gene, i.e., to the level observed in the absence of Tat-dependent *trans*-activation. However, the effect was the same as that observed following the addition of a TAR decoy in spite of a 100-fold higher affinity of RNA^{Tat} for Tat, suggesting that part of the inhibition induced by the TAR decoy was due to the depletion of essential cellular factors; obviously such a mechanism cannot account for the inhibitory effect induced by RNA^{Tat}. Indeed, RNA^{Tat} led to a much lower inhibition of *in vitro* general transcription than the TAR decoy, underlining the specificity provided by the aptamer. RNA^{Tat} was also demonstrated to inhibit the Tat-dependent *trans*-activation of transcription in HeLa cells transfected with a construct expressing a nuclear transcript by 50–70% (Yamamoto *et al.*, 2000).

The Rev protein of HIV-1 facilitates the nuclear export of incompletely spliced viral mRNAs and plays, therefore, an important role in the production of viral structural proteins. Rev specifically binds to a responsive element which folds into a stem-internal loop-stem secondary structure, the Rev-binding element (RBE) located into the *rev* gene. *In vitro* selection has been used to determine interactions between Rev and the RBE. RNA motifs which could bind Rev up to ten-fold better than the wild-type sequence have been isolated either from an RNA library constituted of partly randomized RBE (Bartel *et al.*, 1991) or from completely random sequence pools, based on the RBE secondary structure (Giver *et al.*, 1993; Tuerk and MacDougal-Waugh, 1993). Novel RNA sequences and secondary structural motifs have been selected. In particular, a wild-type G:G pair is frequently replaced by an A:A or even by a C:A pair which are isosteric (Giver *et al.*, 1993).

The binding properties of the selected elements encouraged Symensma *et al.* (1996) to investigate the responsiveness of these aptamers in a functional assay. A CAT reporter gene was placed adjacent to the natural Rev responsive element within an HIV intron. Co-transfection of the reporter plasmid together with a Rev expression plasmid potentiated CAT activity in CV-1 African green monkey kidney cells, indicating that Rev-mediated pre-mRNA transport competed with splicing and allowed translation into an active CAT protein. A similar effect was observed when the authentic RBE was substituted for an anti-Rev aptamer, demonstrating that the selected sequence was functionally equivalent to the wild-type sequence. The efficiency was even better with the aptamer construct when Rev was limiting in agreement with the increased affinity of Rev for the aptamer compared to the wild-type RBE. This study suggests that the RBE may mutate and retain its functionality, for instance in response to drugs targeting the Rev-RBE complex. The Rex protein of the human T-cell leukemia virus plays a role similar to that of Rev for HIV-1: the appearance of unspliced messages in the cytoplasm is mediated in part by the binding of Rex to the Rex-responsive element (XRE). RNA aptamers raised to Rex compete with the wild-type XRE for binding to Rex and can functionally substitute for the XRE *in vivo* (Baskerville *et al.*, 1995, 1999).

APTAMERS TO NUCLEIC ACIDS

At first sight it may seem curious to use *in vitro* selection to identify RNA or DNA sequences that are able to interact with another nucleic strand. SELEX has been used in at least two cases: first, in an attempt to extend the repertoire of triple-stranded structures, and second, to recognize folded RNA structures. Triple helices cannot be generated from any double-stranded sequence but are restricted to the recognition of an homopurine–homopyrimidine duplex by a third strand which engages Hoogsteen (or reverse-Hoogsteen) hydrogen bonds with the purine strand of the duplex (Thuong and Hélène, 1993). Due to the potential of the triplex strategy for the regulation of transcription, it is of interest to generate oligonucleotides that are able to selectively bind to any double-stranded sequence. SELEX experiments have been carried out to identify new triple helical motifs (Hardenbol and van Dyke, 1996; Pei *et al.*, 1991; Soukup *et al.*, 1996). However, the selection performed against different sequences under various conditions did not reveal an alternative to the known canonical triplets for the binding to double-stranded DNA.

A particular case was considered when targeting the double-stranded stem of a nucleic acid hairpin structure. In a model study, *in vitro* selection was used against a DNA hairpin with a 3' overhang (Mishra *et al.*, 1996; Mishra and Toulmé, 1994). The library was composed of DNA candidates with a fixed motif complementary to the 3' single-stranded region of the target hairpin and a randomized region, 16 nucleotides long. Four selection rounds led to the characterization of sequences able to bind to the DNA hairpin. Footprinting studies revealed an interaction between the double-stranded stem and the selected sequence even though a canonical triple helix could not be expected, as the sequences did not match the known motifs. The complex was stable at neutral pH and prevented the cleavage of the stem by a restriction endonuclease (Mishra *et al.*, 1996). Moreover a 2'-*O*-methyloligoribo analogue of the selected sequence was able to recognize the RNA version of the DNA hairpin. This chemically-modified aptamer prevented the translation of a mRNA in a cell-free extract, in which the target hairpin was placed upstream of the AUG start codon (Le Tinévez *et al.*, 1998).

RNA structures constitute one of the limitations to the use of the antisense strategy. Intramolecular base-pairing competes with the intermolecular assocation between the antisense sequence and the sense RNA strand, and thus weakens or even abolishes the effect of the regulatory sequence. A number of studies have been devoted to the identification of accessible sites in target RNA (Sczakiel, 2000; Sohail and Southern, 2000) or to the optimization of the hybridization site for minimizing the penalty to be paid to unfold the target structure (Ecker, 1993; Freier, 1993).

The increasing number of RNA structures playing a major role in the regulation of gene expression suggests that they may constitute targets of interest for artificially controlling these particular genes. A ligand of high affinity which would selectively bind to such a regulatory RNA motif would perturb its function and consequently the synthesis of the protein encoded by the gene under its control. Even though successful results were obtained with antisense oligomers targeted to structured RNA regions (Compagno *et al.*, 1999; Ecker *et al.*, 1992), alternative strategies should be considered (Toulmé *et al.*, 2001). Alternative strategies include *in vitro* selection of oligonucleotides that are able to recognize a folded RNA sequence.

The numerous interactions responsible for the building of tertiary RNA structure suggests that it should be possible to identify oligonucleotides that could give rise to stable complexes involving only a few base pairs in those regions (loops, bulges) not engaged in intramolecular Watson-Crick hydrogen bonding. Additional interactions (such as stacking) would bring an extra-contribution to the free energy of binding.

In vitro selection of RNA candidates targeted to the TAR RNA hairpin of HIV-1 has been carried out starting from a library of sequences with a 60 nt random region, displaying a molecular diversity of about 10^{11} different species. The TAR RNA is an imperfect hairpin generated by the 59 first nucleotides of the HIV-1 RNA. It contains a 6 nt structured loop (Colvin *et al.*, 1993) and a tripyrimidine bulge on the 5′ side of the upper part of the stem. This bulge is part of the site recognized by the retroviral protein Tat which recruits the positive transcription elongation factor (P-TEFb) complex, through the cyclin T1. The TAR-Tat-PTEFb complex, which includes specific contacts with the TAR apical loop, is essential for RNA synthesis and actually constitutes a *trans*-activation transcription complex. The disruption of this complex leads to abortive viral RNA synthesis (Jones, 1997; Karn, 1999). RNA sequences from the library, bound to the 3′ end-biotinylated TAR RNA were captured by magnetic streptavidin beads, washed out and amplified by PCR prior to further selection. After nine selection rounds the cloned sequences revealed an octameric consensus 5′ GUCCCAGA corresponding to the apical part of a hairpin, closing a G, C rich double-stranded upper stem (Figure 6.2). Interestingly, the six central nucleotides of the consensus motif were fully complementary to the terminal loop of the TAR hairpin (Ducongé and Toulmé, 1999). Footprinting studies revealed that TAR RNA-aptamer–RNA complexes involved loop-loop (so-called 'kissing') interaction. Such loop-loop RNA complexes are known to mediate several natural processes, such as the control of plasmids Col E1 or R1 copy number (Persson *et al.*, 1990; Tomizawa, 1986) and the dimerization of retroviral genomes (Muriaux *et al.*, 1996; Paillart *et al.*, 1996).

The best anti-TAR RNA aptamer (R06) displays a Kd of a few nanomolar under the selection conditions (140 mM K^+, 20 mM Na^+, 3 mM Mg^{2+} at room temperature). Systematic analysis of a series of aptamer R06 variants identified the sequence and structural determinants of the highly stable complex formed with TAR RNA. Of course, a perfect match between the aptamer and the TAR loops is required: a point mutation in the R06 loop is detrimental to the binding. A compensatory mutation introduced in the TAR sequence restores the association capacity. However, Watson-Crick base-pairing did not fully account for the tight binding of the aptamer to TAR: the selected octameric sequence which retains the hydrogen-bonding capacity of R06 behaved as a very poor ligand, characterized by an association constant about two to three orders of magnitude lower than the full-length aptamer (Ducongé *et al.*, 2000; Ducongé and Toulmé, 1999). A series of deletions identified the boundary for an active anti-TAR

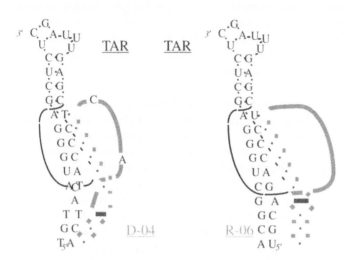

Figure 6.2 Structure of *trans*-activation response (TAR)-aptamer kissing complexes. The DNA D-04 (left) and the RNA aptamer R-06 (right) are shown in green. The crucial non-canonical base pairs are indicated in red (Collin *et al.*, 2000; Ducongé and Toulmé, 1999). (*see Color Plate 5*)

aptamer: a 3 base pair stem leading to a 14 nt long oligomer conferred to the kissing hairpin an affinity similar to the originally selected 98 mer (Darfeuille, unpublished results), underlining the role of the secondary structure in the complex stability.

A last feature was demonstrated to be of key importance for the formation of the kissing TAR-R06 complex. Although the first and last base of the octameric consensus are not likely to be engaged in a direct interaction with TAR, a G and an A residues were systematically selected at these positions, respectively (Figure 6.2). A systematic variation at the two positions demonstrated that purine–purine pairs were by far the best combinations, whereas C,A or C,U were very poor loop closing 'pairs' (Ducongé *et al.*, 2000). Surface plasmon resonance studies demonstrated that the major difference between high and low affinity aptamers, i.e., loops closed by G,A or C,U pairs for instance, originated in the dissociation rate constant k_{off}, whereas k_{on}, the association rate constant, remained essentially invariant. Of note, the G,A closing pair allows the aptamer to bind at low (3 mM) magnesium concentration, in contrast to a few other pairs such as U,A which requires a higher (10 mM) concentration, suggesting that the G,A pair might lead to a larger interchain distance, thus minimizing phosphate-phosphate repulsion (Ducongé *et al.*, 2000). Interestingly, the TAR-R06 complex is recognized by Rop (Darfeuille *et al.*, 2001), a 63 amino acid protein encoded by the Col E1 plasmid from *E. coli* which stabilizes loop–loop RNA–RNA interactions involved in the regulation of the plasmid replication. This Rop protein is known to show structure rather than sequence specificity (Predki *et al.*, 1995). This characteristic definitely demonstrates that the TAR-R06 complex is actually a 'kissing' complex.

In vitro selection targeted to two different RNA hairpins, the dimerization initiation site (DIS) of the HIV-1 genome and the yeast tRNA[Phe], also led to the identification of RNA hairpins, interacting with their relative target through loop–loop interactions and involving purine–purine closing pairs (Lodmell *et al.*, 1998, 2000; Scarabino *et al.*, 1999).

Generally, post-selection chemical modifications of aptamers weaken the binding properties of the selected sequences, as the chemically-modified oligomer does not retain the shape of the parent molecule (see next section). Indeed, the DNA homolog of the anti-TAR RNA aptamer R06 does not bind to its target even at concentrations higher than several micromolar, indicating that the binding constant of this DNA hairpin is more than three orders of magnitude lower than that of the RNA one. Selection of DNA candidates against the TAR RNA stem-loop was undertaken under two different magnesium concentration (10 mM and 3 mM). Both selections identified DNA hairpins whose loops, 8 and 11 nucleotide long, respectively contained a sequence complementary to the TAR loop (Boiziau *et al.*, 1999; Darfeuille *et al.*, submitted; Sekkai *et al.*, unpublished); the consensus obtained at high magnesium (5′ACTCCCATT) was included in the one identified at low magnesium concentration (5′ACACTCCCATTC). The DNA hairpins with the short consensus sequence, selected at 10 mM Mg^{2+}, did not bind at 3 mM, suggesting that the additional consensus bases identified under low magnesium conditions gave some freedom or allowed peculiar local conformation of the aptamer, minimizing phosphate-phosphate repulsions in the aptamer–TAR complex.

The structure of the complex formed by a TAR-derived hairpin and a truncated form of DNA aptamer (D04) selected at 10 mM magnesium was investigated by NMR (Collin *et al.*, 2000) (Figure 6.2). Even though the structure is not solved yet, this study brought interesting information. First, the TAR-D04 loop–loop interaction involved only five base pairs, in contrast to the six Watson-Crick pairs engaged in the TAR-R06 complex. Second, in spite of a bulged residue in the 3′ strand of the D04 stem, stacking was maintained through the formation of a non canonical T–T pair. This is, to our knowledge, the first example of a DNA–RNA kissing complex; this implies that the association of these two molecules results in a quasi-continuous stack, starting with a DNA helix (the aptamer stem) and ending with an RNA helix (the TAR stem) through an RNA–DNA hybrid helix (the loop–loop interaction) (Collin *et al.*, 2000). The geometry of DNA and RNA helices differs in many ways and, therefore, the connectors and the junctions between these helices should accomodate the differences. In contrast to the TAR-R06 complex for which the connectors were reduced to a single phosphodiester linkage, the linkers for the TAR-D04 complex correspond to one RNA and two DNA residues (Figure 6.2). Interestingly, the connecting nucleotides on the aptamer side were not random but belonged to the selected consensus. Exchanging the selected bases for any other one resulted in the abolition of the complex, suggesting a contribution to the interaction (Darfeuille *et al.*, unpublished results).

CHEMICALLY-MODIFIED APTAMERS

RNA and DNA aptamers present remarkable properties of selectivity and affinity. However, they suffer a number of limitations, some of which are shared with antisense oligomers. In particular, nuclease resistant aptamers would be more attractive for therapeutic and diagnostic purposes. Moreover, increasing their affinity and reducing their size is also of interest from these standpoints. Chemically-modified aptamers have been designed in order to fullfil these criteria. In addition, the introduction of synthetic nucleotides on which non-natural chemical entities have been tethered will increase the molecular diversity of the starting pool and might lead to the identification of shapes better adapted to the target of interest.

Two different strategies can be considered for generating modified aptamers. The first one introduces modified triphosphates in the SELEX process, whereas in the second one the modifications are introduced *a posteriori*, once the aptamers are selected and characterized. This latter approach is at first sight simpler but it is also more risky, as the chemical modifications may alter the shape and consequently the binding properties of the selected sequences. An example is provided by the DNA version of the anti-TAR RNA aptamer R06 discussed in the previous section: the desoxy analogue of this high affinity aptamer is a very poor ligand of the TAR hairpin, likely due to the fact that the RNA to DNA conversion results in a A- to B-type conformational change. Starting from this working hypothesis it was tempting to imagine that nucleic acid analogs that would retain the A-type geometry might constitute interesting alternatives to natural RNA. 2′-*O*-methyl oligoribo- (2′*O*Me) and 3′ → 5′ phosphoramidate oligodeoxyribo-nucleotides (NP) are known to generate A-type double helices. Not surprisingly 2′*O*Me and NP derivatives of the aptamer R06 displayed TAR binding properties similar to that of the parent aptamer. The NP-R06 aptamer was even a stronger binder than the RNA one (K_d = 1.5 and 6.2 nM, respectively [Darfeuille *et al.*, 2001]). Moreover, this nuclease-resistant aptamer retained the characteristics of the selected RNA sequence: firstly, it did not bind to a TAR variant containing a A to G point mutation in the loop. Secondly, exchanging the G,A loop–closing pair for a C,U pair resulted in a 100-fold decreased affinity of the mutated NP aptamer for TAR, similar to what was observed for the parent R06 aptamer. This decreased affinity suggests that the NP aptamer-TAR RNA kissing complex preserves the interactions providing the additional stability to the Watson–Crick base-pairing, as in the original RNA–RNA complex.

A Tat-peptide containing the amino-acid residues 37–72 mimicking the binding properties of the intact viral protein (Churcher *et al.*, 1993) was selectively competed out by the phosphoramidate aptamer, even though the magnesium concentration set at 3 mM in the selection procedure had to be decreased to 20 µM to allow the peptide to bind to TAR. This competition was likely related to the formation of the aptamer-TAR complex, as the phosphoramidate derivative of the aptamer with a C,U pair closing the loop, which did not bind to TAR, did not compete with Tat either (Darfeuille *et al.*, submitted). As the binding sites of the aptamer and of the peptide do not overlap this suggests that either the aptamer induced a teleo-conformational change which prevents the binding of Tat or that the aptamer–TAR complex inhibits the structural rearrangements of the TAR RNA which have been demonstrated to take place upon Tat binding (Karn, 1999; Puglisi *et al.*, 1992). In any case this competition demonstrates the potential interest of aptamers targeted to an RNA structure for controlling gene expression.

A very clever way to generate nuclease resistant aptamers rests upon the use of enantiomeric ligands, taking advantage of the observation that enantiomers display identical binding properties. The process involves standard SELEX procedure, i.e., the use of natural D enantiomers of RNA or DNA sequences, against the mirror-image of the target. Consequently the mirror-image of the aptamer (i.e., L-RNA or L-DNA sequences) will bind to the natural target (Figure 6.3). This approach circumvents both the problems inherent to post-selection modifications and of the compatibility between chemically-modified synthons and polymerases (see below). The mirror-design of RNA and DNA aptamers has been successfully used against small ligands (L-arginine, D-adenosine) and against vasopressine (Klussmann *et al.*, 1996; Nolte *et al.*, 1996; Williams *et al.*, 1997). The aptamers identified displayed a rather low affinity ($K_d \approx 1\mu M$).

We used this strategy to identify L-DNA ligands of the TAR RNA motif. To this end a truncated TAR hairpin was chemically synthesized in the L-series. This L-TAR RNA likely folded as a stem-loop structure as shown by the cooperative transition of the melting curve (Santamaria *et al.*, unpublished) similar to the one displayed by the natural D-TAR hairpin. We first validated the assumption that enantiomers display similar properties: indeed, the L enantiomer of a DNA aptamer (D04) targeted to TAR recognized the L-TAR RNA. The stability of the L-TAR-L-D04 and D-TAR-D-D04 complexes were identical (Figure 6.3). We then carried out a SELEX experiment against L-TAR with a DNA library containing candidates with a 50 nucleotide randomized sequence: the candidates bound to biotinylated L-TAR were affinity-captured by magnetic streptavidin beads. In spite of a systematic counter-selection step with beads in the absence of TAR, a number of streptavidin aptamers were selected but no sequence able to recognize L-TAR with a K_d lower than 100 μM was detected. Actually, every sequence identified through *in vitro* selection against RNA structures engaged a few Watson–Crick base pairs (Boiziau *et al.*, 1999; Duconge and Toulmé, 1999; Scarabino *et al.*, 1999). It has been demonstrated that L-oligomers bind with a very weak affinity to natural DNA or RNA sequences (Garbesi *et al.*, 1993). Therefore, one might think that there is no way to generate high affinity nucleic acid ligands out of Watson–Crick complementarity. Nevertheless, it would be worth exploring longer sequences able to generate more complex shapes which might be adapted to the recognition of L-RNA hairpins and to form complexes without Watson–Crick base-pairing.

The above example cannot be generalized; as stated at the beginning of this section, post-selection modifications weaken the affinity of the aptamers for their target. An example is provided by the RNA pseudo-knot which was selected against the HIV-1 reverse-transcriptase (Tuerk *et al.*, 1992). The fully-modified 2'-*O*-methyl oligoribonucleotide aptamer poorly bound the RT compared to the selected RNA sequence (Green *et al.*, 1995a). To evaluate which nucleotides and positions are critical for interacting with the RT, they performed a careful analysis involving chemical modifications and substitutions. In particular, they investigated the binding properties of a mixture of aptamers in which each position could be either 2'-*O*-methyl or 2'-hydroxyl. Following binding to RT; the selected oligomers were subjected to alkaline hydrolysis, a treatment which cleaves RNA but does not cleave 2'-*O*-substituted sequences. The electrophoretic analysis of hydrolysed products identified the two positions showing increased cleavage, corresponding to an enrichment for 2' hydroxyl groups, in other words, the two positions where 2'-*O*-methyl groups interfered with binding. This procedure comprehensively generated a nuclease-resistant aptamer in which 24 out of the 26

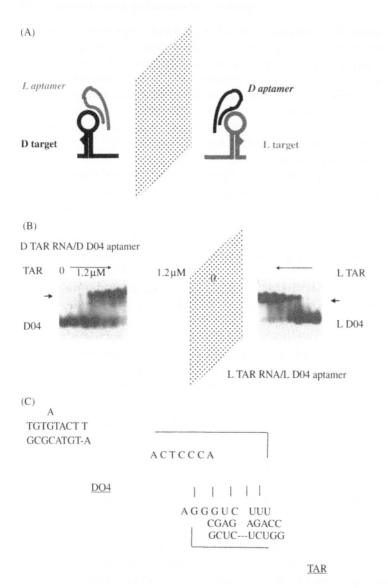

(A)

L aptamer

D target

D aptamer

L target

(B)

D TAR RNA/D D04 aptamer

TAR   0   1.2 µM   1.2 µM   0   ←   L TAR

D04   L D04

L TAR RNA/L D04 aptamer

(C)
              A
TGTGTACT T
GCGCATGT-A
                        ACTCCCA

    DO4

                        | | | | |
                    A G G G U C   U U U
                        CGAG   AGACC
                        GCUC---UCUGG

                                        TAR

Figure 6.3 (A) Schematic representation of the enantiomeric complex formed by a regular (D) aptamer with the mirror-image of a target (right) and vice versa by the mirror-image (L) of the selected aptamer with the natural target (left). (B) Electrophoretic mobility shift assay of a DNA aptamer (D04) targeted to a truncated form of the *trans*-activation responsive (TAR) RNA element of HIV-1 (TAR). *Left*: increasing amounts of the natural TAR (D-Tar) were added to the ^{32}P 5′ end-labeled natural aptamer D-D04 in a 10 mM Tris-HCl buffer, pH 7.5 containing 10 mM MgCl$_2$, 50 mM NaCl and 1 mM dithiotheitol. The samples were run on a 10% polyacrylamide gel at 4 °C. The arrow indicates the D-D04-D-TAR complex. *Right*: similar experiment performed with the L enantiomers of both the aptamer (L-D04) and the target RNA (L-TAR). (C) The structure of TAR and of D04 are shown. The complementarity between the apical loops of the two partners is indicated (Boiziau *et al.*, 1999; Collin *et al.*, 2000). (*see Color Plate 6*)

residues could be substituted by 2'-O-methyl-ribonucleotides, the two unmodified positions corresponding to essential ribonucleotides (Green *et al.*, 1995a).

Other strategies which have been previously suggested to extend the lifetime of antisense oligonucleotides can be used to stabilize aptamers. As the major serum nuclease is a 3' exonuclease, protection can be afforded by the 3' end capping. This can be achieved either by inverting the last 3' nucleotide, thus generating a 3'-3' linkage with the penultimate base, or by adding various 3' substituents. For instance, the lifetime of an anti-thrombin aptamer has been extended by a 3'-biotin-streptavidin substitution (Dougan *et al.*, 2000). The above examples demonstrate that post-SELEX modifications may lead to improved aptamers. But, generally, determining the positions within a selected sequence, which are amenable to modifications, is far from trivial.

Alternatively, chemically-modified aptamers can be obtained starting from a library containing modified oligonucleotide sequences. This means that modified nucleoside triphosphates (NTPs) introduced in the SELEX process should be incorporated efficiently and with a high fidelity by polymerases. Several hundreds of nucleotide derivatives have been synthesized in the frame of antisense investigations (Hélène and Toulmé, 1990), including promising high affinity analogues (Toulmé, 2001). However, a limited number can be incorporated enzymatically and only a few possibilities remain for selecting nuclease-resistant aptamers (Eaton, 1997). Oligomers showing an increased lifetime in nuclease-containing media are modified either on the backbone or on the nucleoside moiety. Phosphorothioate (Figure 6.4) NTPs can be readily incorporated into nucleic acids by polymerases (Ueda *et al.*, 1991). However, the efficiency of polymerization significantly diminishes with the number of modified triphosphates: the incorporation of phosphorothioate by the T7 RNA polymerase is reduced about three-fold when three phosphorothioate NTPs are used, compared to phosphodiester molecules (Ciafrè *et al.*, 1995). Conditions for polymerizing phosphorothioate NTPs have been optimized for enzymes used in the SELEX process to ensure both efficient incorporation and fidelity (Andréola *et al.*, 2000). To improve nuclease resistance of

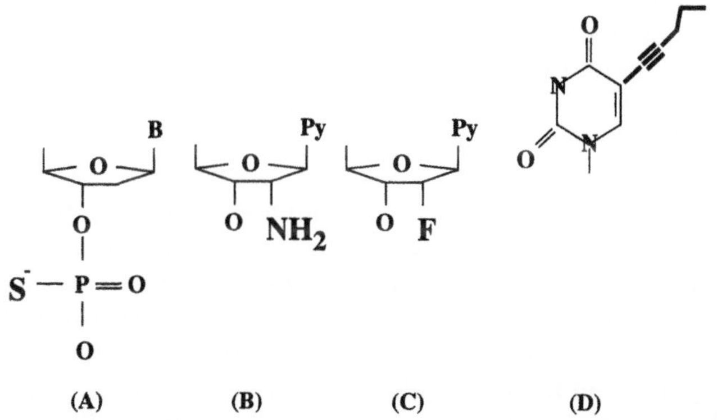

Figure 6.4 Aptamer building blocks incorporated by polymerases: (A) phosphorothioate, (B) 2'-aminodeoxyribopyrimidine, (C) 2'-fluoro-pyrimidine, (D) 5-1-pentynyl-2-deoxyuridine. The modifications are shown in bold.

the selected sequences and to minimize the decrease of incorporation, *in vitro* selection has been performed with three regular dNTPs and a phosphorothioated dA residue (King *et al.*, 1998). The authors identified aptamers that bind tightly ($K_d \approx 2$ nM) to the nuclear factor for IL-6, a transcription factor involved in the induction of acute phase responsive and cytokine gene promotors in response to inflammation. The A-phosphorothioated selected sequences showed a different consensus and displayed a slightly increased lifetime compared to the unmodified DNA aptamers. *In vitro* selection has also been carried out with a phosphor-othioated RNA pool against basic fibroblast growth factor (bFGF) (Jhaveri *et al.*, 1998). However, the binding specificity of this aptamer was questionable as phos-phorothioate antisense oligomers have been shown to bind to multiple non-nucleic acid targets (Stein and Cheng, 1993). Indeed, the anti-bFGF phosphorothioate aptamer did bind to several related proteins (but not to an unrelated one). Furthermore, about 30% of the sequences within the starting pool were retained in the presence of an eight-fold excess of bFGF, compared to 68% after the 11th selection round, indicating a limited improvement of the binding properties (Jhaveri *et al.*, 1998).

Until recently, the phosphorothioate linkage had been the only modified linkage compatible with SELEX enzymes. But certain modifications at the 2′ position, making RNA nuclease resistant, are accepted by polymerases. In par-ticular, 2′-amino- and 2′-fluoro-ribopyrimidines (Figure 6.4) are substrates for the enzymes used in *in vitro* selection (Aurup *et al.*, 1992). Several reports describe the identification of 2′-fluoropyrimidine (Biesecker *et al.*, 1999; Pagratis *et al.*, 1997; Ruckman *et al.*, 1998), 2′-amino-pyrimidine (Green *et al.*, 1995a; Jellinek *et al.*, 1995; Lee and Sullenger, 1997; Lin *et al.*, 1994) or even mixed 2′-fluoro, 2′-amino-pyrimidine RNA-based aptamers (Kubik *et al.*, 1997). The selection is carried out with a mixture of 2′ modified pyrimidine and of unmodified purine nucleoside triphosphates. The resulting sequences have been shown to display an increased lifetime compared to unmodified ones. RNA containing 2′-amino-U was shown to be 10^6-fold more resistant to RNAse A than the unmodified sequence (Pieken *et al.*, 1991). An aptamer containing 2′-amino-pyrimidines, targeted to the human neutrophil elastase, displayed a lifetime increased from eight minutes to nine hours in urine, compared to the homologous RNA sequence (Lin *et al.*, 1994). Similarly, an aptamer containing 2′-amino-pyrimidines to bFGF was shown to be 1000-fold more stable than the unmodified RNA in 90% human serum (Jellinek *et al.*, 1995). Not unexpectedly, the anti-bFGF 2′-modified sequences and the unmodified RNA aptamers selected previously (Jellinek *et al.*, 1993) were quite dissimilar. In particular, G was over-represented and C under-represented in the 2′-amino-pyrimidine selected sequences. Whether this rep-resentation is related to different efficiencies of nucleotide incorporation or whether it reflects a consequence of the low Tm values of 2′-amino-containing sequences is unknown. 2′-Fluoro-containing oligomers generate structures char-acterized by increased melting temperature compared to RNA (Cummins *et al.*, 1995; Kakiuchi *et al.*, 1982). Several studies allow the direct or indirect compar-ison of 2′-fluoro- and 2′-amino-pyrimidine containing aptamers. Frequently 2′-fluoro RNA display higher affinities than 2′-amino RNA ligands; this was indeed the case for vascular endothelial growth factor (Green *et al.*, 1995b; Ruckman *et al.*, 1998) and for the keratinocyte growth factor (Pagratis *et al.*, 1997). In this latter case the best 2'-fluoro aptamers, which adopted a very stable (Tm ≈ 78 °C) pseudo-knot structure, are characterized by a K_d of about 1 pM, i.e., an affinity 10^2–10^3 higher than the best 2'-amino ligands. The nuclease resistance of aptamers containing 2' modified pyrimidines can be further improved by post-SELEX modification at purine positions, introducing for instance 2'-O-methyl residues where these modifications are tolerated. This introduction generally results in highly modified aptamers which may eventually show improved binding affinity (Green *et al.*, 1995b; Ruckman *et al.*, 1998).

In addition to increasing the nuclease resistance, the substitution at the 2' position of the deoxy-ribose has another interesting property; it increases the molecular diversity of the pool by modifying the hydrogen-bonding capacity of the nucleoside and introducing different proportions of the sugar ring conformation. 2'-Fluoronucleosides show a higher content and 2'-aminonucleoside a lower content of the *3' endo* conformation than ribonucleosides. In addition, the pKa of the $2'NH_2$ group (6.2) suggests that at physiological pH a 2'-amino aptamer might correspond to both protonated and unprotonated forms (Guschlbauer and Jankowski, 1980; Lin *et al.*, 1994). Indeed, independent selections against interferon-γ carried out with 2'-fluoro-, 2'-amino-pyrimidines or a mixture of 2'-fluoroC and 2'-aminoU led to different motifs, indicating that the chemical composition of the library offers unique structural possibilities. The diversity can be further enriched as a number of groups can be tethered to different positions of the nucleic acid bases (Eaton *et al.*, 1997; Eaton and Pieken, 1995). Numerous pyrimidines modified at position five and purines modified at position eight are compatible with SELEX enzymes. For example, aptamers containing 5-(1-pentynyl)-2-deoxyuridine (Figure 6.3) have been isolated against human thrombin (Latham *et al.*, 1994); these ligands were strikingly different from the DNA aptamers selected previously (Bock *et al.*, 1992). In addition, several unnatural bases displaying particular hydrogen-bonding patterns have been shown to be readily incorporated by polymerases, thus expanding the repertoire of intra- and interstrand recognition (Guckian *et al.*, 1998; Piccirilli *et al.*, 1990; Schweitzer and Kool, 1995; Tor and Dervan, 1993) and consequently increasing the probability of finding new shapes.

Of particular interest are libraries in which a modified nucleotide that can be activated by light is incorporated in place of a standard ribo- or deoxyribonucleotide. 5-Halo-modified nucleosides are particularly well suited for this purpose. In particular, 5-bromo-2'-deoxyuridine (BrdU) has been widely used for mapping nucleic acid-protein contacts. Upon UV irradiation at about 310 nm, a wavelength at which nucleic acids and proteins absorb very weakly, BrdU specifically cross-links with aromatic amino acids and cysteine. As the photoreaction requires a close proximity between the excited BrdU residue and the cross-linkable amino acid, and a strict relative orientation of the two partners, the so-called photo-SELEX approach is expected to bring additional specificity to aptamer-target interactions. In such a strategy the modified oligonucleotide library is irradiated in the presence of the protein target. Cross-linked aptamers are partitioned from those which did not and the oligonucleotide protein photoadduct is digested by proteases prior to amplification. This step may require optimisation for efficient regeneration of the library due to the structure of the cross-links, even after efficient digestion. Photo-SELEX has been successfully used to identify aptamers to the Rev protein of HIV-1 (Jensen *et al.*, 1995) and to bFGF (Golden *et al.*, 2000).

Aptamers can also be modified for very different purposes. These purposes can include the derivation of the oligonucleotides with polyethylene glycol to enhance their pharmacokinetic properties (Floege *et al.*, 1999; Tucker *et al.*, 1999) or its conjugation to a group of interest. This may lead to a new functionality for the conjugated molecule. For instance, an efficient inhibitor of the human neutrophil elastase has been generated by conjugating a high affinity DNA aptamer (which was not inhibitory) to a tetrapeptide which was a weak competitive inhibitor of the enzyme (Lin *et al.*, 1995).

CONCLUDING REMARKS

In vitro selection generates RNA and DNA sequences that can bind to target molecules with extremely high affinity and specificity. Aptamers are considered as a promising class of compounds with a wide range of application in therapeutics (Famulok *et al.*, 2000; Toulmé, 2000; White *et al.*, 2000), diagnostics (Brody *et al.*, 1999; Jayasena, 1999) and imaging (Hicke and Stephens, 2000). Any kind of molecule, proteins, nucleic acids, can be targeted. These properties strongly suggest that aptamers can also be used to modulate gene expression, following either their expression into the cells by gene or viral therapies, when natural RNA sequences have been selected, or the administration of chemically-modified oligomers. Up to now only a limited number of studies demonstrate that this concept is actually valid. Furthermore, a few examples have shown that the properties of aptamers selected *in vitro* against Rev, Rex, B52, or RNA Pol II (Baskerville *et al.*, 1999; Shi *et al.*, 1999; Symensma *et al.*, 1996; Thomas *et al.*, 1997) are maintained in eukaryotic cells. These proteins are natural nucleic acid binding proteins. However, as aptamers have been successfully raised against proteins which are not known to bind nucleic acids, it should be possible to generate decoys for trapping any protein involved in a cascade of gene control; Blind *et al.* (1999) have developed an expression cassette from which the aptamer sequence flanked by two hairpins, for increasing the stability of the transcript, is produced. Using such a vector they generated in Jurkat and peripheral blood mononuclear cells an aptamer to the cytoplasmic domain of β2 integrin that prevented cell adhesion.

Another interesting development depends on the use of small molecules for inducible control of gene expression in living cells by aptamers (Werstuck and Green, 1998). The sequence corresponding to aptamers against antibiotics or dyes was introduced in front of a reporter gene into CHO cells. The addition of antibiotics or of the dye resulted in the specific inhibition of the reporter gene expression: the aptamer-dye complex was stable enough to prevent ribosome scanning of the 5' untranslated region of the reporter gene.

The above examples open the way to exciting new developments of aptamers in the field of artificial control of gene expression. Access to automated selection platforms (Cox *et al.*, 1998) should even speed up the identification of natural or modified aptamers of potential interest for biology and medicine.

ACKNOWLEDGMENTS

We are grateful to Marie-Line Andréola, Claudine Boiziau, Christian Cazenave, Fabien Darfeuille, Frédéric Pileur, Carmelo Di Primo and Dalila Sekkai for sharing unpublished results. The work performed in J.J. Toulmé's laboratory was supported by the 'Agence Nationale de Recherche sur le Sida' and the 'Conseil Régional d'Aquitaine.'

REFERENCES

Andréola, M.L., Calmels, C., Michel, J., Toulmé, J.J. and Litvak, S. (2000) Towards the selection of phosphorothioate aptamers Optimizing *in vitro* selection steps with phosphorothioate nucleotides. *Eur. J. Biochem.*, **267**, 5032–5040.

Andréola, M.L., Pileur, F., Calmels, C., Ventura, M., Tarrago-Litvak, L., Toulmé, J.J. and Litvak, S. (2001) DNA aptamers selected against the HIV-1RNase H display *in vitro* antiviral activity. *Biochemistry*, **40**, 10087–10094.

Anwar, A., Ali, N., Tanveer, R. and Siddiqui, A. (2000) Demonstration of functional requirement of polypyrimidine tract-binding protein by SELEX RNA during hepatitis C virus internal ribosome entry site-mediated translation initiation. *J. Biol. Chem.*, **275**, 34231–34235.

Aurup, H., Williams, D.M. and Eckstein, F. (1992) 2'-fluoro and 2'-amino-2'deoxynucleoside 5'-triphosphates as substrates for T7 RNA polymerase. *Biochemistry*, **31**, 9636–9641.

Bartel, D.P., Zapp, M.L., Green, M.R. and Szostak, J.W. (1991) HIV-1 Rev regulation involves recognition of non-Watson-Crick base pairs in viral RNA. *Cell*, **67**, 529–536.

Baskerville, S., Zapp, M. and Ellington, A.D. (1995) High-resolution mapping of the human T-Cell leukemia virus type 1 rex-binding element by *in vitro* selection. *J. Virol.*, **69**, 7559–7569.

Baskerville, S., Zapp, M. and Ellington, A.D. (1999) Anti-rex aptamers as mimics of the rex-binding element. *J. Virol.*, **73**, 4962–4971.

Belikova, A.M., Zarytova, V.F. and Grineva, N.I. (1967) Synthesis of ribonucleosides and diribonucleoside phosphates containing 2-chloroethylamine and nitrogen mustard residues. *Tetrahedron Lett.*, **37**, 3557–3562.

Biesecker, G., Dihel, L., Enney, K. and Bendele, R.A. (1999) Derivation of RNA aptamer inhibitors of human complement C5. *Immunopharmacology*, **42**, 219–230.

Blackwell, T.K., Kretzner, L., Blackwood, E.M., Eisenman, R.N. and Weintraub, H. (1990) Sequence-specific DNA binding by the c-Myc protein. *Science*, **250**, 1149–1151.

Blackwell, T.K. and Weintraub, H. (1990) Differences and similarities in DNA-binding preferences of MyoD and E2A protein complexes revealed by binding site selection. *Science*, **250**, 1104–1110.

Blind, M., Kolanus, W. and Famulok, M. (1999) Cytoplasmic RNA modulators of an inside-out signal-transduction cascade. *Proc. Natl. Acad. Sci. USA*, **96**, 3606–3610.

Bock, L.C., Griffin, L.C., Latham, J.A., Vermass, E.H. and Toole, J.J. (1992) Selection of single-stranded DNA molecules that bind and inhibit human thrombin. *Nature*, **355**, 564–566.

Boiziau, C., Dausse, E., Yurchenko, L. and Toulmé, J.J. (1999) DNA aptamers selected against the HIV-1 TAR RNA element form RNA/DNA kissing complexes. *J. Biol. Chem.*, **274**, 12730–12737.

Brody, E.N., Willis, M.C., Smith, J.D., Jayasena, S., Zichi, D. and Gold, L. (1999) The use of aptamers in large arrays for molecular diagnostics. *Mol. Diagn.*, **4**, 381–388.

Brody, E.N. and Gold, L. (2000) Aptamers as therapeutic and diagnostic agents. *Rev. Mol. Biotech.*, **74**, 5–13.

Brown, D. and Gold, L. (1995) Selection and characterization of RNAs replicated by Qβ replicase. *Biochemistry*, **34**, 14775–14782.

Burd, C.G. and Dreyfuss, G. (1994) Conserved structures and diversity of functions of RNA-binding proteins. *Science*, **265**, 615–621.

Burd, C.G. and Dreyfuss, G. (1994) RNA binding specificity of hnRNP A1: significance of hnRNP A1 high-affinity binding sites in pre-mRNA splicing. *EMBO J.*, **13**, 1197–1204.

Burke, L.H., Scates, L., Andrews, K. and Gold, L. (1996) Bent pseudoknots and novel RNA inhibitors of type 1 human immunodeficiency virus (HIV-1) reverse transcriptase. *J. Mol. Biol.*, **264**, 650–666.

Cech, T.R. and Bass, B.L. (1986) Biological catalysis by RNA. *Ann. Rev. Biochem.*, **55**, 599–629.

Chen, H. and Gold, L. (1994) Selection of high-affinity RNA ligands to reverse transcriptase: inhibition of cDNA synthesis and RNase H activity. *Biochemistry*, **33**, 8746–8756.

Chen, H., Mcbroom, D.G., Zhu, Y.Q., Gold, L. and North, T.W. (1996) Inhibitory RNA ligand to reverse transcriptase from feline immunodeficiency virus. *Biochemistry*, **35**, 6923–6930.

Churcher, M.J., Lamont, C., Hamy, F., Dingwall, C., Green, S.M., Lowe, A.D. *et al.* (1993) High affinity binding of TAR RNA by the human immunodeficiency virus type-1 Tat protein requires base-pairs in the RNA stem and amino acid residues flanking the basic region. *J. Mol. Biol.*, **230**, 90–110.

Ciafrè, S.A., Rinaldi, M., Gasparini, P., Seripa, D., Bisceglia, L., Zelante, L., Farace, M.G. and Fazio, V.M. (1995) Stability and functional effectiveness of phosphorothioate modified duplex DNA and synthetic 'mini-genes'. *Nucleic Acids Res.*, **23**, 4134–4142.

Clusel, C., Ugarte, E., Enjolras, N., Vasseur, M. and Blumenfeld, M. (1993) *Ex vivo* regulation of specific gene expression by nanomolar concentration of double-stranded dumbbell oligonucleotides. *Nucleic Acids Res.*, **21**, 3405–3411.

Cohen, J.S. (1989) Oligodeoxynucleotides: antisense inhibitors of gene expression. In: S. Neidle and W. Fuller (eds) *Topics in Molecular and Structural Biology*. The MacMillan Press, London, **12**, 255.

Collin, D., Heijenoort, C., Boiziau, C., Toulmé, J.J. and Guittet, E. (2000) NMR characterization of a kissing complex formed between the TAR RNA element of HIV-1 and a DNA aptamer. *Nucleic Acids Res.*, **28**, 3386–3391.

Colvin, R.A., White, S.W., Garcia-Blanco, M.A. and Hoffman, D.W. (1993) Structural features of an RNA containing the CUGGGA loop of the human immunodeficiency virus type 1 trans-activation response element. *Biochemistry*, **32**, 1105–1112.

Compagno, D., Lampe, J.N., Bourget, C., Kutyavin, I.V., Yurchenko, L., Lukhtanov, E.A. and Gorn, V.V. (1999) Antisense oligonucleotides containing modified bases inhibit translation of *Leishmania amazonensis* mRNAs by invading the mini-exon hairpin. *J. Biol. Chem.*, **274**, 8191–8198.

Convery, M.A., Rowsell, S., Stonehouse, N.J., Ellington, A.D., Hirao, I., Murray, J.B. *et al.* (1998) Crystal structure of an RNA aptamer protein complex at 2.8 angstrom resolution. *Nature Struct. Biol.*, **5**, 133–139.

Couvreur, P. and Malvy, C. (2000) *Pharmaceutical Aspects of Oligonucleotides*. Taylor & Francis, London, p. 321.

Cox, J.C., Rudolph, P. and Ellington, A.D. (1998) Automated RNA selection. *Biotechnol. Prog.*, **14**, 845–850.

Crooke, S.T. and Lebleu, B. (1993) *Antisense Research and Applications*. CRC, Boca Raton, p. 579.

Crouch, R.J. and Toulmé, J.J. (1998) *Ribonucleases H*. Les Editions INSERM, Paris, p. 265.

Cui, Y., Wang, Q., Stormo, G.D. and Calvo, J.M. (1995) A consensus sequence for binding of Lrp to DNA. *J. Bacteriol.*, **177**, 4872–4880.

Cummins, L.L., Owens, S.R., Risen, L.M., Lesnik, E.A., Freier, S.M., McGee, D., Guinosso, C.J. and Cook, P.D. (1995) Characterization of fully 2'-modified oligoribonucleotide hetero- and homoduplex hybridization and nuclease sensitivity. *Nucleic Acids Res.*, **23**, 2019–2024.

Dang, C. and Jayasena, S.D. (1996) Oligonucleotide inhibitors of Taq DNA polymerase facilitate detection of low copy number targets by PCR. *J. Mol. Biol.*, **264**, 268–278.

Darfeuille, F., Cazenave, C., Gryaznov, S., Ducongé, F., Di Primo, C. and Toulmé, J.-J. (2001) RNA and N3′-P5′ kissing aptamers targeted to the *trans*-activation responsive (TAR) RNA of the Human Immunodeficiency Virus-1. *Nucleosides, Nucleotides and Nucleic Acids*, **20**, 441–449.

Dougan, H., Lyster, D.M., Vo, C.V., Stafford, A., Weitz, J.I. and Hobbs, J.B. (2000) Extending the lifetime of anticoagulant oligodeoxynucleotide aptamers in blood. *Nucl. Med. Biol.*, **27**, 289–297.

Ducongé, F. and Toulmé, J.J. (1999) *In vitro* selection identifies key determinants for loop-loop interactions: RNA aptamers selective for the TAR RNA element of HIV-1. *RNA*, **5**, 1605–1614.

Ducongé, F., Di Primo, C. and Toulmé, J.J. (2000) Is a closing 'GA pair' a rule for stable loop–loop RNA complexes? *J. Biol. Chem.*, **275**, 21287–21294.

Eaton, B.E. and Pieken, W.A. (1995) Ribonucleosides and RNA. *Annu. Rev. Biochem.*, **64**, 837–863.

Eaton, B.E. (1997) The joys of *in vitro* selection: chemically dressing oligonucleotides to satiate protein targets. *Curr. Opin. Chem. Biol.*, **1**, 10–16.

Eaton, B.E., Gold, L., Hicke, B.J., Janjic, N., Jucker, F.M., Sebesta, D.P. *et al.* (1997) Post-SELEX combinatorial optimization of aptamers. *Bioorg. Med. Chem.*, **5**, 1087–1096.

Ecker, D.J., Vickers, T.A., Bruice, T.W., Freier, S.M., Jenison, R.D., Manoharan, M. *et al.* (1992) Pseudo-half-knot formation with RNA. *Science*, **257**, 958–961.

Ecker, D.J. (1993) Strategies for invasion of RNA secondary structures. In: B. Lebleu and S.T. Crooke (eds) *Antisense Research and Applications*. CRC, Boca Raton, pp. 387–399.

Eckstein, F. and Lilley, D.M. (1997) *Catalytic RNA*. Springer, Berlin, p. 417.

Elbashir, S.M., Harborth, J., Lendeckel, W., Yalcin, A., Weber, K. and Tuschl, T. (2001) Duplexes of 21-nucleotide RNAs mediate RNA interference in cultured mammalian cells. *Nature*, **411**, 494–498.

Ellington, A.D. and Szostak, J.W. (1990) *In vitro* selection of RNA molecules that bind specific ligands. *Nature*, **346**, 818–822.

Ellington, A.D. (1994) Aptamers achieve the desired recognition. *Current Biol.*, **4**, 427–429.

Ellington, A.D. and Conrad, R. (1995) Aptamers as potential nucleic acid pharmaceuticals. *Biotechnol. Annl. Rev.*, **1**, 185–215.

Famulok, M. and Jenne, A. (1998) Oligonucleotide libraries-variatio delectat. *Curr. Opin. Chem. Biol.*, **2**, 320–327.

Famulok, M. and Mayer, G. (1999) Aptamers as tools in molecular biology and immunology. *Curr. Top. Microbiol. Immunol.*, **243**, 123–136.

Famulok, M., Mayer, G. and Blind, M. (2000) Nucleic acid aptamers-from selection *in vitro* to applications *in vivo*. *Acc. Chem. Res.*, **33**, 591–599.

Floege, J., Ostendorf, T., Janssen, U., Burg, M., Radeke, H.H., Vargeese, C. *et al.* (1999) Novel approach to specific growth factor inhibition *in vivo* – Antagonism of platelet-derived growth factor in glomerulonephritis by aptamers. *Am. J. Pathol.*, **154**, 169–179.

Freier, S. (1993) Hybridization: considerations affecting antisense drugs. In: B. Lebleu and S.T. Crooke (eds.) *Antisense Research and Applications*. CRC, Boca Raton, pp. 67–82.

Garbesi, A., Capobianco, M.L., Colonna, F.P., Tondelli, L., Arcamone, F., Manzini, G. *et al.* (1993) L-DNAs as potential antimessenger oligonucleotides – A reassessment. *Nucleic Acids Res.*, **21**, 4159–4165.

Giovannangeli, C. and Hélène, C. (2000) Triplex-forming molecules for modulation of DNA information processing. *Curr. Opin. Mol. Ther.*, **2**, 288–296.

116   Jean-Jacques Toulmé et al.

Giver, L., Bartel, D., Zapp, M., Pawul, A., Green, M. and Ellington, A.D. (1993) Selective optimization of the Rev-Binding element of HIV-1. *Nucleic Acids Res.*, **21**, 5509–5516.

Gold, L., Polisky, B., Uhlenbeck, O. and Yarus, M. (1995) Diversity of oligonucleotide functions. *Ann. Rev. Biochem.*, **64**, 763–797.

Golden, M.C., Collins, B.D., Willis, M.C. and Koch, T.H. (2000) Diagnostic potential of photoSELEX-evolved ssDNA aptamers. *J. Biotechnol.*, **81**, 167–178.

Green, L., Waugh, S., Binkley, J.P., Hostomska, Z., Hostomsky, Z. and Tuerk, C. (1995a) Comprehensive chemical modification interference and nucleotide substitution analysis of an RNA pseudoknot inhibitor to HIV-1 reverse transcriptase. *J. Mol. Biol.*, **247**, 60–68.

Green, L.S., Jellinek, D., Bell, C., Beebe, L.A., Feistner, B.D., Gill, S.C. *et al.* (1995b) Nuclease resistant nucleic acid ligands to vascular permeability factor/vascular endothelial growth factor. *Chem. Biol.*, **2**, 683–695.

Guckian, K.M., Krugh, T.R. and Kool, E.T. (1998) Solution structure of a DNA duplex containing a replicable difluorotoluene-adenine pair. *Nat. Struct. Biol.*, **5**, 954–959.

Guschlbauer, W. and Jankowski, K. (1980) Nucleoside conformation is determined by the electronegativity of the sugar substituent. *Nucleic Acids Res.*, **8**, 1421–1433.

Hardenbol, P. and van Dyke, M.W. (1996) Sequence specificity of triplex DNA formation: analysis by a combinatorial approach, restriction endonuclease protection selection and amplification. *Proc. Natl. Acad. Sci. USA*, **93**, 2811–2816.

Hartmann, R., Norby, P.L., Martensen, P.M., Jorgensen, P., James, M.C., Jacobsen, C. *et al.* (1998) Activation of 2′-5′ oligoadenylate synthetase by single-stranded and double-stranded RNA aptamers. *J. Biol. Chem.*, **273**, 3236–3246.

Hélène, C. and Toulmé, J.J. (1990) Specific regulation of gene expression by antisense, sense and antigene nucleic acids. *Biochim. Biophys. Acta*, **1049**, 99–125.

Henderson, B.R., Menotti, E., Bonnard, C. and Kuhn, L.C. (1994) Optimal sequence and structure of iron-responsive elements. Selection of RNA stem-loops with high affinity for iron regulatory factor. *J. Biol. Chem.*, **269**, 17481–17489.

Hicke, B.J. and Stephens, A.W. (2000) Escort aptamers: a delivery service for diagnosis and therapy. *J. Clin. Invest.*, **106**, 923–928.

Hornung, V., Hofmann, H.P. and Sprinzl, M. (1998) *In vitro* selected RNA molecules that bind to elongation factor Tu. *Biochemistry*, **37**, 7260–7267.

Jaeger, J., Restle, T. and Steitz, T.A. (1998) The structure of HIV-1 reverse transcriptase complexed with an RNA pseudoknot inhibitor. *EMBO J.*, **17**, 4535–4542.

Jayasena, S.D. (1999) Aptamers: An emerging class of molecules that rival antibodies in diagnostics. *Clin. Chem.*, **45**, 1628–1650.

Jayasena, V.K., Brown, D., Shtatland, T. and Gold, L. (1996) *In vitro* selection of RNA specifically cleaved by bacteriophage T4 RegB endonuclease. *Biochemistry*, **35**, 2349–2356.

Jellinek, D., Green, L., Bell, C., Lynott, C.K., Gill, N., Vargeese, C. *et al.* (1995) Potent 2′-amino-deoxypyrimidine RNA inhibitors of basic fibroblast growth factor. *Biochemistry*, **34**, 11363–11372.

Jellinek, D., Lynott, C.K., Rifkin, D.B. and Janjic, N. (1993) High-affinity RNA ligands to basic fibroblast growth factor inhibit receptor binding. *Proc. Natl. Acad. Sci. USA*, **90**, 11227–11231.

Jensen, K.B., Atkison, M.C., Willis, M., Koch, T.H. and Gold, L. (1995) Using *in vitro* selection to direct the covalent attachment of human immunodeficiency virus type 1 Rev protein to high-affinity RNA ligands. *Proc. Natl. Acad. Sci. USA*, **92**, 12220–12224.

Jhaveri, S., Olwin, B. and Ellington, A.D. (1998) *In vitro* selection of phosphorothiolated aptamers. *Bioorg. Med. Chem. Lett.*, **8**, 2285–2290.

Jones, K.A. (1997) Taking a new TAK on tat transactivation. *Genes Develop.*, **11**, 2593–2599.

Kakiuchi, N., Marck, C., Rousseau, N., Leng, M., De Clerq, E. and Guschlbauer, W. (1982) Polynucleotide helix geometry and stability. Spectroscopic, antigenic and interferon-inducing properties of deoxyribose-, ribose-, or 2'-deoxy-2'-fluororibose-containing duplexes of poly(inosinic acid), poly(cytidylic acid). *J. Biol. Chem.*, **257**, 1924–1928.

Karn, J. (1999) Tackling Tat. *J. Mol. Biol.*, **293**, 235–254.

Kensch, O., Connolly, B.A., Steinhoff, H.J., McGregor, A., Goody, R.S. and Restle, T. (2000) HIV-1 reverse transcriptase-pseudoknot RNA aptamer interaction has a binding affinity in the low picomolar range coupled with high specificity. *J. Biol. Chem.*, **275**, 18271–18278.

King, D.J., Ventura, D.A., Brasier, A.R. and Gorenstein, D.G. (1998) Novel combinatorial selection of phosphorothioate oligonucleotide aptamers. *Biochemistry*, **37**, 16489–16493.

Klug, S.J., Huttenhofer, A. and Famulok, M. (1999) *In vitro* selection of RNA aptamers that bind special elongation factor Selβ, a protein with multiple RNA-binding sites, reveals one major interaction domain at the carboxyl terminus. *RNA*, **5**, 1180–1190.

Klussmann, S., Nolte, A., Bald, R., Erdmann, V.A. and Furste, J.P. (1996) Mirror-image RNA that binds D-adenosine. *Nat. Biotechnol.*, **14**, 1112–1115.

Konopka, K., Duzgunes, N., Rossi, J. and Lee, N.S. (1998) Receptor ligand-facilitated cationic liposome delivery of anti-HIV-1 Rev-binding aptamer and ribozyme DNAs. *J. Drug Target.*, **5**, 247–259.

Kubik, M.F., Bell, C., Fitzwater, T., Watson, S.R. and Tasset, D.M. (1997) Isolation and characterization of 2'-fluoro-, 2'-amino-, and 2'-fluoro-/amino-modified RNA ligands to human IFN-gamma that inhibit receptor binding. *J. Immunol.*, **159**, 259–267.

Kubik, M.F., Stephens, A.W., Schneider, D., Marlar, R.A. and Tasset, D. (1994) High-affinity RNA ligands to human α-thrombin. *Nucleic Acids Res.*, **22**, 2619–2626.

Latham, J.A., Johnson, R. and Toole, J.J. (1994) The application of a modified nucleotide in aptamer selection: novel thrombin aptamers containing 5-(1-pentynyl)-2'-deoyuridine. *Nucl. Acids Res.*, **22**, 2817–2822.

Le Tinévez, R., Mishra, R.K. and Toulmé, J.J. (1998) Selective inhibition of cell-free translation by oligonucleotides targeted to a mRNA structure. *Nucleic Acids Res.*, **26**, 2273–2278.

Lee, S. and Sullenger, B. (1997) Isolation of a nuclease resistant decoy RNA that can protect human acetylcholine receptors from myasthenic antibodies. *Nature*, **15**, 41–45.

Lin, Y., Padmapriya, A., Morden, K.M. and Jayasena, S.D. (1995) Peptide conjugation to an *in vitro*-selected DNA ligand improves enzyme inhibition. *Proc. Natl. Acad. Sci. USA*, **92**, 11044–11048.

Lin, Y., Qiu, Q., Gill, S.C. and Jayasena, S.D. (1994) Modified RNA sequence pools for *in vitro* selection. *Nucleic Acids Res.*, **22**, 5229–5234.

Lodmell, J.S., Ehresmann, C., Ehresmann, B. and Marquet, R. (2000) Convergence of natural and artificial evolution an RNA loop-loop interaction: The HIV-1 dimerization initiation site. *RNA*, **6**, 1267–1276.

Lodmell, J.S., Paillart, J.C., Mignot, D., Ehresmann, B., Ehresmann, C. and Marquet, R. (1998) Oligonucleotide-mediated inhibition of genomic RNA dimerization of HIV-1 strains MAL and LAI: A comparative analysis. *Antisense Nucleic Acid Drug Dev.*, **8**, 517–529.

Marozzi, A., Meneveri, R., Giacca, M., Gutierrez, M.I., Siccardi, A.G. and Ginelli, E. (1998) *In vitro* selection of HIV-1 TAR variants by the Tat protein. *J. Biotechnol.*, **61**, 117–128.

Méthot, N., Pickett, G., Keene, J.D. and Sonenberg, N. (1996) *In vitro* RNA selection identifies RNA ligands that specifically bind to eukaryotic translation initiation factor 4B: the role of the RNA recognition motif. *RNA*, **2**, 38–50.

Mishra, R.K., Le Tinévez, R. and Toulmé, J.J. (1996) Targeting nucleic acid secondary structures by antisense oligonucleotides designed through *in vitro* selection. *Proc. Natl. Acad. Sci. USA*, **93**, 10679–10684.

Mishra, R.K. and Toulmé, J.J. (1994) *In vitro* selection of antisense oligonucleotides targeted to a hairpin structure. *C. R. Acad. Sci. Paris*, **317**, 977–982.

Moine, H., Cachia, C., Westhof, E., Ehresmann, B. and Ehresmann, C. (1997) The RNA binding site of S8 ribosomal protein of *Escherichia coli*: SELEX and hydroxyl radical probing studies. *RNA*, **3**, 255–268.

Montgomery, M.K., Xu, S. and Fire, A. (1998) RNA as a target of double-stranded RNA-mediated genetic interference in *C. elegans*. *Proc. Natl. Acad. Sci. USA*, **95**, 15502–15507.

Muriaux, D., Foose, P. and Paoletti, J. (1996) A kissing complex together with a stable dimer is involved in the HIV-1$_{Lai}$ RNA dimerization process *in vitro*. *Biochemistry*, **35**, 5075–5082.

Nazarenko, I.A. and Uhlenbeck, O.C. (1995) Defining a smaller RNA substrate for elongation factor Tu. *Biochemistry*, **34**, 2545–2552.

Nolte, A., Klussmann, S., Bald, R., Erdmann, V.A. and Furste, J.P. (1996) Mirror-design of L-oligonucleotide ligands binding to L-arginine. *Nat. Biotechnol.*, **14**, 1116–1119.

Pagratis, N., Bell, C., Chang, Y., Jennings, S., Fitzwater, T., Jellinek, D. *et al.* (1997) Potent 2'-amino-, and 2'-fluoro-2'-deoxyribonucleotide RNA inhibitors of keratinocyte growth factor. *Nature Biotech.*, **15**, 68–73.

Paillart, J.C., Skripkin, E., Ehresmann, B., Ehresmann, C. and Marquet, R. (1996) A loop-loop 'kissing' complex is the essential part of the dimer linkage of genomic HIV-1 RNA. *Proc. Natl. Acad. Sci. USA*, **93**, 5572–5577.

Pei, D., Ulrich, H.D. and Schultz, P.G. (1991) A combinatorial approach toward DNA recognition. *Science*, **253**, 1408–1411.

Persson, C., Wagner, E.G.H. and Nordström, K. (1990) Control of replication of plasmid R1: structures and sequences of the antisense RNA, CopA, required for its binding to the target RNA, CopT. *EMBO J.*, **9**, 3761–3775.

Piccirilli, J.A., Krauch, T., Moroney, S.E. and Benner, S.A. (1990) Enzymatic incorporation of a new base pair into DNA and RNA extends the genetic alphabet. *Nature*, **343**, 33–37.

Pieken, W.A., Olsen, D.B., Benseler, F., Aurup, H. and Eckstein, F. (1991) Kinetic characterization of ribonuclease-resistant 2'-modified hammerhead ribozymes. *Science*, **253**, 314–317.

Pollock, R. and Treisman, R. (1990) A sensitive method for the determination of protein-DNA binding specificities. *Nucleic Acids Res.*, **18**, 6197–6204.

Predki, P.F., Nayak, L.M., Gottlieb, M.B. and Regan, L. (1995) Dissecting RNA-protein interactions: RNA-RNA recognition by Rop. *Cell*, **80**, 41–50.

Puglisi, J.D., Tan, R., Calnan, B.J., Frankel, A.D. and Williamson, J.R. (1992) Conformation of the Tar RNA-arginine complex by NMR spectroscopy. *Science*, **257**, 76–80.

Rhim, H. and Rice, A.P. (1997) RNAs selected *in vitro* by the HIV-2 Tat protein. *J. Biomed. Sci.*, **4**, 28–34.

Ringquist, S., Jones, T., Snyder, E.E., Gibson, T., Boni, I. and Gold, L. (1995) High-affinity RNA ligands to *Escherichia coli* ribosomes and ribosomal protein S1: comparison of natural and unnatural binding sites. *Biochemistry*, **34**, 3640–3648.

Ruckman, J., Green, L.S., Beeson, J., Waugh, S., Gillette, W.L., Henninger, D.D. *et al.* (1998) 2'-Fluoropyrimidine RNA-based aptamers to the 165-amino acid form of vascular endothelial growth factor (VEGF165). Inhibition of receptor binding and VEGF-induced vascular permeability through interactions requiring the exon 7-encoded domain. *J. Biol. Chem.*, **273**, 20556–20567.

Scarabino, D., Crisari, A., Lorenzini, S., Williams, K. and Tocchini-Valentini, G.P. (1999) tRNA prefers to kiss. *Embo J.*, **18**, 4571–4578.

Schneider, D., Gold, L. and Platt, T. (1993) Selective enrichment of RNA species for tight binding to *Escherichia coli* rho factor. *FASEB J.*, **7**, 201–207.

Schneider, D., Tuerk, C. and Gold, L. (1992) Selection of high affinity RNA ligands to the bacteriophage R17 coat protein. *J. Mol. Biol.*, **228**, 862–869.

Schneider, D.J., Feigon, J., Hostomsky, Z. and Gold, L. (1995) High-affinity ssDNA inhibitors of the reverse transcriptase of type 1 human immunodeficiency virus. *Biochemistry*, **34**, 9599–9610.

Schweitzer, B.A. and Kool, E.T. (1995) Hydrophobic, non-hydrogen-bonding bases and base pairs in DNA. *J. Am. Chem. Soc.*, **117**, 1863–1872.

Sczakiel, G. (2000) Theoretical and experimental approaches to design effective antisense oligonucleotides. *Front. Biosci.*, **5**, D194–D201.

Shi, H., Hoffman, B.E. and Lis, J.T. (1999) RNA aptamers as effective protein antagonists in a multicellular organism. *Proc. Natl. Acad. Sci. USA*, **96**, 10033–10038.

Shi, H., Hoffman, B.E. and Lis, J.T. (1997) A specific RNA hairpin loop structure binds the RNA recognition motifs of the *Drosophila* SR protein B52. *Mol. Cell Biol.*, **17**, 2649–2657.

Singh, R., Valcarcel, J. and Green, M.R. (1995) Distinct binding specificities and functions of higher eukaryotic polypyrimidine tract-binding proteins. *Science*, **268**, 1173–1176.

Sohail, M. and Southern, E.M. (2000) Selecting optimal antisense reagents. *Adv. Drug Deliv. Rev.*, **44**, 23–34.

Soukup, G.A., Ellington, A.D. and Maher, L.J. (1996) Selection of RNAs that bind to duplex DNA at neutral pH. *J. Mol. Biol.*, **259**, 216–228.

Stein, C.A. and Cheng, Y.C. (1993) Antisense oligonucleotides as therapeutic agents – is the bullet really magical. *Science*, **261**, 1004–1012.

Sullenger, B.A., Gallardo, H.F., Ungers, G.E. and Gilboa, E. (1991) Analysis of *trans*-acting response decoy RNA-mediated inhibition of human immunodeficiency virus type 1 transactivation. *J. Virol.*, **65**, 6811–6816.

Sumikura, K., Yano, K., Ikebukuro, K. and Karube, I. (1997) Thrombin-binding properties of thrombin aptamer derivatives. *Nucleic Acids Symp. Ser.*, 257–258.

Symensma, T.L., Giver, L., Zapp, M., Takle, G.B. and Ellington, A.D. (1996) RNA aptamer selected to bind human immunodeficiency virus type 1 are rev responsive *in vitro*. *J. Virol.*, **70**, 179–187.

Thomas, M., Chedin, S., Carles, C., Riva, M., Famulok, M. and Sentenac, A. (1997) Selective targeting and inhibition of yeast RNA polymerase II by RNA aptamers. *J. Biol. Chem.*, **272**, 27980–27986.

Thuong, N.T. and Hélène, C. (1993) Sequence specific recognition and modification of double-helical DNA by oligonucleotides. *Angew. Chem. Int. Ed. Engl.*, **32**, 666–690.

Tian, H. and Kole, R. (1995) Selection of novel exon recognition elements from a pool of random sequences. *Mol. Cell Biol.*, **15**, 6291–6298.

Tomizawa, J.I. (1986) Control of ColE1 plasmid replication: binding of RNA I to RNA II and inhibition of primer formation. *Cell*, **47**, 89–97.

Tor, Y. and Dervan, P.B. (1993) Site-specific enzymatic incorporation of an unnatural base, N6-(6-aminohexyl)isoguanosine, into RNA. *J. Amer. Chem. Soc.*, **115**, 4461–4467.

Toulmé, J.-J. (2000) Aptamers: selected oligonucleotides for therapy. *Curr. Opin. Mol. Ther.*, **2**, 318–324.

Toulmé, J.-J., Di Primo, C. and Moreau, S. (2001) Modulation of RNA function by oligo-nucleotides recognizing RNA structure. *Progr. Nucleic Acid Res. Mol. Biol.* (in press).

Toulmé, J.J. (2001) New candidates for true antisense. *Nat. Biotechnol.*, **19**, 17–18.

Toulmé, J.J. and Tidd, D. (1998) Role of ribonuclease H in antisense oligonucleotide-mediated effects. In: R.J. Crouch and J.J. Toulmé (eds) *Ribonucleases H*. Les Editions INSERM, Paris, pp. 225–250.

Tsai, D.E., Harper, D.S. and Keene, J.D. (1991) U1-snRNP-A protein selects a ten nucleo-side consensus sequence from a degenerate RNA pool presented in various structural contexts. *Nucleic Acids Res.*, **19**, 4931–4936.

Tucker, C.E., Chen, L.S., Judkins, M.B., Farmer, J.A., Gill, S.C. and Drolet, D.W. (1999) Detection and plasma pharmacokinetics of an anti-vascular endothelial growth factor oligonucleotide-aptamer (NX1838) in rhesus monkeys. *J. Chromatogr. B.*, **732**, 203–212.

Tuerk, C. and Gold, L. (1990) Systematic evolution of ligands by exponential enrichment: RNA ligands to bacteriophage T4 DNA polymerase. *Science*, **249**, 505–510.

Tuerk, C., Macdougal, S. and Gold, L. (1992) RNA pseudoknots that inhibit human immuno-deficiency virus type-1 reverse transcriptase. *Proc. Natl. Acad. Sci. USA*, **89**, 6988–6992.

Tuerk, C. and MacDougal-Waugh, S. (1993) *In vitro* evolution of functional nucleic acids: high-affinity RNA ligands of HIV-1 proteins. *Gene*, **137**, 33–39.

Ueda, T., Tohda, H., Chikazumi, N., Eckstein, F. and Watanabe, K. (1991) Phosphorothioate-containing RNAs show mRNA activity in the prokaryotic translation systems *in vitro*. *Nucleic Acids Res.*, **19**, 547–552.

Vasquez, K.M., Narayanan, L. and Glazer, P.M. (2000) Specific mutations induced by triplex-forming oligonucleotides in mice. *Science*, **290**, 530–533.

Weiss, B. (1997) *Antisense Oligodeoxynucleotides and Antisense Agents. Novel Pharmacological and Therapeutic Agents*. CRC Press, Boca Raton, p. 252.

Werstuck, G. and Green, M.R. (1998) Controlling gene expression in living cells through small molecule-RNA interactions. *Science*, **282**, 296–298.

White, R.R., Sullenger, B.A. and Rusconi, C.P. (2000) Developing aptamers into therapeutics. *J. Clin. Invest.*, **106**, 929–934.

Williams, K.P., Liu, X.-H., Schumacher, T.N.M., Lin, H.Y., Ausiello, D.A., Kim, P.S. *et al.* (1997) Bioactive and nuclease-resistant L-DNA ligand of vasopressin. *Proc. Natl. Acad. Sci. USA*, **94**, 11285–11290.

Witherell, G.W., Gott, J.M. and Uhlenbeck, O.C. (1991) Specific interaction between RNA phage coat proteins and RNA. *Prog. Nucleic Acid Res. Mol. Biol.*, **40**, 185–220.

Wyatt, J.R., Vickers, T.A., Roberson, J.L., Buckheit, R.W.J., Klimkait, T., DeBaets, E. *et al.* (1994) Combinatorially selected guanosine-quartet structure is a potent inhibitor of human immunodeficiency virus envelope-mediated cell fusion. *Proc. Natl. Acad. Sci. USA*, **91**, 1356–1360.

Yamamoto, R., Katahira, M., Nishikawa, S., Baba, T., Taira, K. and Kumar, P.K.R. (2000) A novel RNA motif that binds efficiently and specifically to the Tat protein of HIV and inhibits the *trans*-activation by Tat of transcription *in vitro* and *in vivo*. *Genes Cells*, **5**, 371–388.

Zamore, P.D., Tuschl, T., Sharp, P.A. and Bartel, D.P. (2000) RNAi: Double-stranded RNA directs the ATP-dependent cleavage of mRNA at 21 to 23 nucleotide intervals. *Cell*, **101**, 25–33.

7 Enzymes acting on DNA breaks and its relevance in nucleic acid-based therapy

Masahiko S. Satoh and Tetsu M.C. Yung

INTRODUCTION

In nucleic acid-based therapy, oligonucleic acids are used as a drug to treat genetic and acquired diseases. The stability or half-lives of such oligonucleic acids in cells are likely to be affected by cellular enzymes. One group of enzymes, which would interact with the therapeutic oligonucleic acids, are those involved in the process of DNA repair.

DNA repair is one of the fundamental processes essential for the survival of cells. In fact, disruption of DNA repair often leaves damaged DNA bases on DNA strands, leading to cytotoxicity or carcinogenesis, and consequently cancer. Repair of such damaged DNA bases often occurs through the induction of DNA breaks, and thus, most of the DNA repair enzymes act at DNA breaks. Therefore, it is of the utmost importance to unravel the mechanisms involved in DNA repair enzymes in the stability of oligonucleic acids, which often contain DNA break ends.

Clearly, designing biologically stable oligonucleic acids that would be resistant to these repair enzymes would improve the therapeutic effect of oligonucleic acids. This chapter focuses on the characteristics of these enzymes which act on DNA breaks.

DNA BREAKAGE AND REPAIR

Ionizing radiation can be a cause of DNA breaks (Hutchinson, 1985; Ward, 1998). However, DNA breaks are also induced through processes of DNA repair (Friedberg *et al.*, 1995). In mammalian cells, there are two major repair pathways: nucleotide excision repair (NER) and base excision repair (BER) (Friedberg *et al.*, 1995; Lindahl and Wood, 1999). However, DNA breaks produced during the two repair pathways are characteristically different.

NER pathway involves removing damaged bases from the genome of living cells as oligonucleotide fragments. NER repairs DNA damages which cause structural distortions in DNA. UV-induced pyrimidine dimers are one example of such a substrate repaired by NER. In NER, at least 15 polypeptides, including XPA protein (damage binding), XPF-ERCC1 complex (endonuclease), XPG (endonuclease), and TFIIH (bidirectional helicase), are involved. TFIIH contains nine subunits, including XPB protein (*3'* to *5'* helicase) and XPD protein (*5'* to *3'* helicase), and also plays a role in the initiation of transcription. During the process of NER, these repair enzymes form a complex at the damaged site, and then the damaged DNA strand is incised 23 bases upstream and six bases downstream from the damage, resulting in the removal of an oligonucleotide of about 29 bases in length. The 29-base gap is then filled by a DNA polymerase. However, such gaps are less accessible to other enzymes, since the gaps are likely protected by the NER repair complex (Satoh *et al.*, 1993).

Alkylating agents and ionizing radiation-induced DNA damages are repaired by BER (Friedberg *et al.*, 1995; Lindahl and Wood, 1999). However, contrary to NER, DNA breaks generated during BER are not protected. The steps of BER are illustrated in Figure 7.1. First a DNA glycosylase removes a modified base, resulting in the formation of a baseless site (Apurinic/Apyrimidinic site; AP site). The AP site is then incised by an AP endonuclease, which induces a DNA break on the $5'$ side of the AP site, leaving a hydroxyl group on the $3'$ end and a deoxyribose moiety on the $5'$ end. These nicks then become accessible to other repair enzymes. For example, $3'$-exonuclease digests DNA ends in the $3'$ to $5'$ direction while Flap endonuclease-1 (FEN-1) removes nucleotides in the $5'$ to $3'$ direction. At the same time, the gaps are filled in by DNA polymerases, and DNA strand interruptions are sealed by DNA ligases. DNA breaks generated during BER are also accessible to an abundant nuclear enzyme, poly(adenosine diphosphate ribose) polymerase-1 (PARP-1). PARP-1 binds to the breaks, and dissociates from them after the addition of multiple adenosine diphosphate (ADP) ribose moieties onto itself {poly(ADP-ribosyl)ation, automodification} (Althaus and Richter, 1987; Satoh and Lindahl, 1992). PARP-1 has been suggested to play a DNA damage sensing function (de Murcia and Ménissier-de Murcia, 1994). Synthetic oligonucleic acids designed for gene therapy will be exposed to repair enzymes, most likely those of BER.

ENZYMES MODIFYING DNA BREAKS

Although BER occurs in a coordinated manner, enzymes involved in BER are capable of acting on its substrate independently, as illustrated in Figure 7.2. When therapeutic oligonucleotides with internal single-strand breaks and/or double-strand ends encounter FEN-1, $3'$-exonuclease, DNA polymerases, and DNA ligases, the structure of the double-strand oligonucleic acid could be altered. PARP-1 is an enzyme, which acts on DNA breaks without modifying it. PARP-1 binds to both RNA stem-loops and DNA breaks. However, it is only activated by DNA breaks, which results in the induction of cellular damage responses.

Flap endonuclease-1 (FEN-1)

FEN-1 is a 43 kDa metallonuclease, which cleaves $5'$ single-strand DNA flap structures and possesses the capacity to digest DNA ends in the $5'$ to $3'$ direction (Harrington and Lieber, 1994). FEN-1 also cleaves RNA flaps and has a $5'$ to $3'$ exonuclease activity of double-stranded DNA or RNA annealed with DNA (Huang *et al.*, 1996).

The absence of FEN-1 activity causes lethality (Sommers *et al.*, 1995; Vallen and Cross, 1995). In *Saccharomyces cerevisiae*, a temperature sensitive mutant of a FEN-1

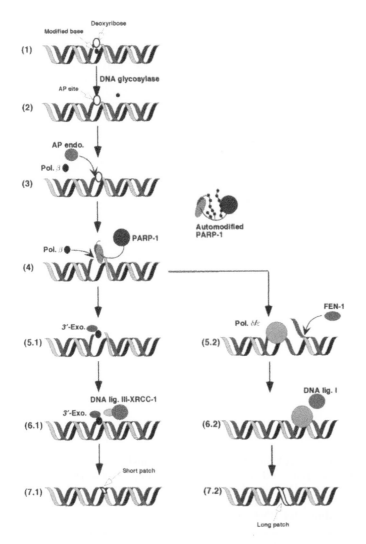

Figure 7.1 Outline for the process of gap filling. Modified DNA bases induced by alkylating agents or ionizing radiation (1) are removed by DNA glycosylase, resulting in the formation of an AP site (baseless site) (2). AP endonuclease (AP endo.) then cleaves the 5′ side of the AP site (3), producing a 3′ hyrdoxy and a 5′ deoxyribose termini. An abundant nuclear enzyme, poly(ADP-ribose) polymerase-1 (PARP-1), binds to the break and dissociates from it as a result of self-poly(ADP-ribosyl)ation (automodification) (4). This binding and dissociation may have a function in damage sensing. DNA polymerase β (Pol. β), which interacts with AP endo., is recruited to the break to initiate DNA polymerization (4)–(5.1). Since Pol. β lacks a proofreading function, 3′-exonuclease (3′-Exo.) may remove misincorporated deoxynucleotides while Pol. β fills in the gap. DNA ligase III(DNA lig. III)-XRCC-1 complex interacts with Pol. β, and seals the DNA nick (6.1). As a result, a one-base repair patch is formed (7.1). Alternatively, when Flap endonuclease-1 (FEN-1) acts on the 5′ termini of DNA breaks, the gap size is expanded (5.2). In this case, DNA polymerase δ or ε (Pol. δ/ε) fills the gap. The resulting DNA nick is then sealed by DNA ligase I (DNA lig. I) (6.2), resulting in the formation of a long repair patch (7.2).

DNA

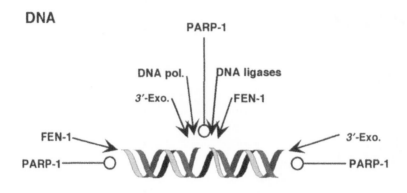

RNA

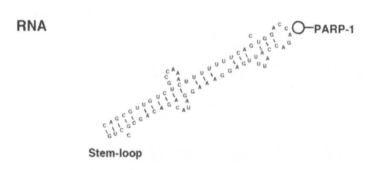

Figure 7.2 Enzymes acting on DNA breaks. FEN-1, *3'*-exonuclease (*3'*-Exo.), DNA polymerases (DNA pol.) and DNA ligases act on single-strand DNA breaks (SSB). Double-strand DNA breaks (DSB) are also susceptible to FEN-1 and *3'*-Exo. PARP-1 is capable of binding to SSB and DSB. In addition, PARP-1 has a binding affinity for RNA stem-loops.

homologue, RAD27/RTH1, enters S-phase arrest at impermissive temperatures. At permissive temperatures, the FEN-1 mutant shows retarded growth due to impaired DNA replication. In addition, the mutant is sensitive to alkylating agents and these observations suggest that FEN-1 is involved in DNA replication and DNA repair. In the case of DNA replication, FEN-1 is required to remove RNA primers in Okazaki fragments (Turchi *et al.*, 1994). In DNA repair, FEN-1 removes deoxy-ribose moieties attached to the 5' ends of DNA breaks (Figure 7.1) (Kim *et al.*, 1998; Klungland and Lindahl, 1997). The lack of such a cleavage activity results in hypersensitivity of cells to DNA damaging agents (Sommers *et al.*, 1995; Vallen and Cross, 1995).

FEN-1's endonuclease activity removes flap substrates by a unique mechanism. As illustrated in Figure 7.2, FEN-1 is first loaded onto the 5' end of flaps (Tom *et al.*, 2000; Wu *et al.*, 1996). It then slides down the flap strand and cleaves the flap at the point of annealing (Tom *et al.*, 2000; Wu *et al.*, 1996). Proliferating cell nuclear antigen (PCNA), a homotrimeric protein primarily found as a cofactor promoting the activity of DNA polymerase δ (Eissenberg *et al.*, 1997), can promote FEN-1's endonuclease activity five- to 50-fold (Eissenberg *et al.*, 1997; Wu *et al.*, 1996).

FEN-1 cleaves regardless of the size of the flap. Pseudo Y-shaped substrates are also cleaved by FEN-1, although the cleavage is less efficient than that for a flap substrate (Figure 7.3) (Harrington and Lieber, 1994). However, substrates with $3'$ tails or loops are not cleaved by FEN-1 due to the lack of FEN-1 loading. Also, certain modifications of $5'$ tails also cause inhibition of FEN-1 activity (Figure 7.3). For example, the attachment of a large complex, such as streptavidin-biotin, to the $5'$ end of flaps (Murante *et al.*, 1994), annealing of short oligonucleotides to the middle or the end of the flaps (Wu *et al.*, 1996), or $5'$ ends which are flipped back, all cause reduced FEN-1 activity (Henricksen *et al.*, 2000), possibly because these modifications prevent the loading of FEN-1 onto flaps. Certain types of DNA damage also cause inhibition of FEN-1 activity. Cisplatin, which is used as an anticancer drug, forms intra-strand cross-linking by targeting G residues. The presence of two cisplatin adducts in the flap strand, in fact, inhibits FEN-1 activity (Bornarth *et al.*, 1999).

In the case of $5'$ to $3'$ exonuclease activity, FEN-1 is capable of initiating digestion of DNA ends from DNA nicks, and the activity is not influenced by the presence or absence of phosphate groups (Wu *et al.*, 1996). In addition, double-strand DNA break ends are also targets of FEN-1 activity (Harrington and Lieber, 1994). Thus, FEN-1 may initiate cleavage of an engineered oligonucleotide if it contains either single-strand or double-strand DNA breaks.

$3'$-Exonuclease

$3'$-exonuclease is a 31 kDa protein that forms homodimers. This enzyme digests DNA ends in the $3'$ to $5'$ direction (Hoss *et al.*, 1999). Based on peptide sequence analysis, homology between this enzyme and human DNA polymerase ε has been found (Hoss *et al.*, 1999). During DNA synthesis, DNA polymerases incorporate incorrect bases with a certain probability (Lindahl and Wood, 1999), and most of DNA polymerases are capable of removing such mismatched nucleotides with its proofreading function, a $3'$ to $5'$ exonuclease activity. DNA polymerase β, however, does not have such a proofreading function (Beard and Wilson, 1998), and, thus, it has been suggested that the $3'$-exonuclease acts as a proofreading exonuclease of DNA polymerase β. In fact, Hoss *et al.* (1999) demonstrated that a mismatched G with A or a T mismatched with G on the $3'$ ends of DNA nicks are removed by $3'$-exonuclease.

In addition to its complementary proofreading role for DNA polymerase β, $3'$-exonuclease has the capacity to remove groups attached to $3'$ ends. Since ionizing radiation often produces phosphoglycolate at the $3'$ terminus (Hutchinson, 1985; Ward, 1998), it has been suggested that one of the functions of $3'$-exonuclease is the trimming of $3'$ ends. However, this enzyme is incapable of digesting ends with RNA (Hoss *et al.*, 1999). Thus, a therapeutic oligonucleotide with RNA ends would be resistant to cleavage by $3'$-exonuclease.

DNA polymerases and DNA ligases

In mammalian cells, at least eight DNA polymerases are present. DNA polymerase α is involved in the initiation of DNA synthesis at DNA replication origins and

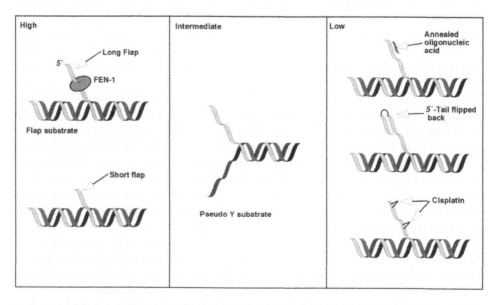

Figure 7.3 Cleavage of DNA flaps and other substrates by FEN-1. A Flap substrate, which is
a duplex DNA containing a floating 5′ single-strand DNA end, is a good substrate of FEN-1. FEN-1 is loaded onto the 5′ tail, tracks down to the points of
annealing, and cleaves such flaps at that point. FEN-1 cleaves at equal efficiencies
regardless of the length of the flap. However, pseudo Y-shaped substrates are
less efficiently cleaved by FEN-1. By annealing of short oligonucleic acids to the
flap by flipping back the tail, or by the attachment of two cisplatin adducts on the
flap, the cleavage activity of FEN-1 is inhibited.

lagging strand synthesis (Wang, 1991). DNA polymerase γ is a mitochondrial DNA
polymerase (Wang, 1991). Recently, bypass polymerases, such as DNA polymerase
η, ι, and ζ have also been identified (Lindahl and Wood, 1999). These DNA
polymerases are capable of continuing DNA synthesis even through bulky DNA
lesions – such as UV-induced pyrimidine-dimers in the template strand (Lindahl
and Wood, 1999).

   Among all the DNA polymerases, β, δ and ε are involved in BER (Lindahl and
Wood, 1999). DNA polymerase β is a 39 kDa monomeric protein (Wang, 1991).
During the process of BER, DNA polymerase β is recruited to DNA breaks by
interacting with AP endonuclease (Figure 7.1), hence DNA polymerase β likely has
more chance of accessing the gap than other DNA polymerases (Bennett *et al.*,
1997). Deoxyribose moieties, which remain at the 5′ ends, are removed by DNA
polymerase β's deoxyribose phosphodiesterase activity (Matsumoto and Kim,
1995), resulting in the formation of ligatable 5′ ends. In addition, DNA polymerase
β forms complex with X-ray cross complementing protein 1 (XRCC-1) (Caldecott
et al., 1994), which also interacts with DNA ligase III, a 100 kDa protein (Lindahl
and Wood, 1999). Thus, DNA gaps produced in BER can be filled in with a small
number of bases (short patch repair) by these enzymes (Figure 7.1).

   If chemical groups, e.g., phosphoglycolate, are attached to the 3′ ends, or if
hydroxyl groups or oxidized deoxyribose are attached to the 5′ ends, these DNA

ends need to be trimmed by $3'$-exonucleases and/or FEN-1, and DNA polymerse δ or ε fills in the gap with over three bases in length (long patch repair, see Figure 7.1) (Lindahl and Wood, 1999). The proliferating cell nuclear antigen (PCNA) acts as an accessory factor for both DNA polymerase δ and ε, and promotes their activity (Figure 7.1) (Eissenberg *et al.*, 1997). The C-terminal domain of PCNA interacts with FEN-1, while other binding domains of PCNA interact with DNA polymerase δ (Hosfield *et al.*, 1998). Thus, PCNA can form complexes with DNA polymerase δ and FEN-1. Furthermore, DNA ligase I, which is the major DNA ligase (Timson *et al.*, 2000), interacts with PCNA (Jonsson *et al.*, 1998). Thus, DNA polymerase δ-mediated long patch repair may be efficiently completed due to an interaction between DNA polymerase δ, DNA ligase I and FEN-1 scored by PCNA.

When therapeutic oligonucleic acids contain DNA breaks, these enzymes likely modify its structure, resulting in the expansion or sealing of DNA breaks or in synthesis of DNA from the breaks. Thus, these enzymes may act as factors affecting the stability of therapeutic oligonucleic acids in cells.

POLY(ADP-RIBOSE) POLYMERASE-1 (PARP-1)

FEN-1, $3'$-exonuclease, DNA polymerases, and DNA ligases directly modify DNA breaks. On the other hand, PARP-1 is an enzyme, which simply binds to DNA breaks and dissociates from them after automodification (Althaus and Richter, 1987; Satoh and Lindahl, 1992). Although functional roles for the binding have not yet been firmly established, PARP-1 has been attributed the role of sensing DNA breaks and regulating cellular damage responses, which ultimately results in either cell survival or cell death. Double-stranded DNA oligomers activate PARP-1 in nuclei (Grube *et al.*, 1991). This activation suggests that PARP-1 is activated by therapeutic oligonucleic acids if it contains DNA ends, and this causes induction of cellular damage responses.

Architecture of PARP-1

Relative to other housekeeping enzymes, PARP-1, a 113 kDa nuclear enzyme found in most eukaryotes (Althaus and Richter, 1987; de Murcia *et al.*, 1991; Lindahl *et al.*, 1995), is highly abundant (5×10^5 molecules/nucleus). As illustrated in Figure 7.4, the N-terminal DNA binding domain of PARP-1 contains two highly homologous zinc finger motifs, I and II (about 90% homologous in humans) (de Murcia *et al.*, 1991). The catalytic (or NAD^+-binding) domain, which is responsible for ADP-ribose polymer formation, is located at the C-terminus (de Murcia *et al.*, 1991). Linking the N-terminal and C-terminal domains of PARP-1 is an automodification site where ADP-ribose polymers are attached to PARP-1 itself (de Murcia *et al.*, 1991). The DNA binding domain of PARP-1 has a high affinity for single-strand or double-strand DNA breaks ($K_D = \sim 10^{-10}$ M) (D'Silva *et al.*, 1999). Upon binding to DNA breaks, PARP-1's catalytic domain is activated, resulting in the synthesis of ADP-ribose polymers from NAD^+ (Figure 7.4) (Althaus and Richter, 1987; de Murcia *et al.*, 1991; Lindahl *et al.*, 1995).

In vitro, various proteins/enzymes, including DNA polymerases, DNA ligases, topoisomerases, and transcription factors, are poly(ADP-ribosyl)ated (Cleaver and

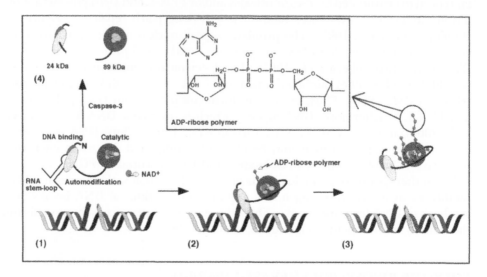

Figure 7.4 Activation of PARP-1 by DNA breaks. PARP-1 is composed of three domains, DNA binding, automodification and catalytic (NAD^+ binding) domains (1). In cells, PARP-1 localizes to nucleoli and actively transcribed regions of chromatin by interacting with RNA. When PARP-1 binds to DNA breaks, PARP-1 initiates the poly(ADP-ribosyl)ation reaction by using NAD^+ as its substrate (2). PARP-1 itself is the main target of the poly(ADP-ribosyl)ation reaction. ADP-ribose polymers are formed on the auto-modification domain of PARP-1 (automodification). As a consequence of automodification, PARP-1 dissociates from DNA breaks (3). When cells are committed to apoptosis, PARP-1 is specifically cleaved by an apoptosis-specific protease, caspase-3, resulting in the formation of a 24 kDa N-terminal and 89 kDa C-terminal fragments (4). (*see Color Plate 7*)

Morgan, 1991). As a consequence, the activities of these enzymes are suppressed, possibly due to the attachment of highly negative charges. However, *in vivo*, there is no clear evidence that these enzymes are actually modified, except for PARP-1's automodification site, which represents more than 90% of poly(ADP-ribosyl)ated substrates (Jump and Smulson, 1980). Histones and high mobility group proteins 1 and 2 (HMG-1 and 2) are also modified, which accounts for the remaining 10% (Aubin *et al.*, 1982). Modification of histones has been proposed to cause an altera-tion in chromatin structure by the neutralization of positive charges of histones by ADP-ribose polymers (Aubin *et al.*, 1982; Poirer *et al.*, 1982). In the case of HMG-1 and 2, functional roles of these proteins are not well known, although HMG-1 and 2 have been reported to regulate transcription initiation activity (Ge and Roeder, 1994; Zappavigna *et al.*, 1996). In gene therapy with liposomes, HMG-1 and 2 are used to promote the level of expression of cloned genes (Isaka *et al.*, 1998; Kaneda *et al.*, 1989), and poly(ADP-ribosyl)ation of HMG-1 and 2 may also affect this type of therapy.

When PARP-1 is poly(ADP-ribosyl)ated (automodified) (Figure 7.4), its DNA binding and poly(ADP-ribosyl)ation activities are suppressed, thereby driving the dissociation of PARP-1 from DNA breaks (Satoh and Lindahl, 1992). The DNA binding domain is also capable of binding to RNA (Vispé *et al.*, 2000; Yung and

Satoh, 2001), although binding to RNA does not catalyze poly(ADP-ribosyl)ation (Vispé *et al.*, 2000; Yung and Satoh, 2001). Between the DNA binding domain and the automodification site is a sequence (Asp-Glu-Val-Asp) recognized by caspase-3, an apoptotic protease (Lazebnik *et al.*, 1994). Activation of caspase-3 during the cell death pathway results in cleavage of PARP-1 and the generation of a 24 kDa N-terminal and 89 kDa C-terminal fragments (Figure 7.4) (Lazebnik *et al.*, 1994).

PARP-1 and DNA breaks

In cells, after one minute of exposure to damaging agents, ADP-ribose polymers are already generated by the binding of PARP-1 to DNA breaks (Affar *et al.*, 1999). After 15 to 60 minutes the amount of polymers reaches maximal levels. The level of polymers returns to basal levels by 90 minutes due to the activity of poly(ADP-ribose) glycohydrolase (Affar *et al.*, 1999). When such polymer formation is suppressed by an inhibitor of PARP-1, the cytotoxic effect of DNA damaging agents is potentiated (Althaus and Richter, 1987). As illustrated in Figure 7.1, PARP-1 binds to DNA breaks but later dissociates from them as a result of automodification, thereby giving DNA repair enzymes access to the break to repair the damage. On the other hand, inhibition of poly(ADP-ribosyl)ation causes persistence of PARP-1 to DNA breaks, and, thus, DNA repair enzymes are incapable of accessing the DNA breaks, resulting in inhibition of DNA repair and increased cytotoxicity (Satoh and Lindahl, 1992). Absence of PARP-1 also causes an abnormal response to DNA damaging agents (Trucco *et al.*, 1998). In this case, however, such abnormal responses may be related to a dysfunctional DNA damage sensing activity of PARP-1, rather than DNA repair (Vodenicharov *et al.*, 2000).

Association of PARP-1 to RNA stem-loops and regulation of transcription in response to DNA damage

In undamaged cells, PARP-1 is found at nucleoli and actively transcribed regions of chromatin (Fakan *et al.*, 1988). When isolated nuclei are treated with RNase, PARP-1 localized to nucleoli is dispersed (Kaufmann *et al.*, 1991). These observations suggest that PARP-1 binds to RNA in cells. The damage sensing function of PARP-1, therefore, should be related to the binding of PARP-1 to RNA.

We demonstrated that PARP-1, in fact, binds to RNA, particularly to RNA stem-loops (Figure 7.4) (Vispé *et al.*, 2000; Yung and Satoh, 2001). Such stem-loops are often found in various transcripts. For example, mRNA from the cystic fibrosis transmembrane conductance regulator gene forms stable stem-loops (Vispé *et al.*, 2000). Transcripts from the HIV-1 gene also form stable RNA stem-loops (Emerman and Malim, 1998). In both cases, these stem-loops are located close to the *5'* end of the mRNA. In general, stem-loops are found at the *3'* end of the mRNA as well, and it has been suggested that these stem-loops are involved in the stability of mRNA (Hentze and Kulozik, 1999). In fact, disruption of either stem-loops in mRNA from the β-globulin gene causes reduced half-lives (Hentze and Kulozik, 1999). Thus, PARP-1 may be involved in the stability of mRNA and rRNA in cells. Alternatively, we demonstrated that the binding of PARP-1 to such stem-loops reduced the rate of mRNA elongation (Vispé *et al.*, 2000). In this case, PARP-1 reduces the overall level of transcription. On the other hand, automodified

PARP-1 is incapable of binding to stem-loops (Vispé *et al.*, 2000). Thus, in damaged cells, transcription should be up-regulated after activation and automodification of PARP-1. Based on these observations, we proposed that the damage-sensing function of PARP-1 plays a role in cell survival by up-regulating transcription.

Cell death and PARP-1

Exposure of cells to DNA damaging agents causes cell death either by necrosis or apoptosis. In necrosis, rapid disruption of the cytoplasmic membrane induces the release of cellular macromolecules as well as some cytotoxic factors, leading to acute immune responses and tissue damage (Lemaire *et al.*, 1998). By contrast, during the apoptotic process, cellular macromolecules, including proteins and DNA, are digested, and the products of digestion are maintained within the cell. Most of these apoptotic cells are removed by phagocytes. PARP-1 is specifically cleaved by an apoptosis-specific protease, caspase-3 (Cryns and Yuan, 1998), resulting in the formation of a 24 kDa N-terminal fragment, containing the DNA binding domain, and an 89 kDa C-terminal fragment, which contains the catalytic domain (Figure 7.4) (Lazebnik *et al.*, 1994). Recently, we investigated the role of the 24 kDa apoptotic fragment of PARP-1 in DNA repair and transcription (Yung and Satoh, 2001). As a result, we found that the 24 kDa fragment has a dominant-negative effect on PARP-1 function, inhibiting DNA repair by persisting on DNA breaks, and also inhibiting the ability of PARP-1 to up-regulate transcription by persisting on RNA stem-loop structures. Thus, the dominant-negative effect of the 24 kDa fragment on PARP-1 function may be required to bias cells from survival to cell death.

CONCLUDING REMARKS

The basic idea for nucleic acid-based therapy is to use oligonucleic acids as a drug. Similar to P450, a drug-metabolizing enzyme, DNA repair enzymes would act as metabolizing enzymes for therapeutic oligonucleic acids. Thus, FEN-1, 3'-exonucleases, DNA polymerases, and DNA ligases would have an influence on the stability of therapeutic oligonucleotides in cells. To date, however, most of the research activities related to these enzymes have been focused on their function in DNA repair. Therefore, virtually no information related to the roles of these enzymes on therapeutic oligonucleic acids has been accumulated, while it is apparent that an understanding of the metabolic processes of therapeutic oligonucleic acids in cells would allow more powerful drug designs for nucleic acid-based therapy.

These enzymes may have an important relevance to DNA type drugs. For RNA type drugs, PARP-1 may have an additional relevance. Although it has been known since 1991 that PARP-1 localizes to nucleoli by binding to RNA (Kaufmann *et al.*, 1991), the functional relevance of PARP-1 binding to RNA has not been closely examined until recently (Vispé *et al.*, 2000; Yung and Satoh, 2001). The investigation of the roles of PARP-1 binding to RNA is still in progress. Considering the abundance of PARP-1 in cells, PARP-1 may play a critical role in maintaining the stability of RNA or in the regulation of transcription. Thus, PARP-1 functions may also influence the therapeutic effects of antisense RNA, RNA aptamers, or ribozymes, which are used in RNA repair.

As an example based on characteristics of the repair enzymes described in this chapter and PARP-1, we designed a modified version of a chimeric oligonucleotide, which is an RNA-DNA hybrid (Cole-Strauss *et al.*, 1996; Gamper *et al.*, 2000). These RNA–DNA hybrids are capable of correcting point mutations in target genes by the transfection of this nucleic acid into cells. For example, a mutation in the β-globulin gene is corrected by this hybrid (Cole-Strauss *et al.*, 1996). As illustrated in Figure 7.5, one strand of this RNA-DNA hybrid is composed from 2′-O-methyl-RNA

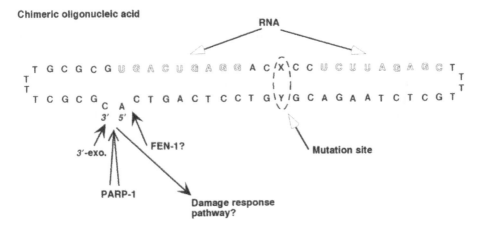

Figure 7.5 Example of a chimeric oligonucleic acid and its modification. Chimeric RNA–DNA hybrids are used for correction of point mutations in target genes. One strand of this oligonucleic acid is composed of O-methyl-RNA (outline) with an interruption of 5 bases of deoxyribonucleic acid. X and Y are target residues for correction. In the complementary strand, there is a DNA nick, and T residues loop both ends. 3′-exonuclease and FEN-1 may act on the nick. PARP-1 possibly binds to and is activated by the nick, resulting in activation of damage response pathways. In the modified version, the 3′ end is replaced by ribonucleic acids. The 5′ end is extended, and the flipped back RNA tail is added. Thus, the nick is expected to be resistant to 3′-exonuclease and FEN-1. In addition, PARP-1 may not be activated by such a nick.

with an interruption of five bases of deoxyribonucleic acid which contains the target residue for correction. In the complementary deoxyribonucleic acid strand, there is a DNA nick. DNA polymerases are apparently incapable of reading this chimeric oligonucleic acid since the complementary strand is RNA. On the other hand, if the 5' end is phosphorylated, DNA ligase may rejoin the nick. 3'-exonuclease is also likely to digest the DNA from the 3' end. FEN-1 may also remove the 5' end, although there is no information on whether FEN-1 can act on such a substrate. PARP-1 is likely activated by the nick. Thus, if several nucleotides from the 3' end are replaced by ribonucleic acid, it would be resistant to digestion by 3'-exonuclease. If the 5' end is extended by several bases and an RNA tail which is flipped back is added, FEN-1 would be incapable of cleaving the 5' end, and sealing of the DNA nick in the chimeric oligonucleic acid by DNA ligase would also be prevented. In addition, this RNA may inhibit activation of PARP-1.

Clearly, it would be necessary to test whether such a modified chimeric oligonucleic acid would be active *in vivo*. Furthermore, one might also envision a pro-drug that could be activated by repair enzymes after delivery into target cells. Finally, such oligonucleic acids could also be useful tools for the study of the mechanisms of DNA repair and damage responses in mammalian cells.

REFERENCES

Affar, E.B., Shah, R.G. and Poirier, G.G. (1999) Poly(ADP-ribose) turnover in quail myoblast cells: relation between the polymer level and its catabolism by glycohydrolase. *Mol. Cell. Biochem.*, **193**, 127–135.

Althaus, F.R. and Richter, C. (1987) *ADP-ribosylation of Proteins: Enzymology and Biological Significance*. Springer-Verlag, Berlin.

Aubin, R.J., Dam, V.T., Miclette, J., Brousseau, Y., Huletsky, A. and Poirier, G.G. (1982) Hyper(ADP-ribosyl)ation of histone H1. *Can. J. Biochem.*, **60**, 1085–1094.

Beard, W.A. and Wilson, S.H. (1998) Structural insights into DNA polymerase β fidelity: hold tight if you want it right. *Chem. Biol.*, **5**, R7–R13.

Bennett, R.A., Wilson, D.M., Wong, D. and Demple, B. (1997) Interaction of human apurinic endonuclease and DNA polymerase beta in the base excision repair pathway. *Proc. Natl. Acad. Sci. USA*, **94**, 7166–7169.

Bornarth, C.J., Ranalli, T.A., Henricksen, L.A., Wahl, A.F. and Bambara, R.A. (1999) Effect of flap modifications on human FEN1 cleavage. *Biochemistry*, **38**, 13347–13354.

Caldecott, K.W., McKeown, C.K., Tucker, J.D., Ljungquist, S. and Thompson, L.H. (1994) An interaction between the mammalian DNA repair protein XRCC1 and DNA ligase III. *Mol. Cell. Biol.*, **14**, 68–76.

Cleaver, J.E. and Morgan, W.F. (1991) Poly(ADP-ribose)polymerase: a perplexing participant in cellular responses to DNA breakage. *Mutat. Res.*, **257**, 1–18.

Cole-Strauss, A., Yoon, K., Xiang, Y., Byrne, B.C., Rice, M.C., Gryn, J. *et al.* (1996) Correction of the mutation responsible for sickle cell anemia by an RNA-DNA oligonucleotide. *Science*, **273**, 1386–1389.

Cryns, V. and Yuan, J. (1998) Proteases to die. *Genes Dev.*, **12**, 1551–1570.

D'Silva, I., Pelletier, J.D., Lagueux, J., D'Amours, D., Chaudhry, M.A., Weinfeld, M. *et al.* (1999) Relative affinities of poly(ADP-ribose) polymerase and DNA-dependent protein kinase for DNA strand interruptions. *Biochim. Biophys. Acta.*, **1430**, 119–126.

de Murcia, G., Ménissier-de Murcia, J. and Schreiber, V. (1991) Poly(ADP-ribose) polymerase: molecular biological aspects. *Bioessays*, **13**, 455–462.

de Murcia, G. and Ménissier-de Murcia, J. (1994) Poly (ADP-ribose) polymerase: a molecular nic-sensor. *Trends Biochem. Sci.*, **19**, 172–176.

Eissenberg, J.C., Ayyagari, R., Gomes, X.V. and Burgers, P.M. (1997) Mutations in yeast proliferating cell nuclear antigen define distinct sites for interaction with DNA polymerase δ and DNA polymerase ε. *Mol. Cell. Biol.*, **17**, 6367–6378.

Emerman, M. and Malim, M.H. (1998) HIV-1 regulatory/accessory genes: keys to unraveling viral and host cell biology. *Science*, **280**, 1880–1884.

Fakan, S., Leduc, Y., Lamarre, D., Brunet, G. and Poirier, G.G. (1988) Immunoelectron microscopical distribution of poly(ADP-ribose)polymerase in the mammalian cell nucleus. *Exp. Cell Res.*, **179**, 517–526.

Friedberg, E.C., Walker, G.C. and Siede, W. (1995). *DNA Repair and Mutagenesis.* ASM Press, Washington, D.C.

Gamper, Jr., H.B., Cole-Strauss, A., Metz, R., Parekh, H., Kumar, R. and Kmiec, E.B. (2000) A plausible mechanism for gene correction by chimeric oligonucleotides. *Biochemistry*, **39**, 5808–5816.

Ge, H. and Roeder, R.G. (1994) The high mobility group protein HMG1 can reversibly inhibit class II gene transcription by interaction with the TATA-binding protein. *J. Biol. Chem.*, **269**, 17136–17140.

Grube, K., Kupper, J.H. and Burkle, A. (1991) Direct stimulation of poly(ADP-ribose) polymerase in permeabilized cells by double-stranded DNA oligomers. *Anal. Biochem.*, **193**, 236–239.

Harrington, J.J. and Lieber, M.R. (1994) The characterization of a mammalian DNA structure-specific endonuclease. *EMBO J.*, **13**, 1235–1246.

Henricksen, L.A., Tom, S., Liu, Y. and Bambara, R.A. (2000) Inhibition of flap endonuclease 1 by flap secondary structure and relevance to repeat sequence expansion. *J. Biol. Chem.*, **275**, 16420–16427.

Hentze, M.W. and Kulozik, A.E. (1999) A perfect message: RNA surveillance and nonsense-mediated decay. *Cell*, **96**, 307–310.

Hosfield, D.J., Mol, C.D., Shen, B. and Tainer, J.A. (1998) Structure of the DNA repair and replication endonuclease and exonuclease FEN-1: coupling DNA and PCNA binding to FEN-1 activity. *Cell*, **95**, 135–146.

Hoss, M., Robins, P., Naven, T.J., Pappin, D.J., Sgouros, J. and Lindahl, T. (1999) A human DNA editing enzyme homologous to the Escherichia coli DnaQ/MutD protein. *EMBO J.*, **18**, 3868–3875.

Huang, L., Rumbaugh, J.A., Murante, R.S., Lin, R.J., Rust, L. and Bambara, R.A. (1996) Role of calf RTH-1 nuclease in removal of 5'-ribonucleotides during Okazaki fragment processing. *Biochemistry*, **35**, 9266–9277.

Hutchinson, F. (1985) Chemical changes induced in DNA by ionizing radiation. *Prog. Nucleic Acid Res.*, **32**, 115–154.

Isaka, Y., Akagi, Y., Kaneda, Y. and Imai, E. (1998) The HVJ liposome method. *Exp. Nephrol.*, **6**, 144–147.

Jonsson, Z.O., Hindges, R. and Hubscher, U. (1998) Regulation of DNA replication and repair proteins through interaction with the front side of proliferating cell nuclear antigen. *EMBO J.*, **17**, 2412–2425.

Jump, D.B. and Smulson, M. (1980) Purification and characterization of the major non-histone protein acceptor for poly(adenosine diphosphate ribose) in HeLa cell nuclei. *Biochemistry*, **19**, 1024–1030.

Kaneda, Y., Iwai, K. and Uchida, T. (1989) Introduction and expression of the human insulin gene in adult rat liver. *J. Biol. Chem.*, **264**, 12126–12129.

Kaufmann, S.H., Desnoyers, S., Ottaviano, Y., Davidson, N.E. and Poirier, G.G. (1991) Specific proteolytic cleavage of poly(ADP-ribose) polymerase: an early marker of chemotherapy-induced apoptosis. *Cancer Res.*, **53**, 3976–3985.

Kim, K., Biade, S. and Matsumoto, Y. (1998) Involvement of flap endonuclease 1 in base excision DNA repair. *J. Biol. Chem.*, **273**, 8842–8848.

Klungland, A. and Lindahl, T. (1997) Second pathway for completion of human DNA base excision-repair: reconstitution with purified proteins and requirement for DNase IV (FEN1). *EMBO J.*, **16**, 3341–3348.

Lazebnik, Y.A., Kaufmann, S.H., Desnoyers, S., Poirier, G.G. and Earnshaw, W.C. (1994) Cleavage of poly(ADP-ribose) polymerase by a proteinase with properties like ICE. *Nature*, **371**, 346–347.

Lemaire, C., Andreau, K., Souvannavong, V. and Adam, A. (1998) Inhibition of caspase activity induces a switch from apoptosis to necrosis. *FEBS Lett.*, **425**, 266–270.

Lindahl, T., Satoh, M.S., Poirier, G.G. and Klungland, A. (1995) Post-translational modification of poly(ADP-ribose) polymerase induced by DNA strand breaks. *Trends Biochem. Sci.*, **20**, 405–411.

Lindahl, T. and Wood, R.D. (1999) Quality control by DNA repair. *Science*, **286**, 1897–1905.

Matsumoto, Y. and Kim, K. (1995) Excision of deoxyribose phosphate residues by DNA polymerase beta during DNA repair. *Science*, **269**, 699–702.

Murante, R.S., Huang, L., Turchi, J.J. and Bambara, R.A. (1994) The calf $5'$- to $3'$-exonuclease is also an endonuclease with both activities dependent on primers annealed upstream of the point of cleavage. *J. Biol. Chem.*, **269**, 1191–1196.

Poirer, G.G., de Murcia, G., Jongstra-Bilen, J., Niedergang, C. and Mandel, P. (1982) Poly(ADP-ribosyl)ation of polynucleosomes causes relaxation of chromatin structure. *Proc. Natl. Acad. Sci. USA*, **79**, 3423–3427.

Satoh, M.S. and Lindahl, T. (1992) Role of poly(ADP-ribose) formation in DNA repair. *Nature*, **356**, 356–358.

Satoh, M.S., Poirier, G.G. and Lindahl, T. (1993) NAD$^+$-dependent repair of damaged DNA by human cell extracts. *J. Biol. Chem.*, **268**, 5480–5487.

Sommers, C.H., Miller, E.J., Dujon, B., Prakash, S. and Prakash, L. (1995) Conditional lethality of null mutations in RTH1 that encodes the yeast counterpart of a mammalian $5'$- to $3'$-exonuclease required for lagging strand DNA synthesis in reconstituted systems. *J. Biol. Chem.*, **270**, 4193–4196.

Timson, D.J., Singleton, M.R. and Wigley, D.B. (2000) DNA ligases in the repair and replication of DNA. *Mutat. Res.*, **460**, 301–318.

Tom, S., Henricksen, L.A. and Bambara, R.A. (2000) Mechanism whereby proliferating cell nuclear antigen stimulates flap endonuclease 1. *J. Biol. Chem.*, **275**, 10498–10505.

Trucco, C., Oliver, F.J., de Murcia, G. and Menissier-de Murcia, J. (1998) DNA repair defect in poly(ADP-ribose) polymerase-deficient cell lines. *Nucleic Acids Res.*, **26**, 2644–2649.

Turchi, J.J., Huang, L., Murante, R.S., Kim, Y. and Bambara, R.A. (1994) Enzymatic completion of mammalian lagging-strand DNA replication. *Proc. Natl. Acad. Sci. USA*, **91**, 9803–9807.

Vallen, E.A. and Cross, F.R. (1995) Mutations in *RAD27* define a potential link between G1 cyclins and DNA replication. *Mol. Cell. Biol*, **15**, 4291–4302.

Vispé, S., Yung, T.M.C., Ritchot, J., Serizawa, H. and Satoh, M.S. (2000) New cellular defense pathway regulating transcription through poly(ADP-ribosyl)ation in response to DNA damage. *Proc. Natl. Acad. Sci. USA*, **97**, 9886–9891.

Vodenicharov, M.D., Sallmann, F.R., Satoh, M.S. and Poirier, G.G. (2000) Base excision repair is efficient in cells lacking poly(ADP-ribose) polymerase 1. *Nucleic. Acids. Res.*, **28**, 3887–3896.

Wang, T.S. (1991) Eukaryotic DNA polymerases. *Annu. Rev. Biochem.*, **60**, 513–552.

Wang, Z.Q., Auer, B., Stingl, L., Berghammer, H., Haidacher, D., Schweiger, M. *et al.* (1995) Mice lacking ADPRT and poly(ADP-ribosyl)ation develop normally but are susceptible to skin disease. *Genes Dev.*, **9**, 509–520.

Ward, J. (1998) Nature of lesions formed by ionizing radiation. In: J. Nickoloff and M. Hoekstra (eds) *DNA Damage and Repair: DNA Repair in Higher Eukaryotes*. Humana Press, Totowa, New Jersey, pp. 65–84.

Wu, X., Li, J., Li, X., Hsieh, C.L., Burgers, P.M. and Lieber, M.R. (1996) Processing of branched DNA intermediates by a complex of human FEN-1 and PCNA. *Nucleic Acids Res.*, **24**, 2036–2043.

Yung, T.M.C. and Satoh, M.S. (2001). Functional competition between poly(ADP-ribose) polymerase and Its 24-kDa apoptotic fragment in DNA repair and transcription. *J. Biol. Chem.*, **276**, 11279–11286.

Zappavigna, V., Falciola, L., Citterich, M.H., Mavilio, F. and Bianchi, M.E. (1996) HMG1 interacts with HOX proteins and enhances their DNA binding and transcriptional activation. *EMBO J.*, **15**, 4981–4991.

8 Compaction and condensation of DNA

Kenichi Yoshikawa and Yuko Yoshikawa

INTRODUCTION

DNA molecules in viral capsids, bacterial nucleoids, and nuclei of eukalyotes occupy a volume 10^{-4}–10^{-6} times less than they do when free in aqueous solution (Livolant, 1991; Reich *et al.*, 1991; Bloomfield, 1996). Whereas living matter has elaborate apparatus for DNA packing, a similar drastic decrease in volume to a compact state can be observed *in vitro* simply by adding various kinds of chemical agents, such as polyamine, multivalent metal cation, hydrophilic polymer, cationic surfactant, or alcohol. Condensation of DNA has served as a simple model system for the packing of DNA in bacteriophage and the cellular environment (Lerman, 1971; Bloomfield, 1991, 1996; Marquet and Houssier, 1991). The transition of conformation from an elongated state into a compact state in DNA has attracted much interest from both physics and physical chemistry. It is of particular interest as an experimental system to examine the intrinsic properties of the coil-globule transition (de Gennes, 1979; Grosberg and Khokhlov, 1994). Extensive studies on such drastic change in the conformation of DNA, known as 'DNA condensation', have actively been carried out. For reviews of 'DNA condensation' and references to earlier works, the articles of Bloomfield (1991, 1996) are recommended. Unfortunately, most of the past studies have dealt with 'DNA condensation' without clearly distinguishing between the transition events occurring on single DNA molecules and those of aggregation and precipitation of multiple DNA molecules. This is due to the limitations of the experimental methodologies of 'DNA condensation', such as light scattering (static & dynamic), sedimentation, viscometry, linear dichroism, and circular dichroism. Although these methodologies afford us useful information on the ensemble of DNA molecules existing in solution, it is very difficult to evaluate the conformational change on each molecular chain.

While electron microscopy is a powerful tool for observing the morphology of compacted forms of DNA, it is unclear whether such morphological features accurately reflect that structure in solution due to the used methods to prepare samples for electron microscopy. Recently developed probe microscopies, such as atomic force microscopy (AFM) and scanning tunnelling microscopy (STM), also give the images only for DNA adsorbed on to a solid surface. Under these circumstances, Bloomfield (1996), the pioneering scientist on 'DNA condensation', has stated, 'Generally, the term "condensation" is reserved for situations in which the aggregate is of finite size and orderly morphology.'

In the literature, 'DNA condensation' was frequently interpreted as a highly cooperative phenomenon, in other words, the transition was regarded as steep but continuous. For example, Widom and Baldwin (1983) concluded, after careful measurement on the 'condensation' of λ-DNA with light scattering; that the transition was not a two-state reaction and the transition for monomolecular condensation was diffuse. A recent account on the conformation of polyelectrolyte by Barrat and Joanny (1996) also stated that the transition of single polyelectrolyte chains should be diffused. Bastolla and Grassberger (1997) reported the second order transition, i.e., continuous nature in the coil-globule transition, on single semistiff polymer chains, using a new Monte Carlo algorithm. Contrary to such interpretation of the diffuse nature in the transition of a single chain, or so called 'coil-globule transition', Post and Zimm (1982) suggested the possibility of an 'all-or-none' transition on the level of single DNA molecules, based on a theoretical consideration under the 'mean field approximation' by ignoring the effect of electronic charge and counter ions. In spite of their idea on the transition, most of the theoretical polymer physicists kept to the continuous coil-globule transition interpretation, except for an 'imaginary polymer chain' with infinite length (de Gennes, 1979; Grosberg and Khokhlov, 1994). This adherence may be partly due to the well-known theoretical problem that 'mean field approximation' does not include the effect of conformational fluctuation and, therefore, the discrete nature predicted under this theoretical framework is rather dangerous.

Owing to a series of studies on the conformational transition of individual DNA molecules based on the experimental techniques for single chain observation (Yanagida *et al.*, 1983; Bustamante, 1991), it has recently been established that the transition is an all-or-none type on the level of single giant DNA (Minagawa *et al.*, 1994; Mel'nikov *et al.*, 1995a,b; Yoshikawa *et al.*, 1996a). Theoretical analysis including the effect of the counter ions reproduces the essential features of the transition into a compact state on isolated chains (Vasilevskaya *et al.*, 1995; Yoshikawa *et al.*, 1996b).

In this chapter, we will focus on recently established knowledge of the folding transition of DNA molecules of size above the order of 10 kbp, as is schematically depicted in Figure 8.1. It is to be noted that a short DNA molecule of less than several hundreds bp cannot fold itself because the persistence length of DNA is around 50 nm, which corresponds to 160 bp. Short DNAs aggregate without the generation of the folding transition. To avoid confusion between the single chain event and multi-chain phenomenon, we will use the term 'folding transition' for the conformational transition on single DNA molecules. When interpreting multi-chain phenomena, we will use the terms assembling or aggregation, depending on the situation. Assembling and aggregation imply the formation of the condensed products from small and large number of DNA molecules, respectively.

SWITCHING ON THE CONFORMATION OF DNA

Figure 8.2a exemplifies the fluorescent images of pig DNA molecules of approximately 60 kbp, coexisting as elongated and folded compact states in Tris-HCl buffer solution containing 0.8 mM of spermidine^{3+}. The DNAs are stained with a fluorescence dye, 4',6-diamidino-2-phenylindole (DAPI), which forms a fluorescent

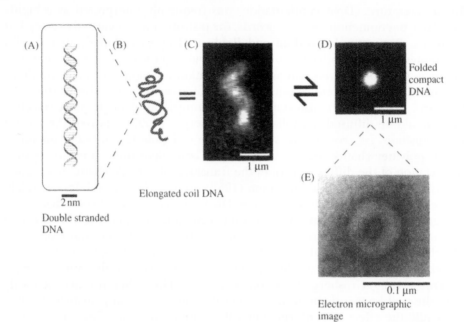

Figure 8.1 Conformational transition between elongated coil (C) and folded compact (D) states of a single duplex T4 DNA in the presence of spermidine[3+] as observed by fluorescence microscopy. Although double stranded DNA is rigid on a microscopic scale (A), long DNA behaves as an elongated coil as a whole (B). Due to a blurring effect the compact DNA (D) looks larger than its actual size. The corresponding electron micrograph of compact DNA is shown (E).

complex by attaching to the groove of the AT-rich regions in DNA. Figure 8.2b shows the dependence of the long-axis length L on the concentration of spermidine[3+]. Figure 8.2c shows the schematic representation of the manner of the folding transition, i.e., individual DNA molecules exhibit the 'all-or-none' transition. However, the transition in physicochemical characteristics on the ensemble average of DNAs should be continuous, both for monodisperse sample, such as T4 DNA (Yoshikawa *et al.*, 1996a), and polydisperse sample as shown in Figure 8.2.

The continuous nature of the transition for the ensemble of DNAs corresponds well to the description in the literature on 'DNA condensation' (Post and Zim, 1982; Bloomfield, 1991; Barrat and Joanny, 1996). Through extensive studies of the folding transition on individual DNA molecules, it has become clear that the discrete nature of the transition is rather general for giant DNAs above the size of 10 kbp. This generality is regardless of the chemicals used for the compaction, e.g., polyamines (Takahashi *et al.*, 1997), metal ions (Yoshikawa *et al.*, 1996b; Yamasaki and Yoshikawa, 1997), neutral flexible polymers (Vasilevskaya *et al.*, 1995), cationic surfactants (Mel'nikov *et al.*, 1995a,b, 1997a,b,c), nonionic surfactant (Mel'nikov *et al.*, 1997d), low polar solvent such as alcohol solution (Ueda and Yoshikawa, 1996; Kramarenko *et al.*, 1997; Mel'nikov *et al.*, 1999; Sergeyev, 1999; Vasilevskaya

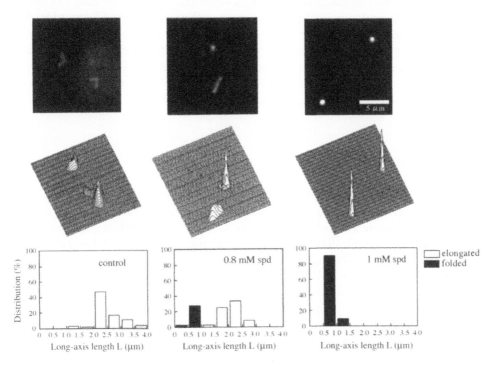

Figure 8.2 Fluorescence microscopic images at different concentrations of spermidine (spd), indicating elongated coil (left), coexistence of coil and compact DNAs (middle), and the folded compact state (right) in pig DNA (ca. 60 kbp). Corresponding quasi-three-dimensional representations of the light intensity distribution are also shown (middle column). Distribution of the long-axis length is given in the bottom column, where the open and closed bars indicate the elongated and compact DNAs, respectively.

et al., 2000), dendrimers (Kabanov *et al.*, 2000), and cationic peptides (Minagawa *et al.*, 1991).

This section will now briefly focus on the effect of fluorescent dyes on the conformation of DNA. From single DNA observation using fluorescence microscopy, it has been confirmed (Yoshikawa *et al.*, 1992; Matsuzawa and Yoshikawa, 1994) that minor groove binders, such as DAPI, decrease the persistence length of DNA but have no effect on the contour length. Conversely, intercalators such as ethidium bromide increase both contour length and the persistence length (Yoshikawa *et al.*, 1992; Matsuzawa and Yoshikawa, 1994; Atwell *et al.*, 1995). As for the folding transition, there is almost no apparent effect with DAPI. On the contrary, an intercalator exhibits a significant effect that prevents the folding transition. In accordance with such effects of intercalators, it was found that daunomycin, an antitumor antibiotic, induces unfolding of compacted single DNA molecules into a thick fibrous structure. (Yoshikawa *et al.*, 1996c).

In the study of DNA condensation by chromium (III) ions, it was reported that Cr(III) inhibits the interaction between ethidium bromide and DNA (Osterberg *et al.*, 1984). This phenomenon can be explained by considering the effect of the intercalator on the compaction of DNA. A different view on the effect of inter-calators on DNA condensation has been reported (Kapuscinski and Darzynkiewicz, 1984). Using light scattering techniques they observed that intercalating aromatic cations, such as the fluorochrome acridine orange or the antitumor drug Mito-xantrone, induced 'condensation' of nucleic acids, DNA and RNA. Further study to examine the actual effects of these intercalators would be necessary to discriminate between the phenomena of the folding of a single chain and the aggregation of multiple chains.

COMPACTION BY MULTI-VALENT CATIONS

Early studies reported that in aqueous solutions at room temperature a cation of valence +3 or greater induces 'DNA condensation', e.g., natural polyamines such as spermidine^{3+} (Gosule and Schellman, 1976; Marquet *et al.*, 1987; Baeza *et al.*, 1987, 1992; Conrad and Topal, 1989; Baeza *et al.*, 1992; Sikorav *et al.*, 1994; Fang and Hoh, 1998; Bottcher *et al.*, 1998), spermine^{4+} (Chattoraj *et al.*, 1978; Gosule and Schell-man, 1978; Raspaud *et al.*, 1998, 1999), metal cations such as cobalt hexamine $(Co(NH_3)_6^{3+})$ (Widom and Baldwin, 1980, 1989; Schwinefus and Bloomfield, 2000), polylysine (Laemmli, 1975), polyethyleneimine (Dunlap *et al.*, 1997; Godbey *et al.*, 1999), dendrimers (Chen *et al.*, 2000) and cationic polysaccharide, chitosan (Erbacher *et al.*, 1998). It was suggested that 'DNA condensation' is induced by multivalent cations where approximately 90% of its charge is neutralized, and that divalent cations have insufficient potency to attain the charge neutralization on such a level (Wilson and Bloomfield, 1979; Bloomfield, 1991, 1996; He *et al.*, 2000; Stevens, 2001).

According to the counter ion condensation theory (Oosawa, 1971; Manning, 1978, 1980, 1985; Dautzenberg *et al.*, 1994) 76% of the DNA phosphate charge is neutralized by territorially bound Na$^+$ ions, in typical aqueous NaCl solutions (less than 1 M). Thus, it was expected that additional neutralization up to 90% is the necessary condition to cause 'DNA condensation', and that, with divalent cations, the maximum value is about 88%, being insufficient for 'condensation'. As an exception to this theory, Mn^{2+} induced 'condensation' of super-coiled plasmid DNA was discussed as the facilitating effect in the supercoiled state (Ma and Bloomfield, 1994). 'Condensation of DNA' on a solid surface in the presence of divalent cations was also reported (Koltover *et al.*, 2000).

In relation to the degree of charge neutralization on 'DNA condensation' with multivalent cations, Manning theorized (Manning, 1980) that neither trivalent spermidine nor tetravalent spermine can, in solution, completely neutralize the phosphate charge on DNA. The theoretically predicted (Manning, 1978) charge neutralization by spermidine bound to saturation was 95%. It is to be noted that such an interpretation under the view of insufficient charge neutralization on DNA condensation (Manning, 1985) was based on the experimental observations for the characteristics of DNA molecule ensembles using methodologies such as light scattering. Theoretical efforts have been made to determine where and how sufficient 'attractive forces' exist to overcome the remaining 10% of the total negative charge in order to induce 'condensation'. It was suggested that electro-static contributions of the multivalent cations can lead to significant attractive forces between 'negatively charged DNA segments' through the effect of correlated counterion fluctuation or distribution (Ray and Manning, 1994; Odijk, 1994; Lyubartsev and Nordenskiold, 1995; Olvera de la Cruz *et al.*, 1995; Rouzina and Bloomfield, 1996; Gronbech-Jensen *et al.*, 1997; Ha and Liu, 1997; Schiessel and Pincus, 1998; Golestanian *et al.*, 1999). Recently Odijk (1998) proposed a different explanation for the dense packing of DNA, which considered the competition between curvature stress and electrostatic repulsive force. From a theoretical approach based on a mean-field approximation, Solis and de la Cruz (2000) studied the transition between fully stretched state and collapsed state in a poly-electrolyte chain. They concluded that practically all multivalent counterions added to the system are condensed into the polymer chain, even before the collapse. Their model seems not to correspond to the actual folding transition between coil and compact states in DNA.

Baumann *et al.* (2000) have performed direct measurements on the stretching force on single collapsed DNA molecules. They have concluded that the intra-molecular attraction is 0.083–0.33 kT/bp in collapsed state through the evaluation of stretching work from the strain-stress curve. Although the obtained result seems interesting, deeper consideration on the interpretation of the observation would be necessary because of the following effect inherent to the single chain measurement. As the stretching process is definitely nonadiabatic throughout the stretching measurement, the work, or apparent free energy difference, evaluated from the strain–stress relationship should be much larger than the real free energy differ-ence between the collapsed state and the stretched state, which is deduced from the Boltzmann distribution. Comparison between these two different free energy differences would shed light on the mechanism of unfolding transition.

Recent measurements on single chain observation have refined the intrinsic properties of the folding transition of DNA molecules induced by multivalent cations (cf. Figure 8.2 and Table 8.1), as follows (Yoshikawa and Yoshikawa, 1995; Yoshikawa *et al.*, 1996b; Takahashi *et al.*, 1997; Yamasaki and Yoshikawa, 1997; Murayama and Yoshikawa, 1999): (1) the folding transition of DNA induced by both bivalent and multivalent cations is largely discrete on the level of individual chains; (2) the compact DNA as the product of the folding transition is sparingly soluble, in other words, it behaves just as a kind of hydrophilic colloid; (3) the cation concentration necessary to induce DNA compaction decreases with an increase in the valence of the cation; the necessary concentrations change as 1,

Table 8.1 Effect of salt and temperature on the folding transition of DNA

	Multivalent cation	*Polymer*
Increase of salt concentration	Inhibition	Promotion
Increase of temperature	Promotion	Inhibition

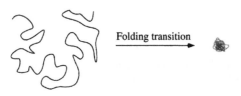

Folding transition

1/10 and 1/100, with the cations of +2, +3 and +4, respectively; (4) the width of the coexisting region between elongated coil and folded compact states is rather large for a bivalent cation and decreases with an increase in the valence of the cation; (5) the change of volume in the transition is larger for cations with a higher valence; (6) the necessary amount of multivalent cation to induce the folding transition increases with the increase of 1:1 salt concentration; In other words, salt has the effect to retard the folding transition, and; (7) at a fixed solution composition in the presence of the multivalent cation, the folding transition is promoted with an increase of temperature.

Theoretical considerations of the above mentioned properties indicate that ion-exchange between monovalent and multivalent cations plays an essential role in stabilising the compact state (Takahashi *et al.*, 1997; Murayama and Yoshikawa, 1999). The temperature effect as mentioned above in (7) indicates that the folded compact state exhibits higher entropy than the elongated coil state, which should be attributed to the ion exchange effect (Figure 8.3). It seems very difficult to explain the observed temperature dependence, i.e., folding at higher temperature, under the theoretical framework of 'correlated counterion fluctuation', because the net attraction should be mostly enthalpic with this theory. If the transition is enthalpic in its thermodynamics, the unfolding of the chain should be induced at a higher temperature. In addition, we have to note the salt effect that retards the folding transition, as mentioned above in (6). Under the theoretical framework of 'correlated counterion fluctuation', salt should have the effect of increasing the

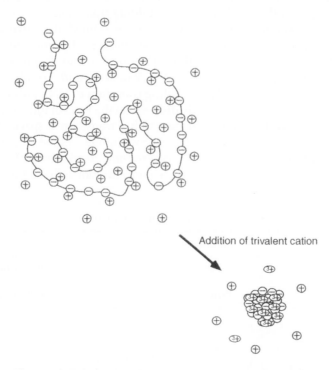

Figure 8.3 Switching of the DNA conformation by trivalent cations. The compact DNA behaves like a soluble colloidal particle.

stability of the compact dense state. This is clearly against the actual experimental trend. Thus, to make the correct interpretation, the effect of ion-exchange should be incorporated as the essentially important factor.

According to the recent study on 'DNA condensation' with titration calorimetry, it was indicated that condensations are entropically driven both by cobalt hexamine and spermidine (Matulis *et al.*, 2000). This result corresponds well to the temperature dependence on the bimodal distribution between coil and compact states obtained with single chain observation (Murayama and Yoshikawa, 1999).

Recently, the net charge of the DNA before and after the folding transition has been studied based on the methodology for single chain observation using fluorescence microscopy and with elecrophoretic measurement by light scattering (Yamasaki *et al.*, 2001). It has been confirmed that the negative charge completely disappears in the compact state except for its surface. This means that the effective attractive interaction can be easily explained by considering the net Coulombic interaction for the system with an equal number of negative and positive charges in the presence of multivalent cations. The origin of the 'attractive interaction' is similar to that in neutral ionic crystals. In other words, the complete charge neutralisation in compact DNA can explain the stability of the compact state, even without delicate consideration of the counterion fluctuation or correlation.

In a study to demonstrate the structure–activity relationship, Jary and Sikorav (1999) reported significant increase on the rate of cyclization reaction of λ-DNA before and after the collapsing transition with spermidine. It has also been found that the relative specificity among the accessible domains with restriction enzyme is largely modulated when accompanied by the folding transition with spermidine (Yoshikawa *et al.*, 1998). Studies to make clear the relationship between the biological activities and the higher order structure of DNA would be a promising research field.

COMPACTION BY POLYMER

Condensation of DNA induced by neutral polymer has been actively studied and is defined in terms of polymer-salt induced condensation, or ψ (psai)-condensation (Lerman, 1971; Ubbink and Odijk, 1995; Evdokimov *et al.*, 1976). Actually, in 1:1 salt solution, such as NaCl solution, DNA molecules are condensed by the addition of neutral hydrophilic polymers, such as polyethylene glycol (PEG) and polyvinylpyrrolidone. It was suggested that the collapse of the DNA coil was caused by the osmotic pressure of the surrounding polymer solution (Lifshitz *et al.*, 1978; Grosberg and Zhestkov, 1986). Some scientists discuss the 'DNA condensation' in terms of crowding effect (Zimmerman and Murphy, 1996). Here again, it is to be noted that the term 'condensation' has been used without clearly distinguishing between single chain and multi-chain phenomena.

Recent studies of single DNA observation have made clear the basic properties of the folding transition induced by PEG, and are summarized in the following (Minagawa *et al.*, 1994; Vasilevskaya *et al.*, 1995; Kidoaki and Yoshikawa, 1999; Mayama *et al.*, 2000): (1) the folding transition is characterized as 'all-or-none' type with a reduction of the effective volume of order $10^{-4} \sim 10^{-5}$; (2) the folded compact DNA in PEG solution is soluble and they do not stick to each

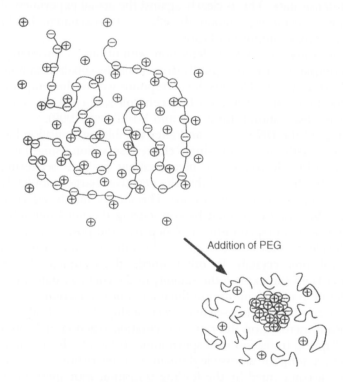

Figure 8.4 Switching of the DNA conformation into compact state with poly(ethylene glycol) (PEG).

other, at least near the critical concentration of PEG necessary to induce the transition, demonstrating the importance of extended volume; (3) PEG with a higher degree of polymerization is more effective for the compaction; (4) an increase in salt concentration promotes the folding transition; (5) increasing temperature tends to unfold compact DNA, and; (6) an increase in PEG concentration above the necessary concentration to induce the folding transition tends to make the compact DNAs assemble or aggregate with multiple DNA chains. With further increases in PEG concentration, the DNAs unfold into the elongated conformation.

It is noted that both the effects of salt and temperature are opposite to those of multivalent cations (Table 8.1). This opposition is explained by taking into account the effect on the enhanced uptake of counter ions accompanied by the folding transition (see Figure 8.4).

Single chain observations have been performed for the folding transitions induced by poly(2-vinylpyrrolidone) (Starodubtsev and Yoshikawa, 1996) and also by a negatively-charged polymer, poly-glutamic acid (Ichiba and Yoshikawa, 1998). In these cases, a phase-segregated state in a single chain is generated, instead of the appearance of the coexistence region between coiled and elongated molecules. In other words, the compact and elongated states coexist along a single DNA molecule, indicating that the correlation length on the phase transition is shorter with these polymers than with PEG (Yoshikawa, 1997).

COMPACTION BY CATIONIC LIPIDS AND SURFACTANTS

Cationic lipid/DNA complexes are known to be effective for gene delivery both *in vitro* and *in vivo*. Among the past reports on the lipid/DNA complexes, some studies have mentioned that the cationic lipid/DNA complexes have no regular morphology (Farhood *et al.*, 1994; Blessing *et al.*, 1998). With the measurement of atomic force microscopy, AFM, on DNAs complexed with neural phospholipid, elongated coiled structures have been reported (Malghani and Yang, 1998). An electron microscopic study indicated that compact DNA is covered with a lipid layer (Gershon *et al.*, 1993). However, a cryo-transmission electroscopic study shows that plasmids are trapped within multilamellar structures of lipids (Gustafsson *et al.*, 1995). Successive studies have confirmed the appearance of lamellar structure on DNA-cationic lipid complexes (Lasic *et al.*, 1997; Salditt *et al.*, 1997, 1998; Harries *et al.*, 1998; Koltover *et al.*, 1998, 1999; Golubovic and Golbovic, 1998; O'Hern and Lubensky, 1998; Artzner *et al.*, 1998). The structure of cationic lipid/DNA complexes seems to be different for different lipids. It is also to be mentioned that the ordered structures detected by x-ray scattering and electron microscopy on large aggregate or precipitate do not necessarily correspond to the structure of the complexes in physiological solutions. As for the interaction of the lipid complexes of DNA with the surface of cell membrane, the surface structure of the complexes should have the significant effect instead of the structure on the inner part of the complexes, even in the case where ordered lamellar structures are generated.

It is known that interactions between ionic surfactants and polyions with the opposite charge lead to the formation of soluble colloidal complexes. The polyelectrolyte chain binds to surfactant molecules through Coulombic attractions, and the hydrophobic moieties of the surfactant molecules stabilize the complexes due to hydrophobic interactions in the aqueous solution (Morris and Jennings, 1976; Satake and Yang, 1976; Osica *et al.*, 1977; Fendler, 1982; Hayakawa *et al.*, 1983; Jonsson *et al.*, 1998).

Single chain observation on the process of complex formation with cationic surfactants has been performed. The conformational change of DNA induced by cationic surfactants is summarized as follows (Mel'nikov *et al.*, 1995a,b, 1997a,b,c; Sergeyev *et al.*, 1999): (1) at levels well below the critical micelle concentration of lipid, the DNA molecule is folded into a compact state by interacting with the lipid; the folding transition is 'all-or-none' on individual DNAs; (2) the compact DNA with cationic surfactant is soluble, indicating the colloidal property of the complex; (3) the volume of the surfactant complex of DNA is about one order larger than the compact state of the same DNA induced by multivalent cations or PEG; this indicates that the DNA chain is folded not in a tightly packed manner but in a rather loosened way; (4) in general, there is a coexistence region between the elongated and compact states, and thus, the transition looks continuous or diffused on the ensemble of DNA molecules; however, when the lipid assembly undergoes structural change; such as a sphere–rod transition, all of the DNA molecules in solution exhibit 'all-or-none' change in a simultaneous manner or, in other words, the transition becomes discrete both on the levels of single chain and of the ensemble of chains, and; (5) the 'all-or-none' nature of the folding transition has also been encountered with the addition of a nonionic surfactant, such as Triton X-100 (Mel'nikov *et al.*, 1997d).

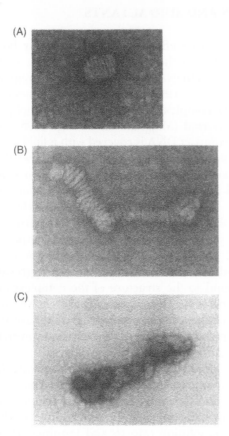

Figure 8.5 Transmission electron microgram on the dioactadodecylaminoglycylsper-
mine (DOGS) complex of pBR322 (A), λ (B) and T4 (C) DNAs, respectively.
The scale bar is 100 nm.

The complex of DNA with dioctadodecylaminoglycylspermine (DOGS) has been
studied by single chain observation with fluorescence microscopy, together with
electron spectroscopic observation (Yoshikawa *et al.*, 1996d). DOGS is a cationic
lipid capable of introducing DNA into various eukaryotic cells and facilitating
relatively high levels of gene expression (Behr *et al.*, 1989; Loeffler and Behr,
1993). On formation of a complex with DOGS, the DNA molecules were found
to be folded into a compact state. Under similar experimental conditions, electron
microscopic measurements were performed on the DOGS complexes of pBR322
(4 kbp), λ (48 kbp) and T4 (166 kbp) DNAs (Figure 8.5). These photographs
indicate that the DNA/DOGS complex is composed of an aggregate core of DOGS
wrapped in DNA strands, resulting in the formation of a spool or a nucleosome-
like structure. A similar spool structure was also reported by Labat-Moleur *et al.*
(1996). In the preceding section, it was mentioned that DNAs complexed with
cationic surfactants, such as cetyltrimethylammonium bromide (CTAB), are soluble colloidal particles. In contrast, it was found that DOGS/DNA complexes tend to
aggregate by forming a network structure. Interestingly, the conditions necessary

to form a network assembly of DOGS complexed with many DNAs correspond to those with the highest transfection efficiency (Yoshikawa *et al.*, 1996d; Promega Technical Bulletin, 1994). In relation to the formation of the assembly, a recent trial to control the size of the DNA–lipid complex through aerobic dimerization of cationic cysteine-detergent was conducted (Blessing *et al.*, 1998).

MORPHOLOGICAL VARIATION IN COMPACT DNA

Figure 8.6 shows the morphologies of DNA molecules compacted under different conditions, as observed by transmission electron microscopy. It has been reported that single long, double stranded DNA, as well as multiple copies of smaller DNAs of several kilo base pairs, can form a toroidal structure as the compact state

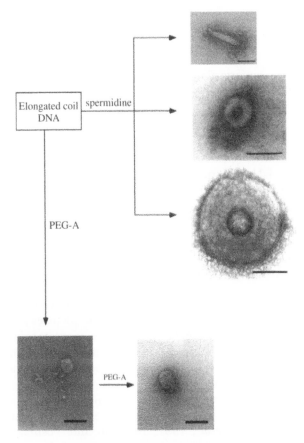

Figure 8.6 Morphological variation of DNA. Transmission electron micrographs of T4 DNA are shown, except for the rod structure where λ DNA is used. The scale bar is 100 nm. The giant toroid is formed under a high concentration of spermidine in the buffer solutions with rather high salt (Yoshikawa *et al.*, 1999). The segregated structure is generated by PEG-A (polyethylene glycol with pendent amino groups; Yoshikawa *et al.*, 1997b). Further explanation on the experimental conditions is available in the text.

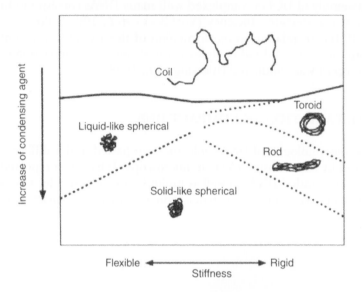

Figure 8.7 Phase diagram of the conformation of a polymer chain, deduced from
theoretical calculations (multicanonical Monte Carlo method; Noguchi
and Yoshikawa, 1998).

(Bloomfield, 1991; Vasilevskaya *et al.*, 1997). The mechanism for the formation of
a toroid has been explained as follows (Grosberg, 1979; Grosberg and Zhestkov,
1986). Due to the stiffness of the DNA chain, DNA usually does not favour tight
bending. To minimize the loss of energy associated with bending accompanied by
folding under poor solvent conditions, DNA wraps itself in a circle. As a result, a
hole is formed in the centre of the compact DNA. The packing of the DNA strands
into this toroidal form can be rather high. It has been reported (Marx and Ruben,
1983, 1986; Arscott *et al.*, 1990; Bloomfield, 1991) that a typical toroid is around
80 nm in outer diameter, almost independent of the length of the DNAs from
400 kbp to 40 kbp.

Figure 8.7 shows an electron micrograph of a toroid of typical size (80 nm in
diameter) and a larger one (200 nm in diameter), where both pictures have
been obtained from a single T4DNA molecule (166 kbp). The giant toroid is
formed under a high concentration of spermidine^{3+} in a buffer solution with a
high salt concentration (Yoshikawa *et al.*, 1999). From physicochemical considerations (Takahashi *et al.*, 1997), it is expected that an increase in sperimidine^{3+}
concentration far above the critical concentration for the folding transition
decreases the effective attraction between the segments in the DNA molecule.
It is theoretically expected (Vasilevskaya *et al.*, 1997; Noguchi and Yoshikawa,
1998, 2000) that the weaker attractive interactions make the size of the toroid
larger, which corresponds well with the experimental trend. It is of interest to
note that a small toroid with an outer diameter of 45 nm and a hole diameter of
10 nm has been successfully generated (Shen *et al.*, 2000) where the DNA is
modified to exhibit a greater curvature through the insertion of A-tracts on a
3 kbp plasmid.

It is also known that a rod structure is generated in compact DNA under some conditions. However, it was not clear whether the rod-like structure is a thermo-dynamically stable state or a kinetically trapped meta-stable state (Chattoraj *et al.*, 1978; Eickbush and Moudrianakis, 1978; Grosberg, 1979; Arscott *et al.*, 1990; Plum *et al.*, 1990; Perales *et al.*, 1994).

A phase diagram of the compact state of a polymer chain, including changes of the chain stiffness, can be seen in Figure 8.7 (Noguchi and Yoshikawa, 1998). From the diagram, together with additional theoretical considerations (Noguchi *et al.*, 1996; Noguchi and Yoshikawa, 1997, 2000), the following aspects can be deduced: (1) when a polymer is rigid enough, a folding transition is induced in a discrete manner, whereas the transition is continuous for a flexible polymer; (2) for a rigid polymer, a toroid or rod solid-like structure is generated in the compact state, depending on the degree of attraction between the segments and the stiffness; (3) for the flexible polymer, the compact state is spherical with liquid-like packing, corresponding to the current interpretation of the compact state in polymer text-books under the term globule, and; (4) when the attractive interaction becomes sufficiently large, spherical solid-like structures are generated, corresponding to the packing structure of chromatin.

The discrete transition for rigid polymers (Noguchi and Yoshikawa, 1997, 1998, 2000; Kuznetsov and Timoshenko, 1999; Liang and Chen, 2000; Ivanov *et al.*, 2000; Jennings *et al.*, 2000) implies that the process of compaction should be similar to crystallization from a supersaturated solution. With respect to the mechanism of crystal formation, it is well known that, in general, nucleation and growth follow a typical kinetic route, so long as the degree of supersaturation or nonequilibricity is small. However, with a large degree of supersaturation, a 'dirty' precipitate is generated through the kinetic route of spinodal decomposition (Chaikin and Lubensky, 1995). By adapting the kinetic process of nucleation and growth, genuine crystals with the regular packing of molecules are obtained. The process of nucleation and growth has been actually observed using single chain observation on long DNA when the concentration of condensing agents was not far from the coexistence region (Yoshikawa and Matsuzawa, 1995, 1996). Matsuzawa *et al.* (1996) found that the nucleation centre is located at the chin ends with rather high frequency, and that GC-rich parts have higher efficiency than AT-rich parts. It is noted that the GC-rich parts are stiffer than the AT-rich parts in double stranded DNA molecules.

Figure 8.8 shows a simulation of the folding process on a polymer chain, indicating the kinetics of nucleation and growth. If the solution conditions are in slight nonequilibricity, a regular toroid is actually obtained in experiments. On the contrary, a large nonequilibricity generates the irregular packing of segments (Kidoaki and Yoshikawa, 1996; Yoshikawa *et al.*, 1997a).

SINGLE CHAIN COMPACTION AND MULTI-CHAIN ASSEMBLING

As mentioned above, compact DNA molecules behave just like a soluble colloid, where the inner part of the compact structure is almost electronically neutralized and the surface is negatively charged. Such colloidal behavior is rather general

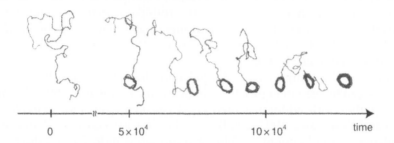

Figure 8.8 Nucleation and growth in a polymer chain (numerical simulation with Brownian dynamics; Sakaue *et al.*, unpublished). After staying for a long time in an elongated state, a nucleation centre appears spontaneously on a chain. Then, the densely packed region grows quickly to form a toroid. Essentially the same process has been observed in an experiment with single DNA observations (Yoshikawa and Matsuzawa, 1995, 1996).

regardless of the chemical nature of the condensing agents, such as multi-valent cations, hydrophilic polymer, and cationic surfactants. The soluble compact DNAs rarely associate with each other even through the occasional collision under thermal motion. With an increase of the concentration of condensing agents, the compact DNAs stick to each other. As a result, multi-chain assembly is induced in moderate concentrations of condensing agents. Recently, the assembling process of toroidal and rod-like DNA molecules has been visualized using atomic force microscopy (AFM) (Martin *et al.*, 2000). An understanding of the process of DNA condensation is essential for the optimization of gene delivery systems. When the concentration of DNA molecules becomes high enough in the presence of condensing agents, liquid crystalline phase appears. Systematic studies on the aggregation of DNAs and the formation of liquid-crystalline structure have been performed by several research groups (Livolant *et al.*, 1989; Livolant, 1991; Sikorav *et al.*, 1994; Pelta *et al.*, 1996a,b; Raspaud *et al.*, 1999).

From electron microscopic analysis of DNA complexed with transferrin-polycation conjugates, Wagner *et al.* (1991) suggested a strong correlation between the manner of 'DNA condensation' and the efficiency of cellular DNA uptake. Recently, direct observation of the conformation of individual DNAs in solution with highly sensitive fluorescence microscopy has shed light on the unique characteristics of the compact DNA complexed with poly-arginine (Emi *et al.*, 1997). It has been found that the compact DNAs, if not assembled, are not effective for gene transfection. The experimental conditions necessary to form an assembly of multiple chains are the most effective for transfection. With an excess of the condensing agents, large aggregates or precipitates are generated that are less effective for the transfection. A similar observation on the dependence of the gene expression on the size of DNA complex has been reported (Ogris *et al.*, 1998). The highest transfection efficiency of DOGS/DNA complexes also corresponds to the solution conditions required to form a multichain assembly (Yoshikawa *et al.*, 1996d). Further studies on the structure of lipid/DNA complexes, together with their charged state, are required to find the optimal conditions for gene transfection.

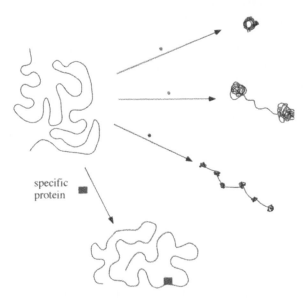

specific
protein

Figure 8.9 Nonspecific interaction induces switching on DNA conformation, whereas specific interaction causes only local perturbation on the conformation (As for the effect of PEG-A, see Figure 8.6).

GENERATION OF LARGE SCALE COOPERATION BY NON-SPECIFIC INTERACTION

Figure 8.9 shows a schematic representation of the changes in the higher order structure of long DNA molecules caused by various kinds of interacting chemicals. In specific binding, as in the case of restriction enzymes, there is almost no change in the conformation of DNA as a whole. On the contrary, with multivalent cations described above, individual DNA molecules undergo a discrete conformational transition accompanied by a change in the volume of the order of 10^4–10^5. Similar large discrete changes in DNA are encountered for the folding transitions induced by PEG, although the temperature and salt have opposite effects to multivalent cations on the transition.

When PEG attached to cationic moieties is added, intrachain segregation is generated where compact and elongated parts coexist along a single DNA molecule, as is exemplified in Figure 8.6 (Yoshikawa *et al.*, 1997b). For a long DNA molecule complexed with histone H1, the 'bead-on-a-string' conformation is generated (Yoshikawa *et al.*, 2001), where the binding interaction would be larger than with multivalent cations. In other words, a number of histone H1 molecules bind to the DNA in a highly cooperative manner by forming compact regions along the DNA chain. The mechanism of formation of the segregated structure and 'bead-on-a-string' conformation is understood with the following scenario.

'All-or-none' behavior, or switching, on the folding transition is a general characteristic in DNA and there exists a rather wide region of coexistence between unfolded coil and folded compact states (Figures 8.1–8.4). The coexistence of the markedly different states for the ensemble of DNA molecules corresponds to 'interchain segregation', i.e., the 'correlation length' is not less than the size of the individual molecular chain (Yoshikawa, 1997). This means that, even using the same solution conditions that induce 'all-or-none' transitions on a DNA molecule (as shown in Figure 8.2), the coexistence of folded and unfolded regions in a single chain would be caused in larger sized DNA molecules. Then, it would be expected that a intermolecular segregated state, i.e., the coexistence between unfolded coil and folded compact states on individual chains, would be induced under conditions of large correlation length, whereas intrachain segregated conformation would be generated when the correlation length was smaller than the size of the individual molecular chains (Iwataki *et al.*, 2000). The next problem would be to know which factor determines the correlation length. In general, the free energy of the conformation, or the higher order structure, of DNA is depicted as a double minima restricted by a barrier. When the free energy profile barrier is high enough, the correlation length is larger than the size of DNA molecule. In such a case, the 'all-or-none' characteristic on whole over a single chain is generated, i.e., there is interchain phase segregation. If the free energy barrier becomes lower, the correlation length becomes shorter. This shortening indicates the appearance of intrachain phase segregation. For both interchain and intrachain segregations, the ratio between the coil and compact states is determined by the Boltzman distribution on the double minimum free energy profile.

It is generally expected that the free energy barrier becomes lower when the negative charge of DNA is shielded. Actually, intrachain segregated conformation is observed for T4 DNA with the addition of alcohol (Ueda and Yoshikawa, 1996). As alcohol solution has lower polarity than water, the negative charge along the DNA chain should be markedly decreased. As for the compaction by multivalent cations, phase-segregated structure is observed in aqueous solutions with high salt concentrations (Takagi *et al.*, 2001; Yamasaki *et al.*, 2001). For the compaction by polymer, phase-segregated structure appears also with a high salt concentration (Vasilevskaya *et al.*, 1995). Roughly speaking, such experimental trends of salt effect on the conformation is explained by consideration of the shielding effect on the negative charge of DNA.

In relation to the intrachain segregated state, several theoretical studies have discussed the stability of necklace structure in polyelectrolytes (Kantor and Kardar, 1994, 1995; Dobrynin *et al.*, 1996; Solis and de la Cruz, 1998; Chodanowski and Stoll, 1999; Lee and Thirumalai, 2000; Micka and Kremer, 2000). Further studies are necessary to make clear the scenario on the conformational variation and stability in the segregated state. Single chain observation has shown that specific strong-binding to DNA induces only local perturbation in the conformation (Oana *et al.*, 1999). On the other hand, non-specific weak-binding induces large-scale changes in the DNA conformation, as in the case with multivalent cations and polymers. In relation, it may be of value to mention the observation that, in the solution containing polyamine, a change in the concentration of ATP induces switching of the conformation of DNA (Makita and Yoshikawa, 1999). A similar observation has been reported by changing the concentration of RNA (Tsumoto and Yoshikawa, 1999). These results suggest the importance of the intracellular environment on the self-regulation of genetic activity (Takagi and Yoshikawa, 1999).

CROSS-TALK BETWEEN FOLDING TRANSITION AND HELIX-COIL TRANSITION

It has been generally assumed that 'condensed DNA' is in the B-conformation (Jordan *et al.*, 1972; Bloomfield, 1996). Nonetheless, several studies (Reich *et al.*, 1991; Duguid *et al.*, 1993; Hud *et al.*, 1995) indicate that there are secondary structural changes accompanying the 'condensation' of DNA. Ma *et al.* (1995) reported that 'condensation' of pUC18 plasmids by the addition of hexamine cobalt is promoted by the insertion of a $(dC\text{-}dG)_n$ (n = 12 and 20) sequence and was accompanied with the conversion of the secondary structure from B form to Z form. The B-Z transition in plasmids pDHf2 and pDHf14 containing $(dA\text{-}dC)_n(dG\text{-}dT)_n$ (n = 23 and 60) sequence inserts in the presence of spermidine^{3+} and spermine^{4+} has also been reported (Thomas and Thomas, 1994).

A recent study has shown that two different kinds of conformational changes, helix-coil transition and the folding transition, mutually interfere with each other in a drastic manner (Mikhailenko *et al.*, 2000). As the melting of the double stranded structure, or helix-coil transition, is an essential process in the genetic activity, further studies on the biological role of the conformational change of DNA are awaited.

MANIPULATING INDIVIDUAL DNA

Figure 8.10 shows the results of optical manipulation of single T4 DNA complexed with histone H1 by using an infrared YAG laser (1064 nm), indicating the change of the conformation at different salt concentrations (Yoshikawa *et al.*, 2000). Here, it is noted that laser trapping is effective for the transportation and conformational regulation of a native DNA molecule without any modification of the molecule, such as avidin-biotin binding to a micrometer-sized plastic bead. Harmless laser manipulation has been shown to be applicable for compact DNA folded by multivalent cation, PEG, and cationic surfactants. The largest attractive potential exerted by the laser is for DNA compacted by a cationic surfactant compared to other condensing agents. In other words, it is rather easy to trap and transport DNA-cationic surfactant complexes by using the laser.

Recently, there has been a marked development in the methodologies to observe and manipulate single biopolymers (Mehta *et al.*, 1999; Arai *et al.*, 1999; Cui and Bustamante, 2000; Liphardt *et al.*, 2001). The key procedure in the successful manipulation of single biopolymers has been the tight attachment of the end of the polymer to a micrometer-sized object. To achieve a wider application of such single-molecular technology, it would be important to manipulate individual macromolecules and control their conformation without any structural modifications (Chiu and Zare, 1996; Brewer *et al.*, 1999). Thus, the manipulation of the compact DNAs without the attachment to a micrometer-sized bead or to any other macroscopic objects is expected to be useful for micrometer-scale laboratory experiments. This manipulation will also be a powerful tool for lab-on-a-chip or lab-on-a-plate (Katsura *et al.*, 1998; Yamasaki *et al.*, 1998; Matsuzawa *et al.*, 1999, 2000). It may of value to refer to a recent study in transporting a compact DNA into a cell-sized liposome (Nomura *et al.*, 2001).

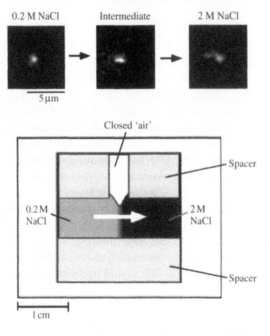

Figure 8.10. Transportation and conformational regulation with laser manipulation. T4 DNA complexed with H1 histone is transported from a high to low salt environment. The distance of the transportation is ca. 1 cm in a cell covered with a glass plate. It is noted that the concentration difference between the places separated by 1 cm is kept almost constant for more than 24 hours, due to the slow rate of the diffusion on the scale of 1 cm.

CONCLUDING REMARKS

Understanding the physical mechanisms of DNA condensation and compaction will be of great help to improve the stability of different nucleic acid delivery systems. Until quite recently, it had been regarded that DNA condensation was a highly cooperative phenomenon, i.e., the transition was steep but continuous. Owing to the development of single DNA observation, it has been confirmed that the transition from an elongated coil into a folded compact state is an 'all-or-none' switching on of its intrinsic nature. Such refinement on the mechanism of compaction is expected to be useful to design a DNA vehicle for gene therapy, and also to make clear the biological significance in the higher order structure of long DNA molecules.

REFERENCES

Arai, Y., Yasuda, R., Akashi, K., Harada, Y., Miyata, H., Kinoshita, Jr., K. and Itoh, H. (1999) Tying a molecular knot with optical tweezers. *Nature*, **399**, 446–448.

Arscott, P.G., Li, A.-Z. and Bloomfield, V.A. (1990) Condensation of DNA by trivalent cations. I. Effects of DNA length and topology on the size and shape of condensed particles. *Biopolymers*, **30**, 619–630.

Atwell, G.J., Denny, W.A., Clark, G., O'Connor, C.J., Matsuzawa, Y. and Yoshikawa, K. (1995) Mono-, bis- and tetra-acridine ligands: synthesis, x-ray structural determination and dynamic fluorescence microscopic studies on the modification of the higher-order structure of DNA. *J. Phys. Org. Chem.*, **8**, 597–604.

Atzner, F., Zantl, R., Rapp, G. and Radler, J.O. (1998) Observation of a rectangular columnar phase in condensed lamellar cationic lipid-DNA complexes. *Phys. Rev. Lett.*, **81**, 5015–5018.

Baeza, I., Gariglio, P., Rangel, L.M., Chavez, P., Cervantes, L., Arguello, C., Wong, C. and Montanez, C. (1987) Electron microscopy and biochemical properties of polyamine-compacted DNA. *Biochemistry*, **26**, 6387–6392.

Baeza, I., Ibanez, M., Wong, C., Chavez, P., Gariglio, P. and Pro, J. (1992) Possible prebiotic significance of polyamines in the condensation, protection, encapsulation, and biological properties of DNA. *Orig. Life*, **21**, 225–242.

Barrat, J.-L. and Joanny, J.-F. (1996) Theory of polyelectrolyte solutions. In: I. Prigogine and S.A. Rice (eds) *Advances in Chemical Physics, XCIV*. John Wiley & Sons, New York, NY, pp. 1–66.

Bastolla, U. and Grassberger, P. (1997) Phase transitions of single semistiff polymer chains. *J. Statist. Phys.*, **89**, 1061–1078.

Baumann, C.G., Bloomfield, V.A., Smith, S.B., Bustamante, C., Wang, M.D. and Block, S.M. (2000) Stretching of single collapsed DNA molecules. *Biophys. J.*, **78**, 1965–1978.

Behr, J.P., Demeneix, B., Loeffler, J.P. and Perez-Mutul, J. (1989) Efficient gene transfer into mammalian primary endocrine cells with lipopolyamine-coated DNA. *Proc. Natl. Acad. Sci. USA*, **86**, 6982–6986.

Blessing, T., Remy, J.-S. and Behr, J.-P. (1998) Monomolecular collapse of plasmid DNA into stable virus-like particles. *Proc. Natl. Acd. Sci. USA*, **95**, 1427–1431.

Bloomfield, V.A. (1991) Condensation of DNA by multivalent cations: consideration on mechanism. *Biopolymers*, **31**, 1471–1481.

Bloomfield, V.A. (1996) DNA Condensation. *Curr. Opin. Struct. Biol.*, **6**, 334–341.

Bottcher, C., Endisch, C., Fuhrhop, J.-H., Catterall, C. and Eaton, M. (1998) High-yield preparation of oligomeric C-type DNA toroids and their characterization by cryoelectron microscopy. *J. Am. Chem. Soc.*, **120**, 12–17.

Brewer, L.R., Corzett, M. and Balhorn, R. (1999) Protamine-induced condensation and decondensation of the same DNA molecule. *Science*, **286**, 120–123.

Bustamante, C. (1991) Direct observation and manipulation of single DNA molecules using fluorescence microscopy. *Ann. Rev. Biophys. Biophys. Chem.*, **20**, 415–446.

Chaikin, P.M. and Lubensky, T.C. (1995) *Principles of Condensed Matter Physics*. Cambridge University Press, Cambridge, pp. 479–494.

Chattoraj, D.K., Gosule, L.C. and Schellman, J.A. (1978) DNA condensation with poly-amines: II. Electron microscopic studies. *J. Mol. Biol.*, **121**, 327–337.

Chen, W., Turro, N.J. and Tomalia, D.A. (2000) Using ethidium bromide to probe the interactions between DNA and dendrimers. *Langmuir*, **16**, 15–19.

Chiu, D.T. and Zare, R.N. (1996) Biased diffusion, optical trapping, and manipulation of single molecules in solution. *J. Am. Chem. Soc.*, **118**, 6512–6513.

Chodanowski, P. and Stoll, S. (1999) Monte Carlo simulations of hydrophobic polyelectro-lytes: Evidence of complex configurational transitions. *J. Chem. Phys.*, **111**, 6069–6081.

Conrad, M. and Topal, M.D. (1989) DNA and spermidine provide a switch mechanism to regulate the activity of restriction enzyme Nae I. *Proc. Natl. Acad. Sci. USA*, **86**, 9707–9711.

Cui, Y. and Bustamente, C. (2000) Pulling a single chromatin fibre reveals the forces that maintain its higher-order structure. *Proc. Natl. Acad. Sci. USA*, **97**, 127–132.

Dautzenberg, H., Jaeger, W., Kotz, J., Philipp, B., Seidel, C.H. and Stscherbina, D. (1994) *Polyelectrolytes: Formation, Characterization and Application*. Hanser Publishers, Munich, pp. 87–129.

de Gennes, P.-G. (1979) *Scaling Concepts in Polymer Physics*. Cornell University Press, N.Y.

Dobrynin, A.V., Rubinstein, M. and Obukhov, S.P. (1996) Cascade of transitions of poly-electrolytes in poor solvents. *Macromolecules*, **29**, 2974–2979.

Duguid, J., Bloomfield, V.A., Benevides, J. and Thomas, Jr., G.J. (1993) Raman spectroscopy of DNA-metal complexes I. Interactions and conformational effects of the divalent cations: Mg, Ca, Sr, Ba, Mn, Co, Ni, Cu, Pd, and Cd. *Biophys. J.*, **65**, 1916–1928.

Dunlap, D.D., Maggi, A., Soria, M.R. and Monaco, L. (1997) Nanoscopic structure of DNA condensed for gene delivery. *Nucleic Acids Res.*, **25**, 3095–3101.

Eickbush, T.H. and Moudrianakis, E.N. (1978) The compaction of DNA helices into either continuous supercoils or folded fibre rods and toroids. *Cell*, **13**, 295–306.

Emi, N., Kidoaki, S. Yoshikawa, K. and Saito, H. (1997) Gene transfer mediated by poly-arginine requires a formation of big carrier-complex of DNA aggregate. *Biochem. Biophys. Res. Commun.*, **231**, 421–424.

Erbacher, P., Zou, S., Bettinger, T., Steffan, A.-M. and Remy, J.-S. (1998) Chitosn-based vector/DNA complexes for gene delivery: Biophysical characteristics and transfection ability. *Pharm. Res.*, **15**, 1332–1339.

Evdokimov, Y.M., Pyatigorskaya, T.L., Polyvtsev, O.F., Akimenko, N.M., Kadykov, V.A., Tsvanki, D.Y. and Marshavsky, Y.M. (1976) A comparative x-ray diffraction and circular dichroism study of DNA compact particles formed in water-salt solutions, containing poly(ethylene glycol). *Nucleic Acids Res.*, **3**, 2353–2366.

Farhood, H., Gao, X., Son, K., Yang, Y., Lazo, J., Huang, L., Barsoum, J., Bottega, R. and Epand, R. (1994) Cationic liposomes for direct gene transfer in therapy of cancer and other diseases. *Ann. NY Acad. Sci.*, **716**, 23–34.

Fang, Y. and Hoh, J.H. (1998) Early intermediates in spermidine-induced DNA conden-sation on the surface of mica. *J. Am. Chem. Soc.*, **120**, 8903–8909.

Fendler, J.H. (1982) *Membrane Mimetic Chemistry*. John Wiley & Sons, New York, pp. 6–47.

Gershon, H., Ghirlando, R., Guttman, S.B. and Minsky, A. (1993) Mode of formation and structural features of DNA-cationic liposome complexes used for transfection. *Biochemistry*, **32**, 7143–7151.

Godbey, W.T., Wu, K.K. and Mikos, A.G. (1999) Tracking the intracellular path of poly(ethylenimine)/DNA complexes for gene delivery. *Proc. Natl. Acad. Sci. USA*, **96**, 5177–5181.

Golestanian, R., Kardar, M. and Liverpool, T.B. (1999) Collapse of stiff polyelectrolytes due to counterion fluctuations. *Phys. Rev. Lett.*, **82**, 4456–4459.

Golubovic, L. and Golubovic, M. (1998) Fluctuations of quasi-two-dimensional smectic intercalated between membrane in multilamellar phases of DNA-cationic lipid complexes. *Phys. Rev. Lett.*, **80**, 4341–4344.

Gosule, L.C. and Schellman, J.A. (1976) Compact form of DNA induced by spermidine. *Nature*, **259**, 333–335.

Gosule, L.C. and Schellman, J.A. (1978) Condensation with polyamines. I. Spectroscopic studies. *J. Mol. Biol.*, **121**, 311–326.

Gronbech-Jensen, N., Mashl, R.J., Bruinsma, R.F. and Gelbart, W.M. (1997) Counterion-induced attraction between rigid polyelectrolytes. *Phys. Rev. Lett.*, **78**, 2477–2480.

Grosberg, A. Yu. (1979) Certain possible conformational states of a uniform elastic polymer chain. *Biopysics.*, **24**, 30–36.

Grosberg, A. Yu. and Zhestkov, A.V. (1986) On the compact form of linear duplex DNA globular state of the uniform elastic (persistent) macromolecule. *J. Biomol. Struct. Dyn.*, **3**, 859–872.

Grosberg, A. Yu. and Khokhlov, A.R. (1994) *Statistical Physics of Macromolecules*. AIP Press, N.Y.

Gustafsson, J., Arvidson, G., Karlsson, G. and Almgren, M. (1995) Complexes between cationic liposomes and DNA visualized by cryo-TEM. *Biochem. Biophys. Acta.*, **1235**, 305–312.

Ha., B.-Y. and Liu, A.J. (1997) Counterion mediated attraction between two like-charged rods. *Phys. Rev. Lett.*, **79**, 1289–1292.

Harries, D., May, S., Gelbart, W. and Ben Shaul, A. (1998) Structure, stability, and thermo-dynamics of lamellar DNA-lipid complexes. *Biophys. J.*, **75**, 159–173.

Hayakawa, K., Santerre, J.P. and Kwak, J.C. (1983) The binding of cationic surfactants by DNA. *Biophys. Chem.*, **17**, 175–181.

He, S., Arscott, P.G. and Bloomfield, V.A. (2000) Condensation of DNA by multivalent cations: Experimental studies of condensation kinetics. *Biopolymers*, **53**, 329–341.

Hud, N.V., Downing, K.H. and Balhom, R. (1995) A constant radius of curvature model for the organisation of DNA in toroidal condensates. *Proc. Natl. Acad. Sci. USA*, **92**, 3581–3585.

Ichiba, Y. and Yoshikawa, K. (1998) Single chain observation on collapse transition in giant DNA induced by negatively-charged polymer. *Biochem. Biophys. Res. Commun.*, **242**, 441–445.

Ivanov, V.A., Stukan, M.R., Vasilevskaya, V.V., Paul, W. and Binder, K. (2000) *Macromol. Theory Simul.*, **9**, 488–499.

Iwataki, T., Yoshikawa, K., Kidoaki, S., Umeno, D., Kiji, M. and Maeda, M. (2000) Cooperativity *vs.* phase transition in a giant single DNA molecule. *J. Am. Chem. Soc.*, **122**, 9891–9896.

Jary, D. and Sikorav, J.L. (1999) Cyclization of globular DNA: Implications for DNA–DNA interactions *in vivo*. *Biochemistry*, **38**, 3223–3227.

Jennings, D.E., Kuznetsov, Y.A., Timoshenko, E.G. and Dawson, K.A. (2000) A lattice model Monte Carlo study of coil-globule and other conformational transitions of polymer, amphiphile, and solvent. *J. Chem. Phys.*, **112**, 7711–7722.

Jonsson, B., Lindman, B., Homberg, K. and Kronberg, B. (1998) *Surfactants and Polymers in Aqueous Solution*. John Wiley & Sons, Chichester.

Jordan, C.F., Lerman, L.S. and Venable, J.H. (1972) Structure and circular dichroism of DNA in concentrated polymer solutions. *Nat. New. Biol.*, **236**, 67–70.

Kabanov, V.A., Sergeyev, V.G., Pyshikina, O.A., Zinchenko, A.A., Zezin, A.B., Joosten, J.G.H., Brackman, J. and Yoshikawa, K. (2000) Interpolyelectrolyte complexes formed by DNA and astramol poly(propylene imine) dendrimers. *Macromolecules*, **33**, 9587–9593.

Kantor, Y. and Kardar, M. (1994) Excess charge in polyampholytes. *Europhys. Lett.*, **27**, 643–648.

Kantor, Y. and Kardar, M. (1995) Instabilities of charged polyampholytes. *Phys. Rev. E.*, **51**, 1299–1312.

Kapuscinski, J. and Darzynkiewicz, Z. (1984) Condensation of nucleic acids by intercalating cations. *Proc. Natl. Acad. Sci. USA*, **81**, 7368–7372.

Katsura, S., Hirano, K., Matsuzawa, Y., Yoshikawa, K. and Mizuno, A. (1998) Direct laser trapping of single DNA molecules in the globular state. *Nucleic Acids Res.*, **26**, 4943–4945.

Kidoaki, S. and Yoshikawa, K. (1996) The folded state of long duplex-DNA chain reflects its solution history. *Biophys. J.*, **71**, 932–939.

Kidoaki, S. and Yoshikawa, K. (1999) Folding and unfolding of a giant duplex-DNA in a mixed solution with polycations, polyanions and crowding neutral polymers. *Biophys. Chem.*, **76**, 133–143.

Koltover, I., Salditt, T., Radler, J.O. and Safinya, C.R. (1998) An inverted hexagonal phase of cationic liposome-DNA complexes related to DNA release and delivery. *Science*, **281**, 78–81.

Koltover, I., Salditt, T. and Safinya, C.R. (1999) Phase diagram, stability, and overcharging of lamellar cationic lipid-DNA self-assembled complexes. *Biophys. J.*, **77**, 915–924.

Koltover, I., Wagner, K. and Safinya, C.R. (2000) DNA condensation in two dimensions. *Proc. Natl. Acad. Sci. USA*, **97**, 14046–14051.

Kuznetsov, Yu. A. and Timoshenko, E.G. (1999) On the conformational structure of a stiff homopolymer. *J. Chem. Phys.*, **111**, 3744–3752.

Kramarenko, E. Yu., Khokhlov, A.R. and Yoshikawa, K. (1997) Collapse of polyelectrolyte macromolecules revisited. *Macromolecules*, **30**, 3383–3388.

Labat-Moleur, F., Steffan, A.-M., Brisson, C., Perron, H., Feugeas, O., Furstenberger, P., Brambilla, E. and Behr, J.-P. (1996) An electron microscopy study into the mechanism of gene transfer wit lipopolyamine. *Gene Ther.*, **3**, 1010–1017.

Laemmli, U.K. (1975) Characterization of DNA condensates induced by poly(ethylene oxide) and polylysine. *Proc. Natl. Acd. Sci. USA*, **72**, 4288–4292.

Lasic, D.D., Strey, H., Stuart, M.C.A., Podgornik, R. and Frederik, P.M. (1997) The structure of DNA-liposome complexes. *J. Am. Chem. Soc.*, **119**, 832–833.

Lee, N. and Thirumalai, D. (2000) Dynamics of collapse of flexible polyelectrolytes and polyamopholyes. *Cond. Mat.*, **0001094**, 1–10.

Lerman, L.S. (1971) A transition to a compact form of DNA in polymer solutions. *Proc. Natl. Acad. Sci. USA*, **68**, 1886–1890.

Liang, H. and Chen, H. (2000) First-order transition of a hompolymer chain with Lennard-Jones potential. *J. Chem. Phys.*, **113**, 4469–4471.

Lifshitz, I.M., Grosberg, A. Yu. and Khokhlov, A.R. (1978) Some problems of the statistical physics of polymer chains with volume interaction. *Rev. Mod. Phys.*, **50**, 683–713.

Liphardt, J., Onoa, B., Smith, S.B., Tinoco, Jr., I. and Bustamante, C. (2001) Reversible unfolding of single RNA molecules by mechanical force. *Science*, **292**, 733–737.

Livolant, F., Levelut, A.M., Doucet, J. and Benoit, J.P. (1989) The highly concentrated liquid-crystalline phase of DNA is columnar hexagonal. *Nature*, **339**, 724–726.

Livolant, F. (1991) Ordered phases of DNA *in vivo* and *in vitro*. *Physica A*, **176**, 117–137.

Loeffler, J.P. and Behr, J.P. (1993) Gene transfer into primary and established mammalian cell lines with lipopolyamine-coated DNA. *Methods Enzymol.*, **217**, 599–618.

Lyubartsev, A.P. and Nordenskiold, L. (1995) Monte Carlo simulation study of ion distribution and osmotic pressure in hexagonally oriented DNA. *J. Phys. Chem.*, **99**, 10373–10382.

Ma, D. and Bloomfiled, V.A. (1994) Condensation of supercoiled DNA induced by $MnCl_2$. *Biophys. J.*, **67**, 1678–1681.

Ma, C., Sun, L. and Bloomfiled, V.A. (1995) Condensation of plasmids enhanced by Z-DNA conformation of d(CG)n inserts. *Biochemistry*, **34**, 3521–3528.

Makita, N. and Yoshikawa, K. (1999) ATP/ADP switches the higher-order structure of DNA in the presence of spermidine. *FEBS Lett.*, **460**, 333–337.

Malghani, M.S. and Yang, J. (1998) Stable binding of DNA to zwitterionic lipid bilayers in aqueous solutions. *J. Phys. Chem. B*, **102**, 8930–8933.

Manning, G.S. (1978) The molecular theory of polyelectrolyte solutions with applications to the electrostatic properties of polynucleotides. *Quarterly Rev. Biophys.*, **11**, 179–246.

Manning, G.S. (1980) Thermodynamic stability theory for DNA doughnut shapes induced by charge neutralization. *Biopolymers*, **19**, 37–59.

Manning, G.S. (1985) Packaged DNA: An elastic model. *Cell Biophys.*, **7**, 57–89.

Marquet, R., Wyart, A. and Houssier, C. (1987) Influence of DNA length on spermine-induced condensation. Importance of the bending and stiffening of DNA. *Biochem. Biophys. Acta.*, **909**, 165–172.

Marquet, R. and Houssier, C. (1991) Thermodynamics of cation-induced DNA condensation. *J. Biomol. Struct. Dyn.*, **9**, 159–167.

Martin, A.L., Davies, M.C., Rackstraw, B.J., Roberts, C.J., Stolnik, S., Tendler, S.J. and Williams, P.M. (2000) Observation of DNA-polymer condensate formation in real time at a molecular level. *FEBS Lett.*, **480**, 106–112.

Marx, K.A. and Ruben, G.C. (1983) Evidence for hydrated spermidine-calf thymus DNA toruses organized by circumferential DNA wrapping. *Nucleic Acids Res.*, **11**, 1839–1854.

Marx, K.A. and Ruben, G.C. (1986) A study of fX-174 DNA torus and lambda DNA torus tertiary structure and the implication for DNA self-assembly. *J. Biomol. Struct. Dyn.*, **4**, 23–39.

Matsuzawa, Y. and Yoshikawa, K. (1994) Change of the higher-order structure in a giant DNA induced by 4',6-diamidino-2-phenylindole as a minor groove binder and ethidium bromide as an intercalator. *Nucleosides & Nucleotides*, **13**, 1415–1423.

Matsuzawa, Y., Yonezawa, Y. and Yoshikawa, K. (1996) Formation of nucleation center in single double-stranded DNA chain. *Biochem. Biophys. Res. Commun.*, **225**, 796–800.

Matsuzawa, Y., Hirano, K., Mori, K., Ktsura, S., Yoshikawa, K. and Mizuno, A. (1999) Laser trapping on an individual DNA molecule folded using various condensing agents. *J. Am. Chem. Soc.*, **121**, 11581–11582.

Matsuzawa, Y., Koyama, Y., Hirano, K., Kanbe, T., Katsura, S., Mizuno, A. and Yoshikawa, K. (2000) Visualization and optical trapping of an individual submicrometer-sized assembly in aqueous solution: Aminated polyethylene glycol (PEG-A) complexed with palmitic acid and DNA in poly(ethylene glycol)(PEG) solution. *J. Am. Chem. Soc.*, **122**, 2200–2205.

Matulis, D., Rouzina, I. and Bloomfield, V.A. (2000) Thermodynamics of DNA binding and condensation: isothermal titration calorimetry and electrostatic mechanism. *J. Mol. Biol.*, **296**, 1053–1063.

Mayama, H., Iwataki, T. and Yoshikawa, K. (2000) Thermodynamics in the folding transition of single T4 DNA molecules in poly(ethylene glycol) solution. *Chem. Phys. Lett.*, **318**, 113–117.

Mehta, A.D., Rief, M., Spudich, J.A., Smith, D.A. and Simmons, R.M. (1999) Single-molecule biomechanics with optical methods. *Science*, **283**, 1689–1695.

Mel'nikov, S.M., Sergeyev, V.G. and Yoshikawa, K. (1995a) Discrete coil-globule transition of large DNA by cationic surfactant. *J. Am. Chem. Soc.*, **117**, 2401–2408.

Mel'nikov, S.M., Sergeyev, V.G. and Yoshikawa, K. (1995b) Transition of double-stranded DNA chains between random coil and compact globule states induced by cooperative binding of cationic surfactants. *J. Am. Chem. Soc.*, **117**, 9951–9956.

Mel'nikov, S.M., Sergeyev, V.G., Yoshikawa, K., Takahashi, H. and Hatta, I. (1997a) Cooperativity or phase transition? Unfolding transition of DNA cationic surfactant complex. *J. Chem. Phys.*, **107**, 6917–6924.

Mel'nikov, S.M., Sergeyev, V.G., Melnikova, Yu.S. and Yoshikawa, K. (1997b) Folding of long DNA chains in the presence of distearyldimethylammonium bromide and unfolding induced by neutral liposomes. *J. Chem. Soc. Faraday Trans.*, **93**, 283–288.

Mel'nikov, S.M., Sergeyev, V.G. and Yoshikawa, K. (1997c) Cooperation between salt induced coil-globule transition in single duplex DNA complexed with cationic surfactant and sphere-rod transition of surfactant micelles. *Prog. Colloid. Polym. Sci.*, **106**, 209–214.

Mel'nikov, S.M. and Yoshikawa, K. (1997d) First-order phase transition in large single duplex DNA induced by a nonionic surfactant. *Biochem. Biophys. Res. Commun.*, **230**, 514–517.

Mel'nikov, S.M., Khan, M.O., Lindman, B. and Jonsson, B. (1999) Phase behavior of single DNA in mixed solvents. *J. Am. Chem. Soc.*, **121**, 1130–1136.

Micka, U. and Kremer, K. (2000) Strongly charged flexible polyelectrolytes in poor solvents – from stable spheres to necklace chains. *Europhys. Lett.*, **49**, 189–195.

Mikailenko, S.V., Sergeyev, V.G., Zinchenko, A.A., Gallyamov, M.O., Yaminsky, I.V. and Yoshikawa, K. (2000) Interplay between folding/unfolding and helix/coil transitions in giant DNA. *Biomacromolecues*, **1**, 597–603.

Minagawa, K., Matsuzawa, Y., Yoshikawa, K., Matsumoto, M. and Doi, M. (1991) Direct observation of the biphasic conformational change of DNA induced by cationic polymers. *FEBS Lett.*, **295**, 67–69.

Minagawa, K., Matsuzawa, Y., Yoshikawa, K., Khokhlov, A.R. and Doi, M. (1994) Direct observation of the coil-globule transition in DNA molecules. *Biopolymers*, **34**, 555–558.

Morris, V.J. and Jennings, B.R. (1976) Electric field light scattering as a mean of studying the effects of additives on bacteria. *J. Coll. Inter. Sci.*, **55**, 143–147.

Murayama, H. and Yoshikawa, K. (1999) Thermodynamics of the collapsing phase transition in a single duplex DNA molecule. *J. Phys. Chem. B.*, **103**, 10517–10523.

Noguchi, H., Saito, S., Kidoaki, S. and Yoshikawa, K. (1996) Self-organized nanostructures constructed with a single polymer chain. *Chem. Phys. Lett.*, **261**, 527–533.

Noguchi, H. and Yoshikawa, K. (1997) First-order phase transition in a stiff polymer chain. *Chem. Phys. Lett.*, **278**, 184–188.

Noguchi, H. and Yoshikawa, K. (1998) Morphological variation in a collapsed single homo-polymer chain. *J. Chem. Phys.*, **109**, 5070–5077.

Noguchi, H. and Yoshikawa, K. (2000) Folding path in a semiflexible homopolymer chain: A Brownian dynamics simulation. *J. Chem. Phys.*, **113**, 854–862.

Nomura, S.M., Yoshikawa, Y., Yoshikawa, K., Dannenmuller, O., Chasserot-Golaz, S., Ourisson, G. and Nakatani, Y. (2001) Towards proto-cells: 'Primitive' lipid vesicles encapsulating giant DNA and its histone complex. *Chem. Bio. Chem.*, 457–459.

Oana, H., Ueda, M. and Washizu, M. (1999) Visualization of specific sequence on a single large DNA molecule using fluorescence microscopy based on a new DNA-stretching method. *Biochem. Biophys. Res. Commun.*, **265**, 140–143.

Odijk, T. (1994) Long-range attraction in polyelectrolyte solution. *Macromolecules*, **27**, 4998–5003.

Odijk, T. (1998) Hexagonally packed DNA within bacteriophage T7 stabilized by curvature stress. *Biophys. J.*, **75**, 1223–1227.

Ogris, M., Steinlein, P., Kursa, M., Mechtler, R. and Wagner, E. (1998) The size of DNA/transferrin-PEI complexes is an important factor for gene expression in cultured cells. *Gene Ther.*, **5**, 1425–1433.

O'Hern, C.S. and Lubensky, T.C. (1998) Sliding columnar phase of DNA-lipid complexes. *Phys. Rev. Lett.*, **80**, 4345–4348.

Olvera de la Cruz, M., Belloni, L., Delsanti, M., Dalbiez, J.P., Spalla, O. and Drifford, M. (1995) Precipitation of highly charged polyelectrolyte solutions in the presence of multi-valent salts. *J. Chem. Phys.*, **103**, 5781–5791.

Oosawa, F. (1971) *Polyelectrolytes.* Marcel Dekker, New York.

Osica, V.D., Pyatigorskaya, T.L., Polyvtsev, O.F., Dembo, A.T., Kliya, M.O., Vasilchenko, V.N., Verkin, B. and Sukharevskya, B.Y. (1977) Preliminary morphological and X-ray diffraction studies of the crystals of the DNA cetyltrimethylammonium salt. *Nucleic Acids Res.*, **4**, 1083–1096.

Osterberg, R., Persson, D. and Bjursell, G. (1984) The condensation of DNA by chromium (III) ions. *J. Biomol. Struct. Dyn.*, **2**, 285–290.

Pelta, J., Livolant, F. and Sikorav, J.L. (1996a) DNA aggregation induced by polyamines and cobalthexamine. *J. Biol. Chem.*, **271**, 5656–5662.

Pelta, J., Durand, D., Doucet, J. and Livolant, F. (1996b) DNA mesophases induced by spermidine: Structural properties and biological implications. *Biophys. J.*, **71**, 48–63.

Perales, J.C., Ferkol, T., Molas, M. and Hanson, R.W. (1994) An evaluation of receptor-mediated gene transfer using synthetic DNA-ligand complexes. *Eur. J. Biochem.*, **226**, 255–266.

Plum, G.E., Arscott, P.G. and Bloomfield, V.A. (1990) Condensation of DNA by trivalent cations. II. Effects of cation structure. *Biopolymers*, **30**, 631–643.

Post, C.B. and Zim, B.H. (1982) Theory of DNA condensation: collapse versus aggregation. *Biopolymers*, **21**, 2123–2137.

Promega Technical Bulletin (1994) Transfectam reagent for the transfection of eukaryotic cells. Madison: WI, No. 116.

Raspaud, E., Olvera de la Cruz, M., Sikorav, J.-L. and Lipovant, F. (1998) Precipitation of DNA by polyamine: a polyelectrolyte behaviour. *Biophys. J.*, **74**, 381–393.

Raspuad, E., Chaperon, I., Leforestier, A. and Lipovant, F. (1999) Spermine-induced aggregation of DNA, Nucleosome, and Chromatin. *Biophys. J.*, **77**, 1547–1555.

Ray, J. and Manning, G.S. (1994) An attractive force between two rodlike polyions mediated by the sharing of condensed counterions. *Langmuir*, **10**, 2450–2461.

Reich, Z., Ghirlando, R. and Minsky, A. (1991) Secondary conformational polymorphism of nucleic acids as a possible functional link between cellular parameters and DNA packaging processes. *Biochemistry*, **30**, 7828–7836.

Rouzina, I. and Bloomfield, V.A. (1996) Macroion attraction due to electrostatic correlation between screening counterions. I. Mobile surface-adsorbed ions and diffuse ion cloud. *J. Phys. Chem.*, **100**, 9977–9989.

Salditt, T., Koltover, I., Radler, J.O. and Safinya, C.R. (1997) Two-dimensional smectic ordering of linear DNA chains in self-assembled DNA-cationic liposome mixtures. *Phys. Rev. Lett.*, **79**, 2582–2585.

Salditt, T., Koltover, I., Radler, J.O. and Safinya, C.R. (1998) Self-assembled DNA-cationic-lipid complexes: two-dimensional smectic ordering, correlations, and interactions. *Phys. Rev. E.*, **58**, 889–904.

Satake, I. and Yang, J.T. (1976) Interaction of sodium decyl sulfate with poly(L-ornithine) and poly(L-lysine) in aqueous solution. *Biopolymers*, **15**, 2263–2275.

Schiessel, H. and Pincus, P. (1998) Counterion-condensation-induced collapse of highly charged polyelectrolytes. *Macromolecules*, **31**, 7953–7959.

Schwinefus, J.J. and Bloomfield, V.A. (2000) The greater negative charge density of DNA in tris-borate buffer does not enhance DNA condensation by multivalent cations. *Biopolymers*, **54**, 572–577.

Sergeyev, V.G., Mikhailenko, S.V., Pyshkina, O.A., Ymainsky, I.V. and Yoshikawa, K. (1999) How does alcohol dissolve the complex of DNA with a cationic surfactant? *J. Am. Chem. Soc.*, **121**, 1780–1785.

Shen, M.R., Downing, K.H., Balhorn, R. and Hud, N.V. (2000) Nucleation of DNA condensation by static loops: formation of DNA toroid with reduced dimensions. *J. Am. Chem. Soc.*, **122**, 4833–4834.

Sikorav, J.-L., Pelta, J. and Livolant, F. (1994) A liquid crystalline phase in spermidine-condensed DNA. *Biophys. J.*, **67**, 1387–1392.

Solis, F.J. and de la Cruz, M.O. (1998) Variational approach to necklace formation in polyelectrolytes. *Macromolecules*, **31**, 5502–5506.

Solis, F.J. and de la Cruz, M.O. (2000) Collapse of flexible polyelectrolytes in multivalent salt solutions. *J. Chem. Phys.*, **112**, 2030–2035.

Starodubtsev, S.G. and Yoshikawa, K. (1996) Intrachain segregation in single giant DNA molecules induced by poly(2-vinylpyrrolidone). *J. Phys. Chem.*, **100**, 19702–19705.

Stevens, M.J. (2001) Simple simulations of DNA condensation. *Biophys. J.*, **80**, 130–139.

Takagi, S. and Yoshikawa, K. (1999) Stepwise collapse of polyelectrolyte chains entrapped in a finite space as predicted by theoretical considerations. *Langmuir*, **15**, 4143–4146.

Takagi, S., Tsumoto, K. and Yoshikawa, K. (2001) Intra-molecular phase segregation in a single polyelectrolyte chain. *J. Chem. Phys.*, **114**, 6942–6949.

Takahashi, M., Yoshikawa, K., Vasilevskaya, V.V. and Khokhlov, A.R. (1997) Discrete coil-globule transition of single duplex DNAs induced by polyamine. *J. Phys. Chem. B*, **101**, 9396–9401.

Thomas, T.J. and Thomas, T. (1994) Polyamine-induced Z-DNA conformation in plasmids containing (dA-dC)n(dG-dT)n inserts and increased binding of lupus autoantibodies to the Z-DNA form of plasmids. *Biochem. J.*, **298**, 485–491.

Tsumoto, T. and Yoshikawa, K. (1999) RNA switches the higher–order structure of DNA. *Biophys. Chem.*, **82**, 1–8.

Ubbink, J. and Odijk, T. (1995) Polymer- and salt-induced toroids of hexagonal DNA. *Biophys. J.*, **68**, 54–61.

Ueda, M. and Yoshikawa, K. (1996) Phase transition and phase segregation in a single double-stranded DNA molecule. *Phys. Rev. Lett.*, **77**, 2133–2136.

Vasilevskaya, V.V., Khokhlov, A.R., Matsuzawa, Y. and Yoshikawa, K. (1995) Collapse of single DNA in poly(ethylene glycol) solutions. *J. Chem. Phys.*, **102**, 6595–6602.

Vasilevskaya, V.V., Khokhlov, A.R., Kidoaki, S. and Yoshikawa, K. (1997) Structure of collapsed persistent macromolecule: toroid *vs.* spherical globule. *Biopolymers*, **41**, 51–60.

Vasilevskaya, V.V., Khokhlov, A.R. and Yoshikawa, K. (2000) Single polyelectrolyte macromolecule in the salt solution: Effect of escaped counter ions. *Macromol. Theory Simul.*, **9**, 600–607.

Wagner, E., Cotton, M., Foisner, R. and Birnstiel, M.L. (1991) Transferrin-polycation- DNA complexes: The effect of polycations on the structure of the complex and DNA delivery to cells. *Proc. Natl. Acd. Sci. USA*, **88**, 4255–4259.

Widom, J. and Baldwin, R.L. (1980) Cation-induced toroidal condensation of DNA: studies with $Co^{3+}(NH_3)_6$. *J. Mol. Biol.*, **144**, 431–453.

Widom, J. and Baldwin, R.L. (1983) Monomolecular condensation of DNA induced by cobalt hexamine. *Biopolymers*, **22**, 1595–1620.

Wilson, R.W. and Bloomfield, V.A. (1979) Counterion-induced condensation of deoxyribonucleic acid. A light-scattering study. *Biochemistry*, **18**, 2192–2196.

Yamasaki, Y. and Yoshikawa, K. (1997) Higher order structure of DNA controlled by the redox state of Fe^{2+}/Fe^{3+}. *J. Am. Chem. Soc.*, **119**, 10573–10578.

Yamasaki, Y., Hirano, K., Morishima, K., Mizuno, A., Arai, F. and Yoshikawa, K. (1998) Optical trapping of single DNA molecule complexed with cationic surfactant. *Forma*, **13**, 397–403.

Yamasaki, Y., Teramoto, Y. and Yoshikawa, K. (2001) Disappearance of the negative charge in giant DNA with a folding transition. *Biophys. J.*, **80**, 2823–2832.

Yanagida, M., Hiraoka, Y. and Katsuya, I. (1983) *Cold Spring Harbor Symp. Quant. Biol.*, **47**, 177–187.

Yoshikawa, K., Matsuzawa, Y., Minagawa, K., Doi, M. and Matsumoto, M. (1992) Opposite effect between intercalator and minor groove binder drug on the higher order structure of DNA as is visualised by fluorescence microscopy. *Biochem. Biophys. Res. Commun.*, **188**, 1274–1279.

Yoshikawa, K. and Matsuzawa, Y. (1995) Discrete phase transition of giant DNA: Dynamics of globule formation from a single molecular chain. *Physica D*, **84**, 220–227.

Yoshikawa, K. and Matsuzawa, Y. (1996) Nucleation and growth in single DNA molecules. *J. Am. Chem. Soc.*, **118**, 929–930.

Yoshikawa, K., Takahashi, M., Vasilevskaya, V.V. and Khokhlov, A.R. (1996a) Large discrete transition in a single DNA molecule appears continuous in the ensemble. *Phys. Rev. Lett.*, **76**, 3029–3031.

Yoshikawa, K., Kidoaki, S., Takahashi, M., Vasilevskaya, V.V. and Khokhlov, A.R. (1996b) Marked discretness on the coil-globule transition of single duplex DNA. *Ber. Bunsen-Ges. Phys. Chem.*, **100**, 876–880.

Yoshikawa, K. (1997) Complexity in a molecular string: Hierarchical structure as is exemplified in a DNA chain. In: *Complexity and Diversity*. Springer-Verlag, Tokyo, pp. 81–90.

Yoshikawa, K., Noguchi, H. and Yoshikawa, Y. (1997a) Folding transition in single long duplex DNA chain. *Progr. Colloid. Polym. Sci.*, **106**, 204–208.

Yoshikawa, K., Yoshikawa, Y., Koyama, Y. and Kanbe, T. (1997b) Highly effective compaction of long duplex DNA induced by polyethylene glycol with pendant amino groups. *J. Am. Chem. Soc.*, **119**, 6473–6477.

Yoshikawa, Y. and Yoshikawa, K. (1995) Diaminoalkanes with an odd number of carbon atoms induce compaction of a single double-stranded DNA chain. *FEBS Lett.*, **361**, 277–281.

Yoshikawa, Y., Yoshikawa, K. and Kanbe, T. (1996c) Daunomycin unfolds compactly packed DNA. *Biophys. Chem.*, **61**, 93–100.

Yoshikawa, Y., Emi, N., Kanbe, T., Yoshikawa, K. and Saito, H. (1996d) Folding and aggregation of DNA chains induced by complexation with lipospermine: formation of a nucleosome-like structure and network assembly. *FEBS Lett.*, **396**, 71–76.

Yoshikawa, Y., Takenaka, A. and Kanbe, T. (1998) Morphological variation of DNA in relation to the sensitivity to restriction enzyme. *Nucleic Acids Symp. Ser.*, **39**, 253–254.

Yoshikawa, Y., Yoshikawa, K. and Kanbe, T. (1999) Formation of a giant toroid from long duplex DNA. *Langmuir*, **15**, 4085–4088.

Yoshikawa, Y., Nomura, S.M., Kanbe, T. and Yoshikawa, K. (2000) Controlling the folding/ unfolding transition of the DNA-histone H1 complex by direct optical manipulation. *Chem. Phys. Lett.*, **330**, 77–82.

Yoshikawa, Y., Velichko, Yu. S., Ichiba, Y. and Yoshikawa, K. (2001) Self-assembled pearling structure of long duplex DNA with histone H1. *Eur. J. Biochem.*, **268**, 2593–2599.

Zimmerman, S.B. and Murphy, L.D. (1996) Macromolecular crowding and the mandatory condensation of DNA in bacteria. *FEBS Lett.*, **390**, 245–248.

9 Structure, dispersion stability and dynamics of DNA and polycation complexes

Alexander V. Kabanov and
Tatiana K. Bronich

INTRODUCTION

Polycation-based non-viral gene delivery systems have recently attracted significant attention. Polyplexes form spontaneously as a result of cooperative electrostatic interactions between phosphate groups of the DNA and oppositely charged groups of the polycation. A number of review manuscripts and book issues have appeared recently that discuss physicochemical, biochemical and therapeutic aspects of these systems (Felgner *et al.*, 1996; Kabanov *et al.*, 1998a; Rolland, 1999; Garnett, 1999; Chesnoy and Huang, 1999). However, the field of non-viral gene therapy is developing extremely fast and requires continuous appraisal. This chapter focuses on the biophysical and polymer aspects of the polyplexes. The biochemical and therapeutic aspects are considered in detail in other chapters of this book. Furthermore, several works are available that discuss the relationship of the physicochemical properties of the polyplexes and their biological performance *in vitro* and *in vivo* (Kabanov and Kabanov, 1995; Kabanov *et al.*, 1998b; Kabanov, 1999). The most important physicochemical properties considered here include: (i) the reactions of polyplex formation; (ii) the colloidal properties and stability of polyplex dispersions; (iii) the effects of the polycation on the structure and properties of the DNA in the complexes, and; (iv) the processes underlying the DNA release from the polyplexes.

POLYCATIONS USED FOR PREPARATION OF POLYPLEXES

Some polycations used for preparation of complexes with DNA are listed in Table 9.1. Figure 9.1 illustrates the different molecular architectures of these polycations. Among the large number of polycations described in gene delivery applications are poly(L-lysine) (PLL) (Wu and Wu, 1987), poly(*N*-alkyl-4-vinylpyridinium) salts (PVP) (Kabanov *et al.*, 1989, 1993), polyamidoamine (PAMAM) dendrimers (Haensler and Szoka, 1993; Kukowska-Latallo *et al.*, 1996), polyethyleneimine (PEI) (Boussif *et al.*, 1995), and poly(2-dimethylaminoethyl methacrylate) (PDEAEM) (Cherng *et al.*, 1996). All these polycations are either homopolymers or random copolymers having linear, branched or dendritic architectures (Figure 9.1a,b,c). To increase the stability of DNA and polycation complexes in dispersion, cationic copolymers were used consisting of a polycation linked to a non-ionic water-soluble polymer, for example, poly(ethylene oxide) (PEO). Several systems with graft and

Table 9.1 Selected polycations used for preparation of polyplexes for gene delivery

Polycation	Structure	Use as of today	Key references[1]
Homopolymers or random copolymers			
Poly(L-lysine) (PLL)	Linear, tends to form secondary structures, primary amino groups	Plasmid and oligonucleotide delivery, *in vitro* and *in vivo*	(Wu and Wu, 1987, Wagner *et al.*, 1991)
Poly(N-alkyl-4-vinylpyridinium) salts (PVP)	Linear, quaternary ammonium salt	*In vitro* transfection in mammalian and bacillus cells	(Kabanov *et al.*, 1989)
Polyamidoamine (PAMAM) dendrimers	Dendrimer, primary amino groups at the dendrimer surface	*In vitro* and *in vivo* transfections	(Haensler and Szoka, 1993; Kukowska-Latallo *et al.*, 1996)
Polyethyleneimine (PEI) (branched)	Randomly branched, primary, secondary, and tertiary amino groups	*In vitro* and *in vivo* transfections, including therapeutic genes	(Boussif *et al.*, 1995)
Poly(2-dimethyl-aminoethyl methacrylate) (PDMAEM)	Linear, tertiary amino groups	*In vitro* transfection	(Cherng *et al.*, 1996)
Polyethyleneimine (PEI) (linear)	Linear, secondary amino groups	*In vitro* and *in vivo* transfections, including therapeutic genes	(Ferrari *et al.*, 1997)
Poly[alpha-(4-aminobutyl)-L-glycolic acid] (PAGA)	Linear, primary amino groups, biodegradable	*In vitro* and *in vivo* transfections, including therapeutic genes	(Koh *et al.*, 2000)
Block and graft copolymers			
Poly(ethylene oxide)-*b*-polyspermine (PEO-*b*-PSP)	Block copolymer, primary and secondary amino groups	Delivery of antisense oligonucleotides *in vitro* and *in vivo*	(Kabanov *et al.*, 1995)
Dextran-*g*-poly(L-lysine) (Dex-*g*-PLL)	Graft copolymer	DNA duplex and triplex stabilization	(Maruyama *et al.*, 1997)
Poly(ethylene oxide)-*b*-poly(L-lysine) (PEO-*b*-PLL)	Block copolymer	*In vitro* transfection, systemic administration of plasmids, encapsulation of oligonucleotides	(Kataoka *et al.*, 1996; Wolfert *et al.*, 1996)
Poly[N-(2-hydroxypropyl)-methacrylamide]-*b*-poly(trimethylam-moniomethyl methacrylate chloride) (PHPMA-*b*-PTMAEM)	Block copolymer, quaternary ammonium salt	*In vitro* transfection	(Wolfert *et al.*, 1996)

Table 9.1 (Continued)

Polycation	Structure	Use as of today	Key references[1]
Poly(ethylene oxide)-*g*-polyethyleneimine (PEO-*g*-PEI)	Graft copolymer, branched PEI segment	Delivery of oligonucleotides and plasmids *in vitro* and *in vivo*	(Vinogradov *et al.*, 1998; Ogris *et al.*, 1999)
Poly(ethylene oxide)-*g*-poly (L-lysine) (PEO-*g*-PLL)	Graft copolymer	*In vitro* and *in vivo* transfection, delivery of oligonucleotides	(Choi *et al.*, 1998)
Poly(ethylene oxide)-*b*-poly (L-lysine) dendrimer (PEO-*b*-dendrPLL)	Block copolymer, dendrimer PLL segment	Encapsulation of plasmids and oligonucleotides	(Choi *et al.*, 1999)
Pluronic-*g*-polyethyleneimine (Pluronic-*g*-PEI)	Graft-copolymer, branched PEI segment grafted with nonionic triblock copolymer	*In vitro* and *in vivo* transfections and oligonucleotide delivery	(Nguyen *et al.*, 2000)
Poly(ethylene oxide)-*b*-polyethyleneimine (PEO-*b*-PEI)	Block copolymer, linear PEI segment	Synthesis of carrier	(Akiyama *et al.*, 2000)
Poly(ethylene oxide)-*b*-poly (*N*-methyl-4-vinylpyridinium) salt (PEO-*g*-PVP)	Block copolymer	DNA topology recognition	(Bronich *et al.*, 2000)
N-Ac-poly (L-histidine)-*g*-poly(L-lysine)	Graft copolymer, pH-sensitive poly(L-histidine) grafts	*In vitro* transfection	(Benns *et al.*, 2000)
Cross-linked networks			
Poly(ethylene oxide)-*cl*-polyethyleneimine (PEO-*cl*-PEI)	Cross-linked nanoscale network	Delivery of antisense oligonucleotides *in vitro*	(Vinogradov *et al.*, 1999a,b)

Note

1 The list of references and contributors is not exhaustive. The authors tried to provide the earliest references known to them that describe preparation of the polyplexes specifically for gene delivery. In most cases these papers were followed by advanced work from the same and other laboratories. Furthermore, in several cases, such as PLL, there are earlier references available that describe the biophysical studies on DNA/polycation complexes. Many of these papers are cited in the text when appropriate.

block copolymer architectures (Figure 9.1D) have recently been described including poly(ethylene oxide)-block-polyspermine (PEO-*b*-PSP) (Kabanov *et al.*, 1995), poly(ethylene oxide)-graft-poly(ethyleneimine) (PEO-*g*-PEI) (Vinogradov *et al.*, 1998, 1999a,b; Ogris *et al.*, 1999), poly(ethylene oxide)-block-poly(L-lysine) (PEO-*b*-PLL) (Wolfert *et al.*, 1996; Kataoka *et al.*, 1996), and PEO-*g*-PLL (Choi *et al.*, 1998),

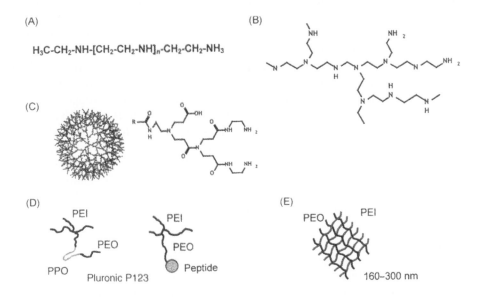

Figure 9.1 Schematic illustration of various polycation structures used for preparation
of polyplexes: (A) linear (PEI); (B) randomly branched (PEI); (C) dendrimer (PAMAM); (D) *block and graft copolymers* (Pluronic-*g*-PEI and PEO-*g*-PEI
modified with a targeting moiety by one PEO end); (E) nanoscale cross-
linked network (PEO-*cl*-PEI).

poly[*N*-(2-hydroxypropyl)-methacrylamide]-*b*-poly(trimethylammoniomethyl
methacrylate chloride) (PHPMA-*b*-PTMAEM) (Wolfert *et al.*, 1996), and dextran-
graft-poly(L-lysine) (Dex-*g*-PLL) (Maruyama *et al.*, 1997). Finally, to increase the
stability of the polyplex, the polycation chains can be cross-linked with each other,
forming a network in which the DNA molecules are trapped (Figure 9.1E). For
example, small hydrogel particles synthesized by cross-linking of PEI with double
end activated PEO (PEO-*cl*-PEI) were recently developed for the delivery of antisense oligonucleotides (Vinogradov *et al.*, 1999a,b). This list of structures is not
complete and is presented here only as an illustration of some early studies. Many
more new cationic polymers have recently been synthesized for gene delivery.

FORMATION OF THE COMPLEXES

Polyion coupling reaction

Complexes between DNA and polycations are spontaneously produced as a
result of polyion coupling reactions after mixing the DNA and polycation solutions. During these reactions polycations condense DNA and counterions are
released in the external media, and a system of salt bonds between DNA and
polycation repeating units is formed. The binding of polycations to DNA is
usually nonspecific and electrostatic. The release of the counterions results in
an entropy gain, which is a driving force of the complex formation (Manning,

1978; Record *et al.*, 1976; Ross and Shapiro, 1974). The contribution of the ion pair formation between polycation and DNA into the enthalpic term of the free energy is minimal, because both polyions are already involved in ionic interaction with the small counterions. A recent study reported complete thermodynamic characterization of the binding of PEO-*g*-PEI copolymer with synthetic DNA, poly[d(AT)]•poly[d(AT)] (Bronich *et al.*, 2000a, 2001). The thermodynamic profiles determined in this work exhibit typical salt effects, which suggest that the interaction is electrostatic. Since the interactions between the copolymer and DNA occurred spontaneously ($\Delta G_b^o < 0$), the small ΔH_b values observed in this work confirmed that the binding phenomenon is primarily entropic in origin. However, the contribution of other interactions like specific H-bonding or van der Waals forces into the complex formation in addition to the changes in the hydration state of the two polymers involved, is also possible. The authors suggested that the small exothermic term of the binding heat might be the result of both exothermic contributions from van der Waals interactions and endothermic contributions from the removal of water molecules of the charged and polar atomic groups participating in binding (Bronich *et al.*, 2001).

The stability of polyelectrolyte complex critically depends on the number of salt bonds between the interacting polyions (Papisov and Litmanovich, 1989). Normally, it takes at least six to ten salt bonds to form a stable system. Therefore, with some short polyions (both DNA and polycation) the binding affinities can be low. One example is the complexes formed by spermine or spermidine, which are characterized by relatively low binding constants (Marx and Reynolds, 1983). With an increase in the lengths of the interacting polyions the cooperation of the binding and the stability of the complex increases (Papisov and Litmanovich, 1989). Furthermore, by increasing the length of the interacting polyions the long-range electrostatic effects become significant. The experimental and theoretical results were presented that the polyelectrolyte character of a DNA makes a large contribution to both the magnitude and the salt concentration dependence of DNA binding with oligocationic ligands (Zhang *et al.*, 1996).

The charge density of polyions determines the amount of the counterions condensed with these polyions (Manning, 1978). Consequently, binding of the polycation to the DNA should increase with an increase in the charge density of the polycation. For example, the complexes of oligonucleotides with PEO-*b*-PSP, having lower charge density, are less stable than the complexes of thee oligonucleotides with PEO-*g*-PEI, having higher charge density (Vinogradov *et al.*, 1998). Possible contributions of the charge density in the polycation interaction with the DNA will be further discussed in the section considering polyion interchange and recognition phenomena.

The role of the complementarity of the configurations of the polycation and DNA chains in the polyion complex formation has been little explored. The structure of the polycation should affect its ability to form arrays of matching ion bridges with DNA. A recent work presented data on the binding of DNA with cationic polypropyleneimine dendrimers (Astramol™), which were synthesized by starting with a diaminobutane core and adding polypropylene branches (Kabanov *et al.*, 2000). The study suggests that the dendrimers of high generation (G4, G5) and DNA assemble into complexes in which a part of the amino groups do not form ion pairs with the DNA. This aspect is explained by the structural rigidity of the DNA and dendrimer that limits the extent of mutual availability of the oppositely charged polymer ionic groups. In contrast, in the case of the flexible polycation chain such as branched PEI, the ionic groups are more available to form salt bonds with DNA. Indeed, the study of binding of PEO-*g*-PEI copolymer with DNA suggests that practically all charged amino groups of the copolymer are involved in the formation of salt bonds in the complex (Bronich *et al.*, 2001).

In the case of the relatively weak polybases that are commonly used for the synthesis of polyplexes (such as PEI, polyspermine, etc.) the degree of ionization, α, and the charge density vary as the pH of the media is changed. Therefore, the polyion coupling reactions between such polycations and DNA strongly depend on the pH of the solution. At a given pH the degree of conversion in the polyion coupling reaction, θ, is determined as the fraction of the polycation repeating units that form ionic pairs with the DNA phosphate groups. The values of θ were determined from the potentiometric titration curves assuming that all acid is consumed only for ionization of secondary amino groups which then form ionic pairs with DNA phosphates (Figure 9.2). Usually, the θ-pH curve is shifted in the alkaline area compared to the ionization curve, α-pH, of the polycation in the absence of DNA. The reason for such a shift is the stabilization of the ionized form of the polycation due to the cooperative electrostatic interaction between the polycation and DNA. The pH difference between θ-pH curve and α-pH curve at each $\theta = \alpha$, ΔpH($\theta = \alpha$), provides a thermodynamic characteristic of the impact of

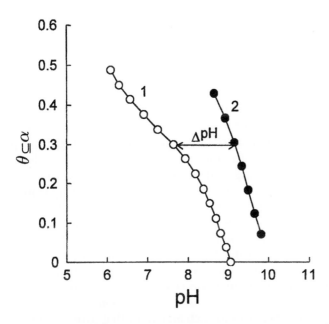

Figure 9.2 pH-Dependencies of the degree of conversion (θ) in the polyion coupling reactions ($\bullet$, $\blacksquare$) and degree of ionization (α) of polybase samples (o, □) for the following systems: PEO-*g*-PEI (curve 1, o); PEO-*g*-PEI and 24-mer phosphorothioate oligonucleotide (curve 2, $\bullet$). The pH-shift, ΔpH, between the θ-pH and α-pH dependencies is shown as an example. Based on the data reported by Vinogradov *et al.* (1998).

DNA in ionization of the polycation: $\Delta\Delta G_{st}(\theta = \alpha) = -2.303RT\Delta pH(\theta = \alpha)$, where $\Delta\Delta G_{st}(\theta = \alpha)$ is the difference of free energies of ionization of the polybase in the presence and absence of the DNA, R is the universal gas constant, and T is the absolute temperature.

Composition of the complex

Physicochemical properties of polyplexes greatly depend on the ratio of polycation and DNA units in the mixture: Z = [polycation units]/[DNA bases] referred to as *'composition of the mixture'* (Kabanov and Kabanov, 1995). In the case of polycations containing amino groups, the composition of the mixture is commonly expressed as N/P ratio, i.e., the ratio of the numbers of amino groups of the polycation to phosphate groups of the DNA. It should be emphasized that the composition of the complex formed after mixing of the polycation and DNA solutions, φ, is not always equal to the composition of the mixture, Z. For example, if only a fraction of the polycation added binds to the DNA, than $\varphi < Z$. This situation can be observed when the binding cooperativity is low, such as with spermine and DNA mixtures (Marx and Reynolds, 1983). It is also possible at excess of the polycation when all the binding sites in DNA are saturated and polycation excess does not incorporate into the complex. If all polycation and DNA chains are bound to each other and polycation is uniformly distributed among DNA chains, then $\varphi = Z$. However, this situation is relatively rare and in many cases an uneven distribution of polycation chains in the complexes, termed 'disproportionation', is observed (Kabanov and Kabanov, 1995). When disproportionation behavior takes place the complexes with $\varphi > Z$, $\varphi \leq Z$ and even free DNA can coexist in the same system.

Disproportionation

A typical disproportionation behavior in the mixtures of oppositely charged polyions has been described in a number of studies (Miller and Bach, 1968; Kabanov *et al.*, 1982, 1991). Figure 9.3 presents a schematic diagram illustrating disproportionation behavior in comparison with uniform distribution of the polycation chains among the DNA chains. Binding of the polycation to the DNA neutralizes the phosphate group charges. In the case of polycations with the hydrophobic backbone of the main chain this leads to the formation of hydrophobic sites. The length of such sites is determined by the degree of polymerization of the polycation. The number of sites is determined by the composition of the complex. Initially when polycation is added to the DNA in small amounts the complexes formed are negatively charged due to the excess of the DNA chains. With an increase in the composition of the mixture the charge of the complex decreases and the portion of the hydrophobic sites increases. At some point ($\varphi = \varphi_c < 1$) the hydrophobicity of the complex increases to such an extent that further binding of polycation leads to precipitation of the complex. Under these critical conditions uneven distribution of the polycation chains among the DNA molecules becomes thermodynamically favorable. As a result two types of the complex that differ in composition and solubility are produced simultaneously. One of these types is the non-stoichiometric complex that has a critical composition ($\varphi = \varphi_c$) and remains in

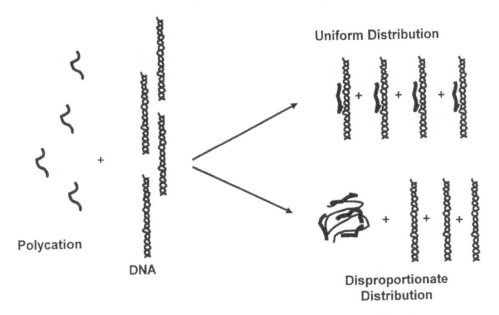

Figure 9.3 Schematic illustration of uniform and disproportionate distributions ('*disproportionation*') of polycation chains between DNA chains.

solution. Another type is the stoichiometric complex ($\varphi = 1$). In this type of the complex all DNA charges are neutralized by the polycation, and the complex species precipitate. The portion of the insoluble complex grows, while that of the soluble one decreases, as the concentration of the polycation increases ($\varphi_c < Z < 1$). Only the stoichiometric complex is present when the concentrations of DNA and the polycation become equal ($Z = 1$).

Disproportionation behavior was observed with many polycations used for the preparation of polyplexes, including linear and branched PEI, PAMAM dendrimer (Superfect^{TM}) and PVP (Gebhart and Kabanov, 2001). Generally, an increase in the hydrophobicity of the polycation main chain or modification of polycations with hydrophobic side groups favours the disproportionation. For example, C_{16} substitution in the repeating units of PVP enhances hydrophobic interactions of the polycation molecules with each other and promotes the disproportionation during interaction of the polycation with DNA (Kabanov *et al.*, 1991). Conversely, one could assume that the hydrophilic modification of a polycation can reduce disproportionation. Indeed, complexes formed in the mixtures of PEO-*g*-PEI copolymer and plasmid DNA did not exhibit disproportionation in the entire N/P range (Bronich *et al.*, 2000b). This is in contrast to the PEI homopolymer that disproportionates during interaction with the plasmid (Gebhart and Kabanov, 2001). However, the effect of the hydrophilic modification is dependent on the structure of the polycations. The mixtures of the plasmid and PEO-*b*-PVP copolymer exhibited pronounced disproportionation behavior, which was probably due to a relative hydrophobicity of the PVP backbone (Bronich *et al.*, 2000b).

STABILITY OF THE COMPLEXES IN DISPERSION

A core-shell model for positively charged complexes

Many studies have both characterized the composition of the polyplexes and determined the stability of the complexes in aqueous dispersion using electrophoresis and dynamic light scattering techniques (Sukhishvili *et al.*, 1993; Yaroslavov *et al.*, 1996; Cherng *et al.*, 1996; Tang and Szoka, 1997). These studies suggested that at deficiency of polycation (Z < 1) the particles of the complex were negatively charged. The charge increased with an increase in the polycation concentration. At the equivalency point the stoichiometric complexes ($\varphi = Z = 1$) formed. These complexes were characterized by low stability in dispersion: they formed large aggregates and precipitated. Remarkably, with certain polycations the size of the particles sharply decreased at the polycation excess. For example, such behavior was described for polyplexes formed by poly(*N*-ethyl-4-vinylpyridinium bromide) (PEVP) (Sukhishvili *et al.*, 1993; Kabanov and Kabanov, 1995), poly(2-dimethyl-amino)ethylmethacrylate (PDMAEM) (Cherng *et al.*, 1996), PEI and PAMAM dendrimer (Tang and Szoka, 1997). In these systems, by increasing the concentration of the polycations the dissolution of the aggregates was observed to result in the formation of small and rather homogeneous positively charged particles (average diameter 80–130 nm). Based on these studies a core-shell model of cationic polyplexes has been proposed (Kabanov *et al.*, 1998b). According to this model (Figure 9.4A) the neutralized polycation and DNA chains segregate into a hydrophobic core. This core is surrounded by a hydrophilic shell from charged polycation chains adsorbed at the surface of the particles. The cationic shell stabilizes the particles in dispersion due to the electrostatic repulsion and excluded volume effects. High transgene expression using polyplexes in *in vitro* transfection experiments often correlated with the formation of small cationic particles. Therefore, it has been hypothesized that small cationic particles are the actual transfection

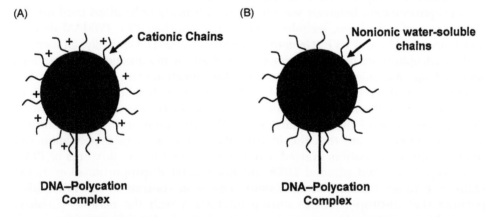

Figure 9.4 Core-shell polyplex structures: (A) cationic particles with a core from neutralized DNA and polycation and a corona from polycation chains adsorbed on the core; (B) electroneutral particles ('polyion complex micelles' or 'block ionomer complex') with a core from neutralized DNA and polycation and a corona from nonionic water soluble polymer.

moiety in the polyplexes formed by the most efficacious polycations, such as PEI, PAMAM dendrimers and other polymers (Kabanov *et al.*, 1998b). In contrast, less active polycations (such as un-conjugated PLL) usually formed large (µm) aggregates with DNA. The differences in the self-assembly of these polycations with DNA is possibly due to the difference in the flexibility of their chains (Kabanov *et al.*, 1998b). More flexible chains, such as PEI, are more likely to form charged 'corona', which surrounds the neutralized DNA/polycation 'core' and stabilizes the particles in solution. Conversely, more rigid molecules, such as PLL, possibly 'bridge' individual DNA molecules into large insoluble clusters, which have lower transfection activity. Although the relationship between the size, charge and transfection activity of the polyplexes is still being debated (Ogris *et al.*, 1998; Ramsay *et al.*, 2000; Gebhart and Kabanov, 2001), it is obvious that stability in dispersion is one major requirement of a successful pharmaceutical formulation of polyplexes (Cherng *et al.*, 1999b; Kabanov, 1999).

Block ionomer complexes

To improve the stability of the polyplexes in aqueous dispersion and prevent their interactions with serum proteins, cationic block and graft copolymers containing segments from polycations and nonionic water-soluble polymers were proposed by several groups of investigators (see Table 9.1). The binding of these copolymers with DNA results in the formation of complexes containing hydrophobic sites from polycation-neutralized DNA and hydrophilic sites from the nonionic water-soluble chains. Despite the charge neutralization the complexes can remain stable in aqueous dispersion due to the solubilizing effect of the nonionic chains. The stable dispersions are usually produced when the nonionic chains are sufficiently long (for example, more than 5 kDa in the case of PEO used as a solubilizing chain). Both double stranded DNA and short oligonucleotides were successfully incorporated into such complexes.

It is important to note that upon the mixing of DNA and cationic copolymers no precipitation was observed over the entire range of Z, including the equivalency point. At the polycation deficiency (Z < 1) some systems such as PEO-*g*-PEI/DNA complexes were negatively charged due to the presence of the DNA parts that were not covered by the polycation chains (Nguyen *et al.*, 2000). In gel electrophoresis experiments these complexes migrated through the gel, but the migration was retarded compared to the free DNA, suggesting gradual neutralization of the DNA charge. Other systems have exhibited typical disproportionation behavior as described in the previous section. It is noteworthy that in many cases the cationic particles did not form even under the conditions of significant excess of cationic copolymers in the mixture (Nguyen *et al.*, 2000). It is likely that formation of the hydrophilic shell from the nonionic polymer prevents the incorporation of excess polycation chains in the complex due to the excluded volume effect.

Overall, these systems belong to a broader class of polyelectrolyte complexes termed 'polyion complex micelles' (Harada and Kataoka, 1995) or 'block ionomer complexes' (Kabanov *et al.*, 1996). They represent a special class of chemical entities with combined properties of amphiphilic block copolymers (micellization, solubilization) and polyelectrolyte complexes (polyion coupling, polyion exchange reactions) (Bronich *et al.*, 1997, 1999, 2000c; Harada and Kataoka, 1997, 1998,

1999b; Stuart *et al.*, 1998; Nishiyama *et al.*, 1999). Such complexes were shown to form micelle-like aggregates in aqueous solution, which contains a hydrophobic core from neutralized polyions and a hydrophilic shell from hydrated nonionic chains (Figure 9.4B). For example, the complexes of oligonucleotides with PEO-*b*-PSP, PEO-*g*-PEI and PEO-*b*-PLL were reported (Kabanov and Kabanov, 1995; Kataoka *et al.*, 1996; Vinogradov *et al.*, 1998, 1999a,b). These complexes spontaneously self-assembled into very small (10 to 40 nm) particles with a hydrophobic core from neutralized polyions and a hydrophilic shell from PEO. These complexes were stable in aqueous dispersion despite complete neutralization of the charge. They could be lyophilized and redissolved or stored in solution for several months without changing size. The simplicity of preparation and long shelf life make these systems attractive as potential pharmaceutical formulations for oligonucleotides. They were used successfully to deliver antisense oligonucleotides into cells *in vitro* and *in vivo* (Kabanov and Kabanov, 1995; Roy *et al.*, 1999; Read *et al.*, 2000). The binding of cationic copolymers to double stranded DNA results in the formation of larger (50 to 200 nm) complexes, which are also stable in aqueous dispersion (Wolfert *et al.*, 1996; Katayose and Kataoka, 1997; Toncheva *et al.*, 1998; Choi *et al.*, 1998; Nguyen *et al.*, 2000). Depending on the structure of the copolymer these systems can have various morphologies, which is discussed in greater detail in one of the following sections. The polyplexes formed by cationic copolymers and plasmid DNA have also been used in both *in vitro* and *in vivo* transfection experiments and are currently being investigated as promising gene delivery vehicles.

Effect of proteins

In the biological milieu polyplexes are exposed to the concentrated solutions of proteins. Therefore, the question about the stability of the polyplex dispersions in the presence of proteins is of practical significance. Numerous studies performed on synthetic polyions have suggested that globular proteins can cooperatively self-assemble with oppositely charged polyelectrolytes (Kabanov and Zezin, 1984). However, the binding of polycations with DNA is usually more efficient than their binding with globular proteins due to better alignment of the DNA and polycation ion pairs compared to protein and polycation ion pairs (Kabanov and Kabanov, 1995). As a result, DNA and polycation complexes are stable in the presence of the serum proteins (Vinogradov *et al.*, 1998; Oupicky *et al.*, 1999a).

The effects of proteins on the dispersion stability of the polyplexes can be more complicated. In the complexes formed by the polycation homopolymers under the excess of the polycations, the negatively charged protein molecules can interact with the positively charged corona, stabilizing polyplexes in the dispersion. Interactions of the low molecular mass electrolytes and serum proteins with the polycation corona can affect the stability of these systems in aqueous dispersion. As a result, these polyplexes are very sensitive to the media composition (Ogris *et al.*, 1998; Nguyen *et al.*, 2000). Very often these complexes aggregate in the presence of the serum proteins. Furthermore, their particle sizes are also sensitive to the mixing order of the DNA and polycation components both with and without serum. In contrast, block ionomer complexes are less sensitive to the order of mixing of the components and are stable in a variety of medium conditions, including the presence of serum proteins (Dash *et al.*, 2000; Nguyen *et al.*, 2000). The improved dispersion stability of these complexes is due to the steric stabilization effect of the hydrophilic nonionic chains that prevent the binding of the serum proteins. Low sensitivity of these complexes to added salts is explained by the electroneutrality of the complexes.

STRUCTURE AND PROPERTIES OF DNA IN THE COMPLEXES

Morphology and conformation in DNA/polycation complexes

A wide variety of multi- and polyvalent cations condense DNA into very compact forms, which commonly represent toroids of ca. 30 to 100 nm (Haynes *et al.*, 1970; Gosule and Schellman, 1976; Marx and Reynolds, 1982; Arscott *et al.*, 1990; Plum *et al.*, 1990; Wagner *et al.*, 1991; Tang and Szoka, 1997). DNA condensation is a result of a superposition of multiple interactions (Bloomfield, 1998). Condensation is opposed by the electrostatic repulsion of DNA charges, DNA bending contribution, effect of the excluded volume of DNA, and a decrease in the conformational entropy of DNA upon its collapse. Furthermore, hydration plays a complex role, which can affect DNA condensation (Leikin *et al.*, 1991). Compressive contributions might be due to the external osmotic pressure or poor solvent quality (Grosberg and Zhestkov, 1986), which explains why DNA condensation is promoted in concentrated polymer solutions as well as water-alcohol mixtures. According to a theoretical prediction by Manning (Manning, 1980, 1981), DNA condensation would occur spontaneously once effective charge neutralization was reached. This conclusion has recently been reinforced by experimental observation that individual DNA chains neutralized by cationic surfactants formed small toroids soluble in low-polar organic solvents, such as chloroform (Sergeyev *et al.*, 1997, 1999). These coils do not condense since the hydrophobically driven aggregation of the surfactant-neutralized chains is excluded in organic solvents. Complexes of synthetic polyanions with oppositely charged surfactants have the extended coil conformation under these conditions. The formation of toroids by DNA/surfactant complexes in organic solvents indicates that some 'driving force' for condensation may be reserved in an extended double helix itself, such as conformational tensions that are relaxed when the DNA is condensed.

Although toroids are the most common morphology in DNA condensation, different manipulations can produce various morphologies, including rods, spherical globules and fibrous networks (Bloomfield, 1998; Eickbush and Moudrianakis, 1978). In water-alcohol mixtures or in the presence of permethylated spermidine, as a condensing agent, a significant portion of rods have been observed along with the toroidal structures (Lang *et al.*, 1976; Plum *et al.*, 1990; Arscott *et al.*, 1990). The extended structures are often observed in the complexes formed between DNA and polycations conjugated with hydrophilic nonionic chains. For example, the formation of rod-shaped or worm-like particles has been reported for the complexes of DNA with cationic copolymers, such as PEO-*b*-PLL (Wolfert *et al.*, 1996), PEO-*g*-PLL (Banaszczyk *et al.*, 1999) or methoxypoly (ethylene glycol)-block-poly(L-lysine) dendrimer (PEO-*b*-*dendr*PLL) (Choi *et al.*, 1999). The formation of spheres was observed in the mixtures of DNA and PHPMA-*b*-PTMAEM (Wolfert *et al.*, 1996). Furthermore, worm-like and spherical structures were observed with PEO-*g*-PEI and Pluronic-*g*-PEI copolymers (Nguyen *et al.*, 2000). It was hypothesized that the steric repulsion of the PEO chains 'grafted' to the complex surface prevented the compaction of polycation-bound DNA into a toroidal structure (Nguyen *et al.*, 2000). Structures formed by DNA and cationic copolymers are critically dependent on the molecular characteristics of the copolymers, including density of grafting, length of the polymer segments, as well as hydrophobicity of the nonionic chains linked to the polycation (Wolfert *et al.*, 1999; Nguyen *et al.*, 2000; Howard *et al.*, 2000). In the case of complexes of DNA with Astramol™ poly(propyleneimine) dendrimers, the morphologies have been shown to depend on the dendrimer generation (Kabanov *et al.*, 2000). The dendrimers of low generation (G1, G2) formed mainly the extended coils, while the dendrimers of higher generation (G4, G5) formed both extended coils and compact particles. In addition, the extent of condensation and structures formed in DNA and polycation mixtures are usually affected by the composition of the mixture (Minagawa *et al.*, 1991; Wagner *et al.*, 1991). The complexes of plasmid DNA with the transferrin-PLL conjugate represented either dense toroids or larger structures with a dense core surrounded with DNA chains, depending on the polycation/DNA ratio (Wagner *et al.*, 1991). While several authors suggest that condensed DNA forms might contain only one or a few molecules (Bloomfield, 1998; Sergeyev *et al.*, 1999), it is quite possible that some of the structures described above are formed by multiple DNA chains (Tang and Szoka, 1997; Nguyen *et al.*, 2000).

The collapse of extended DNA chains commonly proceeds without dramatic changes in the local conformations of the double helix (Bloomfield, 1996). Many studies demonstrated that the B-conformation of the DNA is preserved upon its interaction with polycations (Maruyama *et al.*, 1998; Bronich *et al.*, 2001). However, the formation of the condensed DNA phases is commonly accompanied with a large increase in the magnitude of the positive or negative bands of the DNA CD spectrum (Shapiro *et al.*, 1969; Huey and Mohr, 1981). These condensed forms, designated as $\psi(+)$ or $\psi(-)$, depending on the changes of the CD spectrum, are characterized as cholesteric liquid crystalline phases and suggest long-range ordering of DNA strands (Huey and Mohr, 1981).

Stabilization of DNA secondary structures by polycations

In terms of physiological conditions, DNA exists almost totally in the double-helical conformation. Certain oligonucleotides also exhibit the ability to form triple-helixes with the DNA double strands. The stability of DNA secondary structures strongly depends on the environmental conditions, such as ionic strength, pH, temperature and solvents. Temperature is the most widely used environmental variable for the quantitative characterization of the helix-coil transitions. A commonly accepted characteristic of the thermal stability of DNA secondary structures is melting temperature, T_m. The binding of cationic species, such as multivalent cations, polyamines and polypeptides, has long been known to result in a substantial elevation of the melting temperatures for DNA duplexes (Von Hippel and McGhee, 1972). In general, DNA exhibits extended monophasic melting transitions in the presence of small multivalent cations such as spermidine (Thomas and Bloomfield, 1984), or trivalent cations (Plum *et al.*, 1990). This melting transition was attributed to a relatively weak, reversible binding of these cations to the DNA helix. In contrast, the melting behavior of DNA in the presence of polypeptides is usually biphasic and depends upon the methods of preparation of the complexes (Shapiro *et al.*, 1969; Inoue and Ando, 1970; Minagawa *et al.*, 1991). These systems commonly disproportionate below the saturation conditions, which results in the observation of the melting of the base pairs corresponding to the free and bound DNA. Overall, these studies were complicated by the precipitation of the complexes, particularly, in the conditions close to charge equivalence (Von Hippel and McGhee, 1972).

The development of cationic block and graft copolymers that form stable and transparent dispersions upon binding with the DNA allows investigating helix-coil transitions in the entire range of the compositions of the mixture. Particularly, the thermal stability of DNA duplexes is characterized for the complexes of DNA with PEO-*b*-PLL (Katayose and Kataoka, 1997), Dex-*g*-PLL (Maruyama *et al.*, 1998) and PEO-*g*-PEI (Bronich *et al.*, 2000a, 2001). These studies demonstrated significant elevation of the melting temperatures of the DNA duplexes, accompanied by a decrease in the cooperativity of the helix-coil transitions the presence of the copolymers. Like in the case of the complexes formed by PLL homopolymer, the melting curves of the complexes formed by PLL-based copolymers revealed biphasic behavior in the deficiency of the polycation, obviously due to the disproportionation. In contrast, some studies have shown that the monophasic melting transitions have been observed for PEO-*g*-PEI/poly[d(AT)]•poly[d(AT)] complexes that do not disproportionate (Bronich *et al.*, 2001). In this case, the stabilization effect could not be attributed to any substantial alteration of the base-pairing and base-pair stacking interactions in the polynucleotide duplex because the unfolding enthalpies were practically the same for the free and PEO-*g*-PEI bound DNA. Similar conclusions have been derived from the fact that the absorbance of the free DNA at 260 nm did not change upon binding of PEO-*g*-PEI. In contrast, the absorbance of DNA decreased upon binding of PLL (van Genderen *et al.*, 1990) and Dex-*g*-PLL (Maruyama *et al.*, 1998). Such behavior was attributed to a conformational change of the DNA to a dense globular structure triggered by the polycationic backbone (Maruyama *et al.*, 1998). Additionally, changes in the interior array of stacked base-pairs, due to incorporation of polycation into the grooves of DNA, might contribute to the change of its spectral characteristics (van Genderen *et al.*, 1990). PEI backbone has a higher conformational flexibility compared to the relatively rigid PLL molecules. Furthermore, in contrast to PLL, PEI does not form intramolecular secondary structures. This might explain why PEO-*g*-PEI causes less spatial-perturbation of the DNA duplex compared to the effect of the PLL-based copolymers.

Overall, the effects of polycations on the helix-coil transition of DNA are similar to those exhibited by the small cations: both of them induce thermal stabilization of DNA duplex and decrease the cooperativity of the helix-coil transition. In both cases the reasons for the stabilization effects are the screening of the negatively charged phosphate groups of the DNA, which reduces their electrostatic repulsion

(Schildkraut, 1965). However, the effective concentration of a simple salt at which the same stabilization effect is achieved is ca. 10^3 times higher than the effective concentrations of a polycation. Consequently, polycations provide for a much more efficient screening of the DNA phosphate groups than the small cations.

Pronounced stabilization of the DNA triplexes has also been observed in the presence of cationic oligopeptides and polyamines, such as spermine and spermidine (Hampel *et al.*, 1991; Thomas and Thomas, 1993; Potaman and Sinden, 1995). Recent work has reported that Dex-*g*-PLL significantly promotes DNA triplex formation under physiological pH and ionic conditions (Ferdous *et al.*, 1998). It is noteworthy that the stabilization effect was demonstrated for both purine and pyrimidine motif triplex DNA (Ferdous *et al.*, 1998). The pyrimidine triplexes are known to be extremely unstable at the physiological pH due to deprotonation of the cytosine bases. However, in the presence of Dex-*g*-PLL the association constant of the pyrimidine motif triplex increased about 100 times, which led to the formation of this triplex under physiological pH. Furthermore, this study demonstrated that triplex-promoting efficiency of the copolymer was considerably higher than that of spermine. This result suggests that the use of polyplex technology could provide a successful approach to create efficient triplex stabilizers.

Stabilization of DNA against nuclease digestion

Condensation of the DNA chains and masking of the DNA surface by the polycations usually decrease the rate of the enzymatic degradation. Indeed, it has been demonstrated that incorporation of DNA in various polyplexes decreases accessibility of the DNA to nucleases (Marx and Reynolds, 1982; Kabanov *et al.*, 1991; Katayose and Kataoka, 1998; Vinogradov *et al.*, 1998; Choi *et al.*, 1999; Oupicky *et al.*, 1999b; Harada *et al.*, 2001). This decreased accessibility results in a considerable increase in the stability of plasmid and oligonucleotide DNA in biological fluids. The extent of protection depends on the length of the polycation chain. For example, in the mixtures of plasmid DNA with PEO-*b*-PLL, having relatively short polymer segments, the degradation rate of DNA decreased with an increase in the degree of polymerization of the polycation (Katayose and Kataoka, 1998). Furthermore, in the case of nonstoichiometric DNA/polycation complexes, formed in the deficiency of the polycation, the nuclease resistance of the DNA strongly depended on the composition of the mixture (Kabanov *et al.*, 1991). In such systems, the kinetic curves of DNA degradation revealed two distinctive stages of digestion. The first stage involved rapid cleavage of DNA at the sites that were not covered by the polycation chains. The second stage consisted of slow restriction of the remaining DNA. Meanwhile, the products of restriction were found to be the same for both native and polycation-bound DNA. This result suggested that the bound polycation did not hinder specific recognition of the DNA chain by the nucleases but only decelerated the digestion process. This finding was in agreement with the well-known dynamic properties of the nonstoichiometric polyelectrolyte complexes. The polycation chains are not rigidly fixed on the DNA chains: they migrate from one DNA region to another opening the sites for restriction.

At these sites, the reaction rate is limited by vacation of the restriction sites due to the migration of the polycation from one DNA chain to another.

POLYION INTERCHANGE AND RECOGNITION PHENOMENA

Polyion interchange reactions in DNA containing complexes

Reactions of polyion interchange involve the transfer of the polyion chain, incorporated in the polymer complex, to another polyion present in the solution (Kabanov *et al.*, 1985). These processes are thermodynamically and kinetically controlled by the structure of the reacting species and environmental characteristics, including pH, ionic strength and temperature (Kabanov *et al.*, 1985; Izumrudov *et al.*, 1988; Harada and Kataoka, 1999a). Miller and Bach (1968) were the first to report that exchange reactions (Figure 9.5A) might occur in systems containing DNA complexes. The kinetic and equilibrium behavior in the interchange reactions involving DNA and synthetic polyions, poly(*N*-alkyl-4-vinylpyridinium) cation (PEVP), and polymethacrylate anion (PMA), have been studied in detail (Izumrudov *et al.*, 1995). This work examined the transfer of the polycation chains between two soluble nonstoichiometric polyelectrolyte complexes:

$$\text{Complex}\{\text{PEVP}\cdot\text{PMA}\} + \text{DNA} \rightleftharpoons \text{Complex}\{\text{PEVP}\cdot\text{DNA}\} + \text{PMA} \qquad (I)$$

This reaction was reversible: the equilibrium was attained irrespective of the order in which the reagents were mixed. The ionic strength and the nature of the salt present in solution strongly affected the reaction rate and position of equilibrium. In certain cases (e.g., the presence of lithium cations in the media) there was a

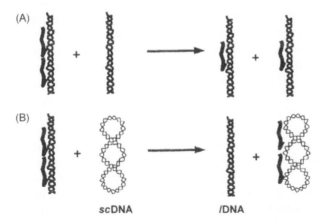

scDNA   *l*DNA

Figure 9.5 Reactions of polyion interchange: (A) polyion exchange resulting in uniform distribution of polycation among DNA chains; (B) polyion substitution resulting in recognition of the *sc*DNA and release of the *l*DNA in a free form.

marked difference in the directionality of reaction involving native and denatured DNA. This phenomenon was explained by the difference in the energy of electrostatic interaction of the counterions with the chains of native and denatured DNA (Izumrudov *et al.*, 1995). The position of equilibrium in the polyion interchange reactions is usually also sensitive to the structure and length of participating polyions (Izumrudov *et al.*, 1988; Harada and Kataoka, 1999a). Particularly, in the case of the reaction (I) it was found that the ability of DNA to displace PMA from {PEVP·PMA} complex was determined by the ratio of the lengths of the polyions (Izumrudov *et al.*, 1995). This behavior has been explained by the contribution of the entropy term in the free energy of the reaction. This contribution increases when the number of the polymer species formed in the process (I) increases. Consequently, for the complexes having the same overall composition the entropy term is a complex function of the ratio of the chains of the polyions involved in the reaction. For example, reaction (I) was examined under the conditions when the PMA chains were shorter than the PEVP chain. In this case, the decrease in the length of PMA resulted in the increase of the number of the free PMA chains released and the equilibrium in the reaction (I) was shifted to the right.

The use of cationic copolymers for the preparation of polyplexes recently facilitated the examination of the polyion interchange reactions, even at the stoichiometric conditions when these complexes formed stable dispersions. A number of studies suggested that various polyanions could displace DNA in the stoichiometric complexes formed by block and graft copolymers, such as PEO-*b*-PLL (Katayose and Kataoka, 1997, 1998), Dex-*g*-PLL (Maruyama *et al.*, 1998), PHPMA-*b*-PTMAEM (Oupicky *et al.*, 1999a) and PEO-*g*-PEI (Bronich *et al.*, 2000b). These studies suggested that hydrophilic nonionic polymer chains in the corona of the block ionomer complexes do not prevent the interaction and the transfer of the reacting polyions. However, it remains to be studied whether the length and the density of the nonionic polymer chains in the corona of the block ionomer complexes can affect the kinetics and equilibrium of the interchange reactions. The effects of the lengths of the polyion chains on the rate of interchange reactions in block ionomer complexes have been reported. Particularly, the rate of release of the DNA from PEO-*b*-PLL/DNA complex in the presence of potassium polyvinylsulfonate increased as the degree of polymerization of the PLL segment decreased (Katayose and Kataoka, 1998). While most of the studies so far have been conducted using synthetic polyanions for DNA displacement, the processes involving transfer of polycation between different polynucleotide molecules have also been reported. For example, the substitution of oligonucleotides from its complex with Dex-*g*-PLL by the excess of calf thymus DNA has been observed (Maruyama *et al.*, 1998). Furthermore, polyion interchange reactions involving double stranded DNA molecules with various structures and topologies, such as synthetic DNA, salmon testes DNA and plasmids were also studied for the block ionomer complexes formed by PEO-*b*-PVP and PEO-*g*-PEI (Bronich *et al.*, 2000b). First, the results of this study reinforced the conclusion that the DNA interchange reactions can proceed in the block ionomer complexes of various compositions, including stoichiometric complexes. Second, the mutual substitution of structurally different DNA molecules in the complexes has been documented. Finally, and probably most importantly, this study uncovered the phenomenon of recognition of a DNA tertiary structure by the polycation molecules during the reactions of the polyion interchange. The recognition phenomenon is discussed in greater detail in the next section.

Recognition of DNA topology by cationic copolymers

The effects of DNA topology in the reactions of polyion coupling and interchange were examined using the supercoiled and linearized forms of plasmid DNA (*sc*DNA and *l*DNA) (Bronich *et al.*, 2000b). Two cationic copolymers, PEO-*b*-PVP and PEO-*g*-PEI were compared in this study. Polyion exchange reactions were observed when *l*DNA was added to the {PEO-*g*-PEI·*sc*DNA} complex or *sc*DNA was added to the {PEO-*g*-PEI·*l*DNA} complex. In this system the direction of the reaction did not depend on the order of mixing of DNA samples, and PEO-*g*-PEI chains were evenly distributed between DNA chains. Totally different behavior was observed in the case of PEO-*b*-PVP. The *sc*DNA added to the {PEO-*b*-PVP·*l*DNA} complex displaced *l*DNA, which was released in the free form. In contrast, no release of the free *sc*DNA was observed when *l*DNA was added to the {PEO-*b*-PVP·*sc*DNA} complex. Therefore, the polyion exchange reaction involving *sc*DNA and *l*DNA complexes was shifted completely towards the formation of the {PEO-*b*-PVP·*sc*DNA} complex:

$$\text{Complex}\{\text{PEO-}b\text{-PVP}\cdot l\text{DNA}\} + sc\text{DNA} \rightarrow \text{Complex}\{\text{PEO-}b\text{-PVP}\cdot sc\text{DNA}\}$$
$$+ l\text{DNA} \qquad\qquad (\text{II})$$

In other words, the recognition of the supercoiled conformation of the DNA was achieved with PEO-*b*-PVP copolymer (Figure 9.5B). The recognition behavior was further demonstrated by adding the copolymers to the mixtures of *l*DNA and *sc*DNA. In this case, PEO-*b*-PVP selectively bound to *sc*DNA, while *l*DNA remained free. In contrast, PEO-*g*-PEI interacted with both forms of the DNA present in the mixture. The distinct behavior of the two copolymers was attributed to the differences in their structure, particularly to the charge density of the polycation segments. A relatively small variation in the polycation ionization state resulted in drastic changes in its behavior upon interaction with DNA. Particularly, the change of pH from 7.0 to 5.0 increased the charge density of PEI block in PEO-*g*-PEI and was also accompanied by the appearance of the recognition phenomena.

The dependence of the direction and equilibrium of the polyion coupling and interchange reactions on the charge density of the reacting species may be due to two major reasons. These reasons include: (i) the effect of the charge density of DNA on the release of counterions condensed with DNA, and; (ii) the effect of the charge density of cationic copolymer on the release of counterions condensed with DNA. It was suggested that the recognition phenomenon is dependent on electrostatic complementarity of the interacting chains. It is known that *sc*DNA has higher charge density than *l*DNA (Manning, 1978; Rolland and Tomlinson, 1996). Consequently, more counterions are condensed with *sc*DNA and can be released upon binding with the polycations. This binding should result in a more favorable interaction of polycations with *sc*DNA than with *l*DNA, i.e., topology recognition. Finally, the release of the counterions condensed with DNA can depend on the charge density of the copolymer. Indeed, it is possible that displacement of counterions condensed with DNA from the site of binding of a cationic copolymer with low charge density is incomplete. In other words, the system of salt bonds formed between DNA and the polycation block have 'mismatches' containing unpaired phosphates with some remaining condensed counterions. Conversely, polycation with high charge density, at the same number of salt bonds formed, should displace a greater portion of DNA counterions due to lower number of mismatches. As a result, the recognition phenomenon should be more pronounced in the case of polycations with high charge density, since a greater portion of the counterions condensed with the DNA are released in this case. In contrast, in the case of the polycations with low charge density the portion of the counterions released from the site of polycation binding with the DNA might be too low to provide for substantial distinction between the two forms of plasmid.

Overall, the polyion interchange reactions may play a significant role in the manifestation of the biological activity of the polyplexes (Kabanov and Kabanov, 1995). Particularly, these reactions may account for the release of the DNA in an active form inside cells. The finding of the phenomenon of recognition of a DNA tertiary structure by the synthetic polycation uncovers possibilities for the control of the DNA retention in the polyplexes, which may have practical significance in using these systems for gene delivery. Differences in the efficiency of the DNA release from polyplexes within the cell may be responsible for the dependence of the transgene expression on the topology of DNA, which was reported by some authors (Cherng *et al.*, 1999a). It is remarkable that topology recognition is achieved by using relatively simple chemical structures interacting with the DNA and can be controlled by small variations in the polycation ionization state. The refining of the structures of both the DNA and polycation components of the polyplexes may be useful for the optimization of the DNA incorporation and release behavior and, ultimately, can result in the improvement of the therapeutic effects of the current non-viral gene delivery systems.

CONCLUDING REMARKS

To be useful for gene delivery, polyplex systems should meet many requirements. First of all there should be a way for the efficient and complete incorporation of DNA in the complex. Second, the resulting complexes need to form stable dispersions of nanoscale size at the physiological values of pH and ionic strength. Third, this dispersion needs to be stable in the presence of macromolecular components of biological fluids. Fourth, the DNA chains incorporated into the polyplexes need to be protected from digestion by nucleases present in these fluids. Fifth, the polyplexes should be transported within the cell and DNA should be released there to exhibit its biological function. These requirements are by no means exhaustive and serve only as an illustration of the multiple properties of polyplexes that are essential for successful gene delivery. Each of these requirements relate to specific aspects of physicochemical behavior of DNA and polycation complexes. As discussed in this chapter, relevant physicochemical properties strongly depend on the structure of both polycation and the DNA components of the complexes. Although significant amount of data on polycation and DNA complexes has been accumulated during recent decades, these studies are far from complete. Specifically, the issues of the balance between the stability of the polyplexes in the extracellular media and efficiency of DNA release within the cell are poorly understood. Furthermore, new aspects have emerged as a result of the development of new polycation structures for gene delivery. These studies have resulted in the design of the polycations of different molecular architecture, including some more complex structures such as dendrimers and block and graft copolymers. It is unclear how the structure of these polymers will affect the performance of polyplexes. While many issues of performance of polyplexes as gene delivery systems should be addressed using relevant cellular and animal models the rational design of these systems is impossible without the knowledge of the fundamentals of their biophysical behavior. One should expect that successful gene therapy research in the future would employ multidisciplinary teams of investigators, which will be able to obtain a comprehensive picture accounting for all of biophysical, biochemical, and pharmaceutical aspects of gene delivery vectors.

ACKNOWLEDGMENTS

Our work cited in this review was supported in parts by NSF (BES-9712657, BES-9986393, DMR-9502807), Nebraska Research Initiative Gene Therapy Program, and Supratek Pharma Inc. AVK serves as a consultant to Supratek Pharma Inc. We are grateful to Prof. V.A. Kabanov (Moscow State University) and Prof. L.A. Marky (University of Nebraska Medical Center) for very fruitful discussions.

REFERENCES

Akiyama, Y., Harada, A., Nagasaki, Y. and Kataoka, K. (2000) Synthesis of poly(ethylene glycol)-block-poly(ethyleneimine) possessing an acetal group at the PEG end. *Macromolecules*, **33**, 5841–5845.

Arscott, P.G., Li, A.Z. and Bloomfield, V.A. (1990) Condensation of DNA by trivalent cations. 1. Effects of DNA length and topology on the size and shape of condensed particles. *Biopolymers*, **30**, 619–630.

Banaszczyk, M.G., Lollo, C.P., Kwoh, D.Y., Phillips, A.T., Amini, A., Wu, D.P., Mullen, P.M., Coffin, C.C., Brostoff, S.W. and Carlo, D.J. (1999) Poly-L-lysine-graft-PEG comb-type polycation copolymers for gene delivery. *J. Macromol. Sci., Pure Appl. Chem.*, **A36**, 1061–1084.

Benns, J.M., Choi, J.S., Mahato, R.I., Park, J.S. and Kim, S.W. (2000) pH-sensitive cationic polymer gene delivery vehicle: *N*-Ac-poly(l- histidine)-graft-poly(l- lysine) comb shaped polymer. *Bioconjug. Chem.*, **11**, 637–645.

Bloomfield, V.A. (1996) DNA condensation. *Curr. Opin. Struct. Biol.*, **6**, 334–341.

Bloomfield, V.A. (1998) DNA condensation by multivalent cations. *Biopolymers*, **44**, 269–282.

Boussif, O., Lezoualc'h, F., Zanta, M.A., Mergny, M.D., Sherman, D., Demeneix, B. and Behr, J.P. (1995) A versatile vector for gene and oligonucleotide transfer into cells in culture and *in vivo* – polyethyleneimine. *Proc. Natl. Acad. Sci. USA*, **92**, 7297–7301.

Bronich, T.K., Kabanov, A.V., Kabanov, V.A., Yu, K. and Eisenberg, A. (1997) Soluble complexes from poly(ethylene oxide)-block-polymethacrylate anions and *N*-alkylpyridinium cations. *Macromolecules*, **30**, 3519–3525.

Bronich, T.K., Nehls, A., Eisenberg, A., Kabanov, V.A. and Kabanov, A.V. (1999) Novel drug delivery systems based on the complexes of block ionomers and surfactants of opposite charge. *Colloids Surf. B*, **16**, 243–251.

Bronich, T.K., Kankia, B.I., Kabanov, A.V. and Marky, L.A. (2000a) A thermodynamic investigation of the interaction of polycations with DNA. *Polym. Prepr.*, **41**, 1611–1612.

Bronich, T.K., Nguyen, H.-K., Eisenberg, A. and Kabanov, A.V. (2000b) Recognition of DNA topology in reactions between plasmid DNA and cationic copolymers. *J. Am. Chem. Soc.*, **122**, 8339–8343.

Bronich, T.K., Popov, A.M., Eisenberg, A., Kabanov, V.A. and Kabanov, A.V. (2000c) Effects of block length and structure of surfactant on self-assembly and solution behavior of block ionomer complexes. *Langmuir*, **16**, 481–489.

Bronich, T.K., Kabanov, A.V. and Marky, L.A. (2001) A thermodynamic characterization of the interaction of a cationic copolymer with DNA. *J. Phys. Chem. B*, **105**, 6042–6050.

Cherng, J.Y., van de Wetering, P., Talsma, H., Crommelin, D.J. and Hennink, W.E. (1996) Effect of size and serum proteins on transfection efficiency of poly((2-dimethylamino) ethyl methacrylate)-plasmid nanoparticles. *Pharm. Res.*, **13**, 1038–1042.

Cherng, J.Y., Schuurmans-Nieuwenbroek, N.M., Jiskoot, W., Talsma, H., Zuidam, N.J., Hennink, W.E. and Crommelin, D.J. (1999a) Effect of DNA topology on the transfection efficiency of poly((2-dimethylamino)ethyl methacrylate)-plasmid complexes. *J. Control. Release*, **60**, 343–353.

Cherng, J.Y., van de Wetering, P., Talsma, H., Crommelin, D.J. and Hennink, W.E. (1999b) Stabilization of polymer-based gene delivery systems. *Int. J. Pharm.*, **183**, 25–28.

Chesnoy, S. and Huang, L. (1999) DNA condensed by polycations and lipids for gene transfer. *S.T.P. Pharma. Sci.*, **9**, 5–12.

Choi, J.S., Lee, E.J., Choi, Y.H., Jeong, Y.J. and Park, J.S. (1999) Poly(ethylene glycol)-block-poly(L-lysine) dendrimer: novel linear polymer/dendrimer block copolymer forming a spherical water-soluble polyionic complex with DNA. *Bioconjug. Chem.*, **10**, 62–65.

Choi, Y.H., Liu, F., Kim, J.-S., Choi, Y.K., Park, J.S. and Kim, S.W. (1998) Polyethylene glycol-grafted poly-L-lysine as polymeric gene carrier. *J. Contr. Release*, **54**, 39–48.

Dash, P.R., Read, M.L., Fisher, K.D., Howard, K.A., Wolfert, M., Oupicky, D., Subr, V., Strohalm, J., Ulbrich, K. and Seymour, L.W. (2000) Decreased binding to proteins and cells of polymeric gene delivery vectors surface modified with a multivalent hydrophilic polymer and retargeting through attachment of transferrin. *J. Biol. Chem.*, **275**, 3793–3802.

Eickbush, T.H. and Moudrianakis, E.N. (1978) The compaction of DNA helices into either continuous supercoils or folded-fiber rods and toroids. *Cell*, **13**, 295–306.

Felgner, P.L., Heller, M.J., Lehn, P., Behr, J.P. and Szoka, Jr., F.C. (eds) (1996) *Artificial Self-Assembling Systems for Gene Delivery*. Washington, D.C.: American Chemical Society.

Ferdous, A., Watanabe, H., Akaike, T. and Maruyama, A. (1998) Poly(l-lysine)-graft-dextran copolymer: amazing effects on triplex stabilization under physiological pH and ionic conditions (*in vitro*). *Nucleic Acids Res.*, **26**, 3949–3954.

Ferrari, S., Moro, E., Pettenazzo, A., Behr, J., Zacchello, F. and Scarpa, M. (1997) ExGen 500 is an efficient vector for gene delivery to lung epithelial cells *in vitro* and *in vivo*. *Gene Therapy*, **4**, 1100–1106.

Garnett, M.C. (1999) Gene-delivery systems using cationic polymers. *Crit. Rev. Ther. Drug Carrier Syst.*, **16**, 147–207.

Gebhart, C.L. and Kabanov, A.V. (2001) Evaluation of polyplexes as gene transfer agents. *J. Contr. Release*, **73**, 401–416.

Gosule, L.C. and Schellman, J.A. (1976) Compact form of DNA induced by spermidine. *Nature*, **259**, 333–335.

Grosberg, A.Y. and Zhestkov, A.V. (1986) On the compact form of linear duplex DNA: globular states of the uniform elastic (persistent) macromolecule. *J. Biomol. Struct. Dyn.*, **3**, 859–872.

Haensler, J. and Szoka, F.C. (1993) Polyamidoamine cascade polymers mediate efficient transfection of cells in culture. *Bioconjug. Chem.*, **4**, 372–379.

Hampel, K.J., Crosson, P. and Lee, J.S. (1991) Polyamines favor DNA triplex formation at neutral pH. *Biochemistry*, **30**, 4455–4459.

Harada, A. and Kataoka, K. (1995) Formation of polyion complex micelles in an aqueous milieu from a pair of oppositely-charged block copolymers with poly(ethylene glycol) segments. *Macromolecules*, **28**, 5294–5299.

Harada, A. and Kataoka, K. (1997) Formation of stable and monodispersive polyion complex micelles in aqueous medium from poly(L-lysine) and poly(ethylene glycol)-poly (aspartic acid) block copolymer. *J. Macromol. Sci., Pure Appl. Chem.*, **A34**, 2119–2133.

Harada, A. and Kataoka, K. (1998) Novel polyion complex micelles entrapping enzyme molecules in the core: preparation of narrowly-distributed micelles from lysozyme and poly(ethylene glycol)-poly(aspartic acid) block copolymer in aqueous medium. *Macromolecules*, **31**, 288–294.

Harada, A. and Kataoka, K. (1999a) Chain length recognition: core-shell supramolecular assembly from oppositely charged block copolymers. *Science*, **283**, 65–67.

Harada, A. and Kataoka, K. (1999b) Novel polyion complex micelles entrapping enzyme molecules in the core. 2. Characterization of the micelles prepared at nonstoichiometric mixing ratios. *Langmuir*, **15**, 4208–4212.

Harada, A., Togawa, H. and Kataoka, K. (2001) Physicochemical properties and nuclease resistance of antisense-oligodeoxynucleotides entrapped in the core of polyion complex micelles composed of poly(ethylene glycol)-poly(L-Lysine) block copolymers. *Eur. J. Pharm. Sci.*, **13**, 35–42.

Haynes, M., Garrett, R.A. and Gratzer, W.B. (1970) Structure of nucleic acid-poly base complexes. *Biochemistry*, **9**, 4410–4416.

Howard, K.A., Dash, P.R., Read, M.L., Ward, K., Tomkins, L.M., Nazarova, O., Ulbrich, K. and Seymour, L.W. (2000) Influence of hydrophilicity of cationic polymers on the biophysical properties of polyelectrolyte complexes formed by self-assembly with DNA. *Biochim. Biophys. Acta.*, **1475**, 245–255.

Huey, R. and Mohr, S.C. (1981) Condensed states of nucleic acids. III. psi(+) and psi(−) conformational transitions of DNA induced by ethanol and salt. *Biopolymers*, **20**, 2533–2552.

Inoue, S. and Ando, T. (1970) Interaction of clupeine with deoxyribonucleic acid. I. Thermal melting and sedimentation studies. *Biochemistry*, **9**, 388–394.

Izumrudov, V.A., Bronich, T.K., Saburova, O.S., Zezin, A.B. and Kabanov, V.A. (1988) The influence of chain length of a competitive polyanion and nature of monovalent counterions on the direction of the substitution reaction of polyelectrolyte complexes. *Makromol. Chem., Rapid Commun.*, **9**, 7–12.

Izumrudov, V.A., Kargov, S.I., Zhiryakova, M.V., Zezin, A.B. and Kabanov, V.A. (1995) Competitive reactions in solutions of DNA and water-soluble interpolyelectrolyte complexes. *Biopolymers*, **35**, 523–531.

Kabanov, A.V., Kiselev, V.I., Chikindas, M.L., Astafieva, I.V., Glukhov, A.I., Gordeev, S.A., Izumrudov, V.A., Zezin, A.B., Levashov, A.V., Severin, E.S. and Kabanov, V.A. (1989) Increasing of transforming activity of plasmid DNA by incorporating it into an interpolyelectrolyte complex with a carbon chain polycation. *Dokl. Akad. Nauk SSSR (in Russian)*, **306**, 226–229.

Kabanov, A.V., Astafyeva, I.V., Chikindas, M.L., Rosenblat, G.F., Kiselev, V.I., Severin, E.S. and Kabanov, V.A. (1991) DNA interpolyelectrolyte complexes as a tool for efficient cell transformation. *Biopolymers*, **31**, 1437–1443.

Kabanov, A.V., Astafieva, I.V., Maksimova, I.V., Lukanidin, E.M., Georgiev, G.P. and Kabanov, V.A. (1993) Efficient transformation of mammalian cells using DNA interpolyelectrolyte complexes with carbon chain polycations. *Bioconjug. Chem.*, **4**, 448–454.

Kabanov, A.V. and Kabanov, V.A. (1995) DNA complexes with polycations for the delivery of genetic material into cells. *Bioconjug. Chem.*, **6**, 7–20.

Kabanov, A.V., Vinogradov, S.V., Suzdaltseva, Y.G. and Alakhov, V.Y. (1995) Water-soluble block polycations as carriers for oligonucleotide delivery. *Bioconjug. Chem.*, **6**, 639–643.

Kabanov, A.V., Bronich, T.K., Kabanov, V.A., Yu, K. and Eisenberg, A. (1996) Soluble stoichiometric complexes from poly(*N*-ethyl-4-vinylpyridinium) cations and poly(ethylene oxide)-*block*-polymethacrylate anions. *Macromolecules*, **29**, 6797–6802.

Kabanov, A.V., Felgner, P.L. and Seymour, L.W. (eds.) (1998a) *Self-Assembling Complexes for Gene Delivery. From Laboratory to Clinical Trial.* Chichester, New York, Weinheim, Brisbane, Singapore, Toronto: John Wiley.

Kabanov, A.V., Szoka, F.C. and Seymour, L.W. (1998b) Interpolyelectrolyte complexes for gene delivery: polymer aspects of transfection activity. In: A.V. Kabanov, P.L. Felgner and L.W. Seymour (eds) *Self-assembling Complexes for Gene Delivery. From Laboratory to Clinical Trial.* Chichester, UK: John Wiley & Sons. pp. 197–218.

Kabanov, A.V. (1999) Taking polycation gene delivery systems from *in vitro* to *in vivo*. *Pharm. Sci. Tech. Today*, **2**, 365–372.

Kabanov, V.A., Zezin, A.B., Rogacheva, V.B. and Ryzhikov, S.V. (1982) Disproportionation of nonstoichiometric polyelectrolyte complexes in water-salt solutions. *Dokl. Akad. Nauk SSSR*, **267**, 862–865.

Kabanov, V.A. and Zezin, A.B. (1984) A new class of complex water-soluble polyelectrolytes. *Macromol. Chem. Phys. Suppl.*, **6**, 259–276.

Kabanov, V.A., Zezin, A.B., Izumrudov, V.A., Bronich, T.K. and Bakeev, K.N. (1985) Cooperative interpolyelectrolyte reactions. *Makromol. Chem. Suppl.*, **13**, 137–155.

Kabanov, V.A., Sergeyev, V.G., Pyshkina, O.A., Zinchenko, A.A., Zezin, A.B., Joosten, J.G.H., Brackman, J. and Yoshikawa, K. (2000) Interpolyelectrolyte complexes formed by DNA and Astramol poly(propyleneimine) dendrimers. *Macromolecules*, **33**, 9587–9593.

Kataoka, K., Togawa, H., Harda, A., Yasugi, K., Matsumoto, T. and Katayose, S. (1996) Spontaneous formation of polyion complex micelles with narrow distribution from antisense oligonucleotide and cationic copolymer in physiological saline. *Macromolecules*, **29**, 8556–8557.

Katayose, S. and Kataoka, K. (1997) Water-soluble polyion complex associates of DNA and poly(ethylene glycol)-poly(L-lysine) block copolymer. *Bioconj. Chem.*, **8**, 702–707.

Katayose, S. and Kataoka, K. (1998) Remarkable increase in nuclease resistance of plasmid DNA through supramolecular assembly with poly(ethylene glycol)-poly(L-lysine) block copolymer. *J. Pharm. Sci.*, **87**, 160–163.

Koh, J.J., Ko, K.S., Lee, M., Han, S., Park, J.S. and Kim, S.W. (2000) Degradable polymeric carrier for the delivery of IL-10 plasmid DNA to prevent autoimmune insulitis of NOD mice. *Gene Ther.*, **7**, 2099–2104.

Kukowska-Latallo, J.F., Bielinska, A.U., Johnson, J., Spindler, R., Tomalia, D.A. and Baker, Jr., J.R. (1996) Efficient transfer of genetic material into mammalian cells using Starburst polyamidoamine dendrimers. *Proc. Natl. Acad. Sci. USA*, **93**, 4897–4902.

Lang, D., Taylor, T.N., Dobyan, D.C. and Gray, D.M. (1976) Dehydrated circular DNA: electron microscopy of ethanol-condensed molecules. *J. Mol. Biol.*, **106**, 97–107.

Leikin, S., Rau, D.C. and Parsegian, V.A. (1991) Measured entropy and enthalpy of hydration as a function of distance between DNA double helices. *Phys. Rev. A*, **44**, 5272–5278.

Manning, G.S. (1978) The molecular theory of polyelectrolyte solutions with applications to the electrostatic properties of polynucleotides. *Q. Rev. Biophys.*, **11**, 179–246.

Manning, G.S. (1980) Thermodynamic stability theory for DNA doughnut shapes induced by charge neutralization. *Biopolymers*, **19**, 37–59.

Manning, G.S. (1981) The possibility of intrinsic local curvature in DNA toroids. *Biopolymers*, **20**, 1261–1270.

Maruyama, A., Ishihara, T., Kim, J.S., Kim, S.W. and Akaike, T. (1997) Nanoparticle DNA carrier with poly(L-lysine) grafted polysaccharide copolymer and poly(D,L-lactic acid). *Bioconjug. Chem.*, **8**, 735–742.

Maruyama, A., Watanabe, H., Ferdous, A., Katoh, M., Ishihara, T. and Akaike, T. (1998) Characterization of interpolyelectrolyte complexes between double- stranded DNA and poly-lysine comb-type copolymers having hydrophilic side chains. *Bioconjug. Chem.*, **9**, 292–299.

Marx, K.A. and Reynolds, T.C. (1982) Spermidine-condensed phi X174 DNA cleavage by micrococcal nuclease: torus cleavage model and evidence for unidirectional circumferential DNA wrapping. *Proc. Natl. Acad. Sci. USA*, **79**, 6484–6488.

Marx, K.A. and Reynolds, T.C. (1983) Ion competition and micrococcal nuclease digestion studies of spermidine-condensed calf thymus DNA. Evidence for torus organization by circumferential DNA wrapping. *Biochim. Biophys. Acta*, **741**, 279–287.

Miller, I.R. and Bach, D. (1968) Interaction of DNA with heavy metal ions and polybases: cooperative phenomena. *Biopolymers*, **6**, 169–179.

Minagawa, K., Matsuzawa, Y., Yoshikawa, K., Matsumoto, M. and Doi, M. (1991) Direct observation of the biphasic conformational change of DNA induced by cationic polymers. *FEBS Lett.*, **295**, 67–69.

Nguyen, H.K., Lemieux, P., Vinogradov, S.V., Gebhart, C.L., Guerin, N., Paradis, G., Bronich, T.K., Alakhov, V.Y. and Kabanov, A.V. (2000) Evaluation of polyether-polyethyleneimine graft copolymers as gene transfer agents. *Gene Ther.*, **7**, 126–138.

Nishiyama, N., Yokoyama, M., Aoyagi, T., Okano, T., Sakurai, Y. and Kataoka, K. (1999) Preparation and characterization of self-assembled polymer-metal complex micelle from *cis*-dichlorodiammineplatinum(II) and poly(ethylene glycol)-poly(α,β-aspartic acid) block copolymer in an aqueous medium. *Langmuir*, **15**, 377–383.

Ogris, M., Steinlein, P., Kursa, M., Mechtler, K., Kircheis, R. and Wagner, E. (1998) The size of DNA/transferrin-PEI complexes is an important factor for gene expression in cultured cells. *Gene Ther.*, **5**, 1425–1433.

Ogris, M., Brunner, S., Schuller, S., Kircheis, R. and Wagner, E. (1999) PEGylated DNA/transferrin-PEI complexes: reduced interaction with blood components, extended circulation in blood and potential for systemic gene delivery. *Gene Ther.*, **6**, 595–605.

Oupicky, D., Konak, C., Dash, P.R., Seymour, L.W. and Ulbrich, K. (1999a) Effect of albumin and polyanion on the structure of DNA complexes with polycation containing hydrophilic nonionic block. *Bioconjug. Chem.*, **10**, 764–772.

Oupicky, D., Konak, C. and Ulbrich, K. (1999b) DNA complexes with block and graft copolymers of N-(2-hydroxypropyl)methacrylamide and 2-(trimethylammonio)ethyl methacrylate. *J. Biomater. Sci. Polym. Ed.*, **10**, 573–590.

Papisov, I.M. and Litmanovich, A.A. (1989) Molecular recognition in interpolymer interactions and matrix polymerization. *Adv. Polym. Sci.*, **90**, 139–179.

Plum, G.E., Arscott, P.G. and Bloomfield, V.A. (1990) Condensation of DNA by trivalent cations. 2. Effects of cation structure. *Biopolymers*, **30**, 631–643.

Potaman, V.N. and Sinden, R.R. (1995) Stabilization of triple-helical nucleic acids by basic oligopeptides. *Biochemistry*, **34**, 14885–14892.

Ramsay, E., Hadgraft, J., Birchall, J. and Gumbleton, M. (2000) Examination of the biophysical interaction between plasmid DNA and the polycations, polylysine and polyornithine, as a basis for their differential gene transfection *in-vitro*. *Int. J. Pharm.*, **210**, 97–107.

Read, M.L., Dash, P.R., Clark, A., Howard, K.A., Oupicky, D., Toncheva, V., Alpar, H.O., Schacht, E.H., Ulbrich, K. and Seymour, L.W. (2000) Physicochemical and biological characterization of an antisense oligonucleotide targeted against the bcl-2 mRNA complexed with cationic-hydrophilic copolymers. *Eur. J. Pharm. Sci.*, **10**, 169–177.

Record, M.T., Jr., Lohman, M.L. and De Haseth, P. (1976) Ion effects on ligand-nucleic acid interactions. *J. Mol. Biol.*, **107**, 145–158.

Rolland, A. and Tomlinson, E. (1996) Controllable gene therapy using nonviral systems. In: P.L. Felgner, M.J. Heller, P. Lehn, J.P. Behr and F.C. Szoka Jr. (eds). *Artificial Self-Assembling Systems for Gene Delivery*. American Chemical Society, Washington, D.C., pp. 86–100.

Rolland, A. (ed.) (1999) *Advanced Gene Delivery: From Concepts to Pharmaceutical Products.* Amsterdam: Harwood.

Ross, P.D. and Shapiro, J.T. (1974) Heat of interaction of DNA with polylysine, spermine, and Mg^{++}. *Biopolymers*, **13**, 415–416.

Roy, S., Zhang, K., Roth, T., Vinogradov, S., Kao, R.S. and Kabanov, A. (1999) Reduction of fibronectin expression by intravitreal administration of antisense oligonucleotides. *Nat. Biotechnol.*, **17**, 476–479.

Schildkraut, C. (1965) Dependence of the melting temperature of DNA on salt concentration. *Biopolymers*, **3**, 195–208.

Sergeyev, V.G., Pyshkina, O.A., Gallyamov, M.O., Yaminsky, I.V., Zezin, A.B. and Kabanov, V.A. (1997) DNA-surfactant complexes in organic media. *Prog. Colloid Polym. Sci.*, **106**, 198–203.

Sergeyev, V.G., Pyshkina, O.A., Lezov, A.V., Mel'nikov, A.B., Ryumtsev, E.I., Zezin, A.B. and Kabanov, V.A. (1999) DNA complexed with oppositely charged amphiphile in low-polar organic solvents. *Langmuir*, **15**, 4434–4440.

Shapiro, J.T., Leng, M. and Felsenfeld, G. (1969) Deoxyribonucleic acid-polylysine complexes. Structure and nucleotide specificity. *Biochemistry*, **8**, 3119–3132.

Stuart, M.A.C., Besseling, N.A.M. and Fokkink, R.G. (1998) Formation of micelles with complex coacervate cores. *Langmuir*, **14**, 6846–6849.

Sukhishvili, S.A., Obol'skii, O.L., Astaf'eva, I.V., Kabanov, A.V. and Yaroslavov, A.A. (1993) DNA-containing interpolyelectrolyte complexes: interaction with liposomes. *Polymer Sci. (translated from Vysokomol. Soedin.)*, **35**, 1602–1606.

Tang, M. and Szoka, F.C. (1997) The influence of polymer structure on the interactions of cationic polymers with DNA and morphology of the resulting complexes. *Gene Therapy*, **4**, 823–832.

Thomas, T. and Thomas, T.J. (1993) Selectivity of polyamines in triplex DNA stabilization. *Biochemistry*, **32**, 14068–14074.

Thomas, T.J. and Bloomfield, V.A. (1984) Ionic and structural effects on the thermal helix-coil transition of DNA complexed with natural and synthetic polyamines. *Biopolymers*, **23**, 1295–1306.

Toncheva, V., Wolfert, M.A., Dash, P.R., Oupicky, D., Ulbrich, K., Seymour, L.W. and Schacht, E.H. (1998) Novel vectors for gene delivery formed by self-assembly of DNA with poly(L-lysine) grafted with hydrophilic polymers. *Biochim. Biophys. Acta*, **1380**, 354–368.

van Genderen, M.H., Hilbers, M.P., Koole, L.H. and Buck, H.M. (1990) Peptide-induced parallel DNA duplexes for oligopyrimidines. Stereospecificity in complexation for oligo(L-lysine) and oligo(L-ornithine). *Biochemistry*, **29**, 7838–7845.

Vinogradov, S., Batrakova, E., Li, S. and Kabanov, A. (1999a) Polyion complex micelles with protein-modified corona for receptor-mediated delivery of oligonucleotides into cells. *Bioconjug. Chem.*, **10**, 851–860.

Vinogradov, S.V., Bronich, T.K. and Kabanov, A.V. (1998) Self-assembly of polyamine-poly(ethylene glycol) copolymers with phosphorothioate oligonucleotides. *Bioconjug. Chem.*, **9**, 805–812.

Vinogradov, S., Batrakova, E. and Kabanov. A. (1999b) Poly(ethylene glycol)-polyethyleneimine NanoGel™ particles: novel drug delivery systems for antisense oligonucleotides. *Colloids and Surfaces B: Biointerfaces*, **16**, 291–304.

Von Hippel, P.H. and McGhee, J.D. (1972) DNA-protein interactions. *Annu. Rev. Biochem.*, **41**, 231–300.

Wagner, E., Cotten, M., Foisner, R. and Birnstiel, M.L. (1991) The effect of polycations on the structure of the complex and DNA delivery to cells. *Proc. Natl. Acad. Sci. USA*, **88**, 4255–4259.

Wolfert, M.A., Schaht, E.H., Tonceva, V., Ulbrich, K., Nazarova, O. and Seymour, L.W. (1996) Characterization of vector for gene therapy formed by self-assembly of DNA with synthetic block copolymers. *Human Gene Ther.*, **7**, 2123–2133.

Wolfert, M.A., Dash, P.R., Nazarova, O., Oupicky, D., Seymour, L.W., Smart, S., Strohalm, J. and Ulbrich, K. (1999) Polyelectrolyte vectors for gene delivery: influence of cationic polymer on biophysical properties of complexes formed with DNA. *Bioconjug. Chem.*, **10**, 993–1004.

Wu, G.Y. and Wu, C.H. (1987) Receptor-mediated *in vitro* gene transformation by a soluble DNA carrier system. *J. Biol. Chem.*, **262**, 4429–4432.

Yaroslavov, A.A., Sukhishvili, S.A., Obolsky, O.L., Yaroslavova, E.G., Kabanov, A.V. and Kabanov, V.A. (1996) DNA affinity to biological membranes is enhanced due to complexation with hydrophobized polycation. *FEBS Lett.*, **384**, 177–180.

Zhang, W., Bond, J.P., Anderson, C.F., Lohman, T.M. and Record, Jr., M.T. (1996) Large electrostatic differences in the binding thermodynamics of a cationic peptide to oligomeric and polymeric DNA. *Proc. Natl. Acad. Sci. USA*, **93**, 2511–2516.

10 Structure and structure-activity correlations of cationic lipid/DNA complexes: supramolecular assembly and gene delivery

Cyrus R. Safinya, Alison J. Lin,
Nelle L. Slack and Ilya Koltover

INTRODUCTION

Following the initial publication of the papers by Felgner *et al.* (1987) and Huang *et al.* (1991), the entire field of gene therapy based on synthetic nonviral delivery systems has enjoyed a renaissance of sorts (Chesnoy and Huang, 2000; Nabel *et al.*, 1993; Miller, 1998). In addition, other groups have demonstrated gene expression *in vivo* in targeted organs (Zhu *et al.*, 1993; Anwer *et al.*, 2000) and in human clinical trials (Nabel *et al.*, 1993; Noone *et al.*, 2000; Laitinen *et al.*, 2000). Felgner *et al.* (1987) hypothesized that cationic liposomes (CLs), when mixed with DNA to form (CL/DNA) complexes with an overall positive charge, should lead to enhanced transfection compared to other synthetic vectors – such as cationic polymers and peptides – because of the enhanced stability and electrostatic interactions between cationic CL/DNA and anionic plasma membranes of mammalian cells. Compared to polymer and peptide-based delivery systems, cationic liposomes tend to mediate higher transfection in most cell lines studied to date.

One of the principle advantages of nonviral over viral methods for gene delivery is the potential of transfecting large pieces of cDNA into cells. The proof of this concept has been clearly demonstrated when partial sections of first-generation human artificial chromosomes (HACs) of order 1 Mbp were transferred into cells with CLs, however inefficiently (Harrington *et al.*, 1997; Wilard, 2000). The future development of HAC vectors will be important for gene therapy applications. Because of their large cDNA insertion capacity HACs would have the ability of delivering not only entire human genes (in many cases exceeding 100 k bp) but also their regulatory sequences which are needed for the spatial and temporal regulation of expression. The development of efficient HAC vectors in the future is a long-range goal in studies designed to characterize chromosome structure and function.

While the transfection efficiencies in many cells have been found to be enhanced using CL/DNA complexes compared to other more traditional nonviral delivery systems, the mechanism of transfection via cationic liposomes remains largely unknown (Zabner *et al.*, 1995; Coonrod *et al.*, 1997; Mortimer *et al.*, 1999). At present, hundreds of plasmid DNA molecules are required for successful gene transfer and expression. The low transfection efficiencies with nonviral methods result from a general lack of knowledge regarding: (i) the structures of CL/DNA complexes, and; (ii) their interactions with cell membranes and events leading to release of DNA in the cytoplasm for delivery within the nucleus. It has only been recently that comprehension of the structures of CL/DNA complexes in different lipid membrane systems has begun (Lasic *et al.*, 1997; Raedler *et al.*, 1997; Salditt *et al.*, 1997; Koltover *et al.*, 1998; Koltover *et al.*, 1999; Salditt *et al.*, 1998). The transfection efficiencies of nonviral delivery methods may be improved through insights into transfection-related mechanisms at the molecular and self-assembled levels. Thus, it is important to elucidate the structures of supramolecular assemblies of CL/DNA complexes and to relate the relevant components of the structure to transfection efficiency.

As described in this chapter, recent synchrotron X-ray diffraction (XRD) has led to the discovery that the supramolecular assembly of CL/DNA complexes may lead to two distinctly different structures (Raedler *et al.*, 1997; Koltover *et al.*, 1998). High resolution small-angle X-ray diffraction has revealed that the structures are different from the hypothesized 'bead-on-string' structure originally proposed by Felgner *et al.* (1987) for CL/DNA complexes in their seminal paper. In this paper the DNA strand decorated with distinctly attached cationic liposomes is pictured. The first type of self-assembled structure, observed in DNA complexed with cationic liposomes consisting of mixtures of neutral (so called 'helper-lipid') dioleoylphosphatidylcholine (DOPC) and cationic lipid dioleoyl trimethylammonium propane (DOTAP), is referred to as the lamellar L_α^C phase of CL/DNA complexes (Figure 10.1, Left) (Raedler *et al.*, 1997; Salditt *et al.*, 1997; Koltover *et al.*, 1999; Salditt *et al.*, 1998), where a multilayer phase of DNA is sandwiched between bilayer membranes. The second type of self-assembled structure, also derived from synchrotron X-ray diffraction experiments (Koltover *et al.*, 1998), consists of DNA strands coated by cationic lipid monolayers and arranged on a 2D inverted hexagonal lattice (H_{II}^C), as shown in Figure 10.1 (right). Two distinct membrane-altering pathways are found to induce the transition from the L_α^C to the H_{II}^C: one where the spontaneous curvature $1/R_o$ of the lipid monolayer is driven negative by the addition of the neutral helper lipid dioleoylphosphatidylethanolamine (DOPE), and another involving a new class of helper lipids consisting of DOPC diluted with co-surfactant molecules, which lowers the membrane bending rigidity κ. The lamellar L_α^C phase and the inverted hexagonal H_{II}^C phase of CL/DNA complexes is also observed with plasmid DNA containing reporter genes (Lin *et al.*, 2000).

LAMELLAR L_α^C PHASE OF CL/DNA COMPLEXES

A recent XRD study of CL/DNA complexes has revealed that the addition of linear lambda-phage DNA (48,502 bp, contour length $= 16.5\,\mu m$) (Raedler *et al.*, 1997) or plasmid DNA (Lin *et al.*, 2000) to binary mixtures of cationic liposomes (mean diameter of 70 nm), consisting of mixtures of neutral lipid DOPC and cationic DOTAP, induces a topological transition from liposomes into collapsed condensates in the form of optically birefringent liquid crystalline (LC) globules with sizes on the order of 1 μm.

Figure 10.2 (A) shows differential interference contrast (DIC) optical images of CL/DNA complexes at four lipid (L) to λ-DNA (D) ratios {L = DOTAP + DOPC(1: 1)}. Similar images are observed with λ-DNA replaced by the pBR322 plasmid (4361 bp)

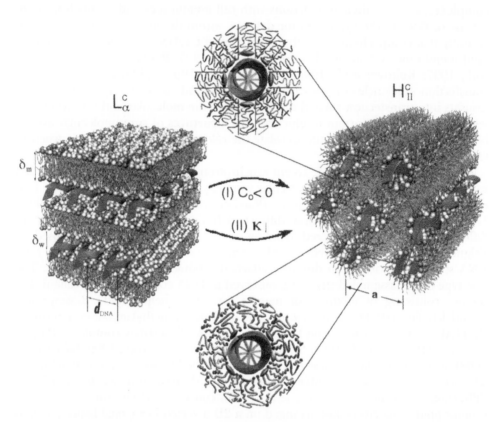

Figure 10.1 Schematic of two distinct pathways from the lamellar L_α^C phase to the columnar inverted hexagonal H_{II}^C phase of cationic liposome/DNA (CL/DNA) complexes. Along Pathway I the natural curvature $C_o = 1/R_o$ of the cationic lipid mono-layer is driven negative by the addition of the helper-lipid DOPE. This is shown schematically (middle top) where the cationic lipid DOTAP is cylindrically shaped while DOPE is cone-like leading to the negative curvature. Along path-way II the L_α^C to H_{II}^C transition is induced by the addition of a new class of helper-lipids consisting of mixtures of DOPC and the cosurfactant hexanol, which reduces the membrane bending rigidity. (*see Color Plate 8*)

DNA. At low DNA concentrations (Figure 10.2A, L/D = 50), in contrast to the pure liposome solution where no objects $> 0.2\,\mu m$ are seen, $1\,\mu m$ large globules are observed. The globules coexist with excess liposomes. As more DNA is added, the globular condensates to form larger chain like structures (Figure 10.2A, L/D = 10). At L/D ≈ 5 the chain-like structures flocculate into large aggregates of distinct globules. For L/D < 5 the complex size is smaller and stable in time again (Figure 10.2A, L/D = 2), and the complexes coexist with excess DNA. Fluorescence micro-scopy of the DNA (labeled with YOYO) and the lipid {labeled with *N*-(Texas Red®) sulfonyl)-1,2-dihexadecanoyl-*sn*-glycero-3-phosphoethanolamine tetraethylammo-nium salt (Texas Red-DHPE)} also shows that the individual globules contain both lipid and DNA. Polarized microscopy also shows that the distinct globules are birefringent, indicating their liquid crystalline nature.

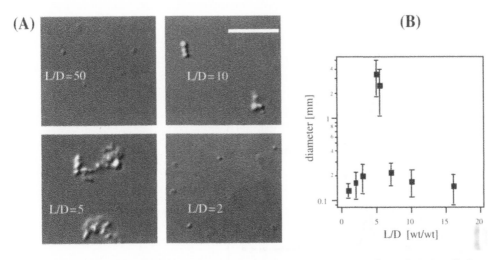

Figure 10.2 (A) High-resolution DIC optical images of CL/DNA complexes forming distinct condensed globules in mixtures of different lipid to DNA weight ratio (L/D). L/D = 4.4 is the isoelectric point, CL/DNA complexes are positively charged for L/D = 50 and 10, and negatively charged for L/D = 2. The positive (negative) regime contains excess lipid (DNA). (B) Average size of the lipid–DNA complexes measured by dynamic light scattering. Bar is 10 μm (Adapted from Raedler *et al.*, 1997).

The size dependence of the complexes as a function of L/D (Figure 10.2B) is measured by dynamic light scattering. The size dependence of the aggregates can be understood in terms of a charge-stabilized colloidal suspension. The charge of the complexes is measured by their electrophoretic mobility in an external electric field. For L/D > 5 (Figure 10.2A; L/D = 50 or 10) the complexes are positively charged, while for L/D < 5 (Figure 10.2A; L/D = 2) the complexes are negatively charged. The charge reversal is in good agreement with the stoichiometrically expected charge balance of the components DOTAP and DNA at L/D ≈ 4.4 (Wt./Wt.) where L = DOTAP + DOPC in equal weights. Thus, the positively and negatively charged globules at L/D = 50 and L/D = 2, respectively, repel each other and remain separate, while as L/D approaches 5 the nearly neutral complexes collide and tend to stick due to van der Waals attraction.

The precise structural nature of the CL/DNA complexes is elucidated in high resolution synchrotron small-angle X-ray scattering (SAXS) experiments carried out at the Stanford Synchrotron Radiation Laboratory (Raedler *et al.*, 1997; Salditt *et al.*, 1997, 1998; Koltover *et al.*, 1999; Lin *et al.*, 2000). Figure 10.3 shows SAXS scans of dilute DOPC/DOTAP – λ-DNA mixtures at the isoelectric point of the complex, where the cationic charge from DOTAP is equal to the anionic charge from DNA. In these experiments the total lipid concentration (L = DOTAP+ DOPC) is increased between L/D = 2.2 and 8.8 (wt./wt.) at the isoelectric point (DOTAP/DNA = 2.20). Equivalently, the weight fraction (Φ_{DOPC}) of DOPC in the DOPC/DOTAP cationic liposome mixtures increases from 0 to 0.75. We see in Figure 10.3 that at $\Phi_{DOPC} = 0.5$ (L/D = 4.4) two sharp peaks are evident at

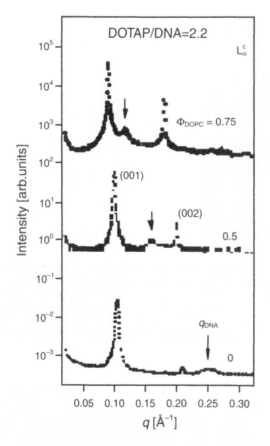

Figure 10.3 SAXS scans of CL/DNA complexes at constant DOTAP/DNA = 2.2 (at the isoelectric point) with increasing DOPC/DOTAP which shows the DNA peak (arrow) moving towards smaller q as L/D (and Φ_{DOPC}) increases. L = DOTAP + DOPC, D = DNA (Adapted from Raedler *et al.*, 1997; Koltover *et al.*, 1999).

$q = 0.099$ and $0.198 \, \text{Å}^{-1}$ which correspond to the (00L) peaks of a layered structure with an interlayer spacing d $(= \delta m + \delta w)$ in the range of $64 \, \text{Å}$. The membrane thickness and the water gap are denoted by δm and δw, respectively (Figure 10.1, left). The middle broad peak q_{DNA} arises from DNA–DNA correlations and gives $d_{DNA} = 2\pi/q_{DNA} = 39 \, \text{Å}$. Thus, the SAXS data lead to a model where the cationic liposomes and DNA condense into a multilayer structure with DNA sandwiched between the bilayers (Figure 10.1, left, denoted L_α^C).

In the absence of DNA, the lamellar L_α phase with membranes comprised of DOPC and cationic lipid DOTAP (1:1) exhibits strong long-range interlayer electrostatic repulsions that overwhelm the van der Waals attraction (Roux and Safinya, 1988; Safinya, 1989). The interlayer spacing d is given by the simple geometric relation $d = \delta_m/(1 - \Phi_W)$ (Φ_W is the volume fraction of water). From d $(= 2\pi/q_{00L})$ at a given Φ_W, we obtain $\delta_m = 39 \pm 0.5 \, \text{Å}$ for membranes with $\Phi_{DOPC} = 0.5$. The DNA that condenses on the CLs screens the electrostatic interaction between lipid

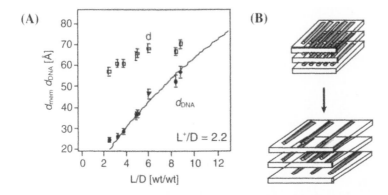

Figure 10.4 (A) The DNA interaxial distance d_{DNA} and the interlayer distance d in the L_α^C phase (Figure 10.2) plotted as a function of Lipid/DNA (L/D) (wt/wt) ratio at the isoelectric point of the complex DOTAP/DNA = 2.2. d_{DNA} is seen to expand from 24.5 Å to 57.1 Å. The solid line through the data is the prediction of a packing calculation where the DNA chains form a space filling one-dimensional lattice. (B) Schematic drawing of DNA-membrane multilayers showing the increase in distance between DNA chains as the membrane charge density is decreased (i.e., as Φ_{DOPC} increases) at the isoelectric point (Adapted from Raedler *et al.*, 1997; Koltover *et al.*, 1999).

bilayers and leads to condensed multilayers. The average thickness of the water gap $\delta_w = d - \delta_m = 64\text{Å} - 39\text{Å} = 26\text{Å}$ is just sufficient to accommodate one monolayer of B-DNA (diameter ≈ 20), including a hydration shell.

The SAXS scans in Figure 10.3, (arrow points to the DNA peak) show that $d_{DNA} = 2\pi/q_{DNA}$ increases with lipid dilution from 24.54 Å to 57.1 Å as the membrane charge density decreases with increasing Φ_{DOPC} between 0 and 0.75 (or equivalently increasing L/D between 2.2 and 8.8). The most compressed interaxial spacing of 24.55 Å at $\Phi_{DOPC} = 0$ approaches the short-range repulsive hard-core interaction of the B-DNA rods containing a hydration layer (Podgornik *et al.*, 1994). Figure 10.4A plots d and d_{DNA} as a function of L/D. The observed behavior is depicted schematically in Figure 10.4B showing that as neutral lipid is added and the membrane charge density decreases at the isoelectric point, the DNA chains also decrease their negative charge density by increasing the DNA inter-chain spacing. The solid line in Figure 10.4A is derived from the simple geometric–packing relationship $d_{DNA} = (A_D/\delta_m)(\rho_D/\rho_L)$ (L/D) which equates the cationic charge density (due to the mixture DOTAP$^+$ and DOPC) with the anionic charge density (due to DNA$^-$). Here, $\rho_D = 1.7$ g/cc and $\rho_L = 1.07$ g/cc denote the densities of DNA and lipid respectively, δ_m the membrane thickness, and A_D the DNA area. $A_D = Wt(\lambda)/(\rho_D L(\lambda)) = 186\text{Å}^2$, $Wt(\lambda) = $ weight of λ-DNA $= 31.5*10^6/(6.022*10^{23})$g and $L(\lambda) = $ contour length of λ-DNA $= 48502*3.4$ Å.

The agreement between the packing relationship (solid line) with the data over the measured interaxial distance from 24.5 Å to 57.1 Å (Figure 10.4A) is quite remarkable given the fact that there are no adjustable parameters. The variation in the interlayer spacing d ($= \delta_w + \delta_m$) (Figure 10.4A, open squares) arises from the increase in the membrane bilayer thickness δ_m as L/D increases (each DOPC

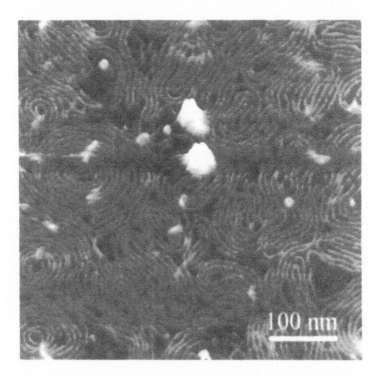

Figure 10.5 High resolution Atomic Force Microscopy image of plasmid DNA adsorbed on a cationic bilayer (DPTAP) coating a freshly cleaved mica surface. The highly packed DNA chains are clearly visible. The measured width of DNA is 2 nm, close to the diameter of B-DNA (Adapted from Mou *et al.*, 1995; Fang and Yang, 1997).

molecule is about 4–6 Å longer than a DOTAP molecule). The variation in the DNA interaxial distance as a function of the lipid to DNA (L/D) ratio in multilayers (Figure 10.4A) unambiguously demonstrates that X-ray diffraction directly probes the DNA behavior in multilayer assemblies. From the line widths of the DNA peaks (Figure 10.3), the 1D lattice of DNA chains is found to consist of domains extending to nearly 10 neighboring chains (Salditt *et al.*, 1997, 1998). This is consistent with observations (Mou *et al.*, 1995; Fang and Yang, 1997) by atomic force microscope (AFM) imaging of DNA adsorbed on a cationic solid lipid bilayer supported on freshly cleaved mica surfaces (Figure 10.5). The success of this AFM preparation is in the direct observation of the periodic helical modulation of the double-stranded DNA molecules measured to be 3.4 nm, which is consistent with the pitch of B-DNA (Mou *et al.*, 1995; Fang and Yang, 1997). Thus, the CL/DNA complex is self-assembled into a new 'hybrid' phase of matter, namely, a two-dimensional smectic phase of DNA chains coupled to a three-dimensional smectic phase of lipid bilayers.

The DNA–lipid condensation can be understood to occur as a result of the release of 'bound' counterions in solution as shown in Figure 10.6. DNA in solution has a bare length l_o between negative charges (phosphate groups), where $l_o = 1.7$Å. This measurement is substantially less than the Bjerrum length in water, $l_B = 7.1$ Å,

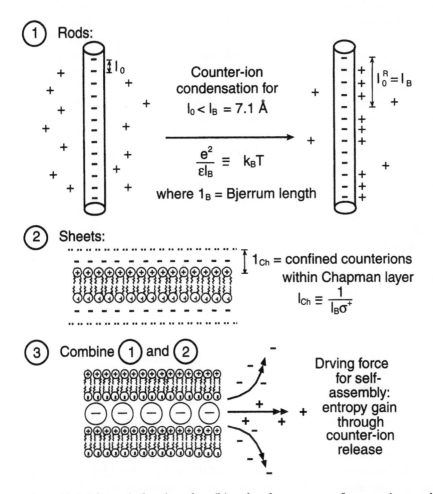

Figure 10.6 Schematic drawings describing the phenomenon of counter-ion condensation near charged rods (1) and sheets (2) and the resulting counter-ion release as the rods and sheets form a complex (3). (1) Schematic of double stranded DNA molecule with a bare distance between negative charges of $l_0 = 1.7 \text{Å}$. From non-linear Poisson-Boltzmann we know that positive counterions condense on DNA until the renormalized distance between the negative charges l_0^R equals the Bjerrum length which is $l_B = 7.1 \text{Å}$ in water. (2) Schematic of a charged lipid bilayer with counter-ions confined within the Chapman layer. (3) Schematic drawing showing that as DNA condenses onto the cationic membrane there is a simultaneous release of counterions and a gain in the entropy of solution when the previously condensed counterions (Na^+ on DNA and Cl^{-1} near the cationic liposome membrane) leave the immediate vicinity of DNA and the cationic membrane respectively.

which corresponds to the distance where the Coulomb energy between two unit charges is equal to the thermal energy $k_B T$. A non-linear Poisson-Boltzmann analysis shows that counterions will condense on the DNA backbone until the Manning parameter $\xi = l_B/l_0^R$ approaches 1 (Manning, 1969), where l_0^R is the renormalized distance between negative charges after counter ion condensation.

A similar analysis shows that counterions also condense near the surface of two-dimensional membranes within the Gouy-Chapman layer $l_{CH} = 1/l_B\sigma^+$, where σ^+ is the membrane charge density (Zimm and Bret, 1983). Through DNA-lipid condensation the cationic lipid tends to fully neutralize the phosphate groups on the DNA, in effect replacing and releasing the originally condensed counterions in solution. Thus, the driving force for higher order self-assembly is the release of counter ions, which are originally one-dimensionally bound to DNA and two-dimensionally bound to cationic membranes into solution.

A series of theoretical papers have recently investigated the structure and thermodynamic stability of CL/DNA complexes (May and Ben-Shaul, 1997; Dan, 1998; Bruinsma, 1998; Bruinsma and Mashl, 1998; Harries *et al.*, 1998; O'Hern and Lubensky, 1998; Golubovic and Golubovic, 1998). Analytical and numerical studies of DNA–DNA interactions bound between membranes show the existence of a novel long-range repulsive electrostatic interaction (Bruinsma, 1998; Bruinsma and Mashl, 1998; Harries *et al.*, 1998). Theoretical work on CL/DNA complexes has also led to the realization of a variety of novel new phases of matter in DNA–lipid complexes (O'Hern and Lubensky, 1998; Golubovic and Golubovic, 1998). In particular, a novel new 'sliding columnar phase', is predicted, where the positional coherence between DNA molecules in adjacent layers is lost without destroying orientational coherence of the chains from layer to layer.

THE INVERTED HEXAGONAL PHASE OF CATIONIC LIPOSOME/DNA COMPLEXES: PATHWAYS FROM LAMELLAR PHASE

The existence of a completely different columnar inverted hexagonal H_{II}^C liquid-crystalline state in CL/DNA complexes (Figure 10.1, right) has been unambiguously demonstrated for the first time using synchrotron small-angle x-ray diffraction. It is found that the commonly used helper-lipid DOPE induces the L_α^C to H_{II}^C structural transition by controlling the spontaneous radius of curvature R_o of the lipid layers (Figure 10.1, pathway I). Further, an entirely new class of helper molecules has been introduced that controls the lipid layer rigidity κ and gives rise to a distinctly different pathway to the H_{II}^C phase (Figure 10.1, pathway II).

The transition from lamellar to the inverted hexagonal phase of complexes along pathway I is shown in SAXS scans in Figure 10.7 for positively charged CL/DNA complexes at DOTAP/DNA (wt./wt.) = 3 as a function of increasing Φ_{DOPE} (weight fraction of DOPE) in the DOPE/DOTAP cationic liposome mixtures (Koltover *et al.*, 1998). The internal structure of the complex changes completely with increasing DOPE/DOTAP ratios. SAXS data of complexes with $\Phi_{DOPE} = 0.26$ and 0.70 clearly show the presence of two different structures. At $\Phi_{DOPE} = 0.26$ SAXS of the lamellar L_α^C complex shows sharp peaks at $q_{001} = 0.099\,\text{Å}^{-1}$ and $q_{002} = 0.198\,\text{Å}^{-1}$ resulting from the lamellar periodic structure ($d = 2\pi/q_{001} = 63.47\,\text{Å}$), with DNA intercalated between cationic lipid analogous to the structure in DOPC/DOTAP–DNA complexes (Figure 10.1, left).

For $0.7 < \Phi_{PE} < 0.85$, the peaks of the SAXS scans of the CL/DNA complexes index perfectly on a two-dimensional (2D) hexagonal lattice with a unit cell spacing of $a = 4\pi/[(3)^{0.5}q_{10}] = 67.4\,\text{Å}$ for $\Phi_{DOPE} = 0.7$. Figure 10.7 at $\Phi_{DOPE} = 0.7$ shows

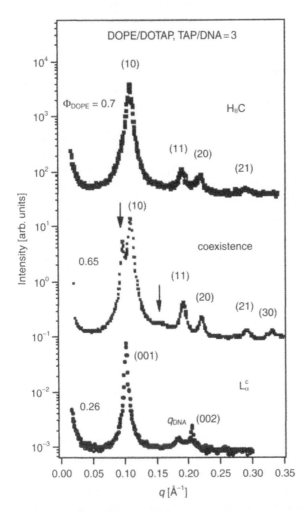

Figure 10.7 Synchrotron SAXS patterns of the lamellar L_α^C and columnar inverted hexagonal H_{II}^C phases of positively charged CL/DNA complexes as a function of increasing weight fraction Φ_{DOPE}. At $\Phi_{DOPE} = 0.41$, the SAXS results from a single phase with the lamellar L_α^C structure shown in Figure 10.5. At $\Phi_{DOPE} = 0.7$, the SAXS scan results from a single phase with the columnar inverted hexagonal H_{II}^C structure shown in Figure 10.9. At $\Phi_{DOPE} = 0.65$, the SAXS shows coexistence of the L_{II}^C (arrows) and H_{II}^C phases (Adapted from Koltover *et al.*, 1998).

the first four order Bragg peaks of this hexagonal structure at $q_{10} = 0.107\,\text{Å}^{-1}$, $q_{11} = 0.185\,\text{Å}^{-1}$, $q_{20} = 0.214\,\text{Å}^{-1}$, and $q_{21} = 0.283\,\text{Å}^{-1}$. Thus, the structure is consistent with a two-dimensional columnar inverted hexagonal structure where the DNA molecules are surrounded by a lipid monolayer with the DNA/lipid inverted cylindrical micelles arranged on a hexagonal lattice (Figure 10.1, right). The structure resembles that of the inverted hexagonal H_{II} phase of pure DOPE in excess water (Seddon, 1989), with the water space inside the lipid micelle filled by

DNA. Assuming once more an average lipid monolayer thickness of $20\,\text{Å}$, the diameter of the micellar void in the H_{II}^C phase is close to $28\,\text{Å}$, again sufficient for a DNA molecule with approximately two hydration shells. For $\Phi_{DOPE} = 0.65$, the L_α^C and H_{II}^C structures coexist as shown in Figure 10.7 (arrows point to the [001] and q_{DNA} peaks of the L_α^C phase) and are nearly epitaxially matched with $a \approx d$. For $\Phi_{DOPE} > 0.85$, the H_{II}^C phase coexists with the H_{II} phase of pure DOPE which has peaks at $q_{10} = 0.0975\,\text{Å}^{-1}$, $q_{11} = 0.169\,\text{Å}^{-1}$, $q_{20} = 0.195\,\text{Å}^{-1}$ with a unit cell spacing of $a = 74.41\,\text{Å}$.

The L_α^C to H_{II}^C phase transition can be induced along a second pathway II (Figure 10.1) by the use of a novel new 'helper lipid mixture'. As a function of increasing hexanol a structural transition is observed in the H_{II}^C phase. To understand the L_α^C to H_{II}^C transition qualitatively along the two pathways (I and II of Figure 10.1), we consider the interplay between the electrostatic and membrane elastic interactions in the complexes. Pure electrostatic interactions are expected to favor the H_{II}^C phase which minimizes the charge separation between the anionic groups on the DNA chain and the cationic lipids (May and Ben-Shaul, 1997). The electrostatic interaction may be resisted by the Helfrich elastic cost (per unit area) of forming a cylindrical monolayer membrane around DNA: $F/A = 0.5\kappa(1/R - 1/R_o)^2$. Here, κ is the lipid monolayer rigidity, R the radius of curvature, and R_o the natural radius of curvature. Along pathway I (Figure 10.1) the membrane consists of the two components DOTAP and DOPE. Cationic DOTAP has a natural curvature $C_o^{DOTAP} = 1/R_o^{DOTAP} = 0$; that is, membranes of pure DOTAP are known to favor the lamellar L_α phase. However, DOPE has a negative natural curvature $C_o^{DOPE} = 1/R_o^{DOPE} < 0$; that is, DOPE has a larger area per two chains than area per head group (Figure 10.1, center top). Pure DOPE in water forms the inverted hexagonal H_{II} phase (Seddon, 1989). Thus, along pathway I the natural curvature of the monolayer mixture of DOTAP and DOPE is driven negative with $C_o = 1/R_o = \Phi_{DOPE}^V C_o^{DOPE}$, where Φ_{DOPE}^V is the volume fraction of DOPE in the lipid mixture monolayer. Hence, as a function of increasing Φ_{DOPE} we expect a softening of the elastic cost of monolayer deformation and the transition to the H_{II}^C phase favored by the electrostatic interactions, as experimentally observed.

Pathway II (Figure 10.1) involves a subtle mechanism and introduces an entirely new class of helper-lipids to the field of nonviral gene therapy. Along this pathway the membrane bending rigidity κ is reduced significantly because of the addition of the membrane-soluble co-surfactant molecule hexanol. Co-surfactant molecules, when mixed in with longer chain 'true' surfactants, can lead to dramatic changes in interface elasticities (Safinya *et al.*, 1989), although they are unable to stabilize an interface separating hydrophobic and hydrophilic regions. Experimental studies have shown that the addition of hexanol to membranes of lamellar phases with a mole ratio of between two to four will lead to a significant decrease of the bending rigidity κ from about 20 k_BT to about 2–5 k_BT. Simple compressional models of surfactant chains show that κ scales with chain length l_n ($\propto \delta_m$, membrane thickness, n = number of Carbons per chain) and the area per lipid chain A_L as $\kappa \propto l_n^3/A_L^5$ (Szleifer *et al.*, 1990). Hexanol affects both l_n and A_L shown schematically in Figure 10.1 (center bottom). First, the membrane thickness δ_m decreases upon addition of the shorter tail co-surfactant molecule hexanol (C_6 chain) to the mixture of DOPC and DOTAP (C_{18} chains). Secondly, the addition of a significant amount of short hexanol chains to the long chains (from DOPC and DOTAP) effectively results in a sudden excess free volume and a significantly larger area per lipid chain. These results will lead to a further strong suppression of κ, making the membrane highly flexible. Thus, a reduction of the elastic cost of curving the membrane due to the reduction of κ, leading to the formation of the H_{II}^C phase favored by the electrostatic interactions and experimentally observed, is expected.

INTERACTIONS BETWEEN LAMELLAR L_α^C AND INVERTED HEXAGONAL H_{II}^C PHASE OF CL/DNA COMPLEXES AND ANIONIC GIANT LIPOSOMES MIMICKING THE CELL PLASMA MEMBRANE

This section will underscore the importance of self-assembled structures to biological function. It is known that transfection efficiency mediated by mixtures of cationic lipids and so-called neutral 'helper-lipids' varies widely and unpredictably (Felgner *et al.*, 1994; Remy *et al.*, 1994). The choice of the helper-lipid has been empirically established to be important. For example, transfection of mammalian cell cultures is efficient in (1:1 and 1:2) mixtures of DOTAP and the neutral helper lipid DOPE, and not in (1:1 and 1:2) mixtures of DOTAP and a similar helper-lipid DOPC (Farhood *et al.*, 1995; Hui *et al.*, 1996). Cationic liposomes comprised of DOPC/DOTAP complexed with DNA form the lamellar (L_α^C) phase (Figure 10.1, left). This formation is seen in quantitative transfection detection carried out using the pGL3-control vector plasmid encoding Luciferase driven by the SV40 promoter-enhancer. Figure 10.8 shows transfection results for the same mixture of DOTAP-containing negative (below dashed line) and positive (above dashed line) complexes as a function of DOTAP/DNA. It can be seen that the DOPE containing complexes are significantly more efficient than CLs with DOPC for the weight fractions of 0.72. DOPE has a high tendency to form the hexagonal phase at acidic pH, whereas DOPC has no such activity (Felgner *et al.*, 1994). Thus, it appears that in (1:1 and 1:2) mixtures of DOTAP/DOPE and DOTAP/DOPC the H_{II}^C phase leads to much higher transfection efficiency than the L_α^C phase of CL/DNA complexes.

To understand why the H_{II}^C phase transfects better than the L_α^C phase in this lipid mixture regime (1:1 and 1:2) the interaction of CL/DNA complexes must be investigated with giant anionic vesicles (G-vesicles) which are models of CL/DNA complex – anionic endosomal vesicles of cells. Recent experiments indicate that the main entry route to the cytoplasm is through endocytosis, where a local inward deformation of the cell plasma membrane leads to a budding off of an internal vesicle forming the early stage endosome (Zabner *et al.*, 1995; Wrobel and Collins, 1995; Legendre and Szoka, 1992; Lin *et al.*, 2000). Thus, at the very early stages of cell transfection, an intact CL/DNA complex is captured inside an endosome, which is known to contain anionic lipids.

In both the H_{II}^C and the L_α^C phases the complexes appear as highly dynamic birefringent aggregates when viewed with video-enhanced optical microscopy in differential interference contrast (DIC) and fluorescence configurations as shown in Figure 10.9A for H_{II}^C ($\Phi_{DOPE} = 0.73$) and Figure 10.9B for L_α^C ($\Phi_{DOPE} = 0.3$) complexes along pathway I (Figure 10.1). The positive complexes (with $\rho = $ DOTAP/DNA $= 3$ [wt./wt.]) are seen to form aggregates consisting of connected blobs, with the aggregates becoming smaller and eventually dissociating

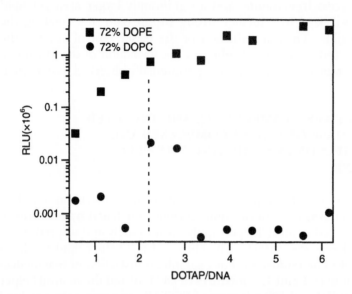

Figure 10.8 Luciferase reporter gene (pGL3-control vector) activity measured in transfected fibroblast L-cells. Transfection efficiencies for positive (DOTAP/DNA > 2.2) and negative (DOTAP/DNA <2.2) CL/DNA complexes. The squares are for DOPE/DOTAP CLs (72% DOPE), the circles are for DOPC/DOTAP CLs (72% DOPC). Cells were transfected with 2 μg of DNA and varying amounts of lipid in 24-well plates where each well had a diameter of 15 mm. 10^6 RLU (relative light units) corresponds to 0.025 ng of luciferase. Background (instrument noise level) done with a control containing no complex is 10 RLU (Adapted from Lin *et al.*, 2000).

into individual blobs with an increasing complex charge. Figure 10.9A shows the distribution of lipid fluorescence (middle) and DNA fluorescence (right) of the same CL/DNA complex in the H_{II}^C phase and Figure 10.9B shows the analogous results for a CL/DNA complex in the L_α^C phase. The observed overlap of lipid and DNA distributions and the precisely identical morphologies in the two fluorescence modes shows that the complexes are indeed highly compact objects with a close association of lipid and DNA consistent with the SAXS data. At these concentrations and volume fractions of DOPE the complexes coexist with excess DNA for $\rho < 2.2$ and with excess lipid when $\rho > 2.2$. Also, the presence of macroscopic lipid aggregates is not observed, which indicates that the only condensed liquid crystalline structures in the CL/DNA mixtures are complexes.

There is a striking difference between positively charged H_{II}^C and L_α^C complexes in their interaction with model anionic lipid membranes even when both types of structures contain DOPE. We show in Figure 10.9 (C and D) typical micrographs of positively charged ($\rho = 4$) complexes attached to the fluid membranes of G-vesicles. The L_α^C (C) complexes attached to the anionic membrane remain stable. The compact complex morphology can be seen in DIC (left) as well as in the lipid (C, middle) and DNA (C, right) fluorescence. Clearly there is no fusion between the complex and the G-vesicle. H_{II}^C complexes behave differently upon attaching to the G-vesicle, rapidly fusing and spreading with it and losing their compact structure

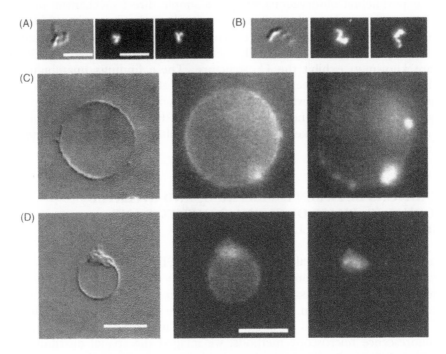

Figure 10.9 Video-microscopy images of positively charged CL/DNA complexes in the (A) H_{II}^C and (B) L_α^C phases, and interacting with negatively charged giant (G) vesicles (C and D). In all cases, complexes were viewed in (DIC) (left), lipid fluorescence (middle), and DNA fluorescence (right). The scale bar for DIC is 3 μm for (A) and (B), and 20 μm for (C) and (D). Fluorescence image is 6 μm for (A) and (B) and 20 μm for (C) and (D). In (C) the L_α^C complexes simply stick to the G-vesicle and remain stable for many hours, retaining their blob-like morphology. The blobs are localized in DIC as well as lipid and DNA fluorescence modes. In (D), the H_{II}^C complexes break up and spread immediately after attaching to G-vesicles, indicating a fusion process between the complex and the vesicle lipid bilayer and release of DNA. The loss of the compact structure of the complex is evident in both lipid and DNA fluorescence modes. (Adapted from Koltover *et al.*, 1998.)

(Figure 10.9D left, DIC). Since the amount of lipid in the complex is comparable with that in the G-vesicle, and since the fusion occurs very quickly, it results in the formation of multiple free lamella which are observed to undergo bilayer fluctuations. The loss of the compact complex structure and the subsequent desorption of DNA molecules from membrane and their Brownian motion between the lamella are seen in fluorescence (Figure 10.9D, right). This behavior is expected following fusion, which results in the mixing of cationic lipid (from the complex) with anionic lipid (from the G-vesicle), effectively 'turning off' the electrostatic interactions (which gave rise to the compact CL/DNA complexes) and releasing DNA molecules *inside* the space between the lamellae and the G-vesicle bilayer. Since the geometry is the inverse of CL/DNA complexes inside anionic endosomal vesicles it is expected, that upon fusion the inverse geometry will occur with DNA released and expelled *outside* the endosome within the cytoplasm.

These experimental observations suggest a simple direct mechanism of DNA release from endosomal membranes into the cytoplasm that is consistent with the higher transfection efficiencies in mammalian cell cultures reported empirically in CL/DNA complexes containing DOPE compared to those containing DOPC, which are known to exhibit the L_α^C structure. These findings unambiguously establish a correlation between the self-assembled structures of CL/DNA complexes and their interactions with model membranes of cellular organelles, paving the way for a fundamental understanding of the early-stage events following the uptake of CL/DNA complexes by mammalian cells in nonviral gene therapy applications.

INTERACTIONS BETWEEN LAMELLAR L_α^C AND INVERTED HEXAGONAL H_{II}^C PHASE OF CL/DNA COMPLEXES AND MOUSE FIBROBLAST CELLS

To date, there are few optical imaging data on CL/DNA complexes inside cells. Biochemical functional data on transfection efficiency cannot independently elucidate the molecular and self-assembled mechanisms involved in the transfer of the complex to the nuclear region. Direct imaging *in vitro* should allow for the elucidation of the various pathways between the plasma membrane and the nucleus. Using fluorescence microscopy methods, we imaged the spatial distribution of complexes at different fixed times in the animal cell. Figure 10.10 shows the optical micrographs where L_α^C CL/DNA complexes were allowed to interact with mouse fibroblast cells for one hour, followed by the fixing of the transfected cells in 1x PBS solution containing 0.1% glutaraldehyde and 4% formaldehyde. Fluorescence labeling of both lipid and DNA allowed for the visualization of complexes, and the lipid was labeled with Texas Red-DHPE (red emission) and the DNA with YOYO-1

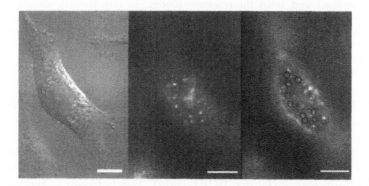

Figure 10.10 Images of mouse fibroblast L-cells mixed with positively charged (L/D = 10) CL/DNA complexes with the L_α^C structure (50%DOPC-50%DOTAP-βgal DNA) and fixed one hour after the transfection experiment. Left: DIC image of transfected cell attached to glass. The positions of the complexes are visualized inside the cells through double-fluorescence, which shows both the YOYO-DNA green fluorescence (center) and the Texas-Red-DHPE (lipid tag) (right). Matching dots imply a complex (e.g., circles in right) (Adapted from Lin *et al.*, 2000).

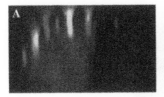 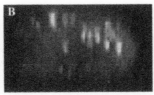 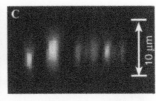

Figure 10.11 Laser scanning 3-dimensional confocal images of mouse L-cells mixed with positively charged CL/DNA complexes with the L_α^C structure (50%DOPC-50%DOTAP-βgal DNA) and fixed one hour after the transfection. Side views looking inside cell. Green is DNA, red is lipid, and the overlap yellow is CL/DNA complex. (A) done at 4 °C (inhibits endocytosis), shows excess lipid and complexes outside on cell surface. (B) done at 37 °C, shows complexes (yellow), DNA aggregates (green blobs), and lipid aggregates (red) inside cell. The large green background in (A) and (B) is due to YOYO not covalently linked to DNA. (C) done at 37 °C, CL/DNA complexes (yellow), lipid aggregates (red) inside cells. The DNA is covalently labeled (Mirus Label IT^{TM}) to reduce the background seen in A and B. (*see Color Plate 9*)

(green emission). Figure 10.10 (left) shows the cells in (DIC). The complexes inside the cell were identified by simultaneously observing the green fluorescence of YOYO-DNA (Figure 10.10, center) and the red fluorescence of Texas Red-DHPE (Figure 10.10, right). The presence of numerous complexes where the two dyes coincide spatially was clearly evident.

Laser scanning three-dimensional confocal images, shown in Figure 10.11 of a similar preparation, enabled us to visualize the complexes inside the cell (B and C). The images showed CL/DNA complexes (yellow) and excess lipid (red), and DNA aggregates (green blobs) in B, which was indicative of DNA that has dissociated from the complex. Our confocal microscopy data also supported other reports (Zabner *et al.*, 1995; Wrobel and Collins, 1995; Legendre and Szoka, 1992) where endocytosis is a major cell entrance route. For example, when transfection was carried out at 4 °C to inhibit endocytosis, the complexes and excess lipid were seen to be mostly attached to the outer plasma membrane surface (Figure 10.11A). It should be noted that positively charged CL/DNA complexes always coexist with excess lipid. The diffuse green background in (A) and (B) was due to YOYO that have escaped from the complexes into the nuclei (YOYO does not attach covalently to DNA). To reduce the background, a recently available DNA marker (Mirus Label IT^{TM}, green emission) was used, which attaches covalently to the DNA in the CL/DNA complex (Figure 10.11C). These preliminary experiments demonstrated that the double-fluorescence technique will allow the imaging of position of CL/DNA complexes inside the cell at different times.

Figure 10.12 shows optical micrographs similar to Figure 10.10 but with H_{II}^C CL/DNA complexes incorporating DOPE. The behavior with H_{II}^C complexes is clearly different where the fusion of lipid with the cell plasma membrane (right, black arrow) was observed. Following endocytosis the H_{II}^C self-assembly enters the cell inside an anionic endosomal vesicles. It may then fuse with the endosomal membrane either completely or partially, releasing DNA into the cytosol. Released lipid from the CL/DNA (both cationic and helper-lipid) would be expected to mix with

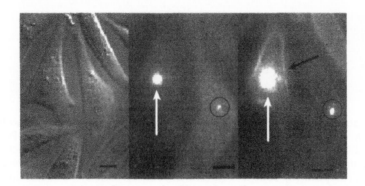

Figure 10.12 Images of mouse fibroblast L-cells mixed with positively charged (L/D = 10) CL/DNA complexes with the H_{II}^C structure (50%DOPE-50%DOTAP-βgal DNA) and fixed for one hour in 1X PBS containing 0.1% glutaraldehyde and 4% formaldehyde after the transfection experiment. Left: DIC image of transfected cells attached to glass. The center is in the YOYO-DNA green fluorescence mode and the Texas-Red-DHPE (lipid tag) in the right. The lipid is seen to have fused with the plasma membrane (right, black arrow). The white arrows (center and right) show the presence of aggregated clusters of CL/DNA complexes. A few isolated complexes are also seen (black circles) (Adapted from Lin *et al.*, 2000).

the plasma membrane (which acts like a large reservoir for free lipid), producing the fused image (Figure 10.12, right).

CONCLUDING REMARKS

There is a growing interest in understanding the nanoscale structures of supramolecular assemblies of nonviral gene delivery systems and in elucidating a relationship between the nano-structure and transfection efficiency. The low transfection efficiencies of synthetic vectors result from our poor understanding of the mechanisms of gene transfer at the molecular and self-assembled levels. A clear understanding between structure and function is necessary to significantly advance the state and reliability of clinical trials with synthetic vectors. Distinct structures have been discovered, including a multilamellar structure with DNA monolayers sandwiched between lipid bilayers, and an inverted hexagonal structure with DNA coated by cationic lipid monolayers and arranged on a two-dimensional lattice. Significantly, recent optical imaging combined with transfection data has revealed that the mechanisms of gene release from complexes in the cell cytoplasm are dependent on the nature of the self-assemblies at the nanoscale.

Direct optical microscopy imaging has revealed that in contrast to the nontransfectant L_α^C complexes, which bind stably to giant anionic vesicles, the transfectant H_{II}^C complexes are unstable upon adhering to vesicles, rapidly fusing and releasing DNA. These observations underscore the importance of structure to 'early-stage' gene delivery mechanisms and provide striking direct experimental support at the microscopic length scale for a mechanism of DNA escape from anionic endosomal vesicles. Anionic endosomal vesicles are generally regarded as the first barrier to the efficient transfection subsequent to the endocytic uptake of CL/DNA complexes by mammalian cells.

DOPE containing CL/DNA complexes in mammalian cell cultures exhibit the H_{II}^C structure rather than the L_α^C found in DOPC containing complexes. As revealed by optical microscopy, L_α^C complexes remained stable inside cells and attached to giant anionic vesicles, whereas H_{II}^C complexes showed fusion of their lipid with the mouse fibroblast cell membranes (Figure 10.12) or giant anionic vesicles that results in DNA release.

Important future goals include discovering all possible self-assembled structures in CL/DNA complexes and achieving an understanding, at the molecular and self-assembled levels, of the critical parameters that control the different structures. Furthermore, it will be crucial to relate the structures to biological function, namely, the interactions of CL/DNA complexes with cellular components inside animal cells which lead to DNA release and gene expression. The broad, long-term objective of this research is to develop a fundamental science base, which will lead to the design and synthesis of optimal nonviral carriers of DNA for gene therapy and disease control. Simultaneously, a major long-term objective is to improve efficiency for delivering large pieces of DNA containing important human genes and their regulatory sequences (>100 k-base pairs), which at present can only be achieved with synthetic vectors. The structure-function data obtained from the research should allow us to begin the formidable task of a rational design of these self assemblies for enhanced gene delivery applications from the ground up, beginning with the chemical structure of the lipids and the correct compositions in mixtures, including functional plasmid.

ACKNOWLEDGEMENTS

We gratefully acknowledge our collaborators Joachim Raedler and Tim Salditt. We would also like to acknowledge Cyril George and Charles Samuel. We have benefited through discussions with Leaf Huang, Philip Felgner, Fyl Pincus, Robin Bruinsma, Tom Lubensky, Bill Gelbart and Avinoam Ben-Shaul. Supported by National Institutes of Health R01 GM59288 and the National Science Foundation DMR-9972246. Also supported by a University of California Biotechnology Research and Education Program Training Grant 99-14 and a Los Alamos-UC collaborative grant CULAR STB-UC:99-216. The synchrotron X-ray experiments carried out at the Stanford Synchrotron Radiation Laboratory were supported by the US. DOE. The Materials Research Laboratory at Santa Barbara is supported by NSF-DMR-0080034.

REFERENCES

Anwer, K., Meaney, C., Kao, G., Hussain, N., Shelvin, R., Earls, R.M. *et al.* (2000) Cationic lipid-based delivery system for systemic cancer gene therapy. *Cancer Gene Ther.*, **7**, 1156–1164.
Bruinsma, R. (1998) Electrostatics of DNA cationic lipid complexes: isoelectric instability. *Eur. Phys. J. B*, **4**, 75–88.

Bruinsma, R. and Mashl, J. (1998) Long-range electrostatic interaction in DNA cationic lipid complexes. *Europhys. Lett.*, **41**(2), 165–170.

Chesnoy, S. and Huang, L. (2000) Structure and function of lipid-DNA complexes for gene delivery. *Annu. Rev. Biophys. Biomol. Struct.*, **29**, 27–47.

Coonrod, A., Li, F.Q. and Horwitz, M. (1997) On the mechanism of DNA transfection: efficient gene transfer without viruses. *Gene Ther.*, **4**, 1313–1321.

Dan, N. (1998) The structure of DNA complexes with cationic liposomes – cylindrical or flat bilayers? *Biochim. Biophys. Acta.*, **1369**, 34–38.

Fang, Y. and Yang, J. (1997) Two-dimensional condensation of DNA molecules on cationic lipid membranes. *J. Phys. Chem., B*, **101**, 441–449.

Farhood, H., Serbina, N. and Huang, L. (1995) The Role of dioleoylphospatidylethanol-amine in cationic liposome mediated gene therapy. *Biochim. Biophys. Acta.*, **1235**, 289–295.

Felgner, P.L., Gadek, T.R., Holm, M., Roman, R., Chan, H.W., Wenz, M. *et al.* (1987) A highly efficient, lipid-mediated DNA-transfection procedure. *Proc. Nat. Acad. Sci. USA*, **84**, 7413–7417.

Felgner, J.H., Kumar, R., Sridhar, C.N., Wheeler, C.J., Tsai, Y.J., Border, R. *et al.* (1994) Enhanced gene delivery and mechanism studies with a novel series of cationic lipid formulations. *J. Biol. Chem.*, **269**, 2550–2561.

Gao, X. and Huang, L. (1991) A novel cationic liposome reagent for efficient transfection of mammalian cells. *Biochem. Biophys. Res. Commun.*, **179**, 280–285.

Golubovic, L. and Golubovic, M. (1998) Fluctuations of quasi-two-dimensional smectics intercalated between membranes in multilamellar phases of DNA cationic lipid complexes. *Phys. Rev. Lett.*, **80**, 4341–4344.

Harries, D., May, S., Gelbart, W.M. and Ben-Shaul, A. (1998) Structure, stability, and thermodynamics of lamellar DNA-lipid complexes. *Biophys. J.*, **75**, 159–173.

Harrington, J.J., Bokkelen, G.V., Mays, R.W., Gustashaw, K. and Williard, H.F. (1997) Formation of de novo centromeres and construction of first-generation human artificial microchromosomes. *Nat. Genet.*, **15**, 345–355.

Hui, S.W., Langner, M., Zhao, Y.L., Ross, P., Hurley, E. and Chan, K. (1996) The role of helper lipids in cationic liposome-mediated gene transfer. *Biophys. J.*, **71**, 590–599.

Koltover, I., Salditt, T., Raedler, J.O. and Safinya, C.R. (1998) An inverted hexagonal phase of DNA-cationic liposome complexes related to DNA release and delivery. *Science*, **281**, 78–81.

Koltover, I., Salditt, T. and Safinya, C.R. (1999) Phase diagram, stability and overcharging of lamellar cationic lipid – DNA self assembled complexes. *Biophys. J.*, **77**, 915–924.

Laitinen, M., Hartikainen, J., Hiltunen, M.O., Eranen, J., Kiviniemi, M. *et al.* (2000) Catheter-mediated vascular endothelial growth factor gene transfer to human coronary arteries after angioplasty. *Hum. Gene Ther.*, **11**, 263–270.

Lasic, D.D., Strey, H.H., Stuart, M.C.A., Podgornik, R. and Frederik, P.M. (1997) The structure of DNA-liposome complexes. *J. Am. Chem. Soc.*, **119**, 832–833.

Legendre, J.Y. and Szoka, F.C. (1992) Delivery of plasmid DNA into mammalian cell lines using pH-sensitive liposomes-comparison with cationic liposomes. *Pharm. Res.*, **9**, 1235–1242.

Lin, A.J., Slack, N.L., Ahmad, A., Koltover, I., George, C.X., Samuel, C.E. and Safinya, C.R. (2000) Structure-function studies of lipid-DNA nonviral gene delivery systems. *J. Drug Target.*, **8**, 13–27.

Manning, G.S. (1969) Limiting laws and counterion condensation in polyelectrolyte solutions. I. Colligative properties. *J. Chem. Phys.*, **51**, 924–933.

May, S. and Ben-Shaul, A. (1997) DNA-lipid complexes: stability of honeycomb-like and spaghetti-like structures. *Biophys. J.*, **73**, 2427–2440.

Miller, A.D. (1998) Cationic liposomes for gene therapy. *Angew. Chem. Intl. Ed.*, **37**, 1768–1785.

Mortimer, I., Tam, P., MacLachlan, I., Graham, R.W., Saravolac, E.G. and Joshi, P.B. (1999) Cationic lipid-mediated transfection of cells in culture requires mitotic activity. *Gene Ther.*, **6**, 403–411.

Mou, J., Czajkowsky, D.M., Zhang, Y. and Shao, Z. (1995) High-resolution atomic-force microscopy of DNA: the pitch of the double helix. *FEBS Lett.*, **371**, 279–282.

Nabel, G.J., Nabel, E.G., Yang, Z.Y., Fox, B.A., Plautz, G.E., Gao, X. *et al.* (1993) Direct gene transfer with DNA liposome complexes in melanoma-expression, biologic activity, and lack of toxicity in humans. *Proc. Nat. Acad. Sci. USA*, **90**, 11307–11311.

Noone, P.G., Hohneker, K.W., Zhou, Z., Johnson, L.G., Foy, C. *et al.* (2000) Safety and biological efficacy of a lipid-CFTR complex for gene transfer in the nasal epithelium of adult patients with cystic fibrosis. *Mol. Ther.*, **1**, 105–114.

O'Hern, C.S. and Lubensky, T.C. (1998) Sliding columnar phase of DNA lipid complexes. *Phys. Rev. Lett.*, **80**, 4345–4348.

Ono, T., Funino, Y., Tsuchiya, T. and Tsuda, T. (1990) Plasmid DNAs directly injected into mouse brain with lipofectin can be incorporated and expressed by brain cells. *Neurosci. Lett.*, **117**, 259–263.

Podgornik, R., Rau, D.C. and Parsegian, V.A. (1994) Parametrization of direct and soft steric-undulatory forces between DNA double helical polyelectrolytes in solutions of several different anions and cations. *Biophys. J.*, **66**, 962–971.

Raedler, J.O., Koltover, I., Salditt, T. and Safinya, C.R. (1997) Structure of DNA-cationic liposome complexes: DNA intercalation in multi-lamellar membranes in distinct interhelical packing regimes. *Science*, **275**, 810–814.

Remy, J.S., Sirlin, C., Vierling, P. and Behr, J.P. (1994) Gene transfer with a series of lipophilic DNA-binding molecules. *Biconjug. Chem.*, **5**, 647–654.

Roux, D. and Safinya, C.R. (1988) A synchrotron X-ray study of competing undulation and electrostatic interlayer interactions in fluid multimembrane lyotropic phases. *J. Physique France*, **49**, 307–318.

Safinya, C.R. (1989) Rigid and fluctuating surfaces: a series of synchrotron x-ray scattering studies of interacting stacked membranes. In: T. Riste and D. Sherrington (eds) *Phase Transitions in Soft Condensed Matter*. Nato ASI Series B, 211, pp. 249–270.

Safinya, C.R., Sirota, E.B., Roux, D. and Smith, G.S. (1989) Universality in interacting membranes: the effect of cosurfactants on the interfacial rigidity. *Phys. Rev. Lett.*, **62**, 1134.

Salditt, T., Koltover, I., Raedler, J.O. and Safinya, C.R. (1997) Two-dimensional smectic ordering of linear DNA chains in self-assembled DNA-cationic liposome mixtures. *Phys. Rev. Lett.*, **79**, 2582–2585.

Salditt, T., Koltover, I., Raedler, J.O. and Safinya, C.R. (1998) Self-assembled DNA-cationic lipid complexes: two-dimensional smectic ordering, correlations, and interactions. *Phys. Rev. E*, **58**, 889–904.

Seddon, J.M. (1989) Structure of the inverted hexagonal phase and non-lamellar phase transitions of lipids. *Biochim. Biophys. Acta.*, **1031**, 1–69.

Szleifer, I., Ben-Shaul, A. and Gelbart, W.M. (1990) Chain packing statistics and thermodynamics of amphilphile monolayers. *J. Phys. Chem.*, **94**, 5081–5089.

Wilard, H.F. (2000) Artificial chromosomes coming to life. *Science*, **290**, 1308–1309.

Wrobel, I. and Collins, D. (1995) Fusion of cationic liposomes with mammalian cells occurs after endocytosis. *Biochim. Biophys. Acta.*, **1235**, 296–304.

Zabner, J., Fasbender, A.J., Moninger, T., Poelinger, K.A. and Welsh, M.J. (1995) Cellular and molecular barriers to gene transfer by a cationic lipid. *J. Biol. Chem.*, **270**, 18997–19007.

Zhu, N., Liggitt, D., Liu, Y. and Debs, R. (1993) Systemic gene expression after intravenous DNA delivery into adult mice. *Science*, **261**, 209–211.

Zimm, B.H. and Bret, M.L. (1983) Counter-ion condensation and system dimensionality. *J. Biomol. Struct. Dyn.*, **1**, 461–471.

11 Cellular uptake, metabolic stability and nuclear translocation of nucleic acids

Delphine Lechardeur and
Gergely L. Lukacs

INTRODUCTION

Genetic material, comprising the information required to maintain the complexity and evolvability of an eukaryotic organism; is largely encoded in the chromosomal DNA and confined to the nucleus. The nuclear envelope and the plasma membrane have an indispensable role in preserving the stability of the nuclear DNA by protecting it from the intrusion of genetic material of pathogenic viruses, bacteria and necrotic or apoptotic cell nuclei. These phospholipid membranes, on the other hand, constitute major obstacles to the nuclear delivery of non-viral vector, which is comprised of an expression cassette, encoded by a therapeutic gene complexed with cationic polymer (polyplex), cationic lipid (lipoplex) or a mixture of these (lipopolyplex). Although the accessibility and specific characteristics of the target organ may impose additional impediments to gene delivery leading to a further decrease in the gene transfer efficiency *in vivo*, both toxicological and immunological considerations favor the application of synthetic vectors over viral delivery systems to alleviate the phenotypic manifestations of genetic or acquired diseases.

Investigations of the cellular itinerary of vectorized DNA in cultured cells have provided insight into the nature of potential barriers to gene transfer. It is estimated that upon exposure of a cultured cell to 10^5–10^6 copies of plasmid molecules, not more than one to ten plasmids can reach the nucleus. This ratio represents a strikingly low transfection efficiency *in vitro*. A large fraction of this filtering effect takes place during the translocation of DNA from the cytoplasm into the nucleus. It was inferred, based on the comparison of the expression of microinjected reporter plasmid DNA into the cytoplasm and nucleus, that not more than 0.1–0.01% of the cytoplasmic plasmid DNA were taken up by and translated in the nucleus (Capecchi, 1980; Pollard *et al.*, 2001). Although we still lack quantitative data regarding the extent of endo-lysosomal entrapment of plasmid DNA, these experiments illustrate that the nucleocytoplasmic transport represents one of the obstacles to nuclear gene delivery.

In this chapter, a brief overview of the cellular barriers to gene delivery is presented. Special emphasis is given to those events that compromise the translocation process of plasmid DNA from the cytosol into the nucleus. In addition, the strategies developed by viruses to efficiently bypass these cellular barriers and target their genomic DNA into the nucleus of infected cells will be discussed.

INTERNALIZATION AND ENTRAPMENT IN
ENDO-LYSOSOMAL COMPARTMENT

Positively charged lipoplex and polyplex adsorb to negatively charged plasma membrane and are internalized by endocytosis, phagocytosis and/or direct fusion. The cellular acceptor site for the complex could be sulfated proteoglycans, cell surface receptors (e.g., scavenger receptor or negatively charged glycoproteins) or phospholipids themselves (Farhood *et al.*, 1995; Labat-Moleur *et al.*, 1996; Simoes *et al.*, 1999). While it is expected that the contribution of the various internalization pathways is dependent upon the cell type, morphological studies at light and electron microscopic levels suggest that clathrin-dependent endocytosis is predominantly responsible for the cellular uptake of DNA (Clark and Hersh, 1999; Meyer *et al.*, 1997). However, the size of the DNA/lipid complex might determine the mechanism of internalization: a large complex (up to 500 nm) would enter the cell by receptor and clathrin independent endocytosis while a smaller complex (200 nm) could be internalized via coated pits through a non-specific clathrin dependent process (Simoes *et al.*, 1999). Electron-dense cationic lipopolylysine containing liposomes could be demonstrated in endosomal compartment within one hour of administration by electron microscopy (Zhou and Huang, 1994). Similar studies showed the localization of gold-labeled DNA complexed with 1,2-dimyristyloxypropyl-3-dimethylhydroxyethylammonium bromide (DMRIE)/ dioleoylphosphatidylethanolamine (DOPE) lipids in cytoplasmic vesicles, presumably representing endosomal vesicles (Zabner *et al.*, 1995). Differentiated primary epithelia or native tissues, in contrast to non-polarized cultured cells, display a slower rate of internalization due to altered cell surface properties and endocytic activity of the apical plasma membrane (Chu *et al.*, 1999; Colin *et al.*, 2000; Fasbender *et al.*, 1997; Matsui *et al.*, 1997). Endocytosis of topically delivered plasmid DNA could be further compromised by mucocilliary clearance and mucus secretion in lung epithelia, implying that internalization per se could be regarded as one of the rate limiting steps of gene delivery (Hillery *et al.*, 1999). Attempts to overcome the apical plasma membrane barrier include the non-specific and specific stimulation of targeting, besides relocating the site of internalization to the basolateral surface by transient disruption of tight junctions, exploiting the enhanced endocytic membrane turnover (Jiang *et al.*, 1998; Matsui *et al.*, 1997).

Little is known about those physico-chemical events and molecular interactions that determine the fate of lipoplex in early endosomes. Endocytosed lipoplex could be routed for recycling to the extracellular compartment, targeted to lysosomes via late endosomes, and released into the cytoplasm (Figure 11.1). Regardless of the subsequent trafficking pathway, penetration of nucleic acid into the cytoplasm appears to be a prerequisite for its nuclear delivery. Cytoplasmic release of internalized lipoplex involves charge neutralization of the cationic complexing agent with anionic macromolecules, such as anionic lipids and proteoglycans, cationic lipid mediated fusion and membrane destabilization by pH-sensitive lipids (Clark and Hersh, 1999; El Ouahabi *et al.*, 1997; Meyer *et al.*, 1997; Wattiaux *et al.*, 2000; Wrobel and Collins, 1995; Xu and Szoka, 1996; Zelphati and Szoka, 1996a). Disruption of the endosomal vesicles occurs through interactions of cationic lipids of the lipoplex by the transbilayer flip-flop of anionic lipids from the external layer of the endosomal membrane (Zelphati and Szoka, 1996a,b). This interaction would

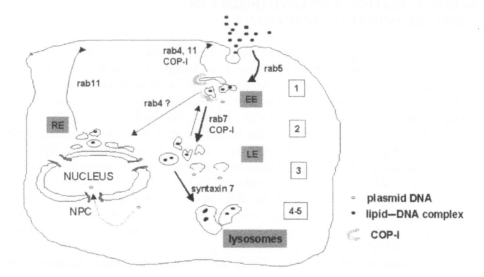

Figure 11.1 The intracellular trafficking pathway of plasmid DNA complexed by polycationic lipid (lipoplex). Critical steps are indicated by numbers: (1) endocytosis, sorting and recycling via vesicular compartments comprising the
early (EE) and sorting endosomes; (2) entrapment and degradation in the
late-endosomes (LE) and lysosomes; (3) destabilization of the endo-lysosomal membrane and release into the cytosol, (the precise location of this
step is not known); (4) diffusion toward the nuclear pore complex (NPC)
and degradation in the cytoplasm, and; (5) nuclear translocation across the
NPC.

eventually induce the destabilization of the endosomal membrane and the release
of the DNA from the lipoplex.

Lipofection efficiency by most of the cationic lipids is enhanced by the addition of
the neutral lipid, dioleoylphosphatidylethanolamine (DOPE). DOPE promotes the
fusion of lipid/DNA particles with the endosomal membrane, inducing their disruption and thus increasing the release of DNA into the cytosol (Mui *et al.*, 2000;
Ross *et al.*, 1998). The high transfection efficacy of the cationic polymer polyethylenimine (PEI) involves its strong buffering capacity, inducing osmotic swelling
of endosomes leading to their rupture.

Nevertheless, accumulating evidences suggest that only a fraction of internalized
lipoplex reaches the cytoplasm, while a larger portion is trapped and degraded in
the endo-lysosomal compartment (El Ouahabi *et al.*, 1997; Godbey *et al.*, 1999;
Plank *et al.*, 1994; Tseng *et al.*, 1997; Wattiaux *et al.*, 2000; Yanez and Porter,
1999). Accordingly, endosome disrupting agents incorporated in lipoplex or polyplex, such as adenoviral particles (Diebold *et al.*, 1999; Wagner *et al.*, 1992), viral
peptides, e.g., the hemagglutinin HA2 peptide from influenza virus (Wagner *et al.*,
1992), synthetic pH-sensitive peptide (Simoes *et al.*, 1999), and diphteria-toxin
subunit (Uherek *et al.*, 1998), are able to enhance the cytoplasmic release of DNA
by destabilizing the endosomal membrane and to facilitate expression of the internalized reporter gene. As a complementary approach, non-specific lysomotropic

agents such as chloroquine (Harbottle *et al.*, 1998; Luthman and Magnusson, 1983; Niidome *et al.*, 1997) or a specific inhibitor of lysosomal nuclease activity, DMI-2, have been shown to potentiate the transfection efficiency by extending the half-life of plasmid DNA within the endo-lysosomal compartment (Ross *et al.*, 1998). Finally, disrupting the microtubulus system, required for endo-lysosome fusion, could enhance gene expression as well, supporting the notion that a significant fraction of internalized plasmid DNA is targeted to and degraded in lysosomes (Chowdhury *et al.*, 1996). While these perturbations are incompatible with therapeutic interventions, they are instrumental in elucidating the intracellular trafficking pathway of plasmid DNA.

CYTOPLASM AS A PHYSICAL AND METABOLIC BARRIER

Following the escape from the endo-lysosomal compartment, the expression cassette has to traverse the cytoplasm and nuclear pore complex (NPC) before transcription can occur. A number of observations suggest that endosomal escape coincides with or is followed by the dissociation of polycation/plasmid DNA complexes. First, microinjection of plasmid DNA complexed with cationic lipids into the cytosol or nucleus failed to induce the expression of reporter genes (Zabner *et al.*, 1995). Second, fluorescence microscopy has shown that dissociation of the lipid/oligonucleotide complexes occurs in the cytosol prior to the nuclear translocation of the nucleic acids (El Ouahabi *et al.*, 1997; Xu and Szoka, 1996; Zelphati and Szoka, 1996a,b). Finally, expression of cytosolic T7 polymerase allowed the transcription/translation of a T7-promoter driven reporter gene in the cytoplasm (Brisson and Huang, 1999; Gao and Huang, 1995; Subramanian *et al.*, 1999). These observations collectively support the notion that naked plasmid DNA is transiently exposed to the cytoplasm during its intracellular trafficking. However, the metabolic stability and diffusional characteristics of plasmid DNA in the cytoplasm remained unknown until recently.

Diffusional constraint of plasmid mobility in cytoplasm

The cellular space, encompassed by the plasma membrane and excluded by organelles and the cytoskeleton, is occupied by the cytoplasm containing macromolecules and small organic and inorganic solutes. Considering that plasmid DNA has to escape from the endocytic vesicles, which are distributed throughout the cytoplasm randomly, it is reasonable to assume that the diffusional mobility of the DNA is an important determinant of the nuclear targeting efficiency of DNA.

The inefficient nuclear uptake of plasmid DNA from the cytoplasm was recognized more than twenty years ago. Comparison of the transfection efficiency of plasmid DNA, encoding the thymidine kinase, introduced into the cytosol or the nucleus showed that not more than 0.1–0.01% of the cytosolically injected DNA could be transcribed (Capecchi, 1980; Page *et al.*, 1995). Similar results were obtained by monitoring the expression of β-galactosidase reporter gene (Dowty *et al.*, 1995; Pollard *et al.*, 1998). While the original interpretation of these studies emphasized that the nuclear envelope represents the major cellular barrier, recent data suggest that restricted lateral mobility and metabolic instability of plasmid

DNA in the cytoplasm contribute to the limited transfection efficiency of plasmid DNA, as well.

Determination of rotational correlation time by time-resolved anisotropy or ratio-imaging of viscosity-sensitive fluorescent probes have revealed that the solvent viscosity of the cytoplasm is comparable to that of aqueous solutions (Fushimi and Verkman, 1991; Luby-Phelps *et al.*, 1993). Nevertheless, the mesh-like structure of the cytoskeleton, the presence of organelles and the relatively high protein concentration (up to 100 mg/ml) impose molecular crowding, which limits the diffusion of macromolecules. Fluorescence recovery after photobleaching (FRAP) of size-fractionated fluorescein isothiocyanate (FITC)-labeled Ficoll and dextran, delivered by microinjection, has demonstrated that the translational mobility of particles smaller than 500–750 kDa was only three to four-fold slower than in water, but was markedly impeded for molecules larger than 750 kDa (Seksek *et al.*, 1997). The anomalous mobility of inert tracers in the cytoplasm appeared at a hydrodynamic radius of 25 nm or greater (Luby-Phelps *et al.*, 1987). Meanwhile, the diffusion of polypeptides is usually slower than inert particles (e.g., Ficoll or dextran), conceivably due to interactions with intracellular components (Luby-Phelps, 2000). Consequently, the diffusion coefficient of large size solutes cannot be correlated to their size or radius. Similar phenomenon was observed by monitoring the diffusion of cytoplasmic vesicles or microinjected beads. The movement of these particles is 500 to 1000 times slower in the cytoplasm than in aqueous solution (Burke *et al.*, 1997; Luby-Phelps, 2000; Steiner *et al.*, 1997), providing an explanation for the active transport required for the intracellular movement of transport-vesicles (Klopfenstein *et al.*, 2000; Rogers and Gelfand, 2000).

Based on these observations, it was predicted that the lateral diffusion of macromolecules with comparable size to expression plasmids (corresponding to 2–10 MDa molecular mass) could be severely impeded in the cytoplasm. The limited lateral diffusion of plasmid or double stranded DNA fragments, larger than 1 kb, could be visualized by injecting FITC-conjugated DNA into the cytosol of Hela cells. In contrast to oligonucleotides (20 bp) or DNA fragments smaller than 250 bp, which rapidly diffuse into the nucleus, nucleic acids larger than 1 kb are excluded from the nuclei following a 45 minutes incubation at 37 °C (Figure 11.2). Since microinjection of oligonucleotides leads to homogenous distribution in the cytoplasm, the size of the plasmid DNA more than interactions with cytoplasmic constituents is thought to be responsible for the poor diffusion of DNA molecules of plasmid size.

To measure the diffusion mobility of FITC-conjugated plasmid DNA (3–6 kb) and DNA fragments (20 bp–2 kb) in living cells, the fluorescence recovery after photo-bleaching technique was utilized. Following the microinjection of FITC-labeled DNA into the cytoplasm or the nucleus, a 0.4 μm diameter spot was bleached with a high intensity laser beam and the time course of fluorescence-recovery was recorded in the spot (Lukacs *et al.*, 2000). The diffusional coefficients of DNA fragments were compared to that measured in aqueous solution. A DNA fragment of 100 bp was fully mobile in the cytoplasm, with a diffusive rate only ~5 times slower than in water, similar to that of a comparably sized FITC-dextran. The diffusion of larger DNA fragments in cytoplasm became remarkably slow, with 250 bp and 2000 bp fragments 17 and >100 times slower, respectively, than diffusion in water (Figure 11.3). The diffusion of larger DNA fragments also

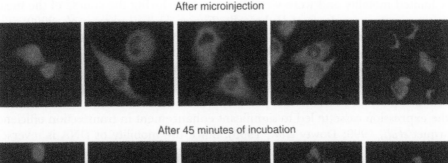

After microinjection

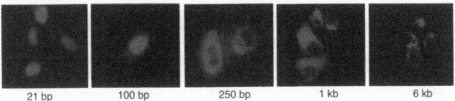

After 45 minutes of incubation

| 21 bp | 100 bp | 250 bp | 1 kb | 6 kb |

Figure 11.2 Subcellular distribution of fluorescein-labeled DNA fragments and plasmid DNA following microinjection into the cytoplasm. Double stranded circular plasmid DNA (3 kb and 6 kb) and DNA fragments (20, 100, 250 and 1 kb) were covalently labeled with fluorescein and microinjected into the cytoplasm of adherent HeLa cells as described in Lukacs *et al.*, 2000. Following microinjection, cells were either fixed or incubated for 45 minutes at 37 °C and the distribution of DNA was visualized by fluorescence microscopy. (*see Color Plate 10*)

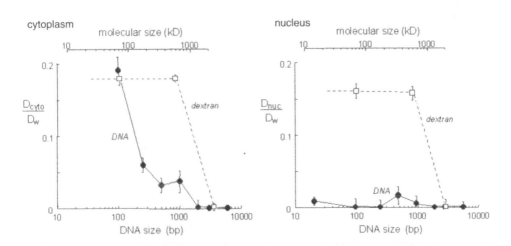

Figure 11.3 DNA size dependence of relative diffusion coefficients in cytoplasm (D_{cyto}/D_w) and nucleus (D_{nuc}/D_w). Apparent diffusional coefficients in the cytoplasm (D_{cyt}) relative to aqueous solution (D_w) were determined from 50% recovery times ($t_{1/2}$) using an experimentally determined calibration relation of $t_{1/2}$ versus D as described in Kao *et al.*, 1993. Each point is the mean ± SE for 5–15 independent measurements for DNA diffusion in cytoplasm (open circles) or nucleus (filled circles). For comparison, D/D_w values for microinjected FITC-dextrans are shown. Reproduced with permission from Lukacs *et al.*, 2000.

became remarkably slower in the cytoplasm. Nucleic acids larger than 2 kb have a very limited mobility and were virtually immobile during the course of the measurements in the cytoplasm of HeLa cells (Figure 11.3) (Lukacs *et al.*, 2000). The restricted mobility of plasmid DNA, relative to a comparable size of dextran, could be explained by molecular crowding, immobile cytoplasmic obstacles or association of the nucleic acids with cytosolic DNA binding proteins.

Consistent with the notion that lateral diffusion may limit nuclear entry, microinjection of plasmid DNA into the proximity of the nucleus or a decrease in the size of the expression cassette led to significant enhancement in transfection efficiency (Darquet *et al.*, 1999; Dowty *et al.*, 1995). Since the mobility of DNA is inversely proportional to the size of the polycation/DNA complex, it is assumed that the faster mobility of condensed DNA could account, at least in part, for enhanced transfection efficiency of the PEI-complexed DNA (Pollard *et al.*, 1998). Intriguingly, double-stranded DNA fragments of 1 kb size could enter the majority of nuclei in digitonin permeabilized cells, but failed to be accumulated after microinjection into the cytoplasm of intact cells (Hagstrom *et al.*, 1997). One possible explanation for these discordant results might be that the cytoskeletal network became disassembled during the permeabilization step (Cook *et al.*, 1983), reinforcing the hypothesis that the cytoplasm constitutes a diffusional barrier to gene transfer.

Metabolic instability of plasmid in cytoplasm

Naked plasmid DNA was not only trapped in the cytoplasm around the site of microinjection, as visualized by fluorescence *in situ* hybridization (FISH) or using FITC-labeled DNA, but was also eliminated rapidly at physiological temperature (Lechardeur *et al.*, 1999). The disposal of the DNA was completely prevented when the cells were kept at 4 °C (Lechardeur *et al.*, 1999). A similar conclusion was reached by monitoring the amount of microinjected expression cassette by the polymerase chain reaction (PCR) (Pollard *et al.*, 2001), suggesting that the metabolic instability of naked DNA contributes to the low efficiency of gene transfer (Lechardeur *et al.*, 1999; Mirzayans *et al.*, 1992; Neves *et al.*, 1999; Pollard *et al.*, 2001).

Quantitative assessment of the decay kinetics of the signal derived from microinjected plasmid DNA measured by FISH and single-cell video image analysis showed that 50% of the DNA is eliminated in one to two hours from HeLa and COS-1 cells (Lechardeur *et al.*, 1999). The rapid turnover rate of plasmid DNA was independent of the copy number (1000–10,000 plasmid/cell), the conformation (linearized versus supercoiled, single- versus double-stranded) of the plasmid and the detection method used (Figure 11.4). Similar turnover rates were measured when the half-life of the biotinylated plasmid or fluorescein-labeled DNA was monitored, implying that the rapid decay of the FISH signal could not be attributed to the inaccessibility of plasmid DNA by the probe. Depletion of the cellular ATP content had no significant effect on the turnover rate of plasmid DNA, suggesting that disposal of cytosolic DNA does not require vesicular transport. When the ambient temperature was reduced to 4 °C the elimination of plasmid DNA was completely prevented, suggesting that disposal DNA is temperature dependent and may be mediated by an enzymatic process.

A large body of evidence favors our hypothesis that cytosolic nucleases are responsible for the rapid degradation of plasmid DNA. First, elimination of

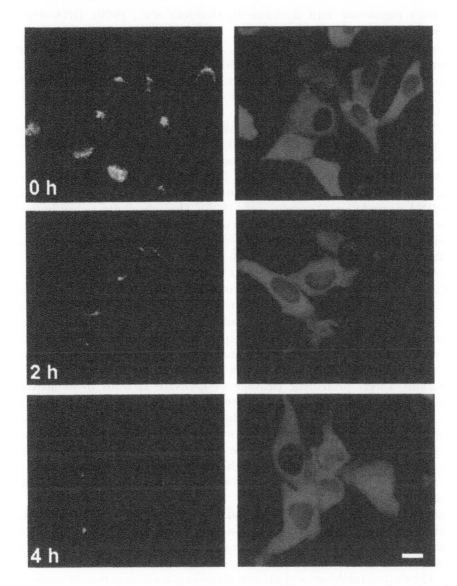

Figure 11.4 Elimination of plasmid DNA from the cytoplasm of microinjected cells. Double stranded fluorescein labeled pGL2 plasmid (0.1 µg/ml) was co-injected with TRITC-dextran into the cytosol of HeLa cells and incubated under tissue culture conditions for the indicated time. Cells were fixed and fluorescence micrographs were taken to visualize the distribution of TRITC-dextran (right column) and fluorescein-labeled pGL2 (left column) of the same field. (*see Color Plate 11*)

plasmid DNA could not be attributed to trafficking to the nucleus, cell division or to the activation or release of nucleases upon microinjection (Lechardeur *et al.*, 1999). Second, disposal of microinjected plasmid DNA was nearly completely inhibited by depletion of the cytosol by selective permeabilization of the plasma membrane with digitonin (Lechardeur *et al.*, 1999). DNA degrad-ation was substantially delayed by the encapsulation of DNA in stabilized phospholipid vesicles (Lechardeur *et al.*, 1999; Wheeler *et al.*, 1999). Third, transient accumulation of free 3'-OH ends of nucleic acids could be detected by the terminal deoxynucleotidyl transferase-mediated dUTP nick end-labeling assay (TUNEL), reflecting the fragmentation of plasmid DNA *in situ* (Lechardeur *et al.*, 1999).

The nucleases, responsible for plasmid DNA degradation in the cytosol, remain to be identified. Numerous cellular endo- and exonucleases have been described, but their physiological function and subcellular localization are still poorly understood (Peitsch *et al.*, 1994; Torriglia *et al.*, 1995; Vanderbilt *et al.*, 1982). Several of them are activated during apoptosis, playing a role in chromo-somal DNA degradation (Torriglia *et al.*, 1995). The subcellular redistribution of DNase I and DNase II from the luminal compartment of the endoplasmic reticu-lum and lysosomes into nucleus via the cytoplasm has been demonstrated (Barry and Eastman, 1993; Polzar *et al.*, 1993; Wyllie, 1980). Other nucleases are expressed as inactive precursors, like the Caspase-Activated Dnase (CAD) and the L-DNase II. While caspase-3 mediated proteolysis of ICAD, the cognate inhibitor of CAD, is required for CAD activation (Enari *et al.*, 1998; Sakahira *et al.*, 1998), our results have demonstrated that the activation process of CAD takes place in the nucleus (Lechardeur *et al.*, 2000). Keeping in line with this observation, over-expression of heterologous ICAD had no impact on the turnover rate of microinjected plasmid DNA in HeLa cells (Lechardeur and Lukacs, unpublished observation). Direct proteolytic cleavage of L-DNase II leads to its activation and subsequent translocation from the cytoplasm into the nucleus (Torriglia *et al.*, 1998). Considering that no sign of apoptosis has been detected in microinjected cells, it is highly unlikely that DNases involved in chromosomal DNA degradation are responsible for the elimination of the microinjected DNA (Lechardeur *et al.*, 1999). This conclusion is consistent with the findings that the activation and inhibitor profiles of the cytosolic nuclease are distinct from that of known DNases (Lechardeur *et al.*, 1999).

Degradation of plasmid DNA is activated by divalent cations such as Ca^{2+}, Mn^{2+} and Mg^{2+} in the cytosolic extract obtained by digitonin permeabilization and monitored by Southern blot analysis and ^{32}P-release from end-labeled DNA (Lechardeur *et al.*, 1999), as well as by agarose gel electrophoresis (Pollard *et al.*, 2001). The distinct inhibitor- and pH-sensitivity-profiles of the cytosolic nuclease(s) are consistent with the notion that neither DNase I nor DNase II contribute to the cleavage of microinjected plasmid (Lechardeur *et al.*, 1999). Based on these find-ings it was concluded that the metabolic instability of plasmid DNA caused by cytosolic nuclease(s) may constitute a previously unrecognized impediment for the nuclear translocation of DNA (Lechardeur *et al.*, 1999; Luo and Saltzman, 2000; Pollard *et al.*, 2001).

While isolation of a specific inhibitor will be necessary to assess the definitive role of the cytosolic nuclease in the low transfection efficiency *in vivo*, circumstantial evidence suggests that the metabolic instability of plasmid DNA represents one of the cellular barriers to gene transfer. Microinjection of DNA complexes with PEI has augmented the transfection efficiency (Pollard *et al.*, 1998). Although the stability of the PEI-complexed DNA has not been determined *in vivo*, it has been demonstrated that the nuclease resistance of plasmid DNA is dramatically increased upon complex formation *in vitro* (Cappaccioli *et al.*, 1993; Chiou *et al.*, 1994; Thierry *et al.*, 1997). Therefore, it is conceivable that faster diffusional mobility and decreased nuclease susceptibility jointly lead to the enhanced nuclear targeting efficiency of the PEI-condensed plasmid DNA.

NUCLEAR UPTAKE OF PLASMID

The nuclear envelope is the ultimate obstacle to plasmid DNA delivery to the nucleus. A large body of evidence indicates that the transductability of mitotic cells is significantly higher than their quiescent counterpart, conceivably due to the disassembly of nuclear envelope during mitosis (Brisson and Huang, 1999). In non-dividing cells, representing most of the target in somatic gene therapy trials, plasmid DNA has to traverse the nuclear envelope. The nuclear envelope is a highly selective barrier, which regulates the trafficking of proteins and ribonucleoproteins between the nucleosol and the cytoplasm (Laskey, 1998). The distribution of proteins between nucleus and cytoplasm depends on their size as well as the presence of specific targeting signals, the nuclear localization sequence (NLS) (Nigg, 1997; Talcott and Moore, 1999). The diffusion and facilitated transport of macromolecules are mediated by the central gated channel of the nuclear pore complex (NPC), allowing the passive transport of molecules smaller than 40–60 kDa but requiring energy for polypeptide larger than 60 kDa (Nigg, 1997; Talcott and Moore, 1999). The rapid uptake of endogenous nucleoproteins (e.g., histones, transcription factors) into the nucleus is achieved by active transport through the NPA. Nucleoproteins include motifs termed nuclear localization signals (NLSs), which interact with cytoplasmic receptors. The classical SV40-T type NLS (-PKKKRKV-) is recognized by the importin-α, which in turn binds through its importin-β binding (IBB) domain to importin-β to form a complex. Unloading of the cargo molecule is triggered by Ran-GTP association in the nucleus (Talcott and Moore, 1999).

Considering that the average size of an expression cassette is 2–10 MDa, the mechanistic aspects of plasmid DNA translocation across the nuclear envelope is still enigmatic. A large body of evidence indicates that nuclear uptake of plasmid DNA is facilitated during the nuclear envelope disassembly. Actively dividing cells displays a higher transfectability compared to their quiescent counterpart (Brunner *et al.*, 2000; Mortimer *et al.*, 1999; Wilke *et al.*, 1996). Blocking the cell cycle progression in the G1 phase by aphidicolin has dramatically reduced reporter gene activity relative to asynchronous cells, while it has no effect on the rate of internalization of lipoplex or on transgene expression in stably transfected cells (Mortimer *et al.*, 1999). In contrast, the level of reporter gene expression was enhanced when cells were exposed to lipoplexes during or just before mitosis (Brunner *et al.*, 2000). Finally, the relatively low rate of cell proliferation of primary cultures of ciliated human airway epithelia was found to be one of the determinants for their low transfectability by lipoplex (Fasbender *et al.*, 1997). These results, however, do not preclude the possibility that DNA can be translocated through nuclear pore complex by a NLS-independent mechanism.

Microinjection of plasmid DNA into the cytoplasm of primary rat myotubes lead to the expression of the reporter gene, indicating that intact plasmid DNA can penetrate postmitotic nuclei by a process sensitive to temperature and wheat germ agglutinin (WGA), an inhibitor of the NPC (Dowty *et al.*, 1995). In addition, gold-labeled plasmid DNA could be detected by electron microscopy at the NPC and in the nucleosol following cytosolic microinjection, suggesting that the NPC is the gateway for plasmid entry (Dowty *et al.*, 1995).

The nuclear translocation of expression cassettes shares some of the pivotal characteristics of the active nuclear entry of polypeptides. The nuclear transloca-tion and expression of reporter plasmid is inhibited by temperature, energy depletion and WGA (Brisson and Huang, 1999). The inhibitory effect of WGA could be reversed by N-acetyl-glucosamine (Dowty *et al.*, 1995), which is consistent with the hypothesis that plasmid DNA penetrates the nucleus, at least in part, through the NPC. Supporting the NPC-mediated uptake mechanism of DNA, attachment of NLS appears to enhance the nuclear accumulation and expression of plasmid DNA (Branden *et al.*, 1999; Ludtke *et al.*, 1999; Sebestyen *et al.*, 1998; Wilson *et al.*, 1999; Zantai, 1999). The coupling of single or multiple classical NLS to plasmid DNA augmented the transfection efficiency up to 30-fold, presumably via the importin-dependent nuclear transport pathway. A similar effect was observed utilizing non-classical NLS (M9 sequence of the human heterogeneous nuclear ribonucleoprotein A1), increasing the transfectability of non-dividing endothelial cells (Subramanian *et al.*, 1999). While condensation of plasmid DNA by the positively charged linker peptide may account, in part, for the stimulatory effect, the majority of the effect was a direct consequence of the activity of NLS and could be abolished by replacing critical amino acid residues in the nuclear target-ing signal (Zanta *et al.*, 1999), providing circumstantial evidence for the nuclear entry process of plasmid DNA.

The possibility that nuclear entry of plasmid DNA is sequence-dependent and influenced by the binding of cytoplasmic polypeptides encompassing NLS, such as transcription factors, has been investigated (Dean, 1997; Dean *et al.*, 1999; Wilson *et al.*, 1999). Engineering binding sites for an endogenous transcription factor in the non-coding region of plasmid DNA demonstrated that the binding of a tran-scription factor with NLS potentiates the expression of reporter molecules in a cell specific manner (Vacik *et al.*, 1999). Although a direct comparison of the efficacy of synthetic peptides and transcription factors is not feasible, these results suggest that the combination of transportin-, importin- and transcription factor-dependent nuclear targeting may influence the nuclear uptake capacity of the non-viral delivery system in an additive manner.

NUCLEOCYTOPLASMIC TRAFFICKING OF OLIGONUCLEOTIDES

The potential therapeutic use of antisense oligonucleotides has provoked intensive studies of their intracellular trafficking, which noticeably differ from plasmid DNA. Oligonucleotides accumulate very rapidly and preferentially in the nucleus after microinjection into the cytosol. Fluorescently tagged 15–25 bp oligomers could be detected in the nucleus within seconds after injection (Figure 11.2) (Leonetti *et al.*,

1991). Nuclear targeting of small size DNA (< 100 bp) is independent of temperature, ATP concentration and is unaffected by the presence of non-labeled oligonucleotide (Leonetti *et al.*, 1991). These observations indicate that oligonucleotides diffuse passively into the nucleus similarly to the nuclear translocation of small polypeptides. Oligonucleotides do not associate with constituents of the cytoplasm, suggesting that cytoplasmic factors are not involved in their nuclear import (Leonetti *et al.*, 1991). Importantly, FRAP measurements have revealed that the mobility of oligonucleotides decreases dramatically in the nucleus, in sharp contrast to their freely mobile nature in the cytoplasm (Lukacs *et al.*, 2000). The diffusional mobility of oligonucleotides in the nucleus is at least two orders of magnitude slower than in the cytoplasm (Lukacs *et al.*, 2000). The efficient nuclear targeting and retention could be explained by the presence of a large number of binding sites for oligonucleotides in the nucleus (Clarenc *et al.*, 1993). In contrast, oligonucleotides complexed by synthetic vectors are trapped in the endo-lysosomal compartment to the same extent as plasmid DNA (Branden *et al.*, 1999; Juliano and Yoo, 2000; Zelphati *et al.*, 1999; Zelphati and Szoka, 1996a,b), decreasing their therapeutic efficacy *in vivo*. Finally, since trafficking of oligonucleotides from the cytoplasm to the nucleus is very efficient, they provide an interesting tool to study the release of DNA from the endocytic compartment independently of the cytoplasmic and nuclear envelope barriers encountered by plasmid DNA (Mui *et al.*, 2000).

NUCLEOCYTOPLASMIC TRANSPORT OF VIRUSES

Viruses are complex particles, entering the cells by fusion of their envelope to the plasma membrane or by endocytosis followed by the escape of the capsid by membrane fusion or lysis (Sodeik, 2000). The diameter of the viral particle could be several hundred nanometers, implying a very inefficient diffusional movement in the cytoplasm, based on those physicochemical considerations that were discussed above (Kasamatsu and Nakanishi, 1998). Despite these limitations, those viruses that replicate in the nucleus have evolved sophisticated mechanisms to ensure a highly efficient nuclear delivery of their genetic material. Since these mechanisms may provide a conceptual framework to design novel non-viral delivery systems, we shall review some of the key elements that account for the nuclear targeting of certain viruses.

Virus trafficking in cytoplasm

The rapid and efficient transport of virus particles in the cytoplasm e.g., Herpes Simplex Virus (HSV), Simian virus 40 (SV40) and adenovirus, takes advantage of the cytoskeleton network. HSV enters the cell by direct fusion of the viral membrane to the plasma membrane. Once inside the cytosol, the virus moves along microtubules (MT) to the microtubule organization center (MTOC) in an ATP and cytosolic factor-dependent manner (Sodeik, 2000; Sodeik *et al.*, 1997). Adenovirus (Ad) enters the cell by endocytosis and undergoes a progressive loss of the capsid as a consequence of dissociation and proteolysis of the coat and matrix proteins. The mildly acidic pH of the endosomal compartment triggers the virus penetration into the cytoplasm. The adenoviral DNA remains associated with some of the capsid proteins in the cytoplasm, which are indispensable for nuclear targeting and their active transport of the viral DNA toward the MTOC, which is in close proximity to the nuclear envelope. Ad2, Ad5 and adeno-associated virus, similarly to HSV, use the microtubule minus-end-directed motor complex dynein/dynactin for retrograde movement towards the MTOC (Leopold *et al.*, 2000; Sodeik, 2000; Suomalainen *et al.*, 1999). After accumulation of the viral particles at the MTOC, their distribution along the nuclear envelope and the translocation mechanism across NPC remain unclear. Reorganization of the actin cytoskeleton may also be involved in the movement of the viral capsid of baculovirus and adeno-associated virus (Ploubidou and Way, 2001).

Nuclear entry of viruses

DNA viruses replicating in the nucleus have to deliver their genome in the nuclear compartment. Depending on the virus type the size of the viral DNA is extremely heterogeneous, ranging from 2.5 kb for hepatitis B virus to 150 kb for HSV. Many viruses deliver their genome through the nuclear pore complex (e.g., adenovirus), while others (e.g., retroviruses) require the breakdown of the nuclear membrane (Kasamatsu and Nakanishi, 1998). Association of the viral DNA to viral proteins not only ensures the tight packing of the genetic material, but also confers efficient cytoplasmic transport and nuclear targeting. For example, the small DNA virus SV40 accesses the nucleus through the NPC following a conformational change of the capsid in the endosomal compartment, which leads to the unmasking of NLS in the Vp3 viral protein (Nakanishi *et al.*, 1996). Nuclear uptake of the viral DNA is followed by uncoating before transcription and replication can resume (Greber *et al.*, 1996; Nakanishi *et al.*, 1996). Accordingly, a functional NLS identified within the integrase protein of the human immunodefficiency virus type-1 (HIV-1) is required for the appropriate nuclear localization of the virus (Bouyac-Bertoia *et al.*, 2001).

Larger DNA viruses, such as adenovirus are submitted to a more extensive un-coating in the endosomal compartment and the cytosol, but still remain associated to capsid proteins until docking at the NPC (Greber, 1997; Greber *et al.*, 1993). Translocation of the viral genome of ~40 kb across the NPC occurs together with the terminal protein, which contains a classical NLS (Greber, 1997). In line with the instrumental role of capsid and matrix proteins in the life cycle of viruses, complete dissociation of polypeptides from the viral genome severely compromised the infectability of viral DNA (Kann *et al.*, 1997). These and other studies have revealed that DNA viruses can successfully bypass the cytoplasmic barrier by packaging their genomes into highly specialized polypeptides, ensuring not only nuclease resistance and transport of the vectors across the cytoplasm, but efficient nuclear translocation, as well. These principles of viral DNA delivery could be utilized in designing synthetic vectors, which are capable of bypassing those serial barriers that impede efficient gene transfer with currently available vector systems.

CONCLUDING REMARKS

In summary, it has become evident during the past few years that extracellular and cellular barriers, with tissue and organ specific characteristics, compromise the transfection efficiency of non-viral vectors (Barron and Szoka, 1999; Clark and Hersh, 1999). The challenge for gene therapy is to pinpoint the rate limiting step(s) in this complex process and implement strategies to overcome the biological, physicochemical and metabolic barriers encountered by therapeutic plasmid DNA during nuclear targeting. A thorough understanding of the differences between plasmid DNA and viral DNA transport will provide us clues on how to manipulate the cytoplasmic and nuclear transport steps in many synthetic gene delivery systems to enhance transfection efficiency.

ACKNOWLEDGMENTS

The work in the laboratory was supported by MRC of Canada and the Canadian Cystic Fibrosis Foundation (Sparx II Program). D.L. was supported in part by a CCFF Postdoctoral Fellowship.

REFERENCES

Barron, L.G. and Szoka, F.C. (1999) The perplexing delivery mechanism of lipoplexes. In: L. Huang, M.-C. Huang and E. Wagner (eds) *Nonviral Vectors for Gene Therapy*. Academic Press, pp. 224–264.

Barry, M.A. and Eastman, A. (1993) Identification of deoxyribonuclease II as an endonuclease involved in apoptosis. *Arch. Biochem. Biophys.*, **300**, 440–450.

Bouyac-Bertoia, M., Devorin, J., Fouchier, R., Jenkins, Y., Meyer, B., Wu, L., Emerman, M. and Malim, M. (2001) HIV-1 infection requires a functional integrase NLS. *Mol. Cell*, **7**, 1025–1035.

Branden, L.J., Mohamed, A.J. and Smith, C.I.E. (1999) A peptide nucleic acid-nuclear localization signal fusion that mediates nuclear transport of DNA. *Nat. Biotech.*, **17**, 784–787.

Brisson, M. and Huang, L. (1999) Liposomes: Conquering the nuclear barrier. *Curr. Opin. Mol. Ther.*, **1**, 140–146.

Brunner, S., Sauer, T., Carotta, S., Cotten, M., Saltik, M. and Wagner, E. (2000) Cell cycle dependence of gene transfer by lipoplex, polyplex and recombinant adenovirus. *Gene Ther.*, **7**, 401–407.

Burke, N., Han, W., Li, D., Takimoto, K., Watkins, S. and Levitan, E. (1997) Neuronal peptide release is limited by secretory granule mobility. *Neuron*, **19**.

Capecchi, M.R. (1980) High efficiency transformation by direct microinjection of DNA into cultured mammalian cells. *Cell*, **22**, 479–488.

Cappaccioli, S., Di Pasquale, G., Mini, E., Wazzei, T. and Quattrone, A. (1993) Cationic lipids improve antisense oligonucleotide uptake and prevent degradation in cultured cells and in human serum. *Biochem. Biophys. Res. Com.*, **197**, 818–825.

Chiou, H.C., Tangco, M.V., Levine, S.M., Robertson, D., Kormis, K., Wu, C.H. and Wu, G.Y. (1994) Enhanced resistance to nuclease degradation of nucleic acids complexed to asialoglycoprotein-polylysine carriers. *Nucleic Acids Res.*, **22**, 5439–5446.

Chowdhury, N.R., Hays, R.M., Bommineni, V.R., Franki, N., Chowdhury, J.R., Wu, C.H. and Wu, G.Y. (1996) Microtubular disruption prolongs the expression of human bilirubin-uridinediphosphoglucuronate glucuronyltransferase-1 gene transferred into Gunn rat livers. *J. Biol. Chem.*, **271**, 2341–2346.

Chu, Q., Tousignant, J., Fang, S., Jiang, C., Chen, L., Cheng, S., Scheule, R. and Eastman, S. (1999) Binding and uptake of cationic lipid:pDNA complexes by polarized airway epithelial cells. *Hum. Gene Ther.*, **10**, 25–36.

Clarenc, J.-P., Lebleu, B. and Leonetti, J.-P. (1993) Characterization of the nuclear binding sites of oligodeoxyribonucleotides and their analogs. *J. Biol. Chem.*, **268**, 5600–5604.

Clark, P.R. and Hersh, E.M. (1999) Cationic lipid-mediated gene transfer: current concepts. *Curr. Opin. Mol. Ther.*, **1**, 158–176.

Colin, M., Maurice, M., Trugnan, G., Kornprobst, M., Harbottle, R.P., Knight, A. and Cooper, R. (2000) Cell delivery, intracellular trafficking and expression of an integrin-mediated gene transfer vector in tracheal epithelial cells. *Gene Ther.*, **7**, 139–152.

Cook, G.A., Gattone, V.H., Evan, A.P. and Harris, R.A. (1983) Structural changes of isolated hepatocytes during treatment by digitonin. *Biochim. Biophys. Acta*, **763**, 356–367.

Darquet, A.-M., Rangara, R., Kreiss, P., Schwartz, B., Naimi, S., Delaere, P., Crouzet, J. and Scherman, D. (1999) Minicircle: an improved DNA molecule for *in vitro* and *in vivo* gene transfer. *Gene Ther.*, **6**, 209–218.

Dean, D.A. (1997) Import of plasmid DNA into the nucleus is sequence specific. *Exp. Cell Res.*, **230**, 293–302.

Dean, D.A., Dean, B.S., Muller, S. and Smith, L.C. (1999) Sequence requirements for plasmid nuclear import. *Exp. Cell Res.*, **253**, 713–722.

Diebold, S.S., Kursa, M., Wagner, E., Cotten, M. and Zenke, M. (1999) Mannose polyethylenimine conjugates for targeted DNA delivery into dendritic cells. *J. Biol. Chem.*, **274**, 18087–19094.

Dowty, M.E., Williams, P., Zhang, G., Hangstrom, J.E. and Wolff, J.A. (1995) Plasmid DNA entry into post-mitotic nuclei of primary rat myotubes. *Proc. Natl. Acad. Sci. USA*, **92**, 4572–4576.

El Ouahabi, A., Thiry, M., Fuks, R., Ruysschaert, J. and Vandenbranden, M. (1997) The role of the endosome destabilizing activity in the gene transfer process mediated by cationic lipids. *FEBS Lett.*, **414**, 187–192.

Enari, M., Sakahira, H., Yokoyama, H., Okawa, K., Iwamatsu, A. and Nagata, S. (1998) A caspase-activated DNase that degrades DNA during apoptosis, and its inhibitors ICAD. *Nature*, **391**, 43–50.

Farhood, H., Serbina, N. and Huang, L. (1995) The role of dioleoyl phosphatidylethanolamine in cationic liposome mediated gene transfer. *Biochim. Biophys. Acta.*, **1235**, 289–295.

Fasbender, A., Zabner, J., Zeiher, B.G. and Welsh, M.J. (1997) A low rate of cell proliferation and reduced DNA limit cationic lipid-mediated gene transfer to primary cultures of ciliated human airway epithelia. *Gene Ther.*, **4**, 1173–1180.

Fushimi, K. and Verkman, A. (1991) Low viscosity in the aqueous domain of cell cytoplasm measured by picosecond polarization microfluorimetry. *J. Cell Biol.*, **112**, 719–725.

Gao, X. and Huang, L. (1995) Cationic liposome-mediated gene transfer. *Gene Ther.*, **2**, 710–722.

Godbey, W.T., Wu, K.K. and Mikos, A.G. (1999) Tracking the intracellular path of poly(ethylenimine)/DNA complexes for gene delivery. *Proc. Natl. Acad. Sci. USA*, **96**, 5177–5181.

Greber, U.F. (1997) The role of the nuclear pore complex in adenovirus DNA entry. *EMBO J.*, **16**, 5998–6007.

Greber, U.F., Webster, P., Weber, J. and Helenius, A. (1996) The role of the adenovirus protease in virus entry into cells. *EMBO J.*, **15**, 1766–1777.

Greber, U.F., Willetts, M., Webster, P. and Helenius, A. (1993) Stepwise dismantling of adenovirus 2 during entry into cells. *Cell*, **75**, 477–486.

Hagstrom, J.E., Ludtke, J.J., Bassik, M.C., Sebestyen, M.G., Adam, S.A. and Wolff, J.A. (1997) Nuclear import of DNA in digitonin-permeabilized cells. *J. Cell Sci.*, **110**, 2323–2331.

Harbottle, R.P., Cooper, R.G., Hart, S.L., Ladhoff, A., McKay, T., Knight, A.M. *et al.* (1998) An RGD-oligolysine peptide: a prototype construct for integrin-mediated gene delivery. *Hum. Gene Ther.*, **9**, 1037–1047.

Hillery, E., Cheng, S.H., Geddes, D.M. and Alton, E. (1999) Effects of altering dosing on cationic liposome-mediated gene transfer to the respiratory epithelium. *Gene Ther.*, **6**, 1313–1316.

Jiang, C., O'Connor, S.P., Fang, S.L., Wang, K.X., Marshall, J., Williams, J.L. *et al.* (1998) Efficiency of cationic lipid-medicated transfection of polarized and differentiated airway epithelial cells *in vitro* and *in vivo*. *Hum. Genet.*, **9**, 1531–1542.

Juliano, R. and Yoo, H. (2000) Aspects of the transport and delivery of antisense oligo-nucleotides. *Curr. Opin. Mol. Ther.*, **2**, 297–303.

Kann, M., Bischof, A. and Gerlich, W.H. (1997) *In vitro* model for the nuclear transport of the hepadnavirus genome. *J. Virol.*, **71**, 1310–1316.

Kao, H., Abney, J. and Verkam, A. (1993) Determinants of the translational mobility of a small solute in cell cytoplasm. *J. Cell Biol.*, **120**, 175–184.

Kasamatsu, H. and Nakanishi, A. (1998) How do animal DNA viruses get to the nucleus? *Annu. Rev. Microbiol.*, **52**, 627–686.

Klopfenstein, D., Vale, R. and Rogers, S. (2000) Motor protein receptors: moonlighting on other jobs. *Cell*, **103**, 537–540.

Labat-Moleur, F., Steffan, A.-M., Brisson, C., Perron, H., Feugeas, O., Furstenberger, P. *et al.* (1996) An electron microscopy study into the mechanism of gene transfer with lipopolyamines. *Gene Ther.*, **3**, 1010–1017.

Laskey, R.A. (1998) Regulatory roles of the nuclear membrane. *Biochem. Soc. Trans.*, **26**, 561–567.

Lechardeur, D., Drzymala, L., Sharma, M., Pacia, J., Hicks, C., Usmani, N. *et al.* (2000) Determinants of the nuclear localization of the heterodimeric DNA fragmentation factor (DFF). *J. Cell Biol.*, **150**, 321–334.

Lechardeur, D., Sohn, K.-J., Haardt, M., Joshi, P.B., Monck, M., Graham, R.W. *et al.* (1999) Metabolic instability of plasmid DNA in the cytosol: a potential barrier to gene transfer. *Gene Ther.*, **6**, 482–497.

Leonetti, J.-P., Mechati, N., Degols, G., Gagnor, C. and Lebleu, B. (1991) Intracellular distribution of microinjected antisense nucleotides. *Proc. Natl. Acad. Sci. USA*, **88**, 2702.

Leopold, P.L., Kreitzer, G., Miyazawa, N., Rempel, S., Pfister, K.K., Rodriguez-Boulan, E. and Crystal, R.G. (2000) Dynein-and microtubule-mediated translocation of adenovirus type 5 occurs after endosomal lysis. *Hum. Gene Ther.*, **11**, 151–165.

Luby-Phelps, K. (2000) Cytoarchitecture and physical properties of cytoplasm: volume, viscosity, diffusion, intracellular surface area. *Int. Rev. Cytol.*, **192**.

Luby-Phelps, K., Castle, P.E., Taylor, D.L. and Lanni, F. (1987) Hindered diffusion of inert tracer particles in the cytoplasm of mouse 3T3 cells. *Proc. Natl. Acad. Sci. USA*, **84**, 4910–4913.

Luby-Phelps, K., Mujumdar, S., Mujumdar, R., Ernst, L., Galbraith, W. and Waggoner, A. (1993) A novel fluorescence ratiometric method confirms the low solvent viscosity of the cytoplasm. *Biophys. J.*, **65**, 236–242.

Ludtke, J.J., Zhang, G., Sebestyen, M.G. and Wolff, J.A. (1999) A nuclear localization signal can enhance both the nuclear transport and expression of 1 kb DNA. *J. Cell Sci.*, **112**, 2033–2041.

Lukacs, G.L., Haggie, P., Seksek, O., Lechardeur, D., Freedman, N. and Verkman, A.S. (2000) Size-dependent DNA mobility in cytoplasm and nucleus. *J. Biol. Chem.*, **275**, 1625–1629.

Luo, D. and Saltzman, W.M. (2000) Synthetic DNA delivery systems. *Nat. Biotech.*, **18**, 33–37.

Luthman, H. and Magnusson, G. (1983) High efficiency polyoma DNA transfection of chloroquine treated cells. *Nucleic Acids Res.*, **11**, 1295–1308.

Matsui, H., Johnson, L.G., Randell, S.H. and Boucher, R.C. (1997) Loss of binding and entry of liposome-DNA complexes decreases transfection efficiency in differentiated airway epithelial cells. *J. Biol. Chem.*, **272**, 1117–1126.

Meyer, K.E.B., Uyechi, L.S. and Szoka, F.C.J. (1997) Manipulating the intracellular trafficking of nucleic acids. In: K.L. Brigham (ed.) *Gene Therapy for Diseases of the Lung*. Marcel Dekker Inc, New York, pp. 135–180.

Mirzayans, R., Remy, A.A. and Malcolm, P.C. (1992) Differential expression and stability of foreign genes introduced into human fibroblasts by nuclear versus cytoplasmic microinjection. *Mut. Res.*, **281**, 115–122.

Mortimer, I., Tam, P., MacLachlan, I., Graham, R.W., Saravolac, E.G. and Joshi, P.B. (1999) Cationic lipid-mediated transfection of cells in culture requires mitotic activity. *Gene Ther.*, **6**, 403–411.

Mui, B., Ahkong, Q., Chow, L. and Hope, M. (2000) Membrane perturbation and the mechanism of lipid-mediated transfer of DNA into cells. *Biochim. Biophys. Acta*, **1467**, 281–292.

Nakanishi, A., Clever, J., Yamada, M., Li, P.P. and Kasamatsu, H. (1996) Association with capsid protein promotes nuclear targeting of simian virus 40 DNA. *Proc. Natl. Acad. Sci. USA*, **93**, 96–100.

Neves, C., Escriou, V., Byk, G., Scherman, D. and Wils, P. (1999) Intracellular fate and nuclear targeting of plasmid DNA. *Cell Biol. Toxicol.*, **15**, 193–202.

Nigg, E. (1997) Nucleocytoplasmic transport: signals, mechanism and regulation. *Nature*, **386**, 779–787.

Niidome, T., Ohmori, N., Ichinose, A., Wada, A., Mihara, H., Hirayama, T. and Aoyagi, H. (1997) Binding of cationic alpha-helical peptides to plasmid DNA and their gene transfer abilities into cells. *J. Biol. Chem.*, **272**, 15307–15312.

Page, R.L., Butler, S.P., Subramanian, A., Gwazdauskas, F.C., Johnson, J.L. and Velander, W.H. (1995) Transgenesis in mice by cytoplasmic injection of polylysine/DNA mixtures. *Transgenic Res.*, **4**, 353–360.

Peitsch, M.C., Mannherz, H.G. and Tschopp, J. (1994) The apoptotic endonucleases: cleaning up after cell death? *Trends Cell Biol.*, **4**, 37–41.

Plank, C., Oberhauser, B., Mechtler, K., Koch, C. and Wagner, E. (1994) The influence of endosome-disruptive peptides on gene transfer using synthetic virus-like gene transfer systems. *J. Biol. Chem.*, **269**, 12918–12924.

Ploubidou, A. and Way, M. (2001) Viral transport and the cytoskeleton. *Curr. Opin. Cell Biol.*, **13**, 97–105.

Pollard, H., Remy, J.S., Loussouarn, G., Demolombe, S., Behr, J.P. and Escande, D. (1998) Polyethylenimine but not the cationic lipids promotes transgene delivery to the nucleus in mammalian cells. *J. Biol. Chem.*, **273**, 7507–7511.

Pollard, H., Toumaniantz, G., Amos, J.-L., Avet-Loiseau, H., Guihard, G., Behr, J.-B. and Escande, J.-B. (2001) Ca^{2+}-sensitive cytosolic nucleases prevent efficient delivery to the nucleus of injected plasmids. *J. Gene Med.*, **3**, 153–164.

Polzar, B., Peitsch, M.C., Loos, R., Tschopp, J. and Mannherz, H.G. (1993) Overexpression of deoxyribonuclease I (DNase I) transfected into COS-cells: its distribution during apoptotic cell death. *Eur. J. Cell Biol.*, **62**, 397–405.

Rogers, S. and Gelfand, V.I. (2000) Membrane trafficking; organelle transport, and the cytoskeleton. *Curr. Opin. Cell Biol.*, **12**, 57–62.

Ross, G.F., Bruno, M.D., Uyeda, M., Suzuki, K., Nagao, K., Whitsett, J.A. and Korfhagen, T.R. (1998) Enhanced reporter gene expression in cells transfected in the presence of DMI-2, an acid nuclease inhibitor. *Gene Ther.*, **5**, 1244–1250.

Sakahira, H., Enari, M. and Nagata, S. (1998) Cleavage of CAD inhibitor in CAD activation and DNA degradation during apoptosis. *Nature*, **391**, 96–99.

Sebestyen, M.G., Ludtke, J.J., Bassik, M.C., Zhang, G., Budker, V., Lukhtanov, E.A. *et al.* (1998) DNA vector chemistry: the covalent attachment of signal peptides to plasmid DNA. *Nat. Biotech.*, **16**, 80–85.

Seksek, O., Biwersi, J. and Verkman, A.S. (1997) Translational diffusion of macromolecule-sized solutes in cytoplasm and nucleus. *J. Cell Biol.*, **138**, 131–142.

Simoes, S., Pedro, P., Duzgunes, N. and Pedrosa de Lima, M.C. (1999) Cationic liposomes as gene transfer vectors: Barriers to successful application in gene therapy. *Curr. Opin. Struct. Biol.*, **1**, 147–157.

Sodeik, B. (2000) Mechanism of viral transport in the cytoplasm. *Trends Microbiol.*, **8**, 465–472.

Sodeik, B., Ebersold, M.W. and Helenius, A. (1997) Microtubule-mediated transport of incoming herpes simplex virus 1 capsids to the nucleus. *J. Cell Biol.*, **136**, 1007–1021.

Steiner, J.A., Hortsmann, H. and Almers, W. (1997) Transport, docking and exocytosis of single secretory granules in live chromaffin cells. *Nature*, **388**, 474–478.

Subramanian, A., Ranganathan, P. and Diamond, S.L. (1999) Nuclear targeting peptide scaffolds for lipofection of non-dividing mammalian cells. *Nat. Biotech.*, **17**, 873–877.

Suomalainen, M., Nakano, M.Y., Keller, S., Boucke, K., Stidwill, R.P. and Greber, U.F. (1999) Microtubule-dependent plus- and minus end-directed motilities are competing processes for nuclear targeting of adenovirus. *J. Cell Biol.*, **144**, 657–672.

Talcott, B. and Moore, M.S. (1999) Getting across the nuclear pore complex. *Trends Cell Biol.*, **9**, 312–318.

Thierry, A.R., Rabinovich, P., Mahan, L.C., Bryant, J.L. and Gallo, R.C. (1997) Characterization of liposome-mediated gene delivery: Expression, stability and pharmacokinetics of plasmid DNA. *Gene Ther.*, **4**, 226–237.

Torriglia, A., Chaudun, E., Chany-Fournier, F., Jeanny, J.-C., Courtois, Y. and Counis, M.-F. (1995) Involvement of DNase II in nuclear dègeneration during lens cell differentiation. *J. Biol. Chem.*, **270**, 28579–28585.

Torriglia, A., Perani, P., Borssas, J., Chaudun, E., Treton, J., Courtois, Y. and Counis, M.-F. (1998) L-DNaseII, a molecule that links proteases and endonucleases in apoptosis, derives from the ubiquitous Serpin Leukocyte Elastase Inhibitor. *Mol. Cell. Biol.*, **18**, 3612–3619.

Tseng, W.-C., Haselton, F.R. and Giorgio, T.D. (1997) Transfection by cationic liposomes using simultaneous single cell measurements of plasmid delivery and transgene expression. *J. Biol. Chem.*, **272**, 25641–25647.

Uherek, C., Fominaya, J. and Wels, W. (1998) A modular DNA carrier protein based on the structure of diphteria toxin mediates target cell-specific gene delivery. *J. Biol. Chem.*, **273**, 8835–8841.

Vacik, J., Dean, B.S., Zimmer, W.E. and Dean, D.A. (1999) Cell-specific nuclear import of plasmid DNA. *Gene Ther.*, **6**, 1006–1014.

Vanderbilt, J.N., Bloom, K.S. and Anderson, J.N. (1982) Endogenous nucleases. *J. Biol. Chem.*, **257**, 13009–13017.

Wagner, E., Plank, C., Zatloukal, K., Cotten, M. and Birnstel, M. (1992) Influenza virus hemagglutinin HA-2 N-terminal fusogenic peptides augment gene transfer by transferrin polylysine-DNA complexes: toward a synthetic virus-like gene-transfer vehicle. *Proc. Natl. Acad. Sci. USA*, **89**, 7934–7938.

Wattiaux, R., Laurent, N., Wattiaux-De Coninck, S. and Jadot, M. (2000) Endosomes, lysosomes: their implication in gene transfer. *Adv. Drug Deliv. Rev.*, **41**, 201–208.

Wheeler, J., Palmer, L., Ossanlou, M., MacLachlan, I., Graham, R., Zhang, Y. *et al.* (1999) Stabilized plasmid-lipid particles: construction and characterization. *Gene Ther.*, **6**, 271–281.

Wilke, M., Fortunati, E., Van den Broek, M., Hoogeveen, A.T. and Scholte, B.J. (1996) Efficacy of a peptide-based gene delivery system depends on mitotic activity. *Gene Ther.*, **3**, 1133–1142.

Wilson, G.L., Dean, B.S., Wang, G. and Dean, D.A. (1999) Nuclear import of plasmid DNA in digitonin-permeabilized cells requires both cytoplasmic factors and specific DNA sequences. *J. Biol. Chem.*, **274**, 22025–22032.

Wrobel, I. and Collins, D. (1995) Fusion of cationic liposomes with mammalian cells occurs after endocytosis. *Biochim. Biophys. Acta*, **1235**, 296–304.

Wyllie, A.H. (1980) Glucocorticoid-induced thymocyte apoptosis is associated with endogenous endonuclease activation. *Nature*, **284**, 555–556.

Xu, Y. and Szoka, F.C. (1996) Mechanism of DNA release from cationic liposome/DNA complexes used in cell transfection. *Biochem.*, **35**, 5616–5623.

Yanez, R.J. and Porter, A.C.G. (1999) Gene targeting is enhanced in human cells over-expressing hRAD51. *Gene Ther.*, **6**, 1282–1290.

Zabner, J., Fasbender, A.J., Moninger, T., Poellinger, K.A. and Welsh, M.J. (1995) Cellular and molecular barriers to gene transfer by a cationic lipid. *J. Biol. Chem.*, **270**, 18997–19007.

Zanta, M.A., Belguise-Valladier, P. and Behr, J.-P. (1999) Gene delivery: a single nuclear localization signal peptide is sufficient to carry DNA to the cell nucleus. *Proc. Natl. Acad. Sci. USA*, **96**, 91–96.

Zelphati, O., Liang, X., Hobart, P. and Felgner, P. (1999) Gene chemistry: functionally and conformationally intact fluorescent plasmid DNA. *Hum. Gene Ther.*, **10**, 15–24.

Zelphati, O. and Szoka, F. (1996a) Intracellular distribution and mechanism of delivery of oligonucleotides mediated by cationic lipids. *Pharm. Res.*, **13**, 1367–1372.

Zelphati, O. and Szoka, F. (1996b) Mechanism of oligonucleotide release from cationic liposomes. *Proc. Natl. Acad. Sci. USA*, **93**, 11493–11498.

Zhou, X. and Huang, L. (1994) DNA transfection mediated by cationic liposomes containing lipopolylysine; characterization and mechanism of action. *Biochim. Biophys. Acta*, **1189**, 195–203.

12 Nucleocytoplasmic trafficking

David A. Dean

INTRODUCTION

Under physiologically relevant conditions, the levels of non-viral gene transfer are low at best. The reason for this is that many barriers exist for the efficient transfer of genes to cells, all of which must be circumvented before any gene expression can occur (Figure 12.1). First, vectors must be targeted to specific cell types while avoiding many others. Second, before the vector can reach any cell, it must make its way through the extracellular matrix. Third, the vector must enter the cell by breaking through the plasma membrane/endosome barrier. Finally, once in the cytoplasm of non-dividing cells, the DNA is confronted by the nuclear membrane, which it must traverse to enter the nucleus. That the DNA must enter the nucleus is self-evident: without localization to the nucleus, no transcription, replication, integration, or maintenance can take place. However, given the importance of the nuclear entry step, there has been surprisingly little attention directed toward either discovering or exploiting the mechanisms used by the cell to direct DNA to the nucleus. In this chapter, I will focus on the nuclear import step of gene delivery, which will hopefully lead to an increased appreciation for this barrier.

BARRIERS TO NUCLEAR TRANSPORT

Mechanisms of nuclear transport

Over 25 years ago, Bonner demonstrated that entry of proteins into the nucleus was not a random event and that there existed within the cell a class of proteins that selectively localized to this compartment (Bonner, 1975a,b). Over the next ten years relatively few studies were directed at understanding how the entry of proteins into (or exit of mRNA from) the nucleus occurred. What was known from these early studies was that nuclear entry was likely signal mediated and size restricted; while small proteins could enter the nucleus, most large proteins could not. Thus, early on it was realized that the nuclear envelope served as a permeability barrier. Further, based on a series of elegant electron micrographic studies by Carl Feldherr, this exchange of molecules between the nucleus and cytoplasm was found to be mediated by the nuclear pore complex (NPC) (Feldherr *et al.*, 1984). In 1984, the first nuclear localization signal (NLS) was identified in the SV40 large T-antigen and progress toward dissecting the mechanisms of nuclear import

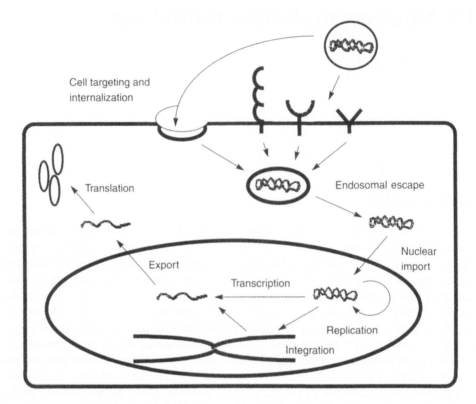

Figure 12.1 Cellular barriers to gene delivery. Extracellular DNA, delivered to cells
in either viral particles, liposomes, or other vehicles, must traverse the
plasma, endosomal, and nuclear membranes before any transcription,
replication, or integration can occur.

quickly followed. With the introduction of a powerful experimental system based
on digitonin-permeabilized cells (Adam *et al.*, 1990), the identification of NLS
receptors and components of the import and export machinery was rapid.

All exchange of macromolecules between the nucleus and cytoplasm occurs
through nuclear pore complexes (NPCs) situated in the nuclear envelope. The pores
are large ($\sim$125 MDa) multiprotein complexes that are composed of upwards of 100
distinct proteins present in multiple copies (Stoffler *et al.*, 1999). At the center of the
NPC is a large pore of 25 nm diameter through which all macromolecular transport
occurs. Studies on the diffusion of proteins across the NPC have shown that proteins
of less than 50 kDa can enter the nucleus in a signal-independent manner at rates
inversely proportional to their size. By contrast, proteins of larger than 50 kDa are
restricted to the cytoplasm unless they possess a nuclear localization signal (NLS).
The first NLS identified was that of the SV40 large T-antigen, which consists of
a central run of basic amino acids (PKKKRKV) flanked be several additional residues
that are not necessary for nuclear import (Kalderon *et al.*, 1984a,b). This sequence
has been named the 'classical' NLS and variations are found in hundreds of nuclear
proteins. A second class of NLS, the 'bipartite' signal, is characterized by the sequence
from the *Xenopus* nucleoplasmin protein in which the classical NLS is broken into two

halves by an intervening group of 5 to 20 amino acids (Robbins *et al.*, 1991). The third best-characterized NLS is that of the heterogeneous nuclear ribonucleoprotein (hnRNP) A1 protein and is termed the M9 sequence. Unlike the other sequences, M9 is not rich in basic amino acids, but functions very efficiently as both a nuclear import and nuclear export signal (NES) (Siomi and Dreyfuss, 1995). Apart from these sequences, many other potential NLSs have been identified, but to date, these secondary sequences have not been well characterized and the mechanisms of their transport have not been completely elucidated.

Proteins containing an NLS are transported into the nucleus through interactions with one or more of a broad family of NLS receptors, termed the 'importins' or 'karyopherins' (Figure 12.2). In the case of classical NLS-mediated nuclear import, the NLS binds to importinα, which in turn binds to importinβ1 in the cytoplasm. The complex is then transported through the NPC into the nucleoplasm. Upon entry into the nucleus, a small ras-like GTP-binding protein, Ran, in its GTP-bound state, interacts with the complex and promotes dissociation (Moroianu *et al.*, 1996; Gorlich *et al.*, 1996; Izaurralde *et al.*, 1997b). Ran is relatively equally distributed throughout the cell, but different nucleotide-bound states predominate in each compartment. In the cytoplasm, Ran-GDP is more abundant, due to the presence of a group of GTPase activating proteins (RanGAP, RanBP1,

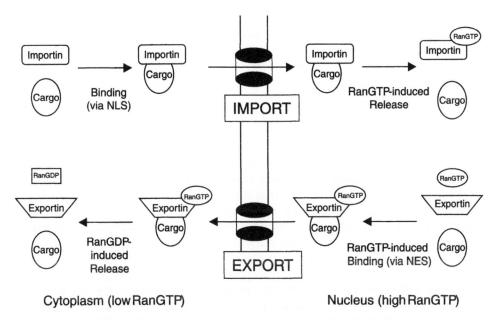

Figure 12.2 Model for importin-mediated nuclear import and export. NLS-containing proteins in the cytoplasm bind to importin family members in the cytoplasm and are translocated through the NPC. Once inside the nucleus, Ran-GTP interacts with the importin-cargo complex to facilitate complex dissociation. Similarly, proteins to be exported from the nucleus interact with one of the exportins, but in contrast to the case with importins, assembly of this complex is promoted by Ran-GTP. As the complex, presumably with Ran-GTP bound, enters the cytoplasm, the GTP is hydrolyzed to GDP, which induces the release of the cargo from exportin.

RanBP2), while Ran-GTP is the predominant species in the nucleus, due to a nuclear GTPase exchange factor, RCC1 (Moore, 1998). Other proteins containing different types of NLSs interact with other members of the importin family. For example, the M9 NLS interacts directly with importinβ2 (also known as transportin), without the need for the importinα subunit (Pollard *et al.*, 1996). Indeed, importinβ1 is the only importin family member that appears to utilize importinα for NLS recognition. To date, over six importinα and 20 importinβ family members have been identified in humans, many of which appear to mediate the nuclear localization of unique families of proteins (Jans *et al.*, 2000). For example, importinβ3 recognizes NLSs present in a subgroup of ribosomal proteins (Yaseen and Blobel, 1997), while importinβ5 and β7 mediate the import of another class of ribosomal proteins (Jakel and Gorlich, 1998), and an importinβ1–β7 heterodimer facilitates transport of histone H1 (Jakel *et al.*, 1999).

The nuclear export of proteins occurs by a remarkably similar mechanism, utilizing other importin family members for the recognition of NESs present on proteins that need to exit the nucleus. Exportin and CAS are two such family members that recognize NESs (Jans *et al.*, 2000). As seen in nuclear import, there is some specificity of binding by the individual family members. Thus, while exportin binds to NESs found on a wide range of proteins, CAS appears to bind uniquely to the NES found in importinα to facilitate its nuclear export after its import in the NLS-importinα-importinβ complex. As in nuclear import, Ran also plays a necessary role in export, but in contrast to its effects on the importinβ-NLS complex, nuclear Ran-GTP promotes binding of exportins to the NES (Izaurralde *et al.*, 1997b). Once the complex is translocated to the cytoplasm, RanGAP hydrolyzes the bound GTP to GDP and the Ran-GDP causes complex dissociation. Again, because of the asymmetric distribution of Ran-GDP and Ran-GTP in the cell, directionality of transport can take place.

The nuclear import and export of small RNAs (e.g., U snRNAs, tRNAs, 5S rRNA) and large RNAs (e.g., mRNA) utilize many of the same proteins as the protein import machinery, including certain importins and Ran (Stutz and Rosbash, 1998). However, RNAs also need additional proteins to facilitate their transport, namely adapter proteins. Although nuclear import and export sequences have been identified on different classes of RNAs, their function is not to bind directly to the importins or exportins, but rather to bind to proteins that in turn contain nuclear import and export sequences. For example, hnRNP A1 binds to hnRNA and mRNA and accompanies the nucleic acids out of the nucleus. As previously discussed, hnRNP A1 contains the M9 NLS/NES. Thus, it is likely that the hnRNP A1 protein acts as an adapter to allow indirect binding of transportin to mRNA (Izaurralde *et al.*, 1997a). In another well-studied example, the Rev protein of HIV binds to the Rev Response Element (RRE) present in the incompletely spliced viral RNAs within the nucleus. Bound to the mRNA, Rev also interacts with exportin (also called CRM1) through its NES to promote the export of the viral RNAs (Fischer *et al.*, 1995). Similar adapter protein-mediated mechanisms will be revisited for DNA nuclear localization.

Nuclear envelope

The nuclear envelope acts as a permeability barrier for a variety of macromolecules, and DNA is no exception. In 1980, Mario Capecchi demonstrated that when a pBR322-derived plasmid expressing thymidine kinase (TK) was micro-injected into the nuclei of TK-deficient mouse fibroblasts, between 50% and 100% of the injected cells showed TK activity at 24 hours post-injection (Capecchi, 1980). By contrast, in over 1000 cytoplasmically injected cells, no gene expression was detected in any cell during the same time frame. Similar results were obtained in another microinjection study using rat TK-deficient cells and a plasmid expressing chloramphenicol acetyl transferase (CAT) driven by a herpes TK promoter. When 1000–2000 copies of the plasmid were injected into the cytoplasm, less than 3% of the activity was seen as compared to cells injected in the nucleus with the same number of plasmids (Graessman *et al.*, 1989). Zabner *et al.* (1995), in a series of elegant experiments, aimed at determining the cellular and molecular barriers to gene transfer using cationic lipids, demonstrated once again, this time in *Xenopus* oocytes, that nuclear injected DNA resulted in high level gene expression, but the same DNA injected into the cytoplasm gave no expression. Nuclear injections of viral DNA genomes have also been shown to be between 10- and 100-times more efficient in producing an infectious virus than similar cytoplasmic injections (Kopchick *et al.*, 1981; Graessman and Graessman, 1981; Nakanishi *et al.*, 1996). Other experiments in a variety of cell systems also have demonstrated the ineffi-cient gene expression of cytoplasmically delivered DNA, leading to the conclusion that the nuclear envelope is a major barrier for gene delivery and expression (Mirzayans *et al.*, 1992; Thornburn and Alberts, 1993).

Cell cycle

Implicit in the previous experiments demonstrating that the nuclear envelope is a permeability barrier is that the cells studied were, for the most part, non-dividing. One of the hallmarks of mitosis is the breakdown of the nuclear envelope. Thus, as the cells go through mitosis there is no longer a barrier between the nuclear and cytoplasmic compartments. Consequently, the main reason that actively dividing cells are much more amenable to gene delivery, transfections, and viral infections, is that one of the major barriers to gene expression has been removed. Perhaps one of the best examples of this is the dependence of retroviral infections on the cell cycle (Miller *et al.*, 1990; Lewis and Emerman, 1994). It is well documented that retroviruses (with the exception of the lentiviruses) can infect cells at any stage of the cell cycle, deposit their RNA genomes into the cytoplasm, and reverse tran-scribe their genome into rtDNA. However, the rtDNA remains in the cytoplasm until the cell undergoes mitosis; if the cells are arrested and do not enter mitosis, the viral genome, now as rtDNA, remains in the cytoplasm until it is likely degraded, never leading to a productive infection. Similarly, it is well appreciated by all researchers that in order for efficient transfections to occur, actively growing populations of cells must be used; confluent, growth-arrested, and terminally differentiated cells are extremely difficult, if not nearly impossible, to transfect with any reasonable success.

The importance of cell division on the nuclear localization and subsequent expression of DNA has been nicely shown in human primary airway epithelial cells (Fasbender *et al.*, 1997). Fasbender and colleagues demonstrated that actively dividing cells, identified by the BrdU incorporation, were ten times more likely to express the transferred gene product than BrdU-negative cells. A more detailed study of the relationship between cell cycle and gene delivery and expression was recently described from Ernst Wagner's group (Brunner *et al.*, 2000). Synchronized cells that were fractionated at different stages of the cell cycle by elutriation were transfected with CMV promoter-driven, luciferase-expressing plasmids using Lipofectamine, transferrin-polyethylenimine, or transferrin-polylysine and evaluated for gene expression. In all cases, cells transfected in G1 expressed 50- to 300-fold less gene product than those transfected in G2 or G2-M.

NUCLEAR TRANSPORT

Nuclear entry of plasmids in the absence of cell division

My laboratory began to study the nuclear entry of DNA with a very simple experiment: microinject protein-free plasmids into the cytoplasm of cells and watch what happens (Dean, 1997). Our initial experiments were performed in African Green monkey kidney epithelial cells using protein-free, purified SV40 DNA (5,243 bp), which was detected post-injection by *in situ* hybridization. The advantage of this approach is that it is direct and does not rely on the transcriptional activity or post-transcriptional processes that must occur in order to detect the expression of a gene product as an indicator of DNA nuclear import. Cells were either synchronized, growth-arrested, or injected when confluent to ensure that all import studies were carried out in the absence of cell division. Further, fluorescent markers that were too large to enter the nucleus in the absence of cell division were co-injected along with the DNA to ensure that only those cells that had not divided were scored. When the cells were fixed immediately after microinjection, the DNA was present throughout the cytoplasm, but by six to eight hours post-injection, the vast majority of the injected DNA had localized to the nucleus. This time course of SV40 DNA nuclear accumulation is in agreement with that observed by Nakanishi *et al.* (1996), who followed nuclear import by measuring large T-antigen expression from the cytoplasmically injected SV40 DNA. By co-injecting agents that block NPC-mediated import, including antibodies against the NPC, and the lectin wheat germ agglutinin, it was shown that the nuclear entry of SV40 DNA was mediated by the NPC (Dean, 1997). Depletion of energy or incubation at low temperature also blocked nuclear import. Using a similar microinjection approach in post-mitotic myotubes, Jon Wolff's group has previously shown the same mechanism of DNA nuclear uptake through the NPC (Dowty *et al.*, 1995). Thus, plasmids are able to gain access to the nuclei of cells in the absence of cell division through the NPC, like all other nuclear-localizing macromolecules.

Sequence specific nuclear uptake

In an attempt to characterize the kinetics of plasmid nuclear entry, we performed a simple competition experiment using one of several bacterial plasmids in the microinjected cell system (Dean, 1997). However, no matter what molar excess of the bacterial plasmid was co-injected, the amount of SV40 DNA that localized to the nucleus remained unchanged. To our surprise, when the location of the bacterial plasmids was determined by *in situ* hybridization in the co-injected cells,

pBR322   SV40

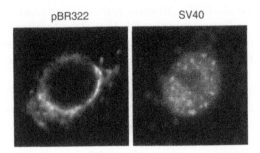

Figure 12.3 Sequence-specific nuclear import of plasmids. Growth-arrrested CV1 cells were cytoplasmically microinjected with either pBR322 or SV40 DNA (5000 copies per cell) as described in Dean, 1997. Eight hours later the location of the DNA was visualized by *in situ* hybridization.

it was found that whereas the SV40 DNA localized entirely to the nucleus, the bacterial DNA remained completely in the cytoplasm (Figure 12.3). By cloning the SV40 genome into the bacterial plasmid, we quickly determined that the nuclear import of plasmid DNA was a sequence specific event. The DNA sequence from SV40 needed for nuclear localization was mapped to the 72 bp SV40 enhancer (Dean, 1997; Dean *et al.*, 1999b). The presence of as little as 50 bp of this sequence in a bacterial plasmid can cause the plasmid to localize to the nucleus with kinetics that are indistinguishable from the entire SV40 genome. Further, we have demonstrated that such sequence-specific nuclear import occurs in all cell types tested to date (Table 12.1). In support of these findings, the origin region of the SV40 genome encompassing the 72 bp enhancer element was shown to lead to increased transcription of a herpes TK promoter-driven reporter gene in actively dividing cells (Graessman *et al.*, 1989). As expected, the presence of the enhancer stimulated transcription when compared to a similar plasmid lacking the enhancer. However, when the plasmids were injected into the cytoplasm, the stimulation by the enhancer was greater than could be accounted for by classic enhancer activity.

Table 12.1   Cells displaying sequence-specific DNA nuclear import

Cell lines	Primary cells	
HeLa	Human cells:	Mouse cells:
A549	Vascular smooth muscle cells	Osteoblasts
TC7	HUVECs	Skin fibroblasts
CV1	Microvascular endothelial cells	Chondrocytes
Cos	Pulmonary artery endothelial cells	Rat cells:
BRL	Corneal epithelial cells	Oligodendrocytes
C2C12	Corneal fibroblasts	Osteoblasts
PC12	Skeletal muscle cells	Skin fibroblasts
NIH3T3	Chicken cells:	Plants:
L929	Vascular smooth muscle cells	Coconut edosperm
CHO	Fibroblasts	*Tradescantia* stamen hairs

Thus, the authors suggested that this element may also lead to increased nuclear localization of the plasmid (Graessman *et al.*, 1989). Moreover, that the increase was seen in dividing populations of cells indicates that the DNA nuclear localization even in dividing cells could be due to a combination of both NPC-mediated, sequence-specific import and localization during mitosis when there is no nuclear envelope.

It is interesting to note that most of the studies that first identified the nuclear envelope as a barrier to gene transfer and expression were performed with plasmids that lacked any SV40 sequences (Graessman *et al.*, 1989; Capecchi, 1980; Thornburn and Alberts, 1993; Zabner *et al.*, 1995). Most of these works utilized plasmids expressing reporter genes driven from one of three promoters: the CMV immediate early promoter, the RSV LTR, or the herpes TK promoter, all of which have been shown to have no import activity (Dean *et al.*, 1999b; Vacik *et al.*, 1999). Thus, it is not surprising that the results obtained were so striking; when these plasmids were introduced into the cytoplasm by either microinjection or transfection, they lacked the sequences necessary for nuclear targeting in the absence of mitosis.

Based on these findings, we developed a model for the nuclear import of plasmids (Figure 12.4). The defining feature of the SV40 enhancer is its ability to bind to multiple transcription factors that are expressed in almost every cell type. Indeed, the SV40 enhancer has been used to identify and characterize many of the general transcription factors utilized by eukaryotic cells, including SP1, AP1, AP2, AP3, AP4, Oct-1, and NF-κB, among others. Like all other proteins in the cell, transcription factors are translated in the cytoplasm. Because they function in the nucleus, they must either contain NLSs or associate with other proteins that

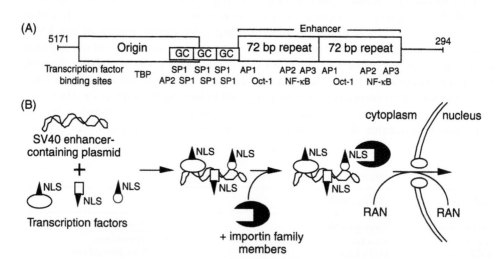

Figure 12.4 Model for SV40 enhancer-mediated sequence-specific plasmid nuclear import. (A) Cartoon of the SV40 origin region, containing two copies of the 72 bp enhancer repeats. As can be seen, multiple transcription factors have been identified to bind to this region (only a few proteins are listed). (B) Model for nuclear import. Newly synthesized NLS-containing transcription factors bind to the SV40 enhancer in the cytoplasm to form a protein-DNA complex. Importin family members can recognize the DNA-bound NLSs to facilitate the nuclear import of the complex.

contain NLSs for their nuclear entry. A second property that the transcription factors must have is a DNA binding domain that recognizes a unique sequence of DNA. Under normal circumstances, after synthesis, a typical transcription factor would be transported into the nucleus, bind to its DNA target sequence in various promoters, and activate or repress transcription. However, if a plasmid containing the transcription factor binding site is present in the cytoplasm, the newly synthesized transcription factor may bind to this site before nuclear import. In the case of the SV40 enhancer, it is known that multiple proteins can bind at once, and this could create a high local concentration of NLSs at a unique site on the plasmid. The NLS import machinery could then bind to the DNA-bound transcription factors and translocate the DNA-protein complex into the nucleus.

In an attempt to identify other DNA sequences that function similarly in nuclear import to the SV40 enhancer, we tested several unrelated viral promoters and enhancers that have been shown to drive substantial gene expression *in vivo*. The long terminal repeat (LTR) promoters from Rous Sarcoma and Moloney Murine Leukemia retroviruses were unable to cause the nuclear localization of pBR322 DNA. This is not surprising since it has been shown that these retroviruses can replicate only in cells that are actively dividing, due to the absence of a nuclear envelope during mitosis allowing nuclear localization of the genome (Miller *et al.*, 1990; Lewis and Emerman, 1994). Similarly, an 800 bp fragment of the CMV immediate early promoter and enhancer was also unable to support nuclear import (Dean *et al.*, 1999b; Vacik *et al.*, 1999). To exclude the possibility that these other promoters may act as cytoplasmic retention signals, the SV40 enhancer was cloned into plasmids containing either the CMV or RSV promoters and shown to cause the nuclear localization of the hybrid plasmids (Dean *et al.*, 1999b).

It should be pointed out that although there is no sequence similarity between the CMV and SV40 promoters, each contains multiple binding sites for transcription factors, in contrast to the structures of the LTR promoters, which contain few such sites. Thus, if our model for nuclear import simply predicts that binding sites for transcription factors on DNA are sufficient for nuclear import, these three additional viral promoters should have been imported. Because this did not happen, three possibilities exist. First, and least attractively, is that the model is wrong. This possibility is unlikely based on a variety of results, both in injected and in permeabilized cells (see below). Second, it is possible that one or more unique transcription factors binds to the SV40 enhancer but do not bind to the other three promoters, and that these proteins are responsible for nuclear import. While this possibility cannot be ruled out, it is unlikely based on two lines of evidence. When the sequences are analyzed for transcription factor binding sites, only one factor, AP2, is found that binds to the SV40 sequence but not to the CMV promoter or the LTRs, suggesting that AP2 may be the 'magic' factor. However, we have shown that another promoter that contains AP2-binding sites is not imported in all cells like the SV40 enhancer and further, plasmids containing tandem synthetic AP2 binding sites are also not imported. Further, using a series of linker scanning mutants that disrupt most of the individual binding sites within the 72 bp enhancer repeat, we found that although disruption of the AP1 site is tolerated, disruption of any and all other sites resulted in plasmids that were no longer able to localize to the nucleus. Finally, the third possibility to account for the lack of nuclear import of various strong promoters, is that the SV40 sequence is somewhat unique in its ability to promote nuclear import in a wide variety of cell types.

Nuclear import in permeabilized cells

In order to characterize the molecular mechanisms of DNA nuclear uptake, a more defined system than intact cells was needed. Digitonin-permeabilized cells offer an attractive system to study nuclear transport events (Adam *et al.*, 1990). Digitonin preferentially solubilizes cholesterol, which is abundant in the plasma membrane. By washing detergent-treated cells, all endogenous cytoplasm can be removed and the requirements for nuclear import can be determined using fractionated extracts and purified recombinant transport proteins (e.g., Ran, importins, etc.). Using this approach, Wolff and colleagues demonstrated that linear fragments of double-stranded DNA are transported into the nucleus through the NPC (based on wheat germ agglutinin [WGA] inhibition) in an energy- and temperature-dependent manner (Hagstrom *et al.*, 1997). DNA nuclear import was also saturable, but was not competed by excess NLS-containing proteins, suggesting that the DNA entered the nucleus through a pathway distinct from that of classic NLS-containing proteins. Interestingly, they found that nuclear uptake of the DNA was size-dependent as well, with DNA fragments of less than 1,000 bp entering the nucleus and those higher (2, 3, and 5 kbp) being excluded. This is in contrast to what is seen in intact cells where 5–10 kbp plasmids readily localize to the nucleus (Dowty *et al.*, 1995; Dean *et al.*, 1999b; Dean, 1997). A somewhat troubling finding of this study was that the fluorescently-labeled linear DNA fragments that localized to the nuclei of permeabilized cells failed to localize to the nuclei of microinjected cells, suggesting that the pathway studied in the *in vitro* system may not be directly relevant to what occurs *in vivo*. Further, the staining pattern of the DNA within the nuclei in these permeabilized cells was different than what has been seen by others in intact cells after microinjection. In this permeabilized cell system, the DNA localized to 10 to 20 spots within the nucleus and showed intense staining at the nuclear rim. In contrast, in liposome-transfected or microinjected cells, nuclear plasmid DNA is much more throughout the nucleoplasm (with the exception of the nucleolus), but with intense foci of DNA in multiple spots as well (Coonrod *et al.*, 1997; Zelphati *et al.*, 1999; Vacik *et al.*, 1999; Dean, 1997; Dean *et al.*, 1999b). It is possible that the difference in staining patterns is simply a matter of the number of molecules transported in the permeabilized cells, suggesting that linear DNA may first localize to these foci before diffusing to the rest of the nucleoplasm. Finally, that this combination of system and substrate may not represent what is happening *in vivo* is suggested by the fact that nuclear import of the DNA was not dependent on cell extracts (as is NLS-dependent protein nuclear import, U snRNA nuclear import or NES-mediated export), but was rather inhibited by the addition of cytoplasmic extracts. However, in a subsequent study from the same laboratory, cytoplasmic extracts were absolutely required for DNA nuclear import when the substrate was not naked DNA, but rather linear or plasmid DNA that was conjugated to multiple NLS peptides (Sebestyén *et al.*, 1998). Again, however, the substrate failed to localize to the nuclei of microinjected cells as determined by fluorescence microscopy, but a slight increase in gene expression from the micro-injected plasmids was seen when NLSs were conjugated. Thus, in order to make any definitive conclusions about the molecular mechanisms of DNA nuclear uptake, the system and substrates must function *in vitro* as they do *in vivo*.

One of the difficulties in studying DNA nuclear localization is the relative inability to produce fluorescently-labeled DNA that remains functional for gene expression and nuclear import. Our laboratory had tried for years to produce a labeled plasmid that still localized to the nucleus. A variety of labeling techniques were tested, including the incorporation of fluorescent nucleotide analogues (e.g., fluorescein-dUTP) by PCR or nick-translation followed by ligation to form intact plasmid DNA, covalent and non-covalent high affinity intercalating dyes (e.g., ethidium bromide monoazide and TOTO-1), and the reaction of supercoiled plasmid with photoactivatable fluorophore conjugates. While all of the methods produced fluorescently-labeled DNA, two problems limited the use of these labeled DNAs as substrates for import reactions. Firstly, several of the techniques produced either linear DNA or low yields of circularized plasmid DNA, making their use impractical. Because we wanted to study the nuclear import of plasmids, we did not want to use linear fragments of DNA in the event that their nuclear import was by different mechanisms. More importantly, all of the labeled DNAs became inactive in both transcription of reporter genes or migration of the DNA to the nucleus in microinjected cells. One approach that was successful was the use of a fluorescently-labeled peptide nucleic acid (PNA) clamp (Wang *et al.*, 1999; Zelphati *et al.*, 1999; Wilson *et al.*, 1999; Zelphati *et al.*, 2000). The advantage of this approach is that the PNA hybridizes to a distinct purine-rich target sequence present in a plasmid with a very high affinity, resulting in a complex that is extremely stable *in vitro* and *in vivo* (Zelphati *et al.*, 1999; Demidov *et al.*, 1994). Thus, the target sequence can be engineered anywhere in a plasmid, preferably away from transcribed genes and nuclear import sequences. Using a fluorescently-labeled PNA, Felgner and colleagues were able to demonstrate that liposomes efficiently delivered fluorescently-labeled PNA-complexed plasmids to cells, and that the plasmids localized to vesicles within the cytoplasm early after transfection (three hours) (Zelphati *et al.*, 1999). Interestingly, no nuclear localization of fluorescent plasmid was observed until after cell division. The plasmids used in this study, however, lacked DNA sequences that we have shown to be necessary for sequence-specific nuclear import (Dean, 1997; Dean *et al.*, 1999b). When the SV40 enhancer was cloned into the plasmid used in the Zelphati study, nuclear import of the fluorescent DNA was observed within six to eight hours, well before cell division (Dean, unpublished observation). Further, using a triplex-forming PNA of our own design, we demonstrated that SV40 enhancer-containing plasmids labeled with this PNA were also able to localize to the nucleus in microinjected cells with the same kinetics as native DNA and showed the same patterns of distribution throughout the nucleus (Wilson *et al.*, 1999).

Using fluorescent PNA-labeled plasmids and the digitonin-permeabilized cell system, we were able to show that plasmid nuclear uptake was time-, energy-, and temperature-dependent and utilized the NPC for translocation (Wilson *et al.*, 1999). Furthermore, nuclear entry of the plasmids, as well as NLS-containing proteins, were absolutely dependent on the addition of cytoplasmic extracts (Figure 12.5). Plasmids up to 14 kbp in size were efficiently transported into the nuclei within four hours, although larger plasmids were not tested. As seen in microinjected cells, DNA nuclear entry was sequence specific: a 4.2 kbp plasmid

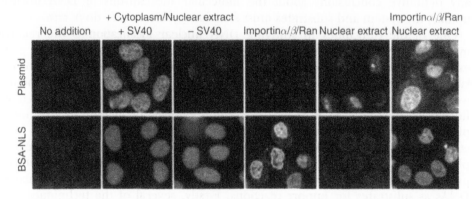

Figure 12.5 Nuclear import in permeabilized cells. HeLa cells were grown on coverslips and permeabilized with digitonin as described in Wilson *et al.*, 1999. Fluorescein-PNA-labeled plasmids (containing the SV40 enhancer, 4.2 kb) or rhodamine-labeled BSA-NLS peptide conjugates were incubated with the cells for four hours at which time they were viewed by fluorescence microscopy. With no additions, neither DNA nor protein was imported, but in the presence of nuclear and cytoplasmic extracts both substrates localized to the nuclei. While plasmids containing the SV40 enhancer were taken up by the nuclei, those lacking the sequence were excluded. The remaining panels demonstrate the need for both the import machinery (importins and Ran) and a source of adapter proteins (nuclear extract) for plasmid nuclear entry, but not for protein nuclear localization.

lacking the SV40 enhancer was excluded from the nuclei while an isogenic plasmid containing the SV40 sequence localized to the nucleus efficiently. Nuclear import of the plasmids was effectively competed by SV40 enhancer-containing plasmids, but not by plasmids lacking the SV40 sequence. To examine the requirements for the cytoplasmic extracts, we reconstituted the NLS-dependent nuclear import machinery using the purified recombinant import factors Ran, importinα, and importinβ. When a fluorescently-labeled NLS-protein was used as substrate, addition of all three import factors was needed for nuclear localization. By contrast, the addition of Ran, importinα and importinβ alone did not support the nuclear import of plasmid DNA. This is in agreement with our model for the nuclear import of plasmids because none of the import factors that bind to the DNA, DNA-binding, NLS-containing adapters are needed. When nuclear extracts were added as a source of transcription factors, import was reconstituted with the purified import factors.

Requirement of nuclear import sequences in the absence of cell division

It is reasonable to assume that the more genes delivered to the nucleus, the more gene expression will be obtained. Indeed, it was demonstrated over 20 years ago that direct injection of plasmids and viral genomes directly into the nucleus caused a profound increase in gene expression versus their cytoplasmic delivery (Kopchick *et al.*, 1981; Graessman and Graessman, 1981; Capecchi, 1980). Thus, the ability of plasmids to localize to the nucleus should greatly increase their expression in both dividing and, more importantly, non-dividing cells. Graessman *et al.* (1989) performed a series of experiments where he microinjected plasmids containing or lacking the SV40 enhancer into the cytoplasm or nuclei of dividing cells. In all experiments, the cells were allowed to undergo between one and two cell doublings. When transfected into cells, the plasmids containing the SV40 sequence showed higher expression, consistent with the enhancer activity on transcription. Further, when injected into the nucleus, enhancer-containing plasmids displayed modestly increased expression versus that found with cytoplasmic injections. However, when plasmids lacking the enhancer sequence were injected into the cytoplasm, they showed 30-fold lower levels of expression than when delivered directly into the nucleus. This effect was more than could be accounted for by the transcriptional effects of SV40 enhancer and it was postulated that the enhancer also had 'helper' activity that may aid nuclear import.

To demonstrate that the helper activity is indeed a nuclear import sequence and that by increasing the concentration of DNA that reaches the nucleus gene expression is also increased, a series of experiments were performed in synchronized cells taking advantage of the inability of the CMV immediate early promoter and enhancer to mediate nuclear import (Dean *et al.*, 1999b). Two enhanced green fluorescent protein (EGFP)-expressing plasmids were used, both of which expressed EGFP from the CMV promoter and one of which contained the SV40 enhancer downstream of the EGFP gene. That both plasmids were transcriptionally equivalent was demonstrated by the fact that both gave similar levels of gene expression when injected directly into the nuclei of the cells. When injected into the cytoplasm of synchronized cells in G1, the SV40 enhancer containing plasmid showed GFP expression within two hours of injection and reached a maximum level by 12 hours (Figure 12.6). By contrast, the plasmid lacking the SV40 sequence showed absolutely no GFP expression until after the cells had divided at around 14 hours, demonstrating the utility of the SV40 sequence for nuclear uptake.

Effect of nuclear import sequences on transfection

Since the ultimate goal is to exploit these nuclear targeting signals to increase gene transfer to cells, we tested whether these DNA sequences also functioned to stimulate gene expression in transfected cells. Using a CMV promoter driven firefly luciferase or LacZ gene construct, plasmids either lacking the SV40 enhancer or carrying it downstream of the reporter gene were transfected into dividing and non-dividing cells. Because the SV40 sequence has classic enhancer activity, any increase in gene expression could be due to a combination of increased nuclear localization and/or transcription. When actively growing KB cells (human nasopharyngeal cancer cells) were transfected using cationic liposomes or dendrimers, a modest two-fold increase in gene expression was detected (Reddy *et al.*, 1999). Since the greatest effect of the nuclear targeting sequences is expected in non-dividing cells, CV1 cells were arrested with aphidicolin prior to and during transfections. When CV1 cells were transfected using the cationic liposomes Lipofectin™, very little activity was detected with the enhancer-lacking plasmid, but when the SV40 promoter/enhancer region was included, gene expression

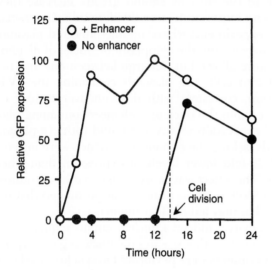

Figure 12.6 Plasmid nuclear localization must precede gene expression. Synchronized TC7 cells were cytoplasmically microinjected with 1000 copies of GFP-expressing plasmids (Dean *et al.*, 1999b). After microinjection, the cells were scored for GFP expression as a function of time. The injected plasmids expressed GFP from the CMV immediate early promoter/enhancer and either contained (open circles) or lacked (closed circles) the SV40 enhancer downstream of the GFP gene. The dotted line represents the time of cell division in this population. As can be seen, plasmids without the SV40 enhancer failed to localize to the nucleus and gave no GFP expression, while plasmids containing the sequence began to express gene product within several hours of cytoplasmic injection.

increased by over 500-fold (Vacik *et al.*, 1999). Similar results were obtained with arrested HeLa cells and HUVECs, as well as confluent primary human corneal epithelial cells and keratocytes (Dean *et al.*, 1999a).

Sequence-specific nuclear import of plasmids *in vivo*

Although the levels of gene transfer and expression in cultured cells is perceived by researchers always to be exceedingly low (hence the constant introduction of new transfection reagents), that in animals is almost always lower. Thus, any method to increase *in vivo* gene delivery and expression would be favorably received by the research community. To determine whether inclusion of these DNA nuclear targeting sequences in plasmids causes increased gene expression in animals, two tissues were chosen: skeletal muscle and the vasculature. Reporter plasmids expressing either GFP, secreted alkaline phosphatase (SEAP), or luciferase from the CMV immediate early promoter/enhancer or the skeletal actin promoter were created. One set of plasmids lacked the SV40 enhancer, while another set contained the enhancer in various places within the plasmid backbone. Plasmids were injected into the CD-1 mouse tibialis muscle, and assayed for gene expression two or seven days later. When the SV40 enhancer was placed upstream of the CMV promoter, a five-fold increase in gene expression was detected at day two (Li *et al.*,

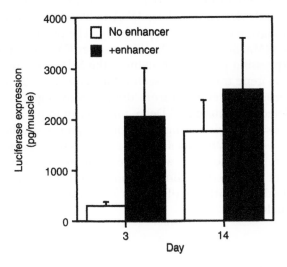

Figure 12.7 Nuclear import sequences increase gene expression in murine muscle. Mouse tibialis muscles were injected with 10 μg of CMV-driven luciferase plasmids either lacking (open bars) or containing (shaded bars) the SV40 enhancer downstream of the luciferase gene. Immediately after injection, the muscles were electroporated (8 pulses, 10 milliseconds each, 200 V/cm) and the animals were allowed to recover. Three or 14 days later, muscles were removed and assayed for luciferase expression (average ± SEM, n = 5).

2001). By day seven, the increase was almost 20-fold. Similarly, when the enhancer was placed upstream of the skeletal actin promoter, in either orientation, the stimulation seen at day two was between 7- and 20-fold. Significant increases in total gene expression were seen when the muscles were electroporated after injection, but the SV40 enhancer had a more modest effect giving roughly a two- to three-fold increase in expression (Li *et al.*, 2001). Using a similar approach in murine skeletal muscle, our laboratory has seen the same stimulation by the SV40 enhancer in CMV-driven luciferase constructs when placed downstream of the reporter gene (Figure 12.7). At day three, the presence of the SV40 enhancer caused an almost ten-fold increase in gene expression that dropped to an only 40% increase at day 14. It should be pointed out that even without an SV40 enhancer, plasmids were able to direct gene expression in skeletal muscle after either injection or injection and electroporation. Indeed, this has been known since the seminal experiments of Wolff and colleagues (Wolff *et al.*, 1990, 1992a,b). In these experiments, both the CMV promoter and the RSV LTR showed robust expression in muscle. This expression implies that in skeletal muscle, plasmids lacking the SV40 enhancer are still able to enter the nucleus, although it is likely that the entry is much slower and less efficient. This entry rate would explain the large difference in gene expression seen at early times after *in vivo* delivery with the SV40 enhancer and the relatively modest effect seen at 14 days; early on the SV40 enhancer stimulates nuclear uptake, but over time even plasmids that take a long time to enter the nucleus will accumulate there and lead to gene expression.

We have also found that the SV40 enhancer leads to increased expression in the vasculature. Using a unique electrode design to deliver DNA to blood vessels, we have demonstrated that up to nanogram levels of gene product can be produced in a 1 cm segment of a 200 μm vessel (Martin *et al.*, 2000). When either CMV promoter driven GFP- or luciferase-expressing plasmids containing the SV40 enhancer are added to vessels, high levels of gene transfer are seen (Martin *et al.*, 2000). By contrast, when the SV40 sequences were removed from the plasmids, significant reductions in expression were detected (Young and Dean, manuscript in preparation). In the case of the GFP vectors, plasmids lacking the import sequence resulted in very weakly- or non-fluorescent vessels. When luciferase was used as the reporter, a 30-fold decrease in gene expression was seen when the SV40 sequence was removed from the vector. Both of these results confirm and extend the findings in skeletal muscle to demonstrate the importance of nuclear targeting of plasmids both in isolated cells and in animals.

Cell-specific nuclear import

Although several very strong viral promoters failed to provide DNA nuclear import activity, it is unlikely that the SV40 enhancer is unique in its ability to target DNA to the nucleus. Based on our model for plasmid nuclear localization, we reasoned that there may exist examples of DNA sequences that promote nuclear import in a cell-specific manner, due to their binding of cell-specific transcription factors (Figure 12.8). To identify such DNA sequences, we screened a number of smooth muscle-specific promoters for their ability to act as import sequences. The smooth muscle gamma actin (SMGA) gene is expressed in vascular and visceral smooth muscle and is regulated at the transcriptional level by a set of smooth muscle specific transcription factors and binding partners (Kovacs and Zimmer, 1993, 1998; Zimmer *et al.*, 1996; Browning *et al.*, 1998). Among these proteins are serum response factor (SRF) and several homeodomain family transcription factors (Browning *et al.*, 1998; Carson *et al.*, 2000). When a plasmid containing the SMGA promoter was microinjected into the cytoplasm of either primary human vascular or chicken visceral smooth muscle cells, it localized to the nucleus within six to eight hours of injection (Vacik *et al.*, 1999). By contrast, when injected into the cytoplasm of CV1 cells or endothelial cells, the SMGA promoter containing plasmids remained in the cytoplasm. In support of our model for nuclear import, we were able to partially reconstitute nuclear import in non-smooth muscle cells by creating an SRF-expressing stable CV1 cell line. In these cells, the SMGA constructs localized to the nucleus at about 30% of the level seen in smooth muscle cells. This suggests that SRF is capable of directing this sequence to the nucleus, but it is likely that other smooth muscle-specific transcription factors are also needed for maximal nuclear localization.

Taking a slightly different approach, we have identified a second cell-specific DNA nuclear import sequence that acts uniquely in endothelial cells (Young *et al.*, 1999). Several endothelial specific promoters were cloned into pCMV-EGFP in place of the SV40 enhancer. To identify which promoters mediated nuclear import, the plasmids were microinjected into the cytoplasm of synchronized cells and GFP expression was scored eight hours after injection, well before cell division. Thus, any GFP expression is the result of enhanced nuclear import of the plasmid

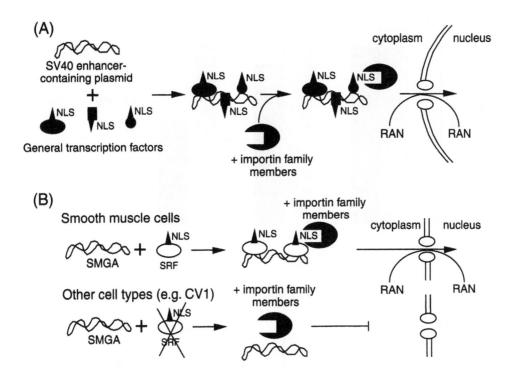

Figure 12.8 Model for general and cell-specific plasmid nuclear import. (A) SV40 enhancer-mediated nuclear import. Because the transcription factors bound by this DNA sequence are ubiquitously expressed, SV40 DNA localizes to the nuclei of all cell types (see Table 12.1). (B) Smooth muscle-specific plasmid nuclear import. Smooth muscle-specific transcription factors, including SRF among others, can bind to their target sites within the SMGA promoter carried on a plasmid and serve to transport the DNA to the nucleus via interactions with the NLS-mediated protein import machinery. Since these factors are not expressed in other cell types, no nuclear import will occur in non-smooth muscle cells.

(Dean *et al.*, 1999b). Using this method, we found that the 553 bp flk-1 promoter (−285 to +268) directed nuclear import in endothelial cells but not CV1 cells or smooth muscle cells (Figure 12.9). These results suggest that (1) the SV40 enhancer is not unique in its ability to target DNA to the nucleus, and that (2) other sequences may be identified to mediate DNA nuclear import in cell-specific, developmental, temporal, and inducible manners.

Nuclear import of exogenous DNA/protein complexes

Although the SV40 enhancer exploits endogenous transcription factors for its nuclear import, examples of similar DNA-NLS containing viral (or bacterial) protein complexes are utilized abundantly in viral and bacterial systems to target their DNA to the nuclei of host cells. However, the major difference between the nuclear targeting of many pathogen genomes and that of SV40 enhancer-containing plasmids is that the SV40 enhancer utilizes only normal host proteins; thus, it will

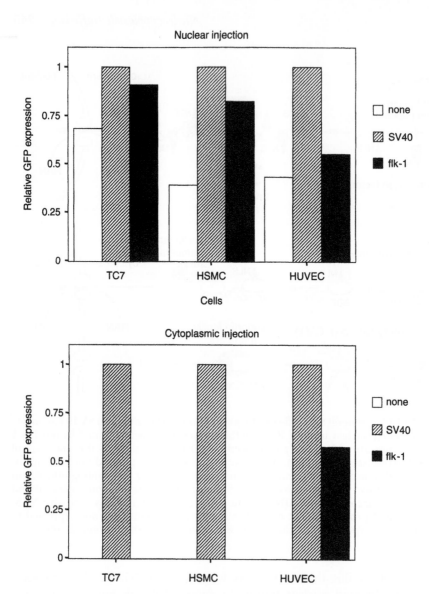

Figure 12.9 Endothelial cell-specific nuclear import of plasmids. Growth-arrested African Green Monkey kidney epithelial cells (TC7), human pulmonary artery smooth muscle cells (HSMCs) and human umbilical vein endothelial cells (HUVECs) were microinjected in the nucleus (top) and cytoplasm with CMV-driven, GFP-expressing plasmids containing either no additional sequences (open bars), the SV40 enhancer (striped bars), or the flk-1 promoter (shaded bars). Eight hours after injection, the cells were visualized for GFP expression by fluorescence microscopy. Whereas all three plasmids supported GFP expression when delivered into the nucleus of all three cell types, only the SV40 enhancer mediated nuclear import and gene expression in all cells when injected into the cytoplasm. As predicted, the flk-1 promoter caused import and expression only in cells in which transcription factors necessary for its expression and import were made, namely endothelial cells.

function autonomously in any given cell type without the need for exogenous viral or bacterial proteins. One of the best-studied examples of a nuclear targeted genome is that of the HIV preintegration complex. Similar to other retroviruses, the incoming viral RNA genome of HIV is reverse transcribed in the cytoplasm into a double stranded DNA molecule of approximately 14 kbp. Complexed with the reverse transcribed DNA is a set of viral proteins that are carried within the virus particle and that remain associated with the viral genome during reverse transcription. Among these are two NLS-containing proteins, matrix (MA) and integrase (IN) and a third viral protein R (Vpr) that is involved either directly or indirectly in the nuclear import process (Bukrinsky *et al.*, 1993). This preintegration complex of proteins and DNA is able to enter the nucleus in the absence of cell division, distinguishing it from the oncoretroviruses (Bukrinsky *et al.*, 1992). Experiments have demonstrated that mutation of the matrix protein NLS can abolish nuclear import of the preintegration complex and subsequent infection by HIV, as does mutation of Vpr (Heinzinger *et al.*, 1994; Popov *et al.*, 1998b; von Schwedler *et al.*, 1994; Vodicka *et al.*, 1998). While the matrix protein appears to function by donating its NLS for DNA nuclear import, the role of Vpr is less well defined, although experiments suggest that it can both promote association of importinα with the matrix NLS and act directly as an importinβ-like protein to facilitate nuclear import of the complex (Popov *et al.*, 1998a,b; Jenkins *et al.*, 1998; Vodicka *et al.*, 1998).

Another well-characterized pathogenic DNA/protein complex that is transported through the nuclear pore complex is the tumor inducing-(Ti) DNA of *Agrobacterium tumefaciens*. In this case a single-stranded linear DNA that is transported into the nucleus in association with two bacterial DNA-binding and NLS-containing proteins, VirD2 and VirE2. VirD2 is covalently attached to the 5′ end of the DNA and VirE2 acts as a ssDNA binding protein to coat the length of the DNA. NLSs on both proteins seem to be needed for the efficient nuclear import in both plant (Sheng and Citovsky, 1996; Zupan *et al.*, 1996) and mammalian systems (Ziemienowicz *et al.*, 1999). Recently, it was shown that the VirE2 protein also has pore-forming activity, suggesting that this activity may aid not in the nuclear import of the DNA complex, but rather in plasma membrane translocation (Dumas *et al.*, 2001).

A third system that has exploited the interactions between a NLS-containing DNA-binding protein and a plasmid containing its DNA target site for increased nuclear import is that of the Epstein-Bar virus EBNA-1/*oriP* interaction. EBNA-1 is a protein involved in EBV genome maintenance and segregation (Aiyar *et al.*, 1998). Rittner and colleagues transfected cells with plasmids either carrying or lacking the *oriP* sequence to which EBNA-1 binds (Langle-Rouault *et al.*, 1998). In cells expressing EBNA-1, 60- to 130-fold increased expression was seen with the *oriP* plasmids, whereas only a 0.6- to 3-fold increase was seen in EBNA-1 lacking cells. When the plasmids were injected into the cytoplasm of EBNA-1 expressing cells, 40- to 100-fold more expression was seen with the *oriP* containing plasmids. When injected into the nucleus of EBNA-1 positive cells, *oriP* plasmids showed 7- to 25-fold more expression than their *oriP*-counterparts. This greater effect in cytoplasmically injected cells lead the authors to conclude that EBNA-1 was aiding in the nuclear transport of the DNA. However, this is only a four-fold difference between nuclear and cytoplasmic injections, and a crucial experiment substantiating this conclusion was never performed: does cytoplasmic injection of an *oriP* plasmid give more expression than the *oriP*-plasmid in an EBNA-1 lacking cell?

Consequently, while suggestive, these results do not unequivocally point to increased nuclear import of DNA as the overriding mechanism.

Alternative pathways of DNA nuclear uptake

Although there is a wealth of data demonstrating that the nuclear import of plasmids is a sequence-specific event, a number of results point to the possibility that alternative mechanisms may also exist for DNA nuclear targeting. It has been known for years that two of the strongest promoters for *in vivo* expression are the CMV immediate early promoter and enhancer and the RSV LTR promoter (Manthorpe *et al.*, 1993; Hartikka *et al.*, 1996; Yew *et al.*, 1997; Wolff *et al.*, 1990). When plasmids carrying these promoters are injected into the post-mitotic myotubes in skeletal muscle from rodents and even primates, robust gene expression is observed, even as quickly as 15 minutes post-injection (Doh *et al.*, 1997). Because these cells are non-dividing, the DNA is somehow gaining access to the intact nucleus, although how remains to be determined. Dowty *et al.* (1995) demonstrated that plasmid nuclear import in myotubes used the NPC for its uptake. Again, in these experiments, a plasmid using the RSV LTR to drive luciferase expression showed very clear nuclear import over a reasonable time frame. One possible explanation is that skeletal muscle represents a tissue unlike any others in the body. While differences in patterns of gene expression are routinely seen in muscle versus other tissues, this is not an adequate explanation. Another, more likely alternative is that plasmid nuclear import is not absolutely sequence-dependent, but rather the presence of certain sequences such as the SV40 enhancer increase the rate of nuclear targeting. Thus, these non-imported promoters may actually allow nuclear import, although at greatly reduced rates. Because the time course for many cell injection studies is 8 to 12 hours, SV40 enhancer-lacking plasmids may not have yet had time to enter the nucleus (Dean, 1997; Dean *et al.*, 1999b). Simple kinetics could then account for the gene expression that is seen within minutes of plasmid injections into muscle: the more plasmid delivered to the cytoplasm, the more likely at least some will be driven into the nucleus. Indeed, it has been shown that 10^6 plasmids (lacking SV40 sequences) are needed to be injected into the cytoplasm of a single myotube *in vivo* to obtain gene expression (Utvik *et al.*, 1999). Similarly, in Dowty's experiments, the minimum concentration of DNA needed for detectable gene expression after cytoplasmic microinjection was 10^{-5} mg/ml for an SV40-containing construct and 10^{-4} mg/ml for an RSV LTR-driven plasmid (on the order or 10 and 100 plasmids/cell, respectively) (Dowty *et al.*, 1995). Since the DNA is much too large to traverse the NPC by diffusion, it probably enters the nucleus as a protein–DNA complex. Once in the cytoplasm, any plasmid will be quickly coated with proteins. That at least some of these DNA-binding proteins have nuclear localization sequences is not surprising. Thus, it is possible that a model similar to that used by SV40 enhancer-containing plasmids can account for the nuclear import of these non-SV40 containing plasmids complexed to fewer and weaker nuclear-localizing proteins.

Studies on the mechanisms of polyethylenimine (PEI) mediated transfections suggest that PEI may promote the nuclear localization of plasmids by alternative mechanisms as well. By injecting increasing copy numbers of free plasmids or PEI-complexed plasmids into the cytoplasm or nucleus, Jean-Paul Behr's laboratory has shown that PEI-condensation increased nuclear targeting by ten-fold (Pollard *et al.*, 1998). Further, unlike the effects seen with cationic lipid-complexed DNA, PEI-complexed plasmids are fully functional for gene expression in the nucleus. They interpreted this to mean that PEI-complexed plasmids, but not cationic lipid–DNA complexes, are targeted to the nucleus with increased efficiency, although no mechanism for this import was suggested. Recently, Godbey *et al.* (1999, 2000) followed the fate of fluorescently-labeled PEI-plasmid complexes in transfected cells and found that although some of the PEI-plasmid complexes dissociated in the cytoplasm, much of the PEI and DNA that entered the nucleus did so as associated complexes. Moreover, the observed nuclear fluorescence of the PEI and DNA (and PEI transfected in the absence of DNA) was in an ordered structure, suggesting that large PEI–DNA complexes entered the nucleus as intact structures. Because of their size and the characteristics of PEI/plasmid complexes, they favor models of PEI fusion with the nuclear envelope for enhanced nuclear entry. Although fusion with the nuclear envelope has been suggested in the past for a number of viral nuclear entry pathways, it has yet to be unequivocally demonstrated. Given the highly structured nuclear lamina that sits below the nuclear envelope, it is doubtful that simple fusion with the nuclear envelope would allow any large molecule to pass through the lamina without major structural rearrangements within the nucleus.

Finally, several experiments from Peter Traub's group have suggested that there exists another pathway for the highly efficient nuclear import of DNA. While studying the ability of oligonucleotides to facilitate the movement of fragments of the intermediate filament protein vimentin from the cytoplasm to the nucleus, they looked for other nucleic acids that would function similarly in nuclear targeting. Alone, vimentin remains cytoplasmic in filaments, but when bound to single- or double-stranded oligonucleotides, the protein targeted to the nucleus where it could function in a variety of nuclear activities (Hartig *et al.*, 1998a). When supercoiled plasmids were bound to vimentin through the DNA-binding activity of this protein, they caused the rapid movement of the protein into the nucleus (Hartig *et al.*, 1998b). By contrast, when the plasmids were relaxed or linearized, they were no longer able to mediate transport into the nucleus. Interestingly, they found that all supercoiled plasmids showed that same activity, regardless of sequence. Although the experiment was not performed, these results suggest that supercoiled DNAs may have the ability to rapidly migrate into the nucleus. However, in all of our experiments, the plasmids we have used for transfections and microinjections have always been at least 70% in the supercoiled form; if supercoiling could promote the nuclear import of any plamsid in a sequence-independent manner, we most likely would have detected it. Thus, these results suggest that the nuclear import of supercoiled DNA/vimentin complexes may be due to the complex rather than either of the parts.

APPROACHES TO INCREASE NUCLEAR TARGETING OF DNA

The goal of all gene therapy approaches is to target enough DNA to cells to obtain sufficient expression for a therapeutic effect. One of the major barriers to this goal is the nuclear envelope and our relative inability to target substantial amounts of DNA to the nucleus. Even using plasmid nuclear targeting sequences such as the SV40 enhancer to exploit the cell's machinery for nuclear import, nuclear import is still inefficient. By microinjecting increasing copy numbers of GFP expressing plasmids that contained the SV40 enhancer into the cytoplasm or nucleus, we found that although gene expression could be detected with as few as ten copies injected into the cytoplasm and one copy in the nucleus, it took almost 100-fold more cytoplasmically delivered DNA to generate the same levels of gene expression as in nuclear injected cells (Dean *et al.*, 1999b). Thus, any methods designed to increase the amount of DNA targeted to the nucleus would be valuable.

Non-covalent attachment of proteins

DNA and certain RNA viruses have developed very efficient strategies for targeting their genomes to the nucleus (Whittaker and Helenius, 1998; Kasamatsu and Nakanishi, 1998). The way they do this is to deliver viral protein-nucleic acid complexes rather than naked DNA or RNA alone (see above). Because these proteins usually contain NLSs and are bound tightly to the incoming genomes, the DNA or RNA (e.g., influenza virus) enter the nucleus through the NLS- and NPC-mediated pathway. Using a similar approach, a number of studies have been reported in which nuclear proteins were complexed with plasmids to facilitate their nuclear localization. Kaneda *et al.* (1989) formed complexes of plasmids with high mobility group-1 (HMG-1) proteins or nucleoplasmin and demonstrated that when incorporated into Sendai virus (HVJ)-liposomes, the HMG-1 proteins increased gene expression in transfected cells by a factor of five within the first 12 hours after transfections. By labeling the DNA with tritium prior to complex formation, they also showed that DNA complexed with HMG-1 localized to the nucleus within four to eight hours, while plasmids complexed with control IgG or BSA were about three-fold less effective at reaching the nucleus and took much longer to get there. Other experiments have also shown that HMG1, HMG17, and histone H1 can lead to increased gene expression (Bottger *et al.*, 1998). Wolff and colleagues took an analogous approach using plasmids complexed to histone H1 and found that the addition of H1 gave a 20-fold stimulation of gene expression versus DNA without H1 when the complexes were transfected into cells using cationic (Fritz *et al.*, 1996) or anionic (Hagstrom *et al.*, 1996) liposomes. However, it does not appear that the incorporated histone is facilitating nuclear import. H1-containing complexes were internalized to a greater extent than DNA-liposomes alone, and when the H1-DNA complexes were microinjected into the cytoplasm, they showed no greater expression than DNA alone (Fritz *et al.*, 1996).

Non-covalent peptide/DNA complexes

NLS peptides are also being used for enhanced gene transfer to the nucleus and subsequent gene expression. Some of the earliest experiments were from Phillippe Collas and Peter Alestrom. When synthetic SV40 T-antigen NLS peptides were complexed with plasmid DNA and microinjected into the cytoplasm of zebrafish embryos, increased nuclear localization of plasmids was observed, as was the increased integration and expression of the transgene (Collas and Alestrom,

1996, 1997a,b; Collas *et al.*, 1996). Using *in vitro* assembled sea urchin nuclei, they were able to demonstrate that DNA nuclear import was energy-dependent, inhibited by agents that block the NPC, and required cytoplasmic extracts (Collas and Alestrom, 1996). Further, the addition of functional NLS peptides was also needed for nuclear binding and uptake of the DNA. Added NLS peptides can also increase gene expression from plasmids delivered to mammalian cells using catioinic liposomes, but in one report the stimulation was a modest three-fold (Aronsohn and Hughes, 1998).

Another approach to non-covalently complex NLS peptides to plasmids taken by David Jans' group was to link the SV40 T-antigen NLS to polylysine and then react this with plasmids (Chan and Jans, 1999). Although polylysine resembles the classical NLS (K_n verses KKKRK), it was shown that polylysine–DNA complexes do not bind to importinα nor do they support nuclear import of DNA to any large extent. By contrast, when an NLS peptide was linked to the polylysine, the complex bound to importinα and accumulated in the nuclei. However, only a two-fold increase in gene expression was observed. Instead of using polylysine to condense the plasmids and act as an anchor for NLS peptides, another study used a scrambled T-antigen NLS to bind to the DNA and linked the M9 NLS from hnRNP A1 to the basic peptide (M9-ScT) (Subramanian *et al.*, 1999). Using permeabilized cells, the M9-ScT conjugate lead to increased nuclear import of the plasmid in a cytosol-dependent manner. Moreover, plasmids complexed with the M9-ScT and transfected using lipoplexes into confluent bovine aortic endothelial cells gave 60-fold increased levels of gene expression over that of transfected plasmid alone and about ten-fold higher levels of expression than the scrambled NLS or scrambled M9 peptides alone.

Covalent attachment of peptides to DNA

Non-covalent linkage between plasmids and peptides may lead to the dissociation of the desired peptides from the plasmids in the cytoplasm, and thus the peptides may not be able to transport the DNA into the nucleus. To circumvent this, Sebestyén *et al.* (1998) used a novel crosslinking reagent to link peptides, through N-terminal cysteine residues, to DNA. Using a digitonin-permeabilized cell system to study nuclear import, they were able to show that the DNA localized to the nucleus in an importin- and NLS peptide-mediated manner, unlike the import of native linear DNA in their system, which did not require cytoplasmic import factors (Sebestyén *et al.*, 1998; Hagstrom *et al.*, 1997). At least 100 NLS peptides/kb conjugated to the plasmid were required for nuclear import to be detected. Unfortunately, such high levels of conjugation to the DNA (one chemical crosslink every 10 bp) have the tendency to abolish transcription and expression of genes on the plasmid. To overcome this tendency, they ligated an unmodified reporter plasmid to a piece of DNA that had been labeled with NLS peptides. However, they detected little benefit to reporter gene expression (less than four-fold), suggesting that this approach may not be suitable for gene delivery. Other studies crosslinking NLS peptides and plasmids also have shown direct interaction of the complex with importins, confirming that these peptide–DNA complexes use the normal nuclear import machinery for their nuclear localization (Ciolina *et al.*, 1999). Another study also failed to detect large increases in gene expression with covalently attached NLS peptides (Neves *et al.*, 1999). Using an NLS peptide linked to a photoactivatable psoralen, they were able to cross-link peptides to the DNA every 35 to 500 bp, depending on labeling ratios. However, only a two-fold enhancement of gene expression was seen when NLS-conjugated plasmids were liposome transfected into cells.

Recently, a single NLS peptide (PKKKRKVEDPYC) fused to a linear piece of DNA that was capped at both ends by DNA hairpins was shown to increase gene expression by a factor of 10 to 1000 when delivered by 25 kDa branched poly-ethylenimine (Zanta *et al.*, 1999). These experiments used an NLS peptide con-jugated to a base within the hairpin at one end of the DNA. Although clearly demonstrating that the addition of an NLS to a piece of DNA will increase gene expression, presumably by increasing the amount of DNA reaching the nucleus, a peptide-free, capped, linear DNA was over 100-fold less transcriptionally active than supercoiled plasmid. Thus, to achieve maximal expression, it appears that supercoiled plasmid should be the form of choice.

Peptide nucleic acids and their use

Peptide nucleic acids (PNAs) are nucleic acid analogs in which the phosphodi-ester backbone has been replaced with a polyamide backbone made up of repeat-ing *N*-(2-amnioethyl)glycine units (for a recent review, see Dean, 2000). The major advantage of this backbone substitution is that the resulting nucleic acid is resistant to both nucleases and proteases (Demidov *et al.*, 1994; Zelphati *et al.*, 1999). Further, it is possible to design triplex forming PNAs if the DNA target sequence is a polypurine tract. One advantage of these triplex-forming PNAs, or 'PNA clamps', is that they bind to defined target sequences on DNA with high affinity (10^{-6} to 10^{-9} M) and the resulting structure is highly stable. Indeed, the addition of 1000-fold molar excess of a target site oligonucleotide does not remove bound PNA from its previously bound DNA (Zelphati *et al.*, 1999; Wilson *et al.*, 1999). A second major advantage of PNAs is that the target site to which they bind can be placed anywhere in a plasmid, close to or removed from promoters, coding sequences, or nuclear import sequences. Thus, these reagents are highly attractive for attaching peptides and other molecules to plasmids at defined sites. Felgner and colleagues have shown that peptides can be linked to PNAs either before PNA hybridization to DNA or after hybridiza-tion (Zelphati *et al.*, 2000). Further, the binding of PNAs to plasmids does not alter the conformation or state of the DNA.

Using PNA technology, several laboratories have linked NLS sequences to plasmids. In one set of experiments, an NLS peptide (PKKKRKV) was linked to a triplex-forming PNA (GCGCTCGGCCCTTCC) and then complexed to either a LacZ- or GFP-expressing plasmid. When PNA–NLS complexed plasmids were transfected into cells by polyethylenimine, they increased gene expression over uncomplexed DNA by between five- and eight-fold (Branden *et al.*, 1999). When 100-fold more free NLS peptide was included in the transfection, the levels of gene expression fell, leading the investigators to conclude that the increase in transfection efficiency afforded by the NLS–PNA was due to increased nuclear import. Thus, while PNA technology is promising, it remains to be exploited.

OTHER OBSTACLES IN TRANSPORT TO NUCLEUS

Although the 'nuclear import' of plasmids or any other macromolecule is usually thought of as the translocation across the NPC into the nucleus, we should be thinking more globally of 'nuclear targeting' instead. It is a long way from the site of release of the DNA into the cytoplasm, either by direct fusion at the plasma membrane or after endosome escape, to the NPC. In most cells this distance is in the order of microns, although in specialized cells such as neurons, the distance can be greater than 1 mm. How then does the DNA migrate through this large distance of cytoplasm to the nucleus? Where does interaction with the nuclear import machinery take place? Is this all just a random process?

The cytoplasm, like the nucleoplasm, is a complex structure with an array of cytoskeletal elements, including actin filaments, microtubules, and intermediate filaments, organized into a lattice-like array. Once thought to be just a viscous gel, it is now appreciated that the cytoplasm has a defined and ever-changing structure. As such, diffusion through the cytoplasm is restricted. It has been shown that macromolecules over 500 kDal are highly restricted in their cytoplasmic diffusion (Luby-Phelps *et al.*, 1987; Provance *et al.*, 1993; Seksek *et al.*, 1997). Lukacs *et al.* (2000) microinjected the cytoplasm of HeLa cells with fluorescently-labeled linear DNA fragments and found that the diffusion of fragments greater than 3000 bp was undetectable, although fragments less than 1000 bp were able to diffuse through the cytoplasm, and fragments less than 500 bp were even able to enter the nucleus. Although these experiments are technically elegant, the results do not make biological sense; plasmids can and do move through the cytoplasm to enter the nucleus, both in dividing and non-dividing cells. The most likely answer to this conundrum is that the productive movement of plasmids and DNAs through the cytoplasm is not primarily by diffusion, but is directed.

Viruses have evolved multiple strategies to target their genomes to the nuclei of cells (Whittaker and Helenius, 1998; Kasamatsu and Nakanishi, 1998). A theme that is becoming evident in the nuclear targeting of many of these viruses is that they travel through the cytoplasm via interactions with the cytoskeleton (Leopold *et al.*, 2000a; Stidwill and Greber, 2000). By fluorescently labeling virus particles or capsids, a number of laboratories have been able to follow the viruses as they traffic to the nucleus. Labeled herpes simplex virus type-1 (HSV) and adenovirus capsids have been shown to target to the NPC using microtubules; depolymerization of the microtubule network abolished intracellular movement of the capsids, but not cell entry (Suomalainen *et al.*, 1999; Sodeik *et al.*, 1997). Using time-lapse fluorescence video microscopy, Phil Leopold was able to detect the directed linear movement of adenovirus capsids toward the nucleus at rates of around 3 µm/s (Leopold *et al.*, 2000b). This transport appeared to utilize the microtubule-associated motor protein dynein, since microinjection of antibodies against dynein, but not kinesin inhibited transport to the nucleus (Leopold *et al.*, 2000b; Sodeik *et al.*, 1997; Suomalainen *et al.*, 1999). By contrast, baculovirus appears to utilize actin filaments for trafficking to the nucleus (van Loo *et al.*, 2001). HIV pre-integration complexes containing the reverse-transcribed genome also have been shown to interact with the actin cytoskeleton (Bukrinskaya *et al.*, 1998), although it is unclear whether the HIV genome trafficks through the cytoplasm along actin filaments or along microtubules (Chicurel, 2000). Whether plasmids, either free or associated with proteins or polycationic delivery agents, also utilize elements of the cytoskeletal network to wind their way to the nuclear envelope remains to be seen, but it would be surprising if the cytoskeleton does not play a role.

CONCLUDING REMARKS

It is difficult to rationally design gene delivery and expression systems unless we know their fate once they enter the cells. After gaining access to the cytoplasm, a principal difficulty facing plasmid DNA is its translocation into the nucleus. A thorough understanding of the mechanisms of cellular uptake and intracellular trafficking of plasmids is crucial if we are to design better gene delivery tools to make gene therapy a realistic treatment option. It is clear that the nuclear envelope is a major barrier to effective gene delivery and expression in cells. This is especially true *in vivo*, where cells either do not divide rapidly or at all. Thus, by characterizing and understanding the mechanisms of cytoplasmic trafficking and nuclear import of DNA, we can begin to exploit these pathways to increase the nuclear targeting and subsequent expression of transgenes.

ACKNOWLEDGMENTS

The author's research was supported in part by NIH grants HL59956 from the NHLBI, EY12962 from the NEI, and AI44567 from the NIAID and by a grant from the National Medical Technology Testbed.

REFERENCES

Adam, S.A., Marr, R.S. and Gerace, L. (1990) Nuclear protein import in permeabilized mammalian cells requires soluble cytoplasmic factors. *J. Cell Biol.*, **111**, 807–816.

Aiyar, A., Tyree, C. and Sugden, B. (1998) The plasmid replicon of EBV consists of multiple *cis*-acting elements that facilitate DNA synthesis by the cell and a viral maintenance element. *EMBO J.*, **17**, 6394–6403.

Aronsohn, A.I. and Hughes, J.A. (1998) Nuclear localization signal peptides enhance cationic liposome-mediated gene therapy. *J. Drug Target.*, **5**, 163–169.

Bonner, W.M. (1975a) Protein migration into nuclei. I. Frog oocyte nuclei *in vivo* accumulate microinjected histones, allow entry of small proteins, and exclude large proteins. *J. Cell Biol.*, **64**, 421–430.

Bonner, W.M. (1975b) Protein migration into nuclei. II. Frog oocyte nuclei accumulate a class of microinjected oocyte nuclear proteins and exclude a class of microinjected oocyte cytoplasmic proteins. *J. Cell Biol.*, **64**, 431–437.

Bottger, M., Zaitsev, S.V., Otto, A., Haberland, A. and Vorob'ev, V.I. (1998) Acid nuclear extracts as mediators of gene transfer and expression. *Biochim. Biophys. Acta.*, **1395**, 78–87.

Branden, L.J., Mohamed, A.J. and Smith, C.I. (1999) A peptide nucleic acid-nuclear localization signal fusion that mediates nuclear transport of DNA. *Nat. Biotechnol.*, **17**, 784–787.

Browning, C.L., Culberson, D.E., Aragon, I.V., Fillmore, R.A., Croissant, J.D., Schwartz, R.J. *et al.* (1998) The developmentally regulated expression of serum response factor plays a key role in the control of smooth muscle-specific genes. *Dev. Biol.*, **194**, 18–37.

Brunner, S., Sauer, T., Carotta, S., Cotten, M., Saltik, M. and Wagner, E. (2000) Cell cycle dependence of gene transfer by lipoplex, polyplex and recombinant adenovirus. *Gene Ther.*, **7**, 401–407.

Bukrinskaya, A., Brichacek, B., Mann, A. and Stevenson, M. (1998) Establishment of a functional human immunodeficiency virus type 1 (HIV-1) reverse transcription complex involves the cytoskeleton. *J. Exp. Med.*, **188**, 2113–2125.

Bukrinsky, M.I., Sharova, N., Dempsey, M.P., Stanwick, T.L., Bukrinsky, A.G., Haggerty, S. *et al.* (1992) Active nuclear import of human immunodeficiency virus type 1 preintegration complexes. *Proc. Natl. Acad. Sci. USA*, **89**, 6580–6584.

Bukrinsky, M.I., Sharova, N., McDonald, T.L., Pushkarskaya, T., Tarpley, W.G. and Stevenson, M. (1993) Association of integrase, matrix, and reverse transcriptase antigens of human immunodeficiency virus type 1 with viral nucleic acids following acute infection. *Proc. Natl. Acad. Sci. USA*, **90**, 6125–6129.

Capecchi, M.R. (1980) High efficiency transformation by direct microinjection of DNA into cultured mammalian cells. *Cell*, **22**, 479–488.

Carson, J.A., Fillmore, R.A., Schwartz, R.J. and Zimmer, W.E. (2000) The smooth muscle gamma-actin gene promoter is a molecular target for the mouse bagpipe homologue, mNkx3-1, and serum response factor. *J. Biol. Chem.*, **275**, 39061–39072.

Chan, C.K. and Jans, D.A. (1999) Enhancement of polylysine-mediated transferrinfection by nuclear localization sequences: polylysine does not function as a nuclear localization sequence. *Hum. Gene Ther.*, **10**, 1695–1702.

Chicurel, M. (2000) VIROLOGY: Probing HIV's elusive activities within the host cell. *Science*, **290**, 1876–1879.

Ciolina, C., Byk, G., Blanche, F., Thuillier, V., Scherman, D. and Wils, P. (1999) Coupling of nuclear localization signals to plasmid DNA and specific interaction of the conjugates with importin alpha. *Bioconjug. Chem.*, **10**, 49–55.

Collas, P. and Alestrom, P. (1996) Nuclear localization signal of SV40 T antigen directs import of plasmid DNA into sea urchin male pronuclei *in vitro*. *Mol. Reprod. Dev.*, **45**, 431–438.

Collas, P. and Alestrom, P. (1997a) Nuclear localization signals: a driving force for nuclear transport of plasmid DNA in zebrafish. *Biochem. Cell Biol.*, **75**, 633–640.

Collas, P. and Alestrom, P. (1997b) Rapid targeting of plasmid DNA to zebrafish embryo nuclei by the nuclear localization signal of SV40 T antigen. *Mol. Mar. Biol. Biotechnol.*, **6**, 48–58.

Collas, P., Husebye, H. and Alestrom, P. (1996) The nuclear localization sequence of the SV40 T antigen promotes transgene uptake and expression in zebrafish embryo nuclei. *Transgenic Res.*, **5**, 451–458.

Coonrod, A., Li, F.Q. and Horwitz, M. (1997) On the mechanism of DNA transfection: efficient gene transfer without viruses. *Gene Ther.*, **4**, 1313–1321.

Dean, B.S., Byrd, Jr., J.N. and Dean, D.A. (1999a) Nuclear targeting of plasmid DNA in human corneal cells. *Cur. Eye Res.*, **19**, 66–75.

Dean, D.A. (1997) Import of plasmid DNA into the nucleus is sequence specific. *Exp. Cell Res.*, **230**, 293–302.

Dean, D.A. (2000) Peptide nucleic acids: versatile tools for gene therapy strategies. *Adv. Drug Deliv. Rev.*, **44**, 81–95.

Dean, D.A., Dean, B.S., Muller, S. and Smith, L.C. (1999b) Sequence requirements for plasmid nuclear entry. *Exp. Cell Res.*, **253**, 713–722.

Demidov, V.V., Potaman, V.N., Frank-Kamenetskii, M.D., Egholm, M., Buchard, O., Sonnichsen, S.H. and Nielsen, P.E. (1994) Stability of peptide nucleic acids in human serum and cellular extracts. *Biochem. Pharmacol.*, **48**, 1310–1313.

Doh, S.G., Vahlsing, H.L., Hartikka, J., Liang, X. and Manthorpe, M. (1997) Spatial-temporal patterns of gene expression in mouse skeletal muscle after injection of *lacZ* plasmid DNA. *Gene Ther.*, **4**, 648–663.

Dowty, M.E., Williams, P., Zhang, G., Hagstrom, J.E. and Wolff, J.A. (1995) Plasmid DNA entry into postmitotic nuclei of primary rat myotubes. *Proc. Natl. Acad. Sci. USA*, **92**, 4572–4576.

Dumas, F., Duckely, M., Pelczar, P., Van Gelder, P. and Hohn, B. (2001) An Agrobacterium VirE2 channel for transferred-DNA transport into plant cells. *Proc. Natl. Acad. Sci. USA*, **98**, 485–490.

Fasbender, A., Zabner, J., Zeiher, B.G. and Welsh, M.J. (1997) A low rate of cell proliferation and reduced DNA uptake limit cationic lipid-meidated gene tranfer to primary cultures of ciliated human airway epithelia. *Gene Ther.*, **4**, 1173–1180.

Feldherr, C.M., Kallenbach, E. and Schultz, N. (1984) Movement of a karyophilic protein through the nuclear pores of oocytes. *J. Cell Biol.*, **99**, 2216–2222.

Fischer, U., Huber, J., Boelens, W.C., Mattaj, I.W. and Luhrmann, R. (1995) The HIV-1 Rev activation domain is a nuclear export signal that accesses an export pathway used by specific cellular RNAs. *Cell*, **82**, 475–483.

Fritz, J.D., Herweijer, H., Zhang, G. and Wolff, J.A. (1996) Gene transfer into mammalian cells using histone-condensed plasmid DNA. *Hum. Gene Ther.*, **7**, 1395–1404.

Godbey, W.T., Barry, M.A., Saggau, P., Wu, K.K. and Mikos, A.G. (2000) Poly-(ethylenimine)-mediated transfection: a new paradigm for gene delivery. *J. Biomed. Mater. Res.*, **51**, 321–328.

Godbey, W.T., Wu, K.K. and Mikos, A.G. (1999) Tracking the intracellular path of poly-(ethylenimine)/DNA complexes for gene delivery. *Proc. Natl. Acad. Sci. USA*, **96**, 5177–5181.

Gorlich, D., Pante, N., Kutay, U., Aebi, U. and Bischoff, F.R. (1996) Identification of different roles for RanGDP and RanGTP in nuclear protein import. *Embo. J.*, **15**, 5584–5594.

Graessman, M. and Graessman, A. (1981) Regulation of SV40 gene expression. *Adv. Cancer Res.*, **35**, 111–149.

Graessman, M., Menne, J., Liebler, M., Graeber, I. and Graessman, A. (1989) Helper activity for gene expression, a novel function of the SV40 enhancer. *Nucleic Acids Res.*, **17**, 6603–6612.

Hagstrom, J.E., Ludtke, J.J., Bassik, M.C., Sebestyen, M.G., Adam, S.A. and Wolff, J.A. (1997) Nuclear import of DNA in digitonin-permeabilized cells. *J. Cell Sci.*, **110**, 2323–2331.

Hagstrom, J.E., Sebestyen, M.G., Budker, V., Ludtke, J.J., Fritz, J.D. and Wolff, J.A. (1996) Complexes of non-cationic liposomes and histone H1 mediate efficient transfection of DNA without encapsulation. *Biochim. Biophys. Acta*, **1284**, 47–55.

Hartig, R., Shoeman, R.L., Janetzko, A., Grub, S. and Traub, P. (1998a) Active nuclear import of single-stranded oligonucleotides and their complexes with non-karyophilic macromolecules. *Biol. Cell.*, **90**, 407–426.

Hartig, R., Shoeman, R.L., Janetzko, A., Tolstonog, G. and Traub, P. (1998b) DNA-mediated transport of the intermediate filament protein vimentin into the nucleus of cultured cells. *J. Cell Sci.*, **111**, 3573–3584.

Hartikka, J., Sawdey, M., Cornefert-Jensen, F., Margalith, M., Barnhart, K., Nolasco, M. *et al.* (1996) An improved plasmid DNA expression vector for direct injection into skeletal muscle. *Hum. Gene Ther.*, **7**, 1205–1217.

Heinzinger, N.K., Bukrinsky, M.I., Haggerty, S.A., Ragland, A.M., Kewalramani, V., Lee, M. *et al.* (1994) The Vpr protein of human immunodeficiency virus type 1 influences nuclear localization of viral nucleic acids in nondividing host cells. *Proc. Natl. Acad. Sci. USA*, **91**, 7311–7315.

Izaurralde, E., Jarmolowski, A., Beisel, C., Mattaj, I.W., Dreyfuss, G. and Fischer, U. (1997a) A role for the M9 transport signal of hnRNP A1 in mRNA nuclear export. *J. Cell Biol.*, **137**, 27–35.

Izaurralde, E., Kutay, U., von Kobbe, C., Mattaj, I.W. and Gorlich, D. (1997b) The asymmetric distribution of the constituents of the Ran system is essential for transport into and out of the nucleus. *Embo J.*, **16**, 6535–6547.

Jakel, S., Albig, W., Kutay, U., Bischoff, F.R., Schwamborn, K., Doenecke, D. *et al.* (1999) The importin beta/importin 7 heterodimer is a functional nuclear import receptor for histone H1. *Embo J.*, **18**, 2411–2423.

Jakel, S. and Gorlich, D. (1998) Importin beta, transportin, RanBP5 and RanBP7 mediate nuclear import of ribosomal proteins in mammalian cells. *Embo J.*, **17**, 4491–4502.

Jans, D.A., Xiao, C.Y. and Lam, M.H. (2000) Nuclear targeting signal recognition: a key control point in nuclear transport? *Bioessays*, **22**, 532–544.

Jenkins, Y., McEntee, M., Weis, K. and Greene, W.C. (1998) Characterization of HIV-1 vpr nuclear import: analysis of signals and pathways. *J. Cell Biol.*, **143**, 875–885.

Kalderon, D., Richardson, W.D., Markham, A.F. and Smith, A.E. (1984a) Sequence requirements for nuclear location of simian virus 40 large-T antigen. *Nature*, **311**, 33–38.

Kalderon, D., Richardson, W.D., Markham, A.F. and Smith, A.E. (1984b) A short amino acid sequence able to specify nuclear location. *Cell*, **39**, 499–509.

Kaneda, Y., Iwai, K. and Uchida, T. (1989) Increased expression of DNA cointroduced with nuclear protein in adult rat liver. *Science*, **243**, 375–378.

Kasamatsu, H. and Nakanishi, A. (1998) How do animal DNA viruses get to the nucleus? *Annu. Rev. Microbiol.*, **52**, 627–686.

Kopchick, J.J., Ju, G., Skalka, A.M. and Stacey, D.W. (1981) Biological activity of cloned retroviral DNA in microinjected cells. *Proc. Natl. Acad. Sci. USA*, **78**, 4383–4387.

Kovacs, A.M. and Zimmer, W.E. (1993) Molecular cloning and expression of the chicken smooth muscle g-actin mRNA. *Cell Motil. Cytoskeleton*, **24**, 67–81.

Kovacs, A.M. and Zimmer, W.E. (1998) Cell specific transcription of the smooth muscle g-actin gene requires both positive and negative acting *cis*-elements. *Gene Exp.*, **7**, 115–129.

Langle-Rouault, F., Patzel, V., Benavente, A., Taillez, M., Silvestre, N., Bompard, A. *et al.* (1998) Up to 100-fold increase of apparent gene expression in the presence of Epstein-Barr virus *ori*P sequences and EBNA1: implications of the nuclear import of plasmids. *J. Virol.*, **72**, 6181–6185.

Leopold, P.L. (2000a) Fluorescence methods reveal intracellular trafficking of gene transfer vectors: the light toward the end of the tunnel. *Mol. Ther.*, **1**, 302–303.

Leopold, P.L., Kreitzer, G., Miyazawa, N., Rempel, S., Pfister, K.K., Rodriguez-Boulan, E. *et al.* (2000b) Dynein- and microtubule-mediated translocation of adenovirus serotype 5 occurs after endosomal lysis. *Hum. Gene Ther.*, **11**, 151–165.

Lewis, P.F. and Emerman, M. (1994) Passage through mitosis is required for oncoretroviruses but not for the human immunodeficiency virus. *J. Virol.*, **68**, 510–516.

Li, S., MacLaughlin, F.C., Fewell, J.G., Gondo, M., Wang, J., Nicol, F. *et al.* (2001) Muscle-specific enhancement of gene expression by incorporation of the SV40 enhancer in the expression plasmid. *Gene Ther.*, **8**, 494–497.

Luby-Phelps, K., Castle, P.E., Taylor, D.L. and Lanni, F. (1987) Hindered diffusion of inert tracer particles in the cytoplasm of mouse 3T3 cells. *Proc. Natl. Acad. Sci. USA*, **84**, 4910–4913.

Lukacs, G.L., Haggie, P., Seksek, O., Lechardeur, D., Freedman, N. and Verkman, A.S. (2000) Size-dependent DNA mobility in cytoplasm and nucleus. *J. Biol. Chem.*, **275**, 1625–1629.

Manthorpe, M., Cornefert-Jensen, F., Hartikka, J., Felgner, J., Rundell, A., Margalith, M. *et al.* (1993) Gene therapy by intramuscular injection of plasmid DNA: studies on firefly luciferase gene expression in mice. *Hum. Gene Ther.*, **4**, 419–431.

Martin, J.B., Young, J.L., Benoit, J.N. and Dean, D.A. (2000) Gene transfer to intact mesenteric arteries by electroporation. *J. Vasc. Res.*, **37**, 372–380.

Miller, D.G., Adam, M.A. and Miller, A.D. (1990) Gene transfer by retrovirus vectors occurs only in cells that are actively replicating at the time of infection. *Mol. Cell Biol.*, **10**, 4239–4242.

Mirzayans, R., Remy, A.A. and Malcom, P.C. (1992) Differential expression and stability of foreign genes introduced into human fibroblasts by nuclear versus cytoplasmic micro-injection. *Mutation Res.*, **281**, 115–122.

Moore, M.S. (1998) Ran and nuclear transport. *J. Biol. Chem.*, **273**, 22857–22860.

Moroianu, J., Blobel, G. and Radu, A. (1996) Nuclear protein import: Ran-GTP dissociates the karyopherin alphabeta heterodimer by displacing alpha from an overlapping binding site on beta. *Proc. Natl. Acad. Sci. USA*, **93**, 7059–7062.

Nakanishi, A., Clever, J., Yamada, M., Li, P.L. and Kasamatsu, H. (1996) Association with capsid proteins promotes nuclear targeting of simian virus 40. *Proc. Natl. Acad. Sci. USA*, **93**, 96–100.

Neves, C., Byk, G., Scherman, D. and Wils, P. (1999) Coupling of a targeting peptide to plasmid DNA by covalent triple helix formation. *FEBS Lett.*, **453**, 41–45.

Pollard, H., Remy, J.S., Loussouarn, G., Demolombe, S., Behr, J.P. and Escande, D. (1998) Polyethylenimine but not cationic lipids promotes transgene delivery to the nucleus in mammalian cells. *J. Biol. Chem.*, **273**, 7507–7511.

Pollard, V.W., Michael, W.M., Nakielny, S., Siomi, M.C., Wang, F. and Dreyfuss, G. (1996) A novel receptor-mediated nuclear import pathway. *Cell*, **86**, 985–994.

Popov, S., Rexach, M., Ratner, L., Blobel, G. and Bukrinsky, M. (1998a) Viral protein R regulates docking of the HIV-1 preintegration complex to the nuclear pore complex. *J. Biol. Chem.*, **273**, 13347–13352.

Popov, S., Rexach, M., Zybarth, G., Reiling, N., Lee, M.A., Ratner, L. *et al.* (1998b) Viral protein R regulates nuclear import of the HIV-1 pre-integration complex. *Embo J.*, **17**, 909–917.

Provance, Jr., D.W., McDowall, A., Marko, M. and Luby-Phelps, K. (1993) Cytoarchitecture of size-excluding compartments in living cells. *J. Cell Sci.*, **106**, 565–577.

Reddy, J.A., Dean, D., Kennedy, M.D. and Low, P.S. (1999) Optimization of folate-conjugated liposomal vectors for folate receptor-mediated gene therapy. *J. Pharm. Sci.*, **88**, 1112–1118.

Robbins, J., Dilworth, S.M., Laskey, R.A. and Dingwall, C. (1991) Two interdependent basic domains in nucleoplasmin nuclear targeting sequence: identification of a class of bipartite nuclear targetting sequence. *Cell*, **64**, 615–623.

Sebestyén, M.G., Ludtke, J.L., Bassik, M.C., Zhang, G., Budker, V., Lukhtanov, E.A. *et al.* (1998) DNA vector chemistry: the covalent attachment of signal peptides to plasmid DNA. *Nat. Biotechnol.*, **16**, 80–85.

Seksek, O., Biwersi, J. and Verkman, A.S. (1997) Translational diffusion of macromolecule-sized solutes in cytoplasm and nucleus. *J. Cell Biol.*, **138**, 131–142.

Sheng, J. and Citovsky, V. (1996) Agrobacterium-plant cell DNA transport: have virulence proteins, will travel. *Plant Cell*, **8**, 1699–1710.

Siomi, H. and Dreyfuss, G. (1995) A nuclear localization domain in the hnRNP A1 protein. *J. Cell Biol.*, **129**, 551–560.

Sodeik, B., Ebersold, M.W. and Helenius, A. (1997) Microtubule-mediated transport of incoming herpes simplex virus 1 capsids to the nucleus. *J. Cell Biol.*, **136**, 1007–1021.

Stidwill, R.P. and Greber, U.F. (2000) Intracellular virus trafficking reveals physiological characteristics of the cytoskeleton. *News Physiol. Sci.*, **15**, 67–71.

Stoffler, D., Fahrenkrog, B. and Aebi, U. (1999) The nuclear pore complex: from molecular architecture to functional dynamics. *Curr. Opin. Cell Biol.*, **11**, 391–401.

Stutz, F. and Rosbash, M. (1998) Nuclear RNA export. *Genes Dev.*, **12**, 3303–3319.

Subramanian, A., Ranganathan, P. and Diamond, S.L. (1999) Nuclear targeting peptide scaffolds for lipofection of nondividing mammalian cells. *Nat. Biotechnol.*, **17**, 873–877.

Suomalainen, M., Nakano, M.Y., Keller, S., Boucke, K., Stidwill, R.P. and Greber, U.F. (1999) Microtubule-dependent plus- and minus end-directed motilities are competing processes for nuclear targeting of adenovirus. *J. Cell Biol.*, **144**, 657–672.

Group I Intron

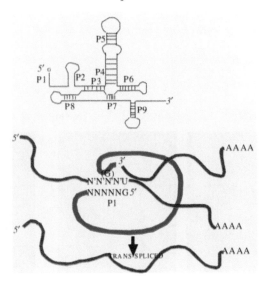

Color Plate 1 Group I intron structure and model for *trans*-splicing. (*see page 56*)

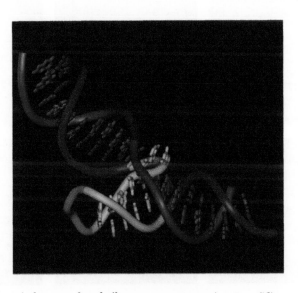

Color Plate 2 Chimeric hammerhead ribozyme structure. (*see page 58*)

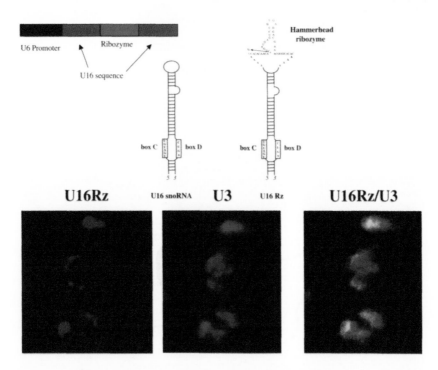

Color Plate 3 Nucleolar localized anti-HIV-1 ribozyme. (see page 61)

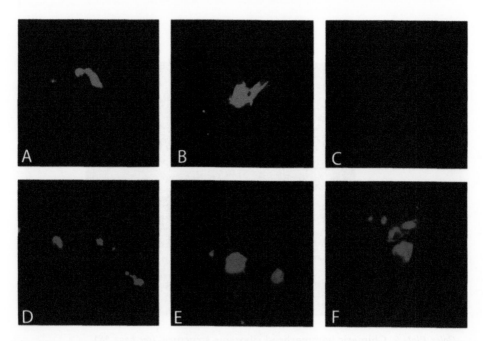

Color Plate 4 Detection of PNA binding-mediated GFP gene expression in CV1 cells. (see page 80)

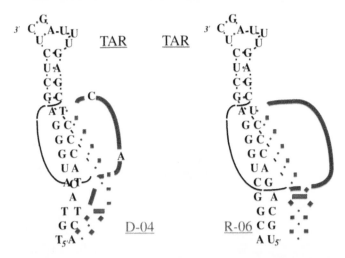

Color Plate 5 Structure of *trans*-activation response (TAR)-aptamer kissing complexes. (*see page 104*)

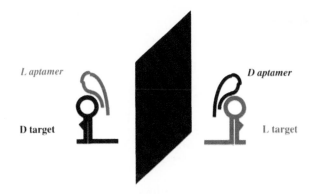

Color Plate 6 Schematic representation of the enantiomeric complex formed by a regular (D) aptamer with the mirror-image of a target (right) and vice versa by the mirror-image (L) of the selected aptamer with the natural target (left). (*see page 108*)

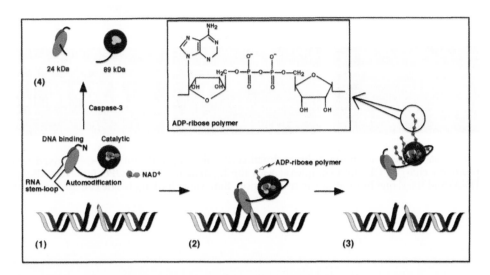

Color Plate 7 Activation of PARP-1 by DNA breaks. (*see page 128*)

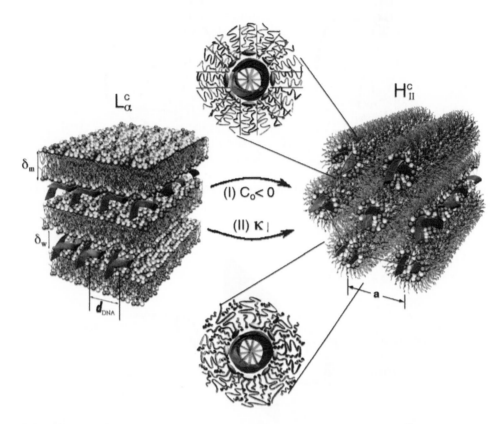

Color Plate 8 Schematic of two distinct pathways from the lamellar L_α^C phase to the columnar inverted hexagonal H_{II}^C phase of cationic liposome/DNA (CL/DNA) complexes. *(see page 192)*

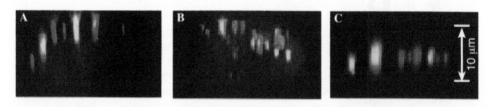

Color Plate 9 Laser scanning 3-dimensional confocal images of mouse L-cells mixed with positively charged CL/DNA complexes with the L_α^C structure (50%DOPC-50%DOTAP-*b*gal DNA) and fixed one hour after the transfection. Side views looking inside cell. *(see page 205)*

After microinjection

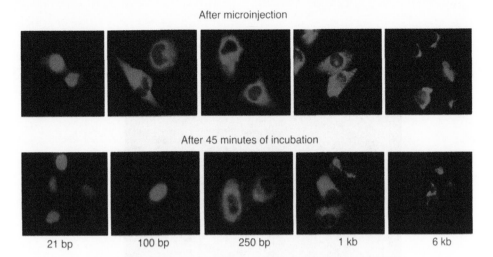

After 45 minutes of incubation

| 21 bp | 100 bp | 250 bp | 1 kb | 6 kb |

Color Plate 10 Subcellular distribution of fluorescein-labeled DNA fragments and plasmid DNA following microinjection into the cytoplasm. (*see page 215*)

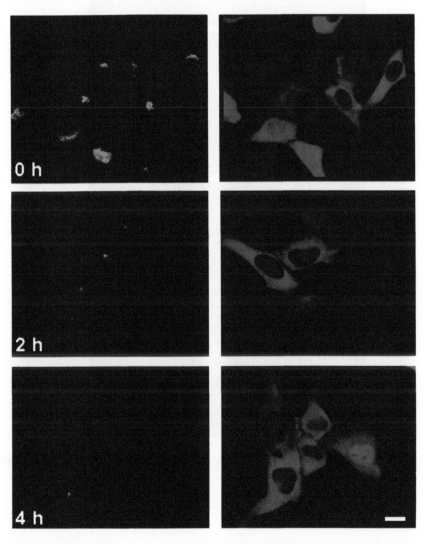

0 h

2 h

4 h

Color Plate 11 Elimination of plasmid DNA from the cytoplasm of microinjected cells. (*see page 217*)

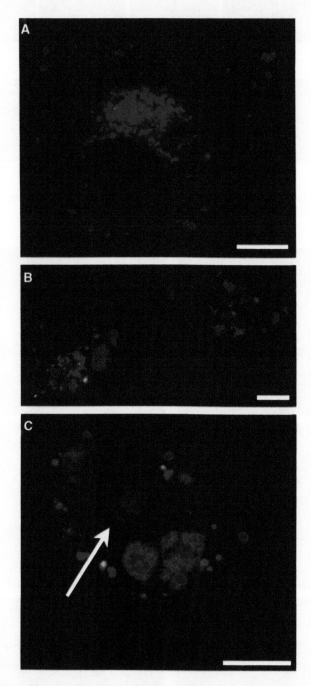

Color Plate 12 Tracking of labeled PEI/DNA complexes (green) in cells with labeled lysosomes (red). (*see page 373*)

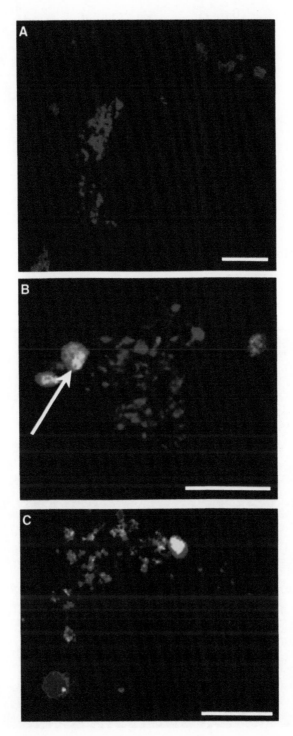

Color Plate 13 Tracking of labeled PLL/DNA complexes (green) in cells with labeled lysosomes (red). (*see page 374*)

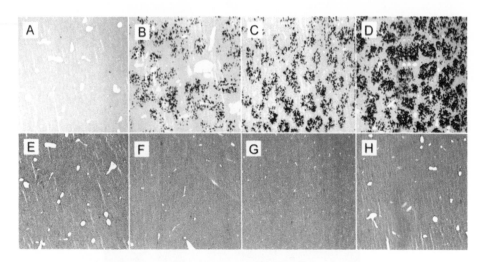

Color Plate 14 Histochemical analysis of *b*-galactosidase gene expression in liver. (*see page 460*)

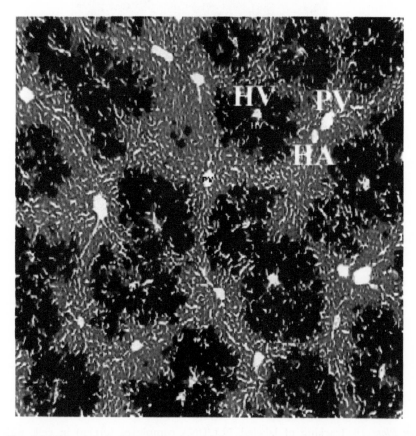

Color Plate 15 Histochemical analysis of *b*-galactosidase gene expression in liver. (*see page 461*)

Thornburn, A.M. and Alberts, A.S. (1993) Efficient expression of miniprep plasmid DNA after needle micro-injection into somatic cells. *Biotechniques*, **14**, 356–358.

Utvik, J.K., Nja, A. and Gundersen, K. (1999) DNA injection into single cells of intact mice. *Hum. Gene Ther.*, **10**, 291–300.

Vacik, J., Dean, B.S., Zimmer, W.E. and Dean, D.A. (1999) Cell-specific nuclear import of plasmid DNA. *Gene Ther.*, **6**, 1006–1014.

van Loo, N.D., Fortunati, E., Ehlert, E., Rabelink, M., Grosveld, F. and Scholte, B.J. (2001) Baculovirus infection of nondividing mammalian cells: mechanisms of entry and nuclear transport of capsids. *J. Virol.*, **75**, 961–970.

Vodicka, M.A., Koepp, D.M., Silver, P.A. and Emerman, M. (1998) HIV-1 Vpr interacts with the nuclear transport pathway to promote macrophage infection. *Genes Dev.*, **12**, 175–185.

von Schwedler, U., Kornbluth, R.S. and Trono, D. (1994) The nuclear localization signal of the matrix protein of human immunodeficiency virus type 1 allows the establishment of infection in macrophages and quiescent T lymphocytes. *Proc. Natl. Acad. Sci. USA*, **91**, 6992–6996.

Wang, G., Xu, X., Pace, B., Dean, D.A., Glazer, P.M., Chan, P. *et al.* (1999) Peptide nucleic acid (PNA) binding-mediated induction of human [gamma]-globin gene expression. *Nucleic Acids Res.*, **27**, 2806–2813.

Whittaker, G.R. and Helenius, A. (1998) Nuclear import and export of viruses and virus genomes. *Virology*, **246**, 1–23.

Wilson, G.L., Dean, B.S., Wang, G. and Dean, D.A. (1999) Nuclear import of plasmid DNA in digitonin-permeabilized cells requires both cytoplasmic factors and specific DNA sequences. *J. Biol. Chem.*, **274**, 22025–22032.

Wolff, J.A., Dowty, M.E., Jiao, S., Repetto, R., Berg, R.K., Ludtke, J.J. *et al.* (1992a) Expression of naked plasmids by cultured myotubes and entry into T tubules and caveolae of mammalian skeletal muscle. *J. Cell Sci.*, **103**, 1249–1253.

Wolff, J.A., Ludtke, J.J., Acsadi, G., Williams, P. and Jani, A. (1992b) Long-term persistence of plasmid DNA and foreign gene expression in mouse muscle. *Hum. Mol. Genet.*, **1**, 363–369.

Wolff, J.A., Malone, R.W., Williams, P., Chong, W., Acsadi, G., Jani, A. *et al.* (1990) Direct gene transfer into mouse muscle *in vivo*. *Science*, **247**, 1465–1468.

Yaseen, N.R. and Blobel, G. (1997) Cloning and characterization of human karyopherin beta3. *Proc. Natl. Acad. Sci. USA*, **94**, 4451–4456.

Yew, N.S., Wysokenski, D.M., Wang, K.X., Ziegler, R.J., Marshall, J., McNeilly, D. *et al.* (1997) Optimization of plasmid vectors for high-level expression in lung epithelial cells. *Hum. Gene Ther.*, **8**, 575–584.

Young, J.L., Byrd, J.N., Wyatt, C.R. and Dean, D.A. (1999) Endothelial cell-specific plasmid nuclear import. *Mol. Biol. Cell*, **10S**, 443a.

Zabner, J., Fasbender, A.J., Moninger, T., Poellinger, K.A. and Welsh, M.J. (1995) Cellular and molecular barriers to gene transfer by a cationic lipid. *J. Biol. Chem.*, **270**, 18997–19007.

Zanta, M.A., Belguise-Valladier, P. and Behr, J.P. (1999) Gene delivery: A single nuclear localization signal peptide is sufficient to carry DNA to the cell nucleus. *Proc. Natl. Acad. Sci. USA*, **96**, 91–96.

Zelphati, O., Liang, X., Hobart, P. and Felgner, P.L. (1999) Gene chemistry: functionally and conformationally intact fluorescent plasmid DNA. *Hum. Gene Ther.*, **10**, 15–24.

Zelphati, O., Liang, X., Nguyen, C., Barlow, S., Sheng, S., Shao, Z. *et al.* (2000) PNA-dependent gene chemistry: stable coupling of peptides and oligonucleotides to plasmid DNA. *Biotechniques*, **28**, 304–316.

Ziemienowicz, A., Gorlich, D., Lanka, E., Hohn, B. and Rossi, L. (1999) Import of DNA into mammalian nuclei by proteins originating from a plant pathogenic bacterium. *Proc. Natl. Acad. Sci. USA*, **96**, 3729–3733.

Zimmer, W.E., Browning, C. and Kovacs, A.M. (1996) Cell-specific regulation of the SMGA gene. *Dev. Biol.*, **175**, 399.

Zupan, J.R., Citovsky, V. and Zambryski, P. (1996) Agrobacterium VirE2 protein mediates nuclear uptake of single-stranded DNA in plant cells. *Proc. Natl. Acad. Sci. USA*, **93**, 2392–2397.

13 Optimizing RNA export for transgene expression

Ileana Popa and Thomas J. Hope

INTRODUCTION

There has been an extensive research effort to develop vectors that efficiently introduce foreign genes into cells. These efforts have lead to the development of a number of viral and non-viral vectors. Following cellular uptake, genes must be transported to the nucleus for efficient gene expression. Among many other factors, it is believed that efficient gene expression depends on the type of promoters used. After transcription, the mRNA must undergo extensive processing before becoming functional, i.e., 5' capping, splicing, and 3' end processing i.e., cleavage and polyadenylation. Once processing is complete, the mature mRNA is exported into the cytoplasm where it undergoes translation. Recently, significant progress has been made in our understanding of mRNA export mechanisms. It is now clear that efficient gene expression will require the optimization of the transgene mRNA export.

In this chapter we will describe the current understanding of mRNA export. First, we will describe the players in this process, including the nuclear pore, the nuclear pore proteins, and the transport receptors. Then, we will discuss the current understanding of the viral and cellular mRNAs export. Finally, we will discuss current efforts to use the new information on mRNA export to increase the efficiency of transgene expression.

FUNDAMENTALS OF RNA EXPORT

To gain insights into gene expression, it is important to realize that transcription, RNA processing, and RNA export are intimately linked. The carboxy-terminal domain of the large subunit of RNA polymerase II (Pol II) directly binds to the factors involved in RNA processing (Bentley, 1999; Hirose and Manley, 2000). Some of these factors bind only when the polymerase is elongating the transcript. Consequently, the transcription unit is considered an RNA processing unit, in which Pol II orchestrates the recruitment of a multitude of factors essential for pre-mRNA processing (Neugebauer and Roth, 1997). While being synthesized, the pre-mRNA associates with a subset of RNA-binding proteins termed heterogeneous nuclear ribonucleoproteins (hnRNPs) to become an mRNP. Formation of the mRNPs ensures that the nascent transcripts are protected from degradation and that their maturation proceeds correctly. hnRNPs have been shown to participate in various processes in the nucleus, such as transcriptional regulation, alternative pre-mRNA splicing, pre-mRNA $3'$ end processing and, probably, mRNA export (Krecic and Swanson, 1999). Hence, within the RNA processing unit, capping, splicing, and polyadenylation can regulate each other. The RNA processing unit provides increased local concentrations of components that must function together, allowing their efficient recruitment at the maturing RNA. It is believed that mRNA transcribed and, at least partially processed at the edge of a transcriptional domain, is released un-tethered into the inter-chromosomal space and, while diffusing, it may further complex with additional nuclear factors, some important for controlling nuclear export. The link between RNA processing and export ensures that only efficiently processed mRNAs are exported. Newly synthesized and processed mRNAs moves throughout interchromatin space until they randomly come across and are captured by the export machinery (Daneholt, 1999; Politz and Pederson, 2000; Singh *et al.*, 1999).

Because the export machinery selectively binds transport-competent mRNPs, i.e., mRNAs associated with the appropriate nuclear proteins, the diffusion-based model for intranuclear RNA movement provides an additional checkpoint for gene expression at the level of mRNA export. This type of control has been demonstrated for tRNA export: only mature tRNAs are transported to the cytoplasm because incompletely processed tRNAs do not efficiently bind to exportin-t, the tRNA-specific export receptor.

hnRNPs

As they are being synthesized, mRNAs become coated with hnRNPs to form messenger ribonucleoprotein complexes (mRNPs) (Figure 13.1). hnRNPs are abundant cellular proteins that localize all over the nucleus. hnRNPs have modular structure, being composed of one or more RNA-binding domains and auxiliary domains that mediate essential functions, such as protein–protein interaction and nuclear localization. Three types of RNA-binding domains have been identified so far: the RNP domain, the RGG box and the K-Homology (KH) motif. The most common RNA-binding domain is the RNP domain, also known as the RNA recognition motif (RRM), the RNP consensus sequence (RNP-CS), and the consensus sequence RNA-binding domain (CS-RBD). The RNP domain is 90–100 amino acids long and it is composed of two short consensus sequences (RNP1 and RNP2) separated by a stretch of 30 amino acids and other interspersed conserved residues (Dreyfuss *et al.*, 1993). RNP1 is a highly conserved octapeptide, Lys/Arg-Gly-Phe/Tyr-Gly/Ala-Phe-Val-X-Phe/Tyr, RNP2 is less well conserved, consisting of a hexapeptide rich in aromatic and aliphatic amino acids (Dreyfuss *et al.*, 1993). The RGG box is a short, 20 to 25 amino acids long sequence, consisting of closely spaced Arg-Gly-Gly repeats often separated by aromatic amino acids. The RGG box is normally found in combination with other types of RNA-binding domains (Weighardt *et al.*, 1996). It is believed that the RGG box is sequence-unspecific and that its role is to facilitate the binding of other RNA-binding domains. However, sequence-specific RNA binding has been demonstrated for hnRNP U in which the RGG box is the only RNA-binding domain (Burd and Dreyfuss, 1994). The KH motif, first identified in the human hnRNP K, is a stretch of approximately 45 amino acids that contains a core sequence (VIGXXGXXI) flanked by a few

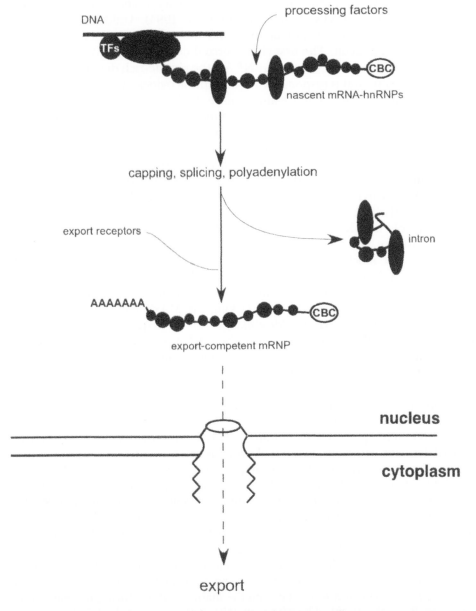

Figure 13.1 Schematic representation of mRNA biogenesis. The nascent mRNA associates with a subset of RNA-binding proteins, termed heterogeneous nuclear ribonucleoproteins (hnRNPs) and splicing. Through specific protein-protein, hnRNPs direct the assembly of processing factors to the newly synthesized mRNA. hnRNPs remain associated with the pre-mRNA until processing is complete and some stay with the mature mRNA during nuclear export.

interspaced conserved residues. The KH domain probably binds RNA directly, as the binding of KH motif-containing proteins to single-stranded RNAs *in vitro* is impaired by mutations of the highly conserved residues (Burd and Dreyfuss, 1994).

In addition to RNA-binding domains, the auxiliary domains are important components of the hnRNPs (Biamonti and Riva, 1994). Unlike RNA-binding domains, these domains are unstructured and have diverse sequences, making their classification difficult. The best characterized domain is the glycine-rich type found in hnRNPs A1 and A2/B1. In hnRNP A1, the glycine-rich domain is localized near the C-terminus and is responsible for multiple activities, such as RNA binding (through a 36 amino acid sequence analogous to an RGG box), nucleocytoplasmic shuttling (through the M9 signal, an ~38 amino acid sequence, located immediately downstream of the RGG box), and protein–protein interactions (Cartegni *et al.*, 1996). Similar to hnRNP A1, hnRNP K also contains a nucleocytoplasmic shuttling domain. This domain of 38 amino acids was termed KNS (for hnRNP K̲ ṉuclear ṣhuttling domain). Competition experiments demonstrated that M9 does not inhibit KNS activity, indicating that the pathways utilized by these two signals are different (Michael *et al.*, 1997). Although the existence of shuttling domains suggested a role in mRNA export for these hnRNPs, this is still a controversial issue. For instance, microinjection of M9-containing fusion proteins into *Xenopus* oocytes does not block mRNA export, while microinjection of the full-length hnRNP A1 does. Moreover, a point mutation in the M9 domain (Gly 274 to Ala) that inactivates the M9 signal did not alter the ability of hnRNP A1 to inhibit mRNA export. Microinjection of truncated A1 lacking the M9 domain did not interfere with the export of mRNA (Izaurralde *et al.*, 1997a). Consequently, M9 alone is not sufficient for the hnRNP A1 to recognize the mRNA export factors. Rather than acting as an export signal, M9 together with other sequences present in the full-length protein may mediate hnRNP A1 association with real export receptors. These results suggest that the nuclear role of hnRNPs is to protect the mRNA from degradation and to recruit the factors necessary for pre-mRNA processing and mRNA export (Figure 13.1).

All hnRNPs have general RNA binding activity mediated, in most of the cases, by the RNP domains. However, individual proteins recognize defined regions in pre-mRNAs that often correspond to sites important for RNA processing (Weighardt *et al.*, 1996). For example, hnRNP A1 has preferential affinity for the sequence UAGGGA/U that resembles both the 3'- and the 5'-splice site consensus. hnRNP C has a strong preference for U-rich substrates. hnRNP I preferentially binds to certain polypyrimidine tracts near 3'-splice sites, hence the name polypyrimidine-tract binding protein (PTB). hnRNP K prefers poly(C). Through specific protein–protein interaction mediated by their auxiliary domains, hnRNPs direct the assembly of processing factors to these sites. hnRNPs remain associated with the pre-mRNA until processing is complete and some stay with the mature mRNA during nuclear export (Stutz and Rosbash, 1998). Therefore, mRNP, rather than naked mRNA, is the substrate for nuclear export (Figure 13.1).

The shuttling of some hnRNPs and their presence in the cytoplasm suggests that they play a role in the cytoplasmic metabolism of mRNA. It appears that the nuclear history of mRNAs influences their cytoplasmic fate, providing the cell with a new level for the control of gene expression (Matsumoto *et al.*, 1998). The possibility exists that the shuttling hnRNPs are important players in this process.

TRANSPORT RECEPTORS

The majority of nucleocytoplasmic transport requires factors belonging to the importin β family of nuclear transport receptors (Gorlich and Kutay, 1999; Mattaj and Englmeier, 1998; Nakielny and Dreyfuss, 1999; Weis, 1998). These receptors shuttle between the nucleus and cytoplasm, interact with nuclear pore complexes (NPC) and bind cargo either directly or via adaptor molecules. An attribute of nucleocytoplasmic transport is its directionality. Regulatory proteins controlling Ran's GTPase activity are critical to maintaining this directionality. These regulatory proteins are asymmetrically distributed across the nuclear envelope (NE). As a result, GTP to GDP hydrolysis occurs in the cytoplasm while the GDP/GTP exchange takes place in the nucleus (Bischoff and Ponstingl, 1991; Matunis *et al.*, 1996), leading to a RanGTP gradient across the NE.

According to the direction in which they carry a cargo, the receptors are classified as importins or exportins. Importins bind their import substrates in the presence of RanGDP in the cytoplasm. Upon RanGTP binding in the nucleus they release their cargo and return to the cytoplasm as RanGTP-importin complexes (Gorlich and Mattaj, 1996; Izaurralde *et al.*, 1997a). In the cytoplasm, RanGTP-importin complexes are disassembled by the combined action of Ran-specific GTPase-activating protein (RanGAP) and Ran-binding protein 1 (RanBP1) or 2 (RanBP2). Importins are then ready for another round of import (Bischoff and Gorlich, 1997; Lounsbury and Macara, 1997). Exportins are regulated in a converse manner. They bind their substrate in the nucleus in the presence of high RanGTP concentrations and exit the nucleus as cargo-exportin-RanGTP complexes (Fornerod *et al.*, 1997; Kutay *et al.*, 1997, 1998). Dissociation of exported complexes occurs in the cytoplasm, where RanGAP and RanBP1 (or RanBP2) are localized (Bischoff and Gorlich, 1997; Kutay *et al.*, 1997). This localization results in cargo release from the exportins and GTP hydrolysis. Exportins shuttle back to the nucleus to mediate other export events.

Importins and exportins constantly export RanGTP from the nucleus. Therefore, the nuclear RanGTP pool has to be replenished. This replenishment is accomplished by two factors: the nuclear transport factor 2 (NTF2) (Ribbeck *et al.*, 1998), that mediates the nuclear import of RanGDP, and Ran-specific guanine nucleotide exchange factor (RanGEF) (Bischoff and Ponstingl, 1991), which recharges Ran with GTP in the nucleus. Two of the importinβ family members, exportin-t and chromosome region maintenance (CRM1), have been shown to play roles in RNA export. Exportin-t directly binds and exports mature tRNA (Arts *et al.*, 1998). The ability of exportin-t to directly bind to RNA is unique among the importinβ family members. The other family member, CRM1 has been shown to mediate viral RNA export. In this case the interaction is not direct, but mediated by an adaptor nuclear export signal (NES)-containing protein.

There are some transport pathways for mRNA export which do not require an importinβ family member. Mex67/TAP is a factor with a direct role in mRNA export (Strasser and Hurt, 2000; Stutz *et al.*, 2000; Nakielny and Dreyfuss, 1999). Mex67/TAP binds RNA and Nups and has the ability to undergo nucleocytoplasmic shuttling. Another factor might be involved (Hodge *et al.*, 1999). How the actions of these factors are coordinated to mediate mRNA export is presently unknown. Once recognized by the export machinery, RNAs must transverse the nuclear pore.

NUCLEAR PORE COMPLEXES (NPC)

The morphology of both yeast and vertebrate NPCs has been the subject of extensive reviews (Stoffler *et al.*, 1999; Yang *et al.*, 1998). NPCs are complex cylindrical proteinaceous structures, about 1200 A in diameter and 700 A thick, that perforate the nuclear envelope (Yang *et al.*, 1998). NPCs have a mass of $\sim$ 125 MDa in higher eukaryotes (Akey and Radermacher, 1993) or 66 MDa in *Saccharomyces cerevisiae* (Yang *et al.*, 1998). NPC is formed from eight spoke-like structures that form a ring in which resides a central plug. Active transport is thought to occur through this central plug or transporter. The presence of the transporter is controversial, as some studies propose the presence of a distinct cylindrical transporter (Akey and Radermacher, 1993; Yang *et al.*, 1998), while another indicates that this feature might be material in transit (Stoffler *et al.*, 1999). In addition, NPCs contain fibers that extend into both cytoplasmic (the cytoplasmic filaments) and the nucleus (the nuclear basket).

A single NPC can mediate both import and export (Keminer *et al.*, 1999). There are two ways to move through the NPC: passive diffusion and facilitated translocation. Passive diffusion does not require specific interactions to take place. For small molecules it is fast, but becomes inefficient as the size of the molecules approach 20–40 kDa (Paine *et al.*, 1975). In contrast, facilitated translocation is a selective process that allows the passage of macromolecules as large as several MDa. This process is facilitated by transport receptors that can specifically interact with NPC components and directly promote cargo translocation through the NPC.

A great deal of information has emerged regarding factors that are essential for RNA export (Nakielny and Dreyfuss, 1999), but the exact mechanism of translocation through the nuclear pore is still unclear. RNAs require extensive processing before becoming mature RNAs ready to be exported to the cytoplasm. Moreover, there is a strong connection between RNA processing and export. Therefore, it is often difficult to make the distinction between factors required for RNA processing and factors that mediate export.

NUCLEAR PORE PROTEINS (NUCLEOPORINS)

The NPC components are called nucleoporins (Nups). Yeast NPCs contain 40 different Nups (Rout *et al.*, 2000), of which only 30 have been identified (Rout *et al.*, 2000). Vertebrate NPCs are composed of $\sim$80 to 100 different Nups. So far 16 to 20 have been cloned (Bayliss *et al.*, 2000; Gorlich and Kutay, 1999). Many Nups are members of the FG repeat family. The two most common repeats are based on GLFG or FxFG cores (where x is usually a small residue such as serine, glycine or alanine). NP domains often contain many copies of these repeats. For example, 19 FxFG repeats in Nsp1p and 33 GLFG repeats in Nup116p. Several data directly implicate these repeats in nuclear transport. Nucleoporins localized at both the cytoplasmic fibers (Nup 358 and Nup214) and the nuclear basket (Nup 153 and Nup98) bind transport factors *in vitro* (Moroianu *et al.*, 1995; Radu *et al.*, 1995a,b).

Binding experiments using isolated yeast nucleoporins demonstrate an interaction between NP domains and import factors, indicating that this interaction could be meaningful for transport (Nehrbass and Blobel, 1996; Strasser *et al.*, 2000; Strawn *et al.*, 2001). Antibodies that recognize FG repeats block nuclear trafficking. For example, the injection of anti-Nup98 into *X. laevis* nuclei blocks the export of snRNAs, 5S RNA, large ribosomal RNA, and mRNA; in contrast, the export of tRNA was unaffected (Powers *et al.*, 1997). Constructs that express FG repeats also block nuclear trafficking. After injection into *X. laevis* oocyte nuclei, several FG repeat domains inhibit the export of both Rev protein and U snRNAs, suggesting that these nucleoproteins participate in Rev-mediated and cellular RNA export (Stutz *et al.*, 1996). Not all FG nucleoporin repeat domains produce the same pattern of RNA export inhibition, suggesting that only selected nucleoporins are involved in these pathways. An mRNA trafficking defect was observed upon the over-expression of Nup153 FxFG repeats in BHK cells (Bastos *et al.*, 1996). Members of the importinβ super-family were shown to interact directly with the FG-containing Nups (Ryan and Wente, 2000). At least two of the factors involved in mRNA export are also associated with FG Nups (Bachi *et al.*, 2000; Strasser *et al.*, 2000). The FG repeat-containing Nups are, therefore; believed to play a crucial role in the translocation process.

MULTIPLE RNA EXPORT PATHWAYS

Different classes of RNAs, including mRNAs, tRNAs, and U snRNAs, are transcribed and processed within the nucleus and then exported to the cytoplasm by multiple pathways. Competition experiments with microinjected *Xenopus* oocytes have revealed that tRNA, mRNA, U snRNA and ribosomal subunits all use saturable pathways, but none of them saturated the export of others (Jarmolowski *et al.*, 1994). For instance, microinjection of excess levels of tRNA inhibits tRNA export, but not U snRNA or mRNA export (Izaurralde and Adam, 1998; Jarmolowski *et al.*, 1994; Nakielny and Dreyfuss, 1997). Further studies indicated that U snRNAs accesses an export pathway that is shared with both 5S RNA and proteins that carry a specific type of nuclear export signal (NES) (Fisher *et al.*, 1995).

Understanding nuclear export is not an easy task. Limitations include lack of an *in vitro* system for studying RNA export, and the fact that RNA export is intimately linked to its processing (Gorlich and Mattaj, 1996; Izaurralde and Mattaj, 1995; Nakielny *et al.*, 1997). Elucidations to date have primarily come from three approaches: *Xenopus* oocytes microinjection experiments, genetic analysis in yeast and studies on export pathways utilized by viruses. Microinjection of proteins or RNAs into the nucleus of *Xenopus* oocytes demonstrated that RNA export is energy-dependent and saturable, and that the export of distinct classes of RNAs (mRNAs, U snRNAs, tRNAs, and rRNAs) takes place through, at least partly, distinct pathways (Jarmolowski *et al.*, 1994). Study of yeast mutants defective in RNA export provided information about potentially relevant genes (Amberg *et al.*, 1992; Kadowaki *et al.*, 1994). A system that has proven to be particularly useful is the analysis of retroviral nuclear RNA export pathways. Viruses hijack their host cell's metabolic processes for replication. These borrowed processes are also essential cellular processes, and thus of great interest to cellular biologists. One such process is the nuclear export of RNA. At present, no complete mechanism can be proposed for the export of any type of RNA, but significant progress has been made in a few specific areas.

REV-MEDIATED EXPORT OF VIRAL RNA

Important insight into RNA export mechanisms has come from studies on the viral Rev protein encoded by the human immunodeficiency virus type-1 (HIV-1) (Fisher *et al.*, 1995). HIV expresses nine different gene products from a relatively small genome. This efficient utilization of coding sequences is accomplished by the use of different splicing events and overlapping reading frames. HIV also expresses genes from RNAs that retain introns. The expression of intron-containing messages is unusual for eukaryotic cells. Splicing must be complete before a message is allowed to exit the nucleus. This checkpoint ensures that only the mature messages reach the cytoplasm, therefore only the correct proteins are expressed. To bypass this checkpoint, HIV encodes a protein called Rev, which is expressed from a fully spliced viral mRNA. Rev is required for the expression of the HIV structural proteins encoded by the various incompletely spliced viral mRNAs (Emmermman *et al.*, 1989; Felber *et al.*, 1989).

HIV-1 Rev is a small, 13 kDa sequence-specific RNA-binding protein that contains at least three functional domains (Hope *et al.*, 1990; Malim *et al.*, 1989a): an arginine–rich domain that functions both as RNA binding domain (RBD) and nuclear localization signal (NLS) (Cochrane *et al.*, 1990; Kjems *et al.*, 1992); a leucine-rich nuclear export signal (NES) (Fisher *et al.*, 1995; Malim *et al.*, 1989a) and; a multimerization domain (Hope *et al.*, 1992; Zapp *et al.*, 1991). The presence of both NLS and NES enables Rev to shuttle continuously between the nucleus and the cytoplasm (Meyer and Malim, 1994). Through the RBD, Rev specifically binds to a 240-base region of complex secondary structure called the Rev response element (RRE) (Malim *et al.*, 1989b) (Figure 13.2A). The RRE is located within the second intron of HIV messages, and therefore is present in all incompletely spliced HIV RNAs. When bound to the RRE, Rev allows the export of un-spliced RNA. Rev NES was shown to function as an autonomous nuclear export signal (NES) (Fisher *et al.*, 1995; Wen *et al.*, 1995).

It is now clear that leucine-rich NESs similar to the one found in Rev play an essential role in the export of many cellular and viral proteins (Gorlich and Kutay, 1999; Mattaj and Englmeier, 1998; Nakielny and Dreyfuss, 1999). Subsequently, it was shown that leucine-rich NESs are binding sites for CRM1 (also known as Xpo1 in budding yeast), a nuclear transport factor belonging to the importinβ family of nuclear transport receptors (Fornerod *et al.*, 1997; Fukuda *et al.*, 1997; Neville *et al.*, 1997; Ossareh-Nazari *et al.*, 1997; Stade *et al.*, 1997). Therefore, nuclear export of Rev-bound HIV-1 mRNAs is dependent on the RanGTP gradient (Figure 13.2A).

An important question was whether CRM1 would also mediate the nuclear export of other classes of cellular RNAs. Experiments designed to address this question, initially using competition assays with *Xenopus* oocytes and subsequently using reagents that specifically inhibit CRM1 function, have revealed that CRM1 is essential for U snRNA and 5S rRNA export, but is not necessary for cellular mRNA, tRNA, and large-rRNA export (Bogerd *et al.*, 1998; Neville and Rosbash, 1999; Otero *et al.*, 1998).

CTE-MEDIATED EXPORT OF VIRAL RNAs

A main candidate as an mRNA export factor has emerged from studies on the retrovirus Mason-Pfizer monkey virus (MPMV). Similar to the other retroviruses,

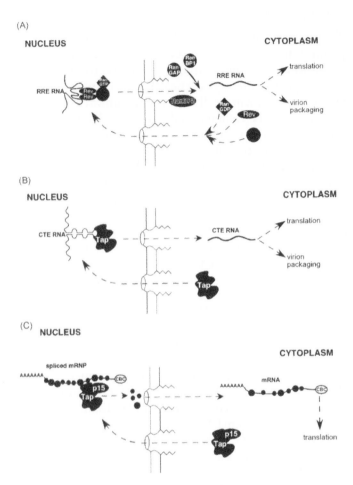

Figure 13.2 Nuclear RNA export pathways. (A) Rev-mediated mRNA export. Rev bridges the interaction between RRE-containing RNA and Ran-GTP-bound CRM1. CRM1 mediates the translocation of the resultant ribonucleoprotein complex to the cytoplasm by directly interacting with nucleoporins. In the cytoplasm, hydrolysis of RanGTP to RanGDP by the combined action of RanGAP and RanBPs induces the dissociation of the complex. The RRE-containing unspliced or incompletely spliced HIV-1 mRNAs can now be translated into viral proteins or, in the case of unspliced mRNA, packaged into viral particles. CRM1 and Rev shuttle back to the nucleus to mediate other rounds of export events. (B) CTE-mediated mRNA export. Unlike RRE, CTE does not use a viral-encoded protein to mediate its interaction with the cellular export receptor Tap. By directly binding to CTE, Tap mediates the nuclear export of intron-containing MPMV RNAs. In the cytoplasm, Tap is released and recycled back to the nucleus. (C) Export of cellular mRNA. Lacking CTE-like sequences, unspliced cellular mRNAs are not able to directly recruit Tap and are retained in the nucleus. However, in a splicing–dependent manner (see text) Tap and its cofactor p15 are recruited to the mature mRNA. It is thought that the role of p15 is to facilitate, by an unknown mechanism, the recruitment of Tap exclusively to the spliced mRNAs. Nonshuttling hnRNPs are released and retained in the nucleus. Spliced mRNAs are now export-competent and undergo translocation through the nuclear pore. After discharging the cargo in the cytoplasm, Tap and p15 shuttle back to the nucleus.

MPMV has to export both spliced and un-spliced variants of the same initial transcript into the cytoplasm of infected cells. However, MPMV is a simple retrovirus that does not encode a Rev equivalent (Cullen, 1998), and therefore has to rely on cellular protein(s) to export its messages. The completely spliced messages are exported to the cytoplasm by the normal cellular export pathways. The intron-containing messages would normally be retained in the nucleus. To overcome this problem, MPMV uses a *cis*-acting structured element located near the 3' end of viral RNA. This element, termed the constitutive transport element (CTE), was demonstrated to induce the export of unspliced MPMV mRNAs (Bray *et al.*, 1994; Ernst *et al.*, 1997a). The CTE is structurally and functionally conserved in the related type D retroviruses (Ernst *et al.*, 1997b; Tabernero *et al.*, 1996; Zolotukhin *et al.*, 1994).

The MPMV CTE is distinct from the HIV-1 RRE in that it must rely on a cellular protein cofactor to function. The next step was to identify this cofactor. Competition and inhibitor experiments revealed that CTE is not dependent on CRM1 nuclear export factor (Bogerd *et al.*, 1998; Otero *et al.*, 1998; Pasquinelli *et al.*, 1997a; Saavedra *et al.*, 1997). In addition, microinjection of high levels of CTE in *Xenopus* oocyte nuclei selectively inhibited mRNA export, while tRNA, U snRNA, and Rev-RRE-dependent RNA export were unaffected (Pasquinelli *et al.*, 1997a; Saavedra *et al.*, 1997). Thus, the CTE cofactor was also likely to be a key participant in cellular mRNA export.

Efforts to identify the cofactor led to the isolation of a protein, termed TAP. TAP was shown to bind specifically to functional forms of the MPMV CTE and to shuttle between the cell nucleus and cytoplasm (Gruter *et al.*, 1998; Kang and Cullen, 1999) (Figure 13.2B). Expression of human TAP enhances CTE function in microinjected *Xenopus* oocyte and rescues CTE function in otherwise non-permissive quail cells (Gruter *et al.*, 1998; Kang and Cullen, 1999). TAP contains a CTE RNA binding motif (Braun *et al.*, 1999; Kang *et al.*, 2000) (Figure 13.3). Recently, the crystal structure of the minimal TAP fragment that binds CTE has been determined (Liker *et al.*, 2000). This fragment includes two independent globular sub-domains (Figure 13.3). One sub-domain is a non-canonical ribonucleoprotein (RNP) domain. Despite the fact that it lacks the canonical conserved sequence motif present in RNP, this sub-domain has general RNA-binding activity. The other sub-domain is a leucine-rich repeat (LRR) domain. LRR does not show general RNA-binding activity, but it is required for specific binding to the CTE. Recognition of CTE requires both RNA and LRR domains present in *cis* in the same polypeptide together with an N-terminal flexible region. Studies performed *in vitro* and *in vivo* with structure-based mutants suggested that LRR might function in the nuclear export of cellular mRNAs. In this case, LRR acts as a protein–protein interaction module for adapter proteins. Thus, the LRR, which acts in *cis* to promote CTE recognition, may generally function in *trans* to interact with other proteins associated with spliced cellular mRNAs (Liker *et al.*, 2000) (see section on nuclear export of mRNAs). TAP also contains an NTF2-like domain that mediates the heterodimerization with the cellular factor p15. p15 is not necessary for the CTE binding by TAP. However, p15 is thought to help recruit TAP exclusively to the fully processed mRNAs (see section on nuclear export of mRNAs).

Besides the CTE binding motif, TAP also contains an essential C-terminal domain that functions as a nucleocytoplasmic shuttle domain (Figure 13.3).

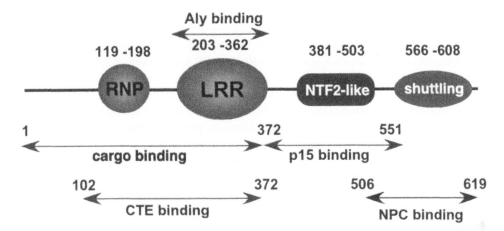

Figure 13.3 Domain organization of Tap. Human Tap is a 619-amino acids protein. The minimal CTE-binding domain is composed of two globular sub-domains (the ribonucleoprotein or RNP domain and the leucine-rich repeat or LRR) and a flexible N-terminal region. Also shown is the localization of the C-terminal nucleocytoplasmic shuttling domain, the cargo-binding domain, and the NTF2-like domain that exhibits p15 binding activity.

The C-terminal domain of TAP was shown to directly and specifically interact with several nucleoporins (Bachi *et al.*, 2000; Kang *et al.*, 2000; Katahira *et al.*, 1999). These latter activities have proven to be mutationally inseparable. Therefore, the ability of TAP to exit the nucleus, and hence to export CTE containing RNAs, seems to be mediated by a direct interaction of TAP with constituents of the NPC (Kang *et al.*, 2000).

NUCLEAR EXPORT OF INTRONLESS VIRAL MESSAGES

A number of intronless messages are found in herpes simplex virus, the human hepatitis B virus (HBV), and the woodchuck hepatitis virus (WHV) (Donello *et al.*, 1998; Huang and Liang, 1993; Huang and Yen, 1995; Otero and Hope, 1998). HBV and WHV are DNA viruses that undergo reverse transcription during its replication cycle and hence they are distantly related to the retroviruses (Ganem and Varmus, 1987). All of the four known HBV and WHV proteins are encoded on one strand of the circular genome, and they are translated from un-spliced transcripts that originate from at least four internal promoters and terminate at a common polyadenylation site (Yen, 1993). Thus, HBV and WHV mRNAs are exported from the nucleus un-spliced.

In contrast to retroviral and cellular messages, much less is known about the expression of intronless messages. Recent studies have indicated that, similar to the type D retroviruses, nuclear export of these RNAs is facilitated by interactions between specific *cis*-acting elements and cellular factors (Donello *et al.*, 1998; Huang and Yen, 1995; Huang *et al.*, 1996; Otero and Hope, 1998). These *cis*-acting elements were named post-transcriptional regulatory element or HPRE (for HBV) and WPRE (for WHV).

Structural studies revealed that the PREs are composed of multiple *cis*-acting sequences, referred to as sub-elements. HPRE and WPRE contain homologous sub-elements, which were designated PREα and PREβ (Donello *et al.*, 1996, 1998). WPRE is significantly more active than HPRE and this correlates with the presence of an additional sub-element, PREγ, which is not found in HPRE (Donello *et al.*, 1998). Studies in our laboratory have not found a cell type in which these PREs are not functional, suggesting that the PRE-binding protein(s) are highly conserved and ubiquitously expressed.

HPRE and WPRE can functionally substitute for Rev/RRE complex in a transient reporter assay (Donello *et al.*, 1998; Huang and Liang, 1993; Huang and Yen, 1995). Given that it can substitute for Rev/RRE in a reporter gene assay, it has been suggested that HPRE may function in a Rev-like manner. However, experiments using reagents that specifically inhibit CRM1 function, have suggested that HPRE does not use CRM1 as an export receptor (Otero *et al.*, 1998; Zang and Yen, 1999). Since Rev/RRE export depends on leucine-rich NES–CRM1 interaction, it appears that the cellular export factor(s) that binds to HPRE and mediates its function does not contain a Rev-type NES. This factor(s) remains to be identified.

The exact mechanism by which the PREs facilitate the cytoplasmic localization of unspliced RNAs remains unknown. Recent data indicate that HPRE could affect many steps in mRNA processing, including the inhibition of splicing, the enhancement of both polyadenylation and mRNA export (Huang *et al.*, 1999). In addition, both can increase the amount of intronless cytoplasmic RNA of a normally intron-dependent β-globin cDNA, which is consistent with the idea that they functionally replace an intron during RNA processing (Huang and Yen, 1995; Schambach *et al.*, 2000).

NUCLEAR EXPORT OF mRNAs

Apart from mediating the export of RRE-containing viral RNAs through Rev, CRM1 is believed to participate in the export of U snRNAs (Fisher *et al.*, 1995; Fornerod *et al.*, 1997) and possibly in mRNA export in yeast (Murphy and Wente, 1996; Stade *et al.*, 1997). The question of whether CRM1 is involved in mRNA export in higher eukaryotes is a controversial issue. While some data argue for a role of CRM1 in mRNA export (Pasquinelli *et al.*, 1997b), several other studies arrived at the opposite conclusion (Clouse *et al.*, 2001; Fisher *et al.*, 1995; Fornerod *et al.*, 1997; Paraskeva *et al.*, 1999). Injection of Rev NES into *Xenopus* oocytes competes with U snRNA export but has no effect on mRNA export. Hence, the mRNA export pathway appears to be distinct from the CRM1-mediated pathway shared by Rev NES and U snRNAs (Fisher *et al.*, 1995; Fornerod *et al.*, 1997). The CRM1-specific inhibitor leptomycin B (LMB) does not inhibit mRNA export in oocytes, whereas it strongly inhibits U snRNA export (Fornerod *et al.*, 1997).

The over-expression of a dominant negative form of CAN/Nup214 (ΔCAN) that inhibits CRM1 interaction with nucleoporins, thus CRM1-mediated export, has no effect on the cellular mRNA export pathway in mammalian cells (Bogerd, 1996). A further argument against a role of CRM1 in mRNA export came from Reed and co-workers (Clouse *et al.*, 2001). Nuclear injection of the Ran mutant RanT24N or RanGAP (normally localized in the cytoplasm) inhibited tRNA and U1 snRNA export, but not the spliced mRNA export. Nuclear co-injection of RanGAP and RanBP1 did not inhibit mRNA export. As CRM1 requires RanGTP to function, the results suggest that this export receptor is not required for spliced mRNA nuclear export.

Circumstantial evidence suggests that TAP, the cellular factor for CTE, also plays an important role in mRNA export. Titration of TAP by microinjection of high levels of CTE RNA inhibits nuclear mRNA export but does not affect the export of other RNAs, such as tRNAs or U snRNAs (Pasquinelli *et al.*, 1997a; Saavedra *et al.*, 1997). Co-injection of human TAP rescues both CTE-dependent and CTE-independent mRNA transport (Gruter *et al.*, 1998). Subsequently, TAP was shown to be associated with global poly(A)$^+$ RNA in human cells and to bind RNA nonspecifically *in vitro* (Katahira *et al.*, 1999; Liker *et al.*, 2000). However, the affinity of TAP for nonspecific RNAs is much lower than its affinity for CTE RNA (Gruter *et al.*, 1998; Kang *et al.*, 1999; Kang and Cullen, 1999; Liker *et al.*, 2000). The mechanism of TAP recruitment to the global poly(A)$^+$ RNA *in vivo* is unclear. More compelling evidence for a role of TAP in mRNA export came from yeast studies (Katahira *et al.*, 1999). Mex67p, the yeast homologue of TAP, was found to directly interact *in vivo* with a second essential yeast mRNA export factor, termed Mtr2p, which promotes the efficient recruitment of Mex67p to the yeast NPCs (Santos-Rosa *et al.*, 1998). Significantly, the Mex67p-Mtr2p heterodimer was found to directly bind to poly(A)$^+$ RNA both *in vivo* and *in vitro*.

The search for the human equivalent to Mtr2p led to the identification of p15, which actually has little or no homology to Mtr2p (Katahira *et al.*, 1999). Even so, p15 seems to be the functional homologue of Mtr2p, as yeast cells lacking Mex67p can be complemented by human TAP plus p15, but not by TAP alone. In fact, TAP and p15 can rescue the viability of yeast cells lacking both Mex67p and Mtr2p. This result demonstrates that the TAP-Mex67p nuclear RNA export pathway has been conserved during evolution, and suggests a role for p15 in TAP-dependent export of cellular mRNA (see Figure 13.2C).

It is difficult to define a role for p15 in vertebrate cells. This difficulty is in part because p15 is not essential for the TAP-dependent nuclear export of CTE-containing RNA (Bachi *et al.*, 2000; Kang *et al.*, 2000). However, p15 enhances TAP binding to CTE and can form a ternary complex with TAP on the CTE (Kang *et al.*, 2000). Therefore, p15 could normally act as a quality control step facilitating the recruitment of TAP exclusively to the mature mRNA (Figure 13.2C). Since it recruits TAP directly, CTE may well avoid the p15-dependent quality control step and hence induce nuclear export of unspliced viral mRNA (Figure 13.2B). Recent experiments demonstrated that TAP is able to mediate the export of RRE-containing messages (Guzyk *et al.*, 2001). The fusion of TAP to an NES-defective Rev gave rise to a chimera that was able to complement Rev function. Notably, co-transfection of p15 dramatically increased the ability of the chimera to mediate the export of RRE-containing RNA. These results are significant, because they demonstrate that TAP is an export protein in mammalian cells, and that p15 is required for its function.

It has been suggested that the recruitment of TAP/p15 complex might be the critical, final step that would induce mRNA export from the nucleus (Gruter *et al.*,

1998) (Figure 13.2C). However, how TAP/p15 is recruited to the mature mRNAs remains unknown. This important issue, i.e., how mRNAs receive an export license from the nucleus, is addressed by Luo and Reed (1999). Their experiments demonstrated that splicing generates specific mRNA-protein (mRNP) complexes that are more competent for nuclear export. Thus, injection of intron-containing pre-mRNAs into the *Xenopus* oocytes nucleus results in the efficient splicing and subsequent nuclear export of these mRNAs. In contrast, nuclear injection of the fully spliced forms of the same mRNAs (Δi-mRNAs) results in very inefficient nuclear export and primarily leads to their nuclear degradation. Moreover, Luo and Reed (1999) demonstrate that mRNA splicing can result not only in the removal of nuclear retention factors, but also in the selective recruitment of nuclear RNA export factors. Incubation of pre-mRNAs in a nuclear extract *in vitro* results in splicing and in assembly of the resultant mature mRNA into a ribonucleoprotein (RNP) complex. However, the RNP complex containing the mRNA spliced *in vitro* was found to migrate significantly slower on a nondenaturing polyacrylamide gel than the RNP formed on the identical Δi-mRNAs. More importantly, microinjection of these isolated RNP complexes into *Xenopus* oocytes nuclei resulted in efficient nuclear export of the spliced mRNAs, whereas the Δi-mRNAs remained almost entirely nuclear. Therefore, the factors assembled onto the spliced mRNA *in vitro*, during the process of splicing, were able to target these mRNAs for nuclear export. In contrast, the equivalent Δi-mRNAs were unable to assemble these factors, as they remained confined to the nucleus. Thus, the process of splicing, either *in vivo* or *in vitro*, was able to confer an export license to the spliced mRNAs. This export license is not available to the, in principle, identical Δi-mRNAs. It is possible that splicing enhances either recruitment of TAP/p15 directly, or it promotes the assembly of proteins that then act to recruit TAP/p15.

There is accumulating evidence supporting an indirect recruitment of the TAP/p15 complex to the spliced mRNA. Le Hir *et al.* (2000b) provided compelling evidence that pre-mRNA splicing indeed alters mRNP protein composition. The end result is the stably deposition of several proteins as a single complex of ∼335 kDa at a conserved position 20–24 nucleotides upstream of the exon-exon junction in mRNA (Le Hir *et al.*, 2000a). Using a novel *in vitro* cross-linking approach, the authors detected several proteins that associate with mRNA exon-exon junctions only as a consequence of splicing. Immunoprecipitation experiments suggested that these proteins are part of a tight complex (or the 'licensing complex') around the junction. Glycerol gradient fractionation showed that a subset of these proteins remained associated with mRNA after its release from the spliceosome. Thus, the spliceosome can leave behind signature proteins at exon-exon junctions. Such proteins could influence downstream metabolic events *in vivo*, such as mRNA export, translation, and nonsense-mediated decay. The licensing complex remains stably bound to mRNA without apparent preference for a particular RNA sequence. Consistent with there being no consensus sequence in the −24 region of the 5' exon, the authors demonstrated that the position of −20/24 protection is determined exclusively by its distance from the exon-exon junction, and not by the exon sequence (Le Hir *et al.*, 2000a).

Specific proteins have been found in this complex, including the splicing-associated factors SRm160, DEK, and RNPS1, the mRNA-associated shuttling protein Y14 and the mRNA export factor Aly (also called REF) (Kim *et al.*, 2001; Le Hir *et al.*, 2000a; Zhou *et al.*, 2000). The Y14 and REF proteins have no known function in the splicing process, but they have both been linked to mRNA export (Kataoka *et al.*, 2000; Stutz *et al.*, 2000; Zhou *et al.*, 2000).

Aly, like its yeast ortholog, Yra1, is required for mRNA export (Strasser and Hurt, 2000; Stutz *et al.*, 2000; Zhou *et al.*, 2000). Aly/Yra1 can bind RNA and simultaneously contact the mRNA export factor TAP (Mex67p in yeast) (Strasser and Hurt, 2000; Stutz *et al.*, 2000). As mentioned above, TAP/Mex67p is a shuttling protein that interacts with components of the nuclear pore complex, and Mex67p is essential for viability in yeast (Bachi *et al.*, 2000; Katahira *et al.*, 1999). Although TAP can bind directly to certain viral RNA export elements (Bear *et al.*, 1999; Gruter *et al.*, 1998), it does not have high affinity for RNA in general (Braun *et al.*, 1999; Stutz *et al.*, 2000). It has been suggested that the principal means of TAP association with cellular mRNAs is through protein–protein interactions (Bachi *et al.*, 2000; Liker *et al.*, 2000; Strasser and Hurt, 2000; Stutz *et al.*, 2000). In addition to Aly, TAP can associate with other RNA binding proteins *in vivo* and *in vitro*. One of these, Y14, binds to TAP, spliced mRNA and hnRNP proteins *in vivo* (Kataoka *et al.*, 2000). The findings that both Aly and Y14 are contained in the licensing complex suggests that these proteins mediate the preferential export of spliced mRNA by recruiting export factors, such as TAP, to spliced mRNPs. Since TAP could not be detected in the licensing complex, it is possible that TAP is recruited at an intermediate stage between splicing and export that is not replicated under *in vitro* conditions.

ROLE OF RNA EXPORT IN GENE THERAPY

The study of viral and cellular mRNA export has provided great insights into cellular functions and how cells and viruses use regulatory elements to facilitate their gene expression. This study generated great interest in gene therapy research. For example, such regulatory elements can be used to improve transgene delivery and expression. Several sequence modifications can be introduced that act at the level of transcription, posttranscriptional processing of mRNAs, or half-life of the encoded protein. Sequences that improve posttranscriptional processing and export of a given mRNA are of great interest because: (i) the majority of transcribed RNA is not efficiently processed and licensed for nuclear export (Jackson *et al.*, 2000), and; (ii) cytoplasmic accumulation and translation of many cellular mRNAs are rate limiting and dependent on the presence of appropriate introns, export signals and/or polyadenylation tails (Huang *et al.*, 1999; Luo and Reed, 1999). At least three different *cis*-acting modules have been shown to play an important role in this context: splice sites (SS), retroviral *cis*-acting elements that are active in the absence of virus-encoded proteins, such as the constitutive RNA transport elements (CTE) and hepadnaviral posttranscriptional regulatory elements, such as WPRE. Several studies have demonstrated the utility of these three groups of elements to increase transgene expression in the context of either plasmids or viral gene vectors (Donello *et al.*, 1998; Luo and Reed, 1999; Matsumoto *et al.*, 1998; Wodrich *et al.*, 2000; Zufferey *et al.*, 1999; Hildinger *et al.*, 1999; Loeb *et al.*, 1999; Schambach *et al.*, 2000).

Viruses had to develop ways to avoid immunosurveillance by infected hosts and to efficiently deliver genes to specific cell types. Several types of viruses have been modified and tested for their efficacy in gene therapy. The ability of retroviruses to insert their genome into the host DNA allows for stable genetic modification of the host cell. This stability is in contrast to gene delivery using certain DNA viruses, such as adenovirus and herpes simplex virus, which remain episomal. Replication of retroviruses occurs through a specific interaction between the viral envelope protein and a cell surface receptor on the target cell, followed by internalization. After internalization, the virus is uncoated and its RNA is reverse-transcribed into double-stranded DNA (dsDNA). The dsDNA is then imported into the nucleus, where it stably integrates into the host genome. Mitosis and, thus, the breakdown of the nuclear envelope are required for dsDNA to reach the nucleus.

From a bio-safety point of view, it is necessary to remove as much of the HIV viral sequences as possible. Rev removal would permit elimination of additional viral sequences from the vector. This removal minimizes the possibilities for recombination events that could lead to a replication-competent virus. With Rev removed, *cis*-acting elements, not requiring viral proteins for function, must be introduced in the vector. RNA export elements derived from simple retroviruses, such as CTE, can be used to replace Rev in exporting intron-containing genomic RNA into the cytoplasm. It was possible to generate a replication-competent CTE-dependent virus that could achieve wild-type levels in certain culture systems (Zolotukhin *et al.*, 1994). The ability of CTE to replace Rev/RRE for HIV replication was exploited to generate lentiviral vector stocks. However, in this case, the titers were slightly lower than those obtained using the Rev/RRE system. Further modifications were used to improve the CTE-based vector system. For example, four CTE were found to be more efficient than a single copy in Rev-independent expression of HIV gag (Wodrich *et al.*, 2000). By incorporating multiple copies of the CTE into a lentiviral vector, the vector titer could be improved. Thus, the titers of Rev-independent lentiviral vectors were improved by using the simian virus 1 (SRV-1) CTE together with mutations in the major splice donor and acceptor sites present in the vector and re-localization of the CTE adjacent to the HIV-1 3'LTR. These modifications have additive beneficial effects in that they generate a system that yields higher titers than those obtained with a Rev-dependent lentiviral vector (Mautino *et al.*, 2000). While CTE-dependent vector is useful for the generation of viral stocks, it does not usually enhance transgene expression (Schambach *et al.*, 2000).

Elements functionally related to CTE, such as HSV-TK, HPRE, and WPRE, have been tested for their ability to boost gene expression. Of these, only WPRE was found to induce a significant increase in gene expression (Loeb *et al.*, 1999; Zufferey *et al.*, 1999). To function, WPRE must be located within the transgene message, consistent with its post-transcriptional function. Results obtained in our laboratory demonstrated that WPRE could further increase the expression of a gene that is already well expressed (Loeb *et al.*, 1999; Zufferey *et al.*, 1999). Due to its efficiency, WPRE has been tested in a variety of contexts. Thus, WPRE can stimulate transgene expression when used in retroviral, adeno-associated virus (AAV) and plasmid-based vectors (Loeb *et al.*, 1999; Zufferey *et al.*, 1999). WPRE can stimulate transgene expression in a variety of primary and cultured cells. In addition, mammalian tissues, such as hematopoietic cells or brain cells, successfully express transgenes when transduced with WPRE-dependent lentiviral vectors (Paterna *et al.*, 2000; Ramezani *et al.*, 2000). The ability of WPRE to stimulate gene expression seems to be transgene-independent, but the extent of stimulation varies (Schambach *et al.*, 2000).

The extent of stimulation by WPRE-dependent HIV vectors was shown to be promoter-dependent (Ramezani *et al.*, 2000). WPRE stimulated transgene expression when the cytomegalovirus (CMV) immediate early region promoter-enhancer, the murine stem cell virus (MSCV) long terminal repeat (LTR), the Gibbon ape leukemia virus (GALV) LTR, or the human phosphoglycerate kinase 1 (PKG) promoter were used. Conversely, the human elongation factor 1α (EF1α) promoter and the composite CAG promoter (CMV immediate early enhancer + the chicken β-actin promoter) only modestly stimulated transgene expression. Likewise, Trono and co-workers have found that WPRE inhibited GFP in the context of a HIV-EF1α vector system (Salmon *et al.*, 2000). Transgene expression from retroviral vectors containing the herpes virus thymidine kinase promoter or the SV40 early promoter was also stimulated by WPRE (Loeb *et al.*, 1999; Zufferey *et al.*, 1999). Consequently, it is advisable to determine whether WPRE enhances transgene expression in the presence of the promoter being used. That WPRE can stimulate transgene expression, while the related HPRE cannot, was unexpected. As previously mentioned, the ability of WPRE to stimulate transgene expression could be due to the presence of an additional *cis*-acting sub-element that is not present in HPRE (Donello *et al.*, 1998).

The mechanism by which WPRE stimulates gene expression is just beginning to be deciphered. Several lines of evidence (Loeb *et al.*, 1999; Zufferey *et al.*, 1999) suggest that WPRE functions posttranscriptionally inside the nucleus to stimulate transgene expression: (i) WPRE increases the level of nuclear transgene mRNA; (ii) the observed increase in protein levels correlates with an increase in RNA levels; (iii) the relative increase in RNA levels induced by WPRE is the same in both nucleus and cytoplasm. Although WPRE does not affect RNA stability, it may facilitate many steps in RNA processing, directing RNAs that would normally be degraded inside the nucleus to be efficiently expressed (Zufferey *et al.*, 1999). WPRE seems to act independently of transcription and splicing, but may improve gene expression by facilitating 3' cleavage and polyadenylation, RNA export, or translation (Donello *et al.*, 1998; Huang *et al.*, 1999). Efficient 3' processing has been shown to stimulate gene expression (Carswell and Alwine, 1989). Consistent with this stimulation, the results obtained in our laboratory suggest that WPRE modulates the length of poly(A) tails in the transgene mRNAs. In general, cellular mRNAs have poly(A) tails that are approximately 250 nucleotides long. We found that transgenes typically have poly(A) tails that are much shorter than these. Nevertheless, in the presence of WPRE, transgenes' poly(A) tails are 250 A long. It is possible that a poly(A) tail with the correct length could signal to the cell that the transgene is a cellular message that should not be degraded in the nucleus, but rather be properly processed, exported and efficiently translated into the cytoplasm.

CONCLUDING REMARKS

Efficient transgene expression is a prerequisite to making gene therapy a reality. Recent studies on cellular and viral RNA export demonstrated the importance of RNA export in gene expression. Significant improvements in the design of gene expression systems have come from the studies on viruses i.e., their ability to transfer and maintain viral gene expression in the infected cell. It is clear now that, to further increase the yield of transgene expression, processing and export of mRNA must be improved. Efficient gene transfer mimics what viruses are doing during their replication. Viruses encode both *cis*- and *trans*-acting factors that efficiently utilize the host cell machinery to promote viral replication. Therefore, it is appropriate that viral-derived *cis*-acting elements, such as WPRE, are being utilized as tools to facilitate efficient gene expression. By increasing the efficiency of transgene expression it is possible to obtain better production of therapeutic proteins per individually delivered genes. If transgene expression can be increased by five-fold, a smaller amount of vector is needed. This would decrease the cost of production of the expression vectors for each treatment. Therefore, it appears that the transgene expression systems of the future will be optimized for RNA export.

REFERENCES

Akey, C.W. and Radermacher, M. (1993) Architecture of the *Xenopus* nuclear pore complex revealed by three-dimensional cryo-electron microscopy. *J. Cell Biol.*, **122**, 1–19.

Amberg, D.C., Goldstein, A.L. and Cole, C.N. (1992) Isolation and characterization of RAT1: an essential gene of *Saccharomyces cerevisiae* required for the efficient nucleocytoplasmic trafficking of mRNA. *Genes Dev.*, **6**, 1173–1189.

Arts, G.J., Kuersten, S., Romby, P., Ehresmann, B. and Mattaj, I.W. (1998) The role of exportin-t in selective nuclear export of mature tRNAs. *EMBO J.*, **17**, 7430–7441.

Bachi, A., Braun, I.C., Rodrigues, J.P., Pante, N., Ribbeck, K., von Kobbe, C. *et al.* (2000) The C-terminal domain of TAP interacts with the nuclear pore complex and promotes export of specific CTE-bearing RNA substrates. *RNA*, **6**, 136–158.

Bastos, R., Lin, A., Enarson, M. and Burke, B. (1996) Targeting and function in mRNA export of nuclear pore complex protein Nup153. *J. Cell Biol.*, **134**, 1141–1156.

Bayliss, R., Corbett, A.H. and Stewart, M. (2000) The molecular mechanism of transport of macromolecules through nuclear pore complexes. *Traffic*, **1**, 448–456.

Bear, J., Tan, W., Zolotukhin, A.S., Tabernero, C., Hudson, E.A. and Felber, B.K. (1999) Identification of novel import and export signals of human TAP, the protein that binds to the constitutive transport element of the type D retrovirus mRNAs. *Mol. Cell. Biol.*, **19**, 6306–6317.

Bentley, D. (1999) Coupling RNA polymerasae II with pre-mRNA processing. *Curr. Opin. Cell Biol.*, **11**, 347–351.

Biamonti, G. and Riva, S. (1994) New insights into the auxiliary domain of eukaryotic RNA binding proteins. *FEBS Lett.*, **340**, 1–8.

Bischoff, F.R. and Gorlich, D. (1997) RanBP1 is crucial for the release of RanGTP from importin β-related nuclear transport factors. *FEBS Lett.*, **419**, 249–254.

Bischoff, F.R. and Ponstingl, H. (1991) Catalysis of guanine nucleotide exchange on Ran by the mitotic regulator RCC1. *Nature*, **354**, 80–82.

Bogerd, H.P., Echarri, A., Ross, T.M. and Cullen, B.R. (1998) Inhibition of human immunodeficiency virus Rev and human T-cell leukemia virus Rex function, but not Mason-Pfizer monkey virus constitutive transport element activity, by a mutant human nucleoporin targeted to Crm1. *J. Virol.*, **72**, 8627–8635.

Bogerd, H.P., Fridell, R.A., Benson, R.E. and Cullen, B.R. (1996) Protein sequence requirements for function of the human T-cell leukemia virus type 1 Rex nuclear export signal delineated by an *in vivo* randomization-selection assay. *Mol. Cell. Biol.*, **16**, 4207–4214.

Braun, I.C., Rohrbach, E., Schmitt, C. and Izaurralde, E. (1999) TAP binds to the constitutive transport element (CTE) through a novel RNA-binding motif that is sufficient to promote CTE-dependent RNA export from the nucleus. *EMBO J.*, **18**, 1953–1965.

Bray, M., Prasad, S., Dubay, J.W., Hunter, E., Jeang, K.T., Rekosh, D. *et al.* (1994) A small element from the Mason-Pfizer monkey virus genome makes human immunodeficiency virus type 1 expression and replication Rev-independent. *Proc. Natl. Acad. Sci. USA*, **91**, 1256–1260.

Burd, C. G. and Dreyfuss, G. (1994) Conserved structure and diversity of functions of RNA-binding proteins. *Science*, **265**, 615–6221.

Cartegni, L., Maconi, M., Morandi, E., Cobianchi, F., Riva, S. and Biamonti, G. (1996) hnRNP A 1 selectively interacts through its Gly-rich domain with different RNA-binding proteins. *J. Mol. Biol.*, **259**, 337–348.

Carswell, S. and Alwine, J.C. (1989) Efficiency of utilization of the simian virus 40 late polyadenylation site: effects of upstream sequences. *Mol. Cell.*, **9**, 4248–4258.

Clouse, K.N., Luo, M.J., Zhou, Z. and Reed, R. (2001) A Ran-independent pathway for export of spliced mRNA. *Nat. Cell Biol.*, **3**, 97–99.

Cochrane, A.W., Perkins, A. and Rosen, C.A. (1990) Identification of sequences important in the nucleolar localization of human immunodeficiency virus Rev: relevance of nucleolar localization to function. *J. Virol.*, **64**, 881–885.

Cullen, B.R. (1998) Retroviruses as model systems for the study of nuclear RNA export pathways. *Virology*, **249**, 203–210.

Daneholt, B. (1999) Pre-mRNA particles: from gene to nuclear pores. *Curr. Biol.*, **9**, R412–R415.

Donello, J.E., Beeche, A.A., Smith, Jr., G., Lucero, G.R. and Hope, T.J. (1996) The hepatitis B virus posttranscriptional regulatory element is composed of two sub-elements. *J. Virol.*, **70**, 4345–4351.

Donello, J.E., Loeb, J.E. and Hope, T.J. (1998) Woodchuck hepatitis virus contains a tripartite postranscriptional regulatory element. *J. Virol.*, **72**, 5085–5092.

Dreyfuss, G., Matunis, M.J., Pinol-Roma, S. and Burd, C.G. (1993) hnRNP proteins and the biogenesis of mRNA. *Annu. Rev. Biochem.*, **62**, 289–321.

Emmermman, M., Vazeux, R. and Pedeu, K. (1989) The *rev* gene product of the human immunodeficiency virus affects envelope-specific RNA localization. *Cell*, **57**, 1155–1165.

Ernst, R.K., Bray, M., Rekosh, D. and Hammarskjold, M.-L. (1997a) Secondary structure and mutational analysis of the Mason-Pfizer monkey virus constitutive transport element. *RNA*, **3**, 219–222.

Ernst, R.K., Bray, M., Rekosh, D. and Hammarskjold, M.-L. (1997b) A structural retroviral element that mediates nucleocytoplasmic export of intron-containing RNA. *Mol. Cell. Biol.*, **17**, 135–144.

Felber, B.K., Hadzopoulou-Cladaras, M., Cladaras, C., Copeland, T. and Pavlakis, G. (1989) Rev protein of human immunodeficiency virus affects the stability and transport of viral mRNA. *Proc. Natl. Acad. Sci. USA*, **86**, 1496–1499.

Fisher, U.J., Huber, J., Boelens, W.C., Mattaj, I.W. and Luhrmann, R. (1995) The HIV-1 Rev activation domain is a nuclear export signal that accesses an export pathway used by specific cellular RNAs. *Cell*, **82**, 475–483.

Fornerod, M., Ohno, M., Yoshida, M. and Mattaj, I.W. (1997) CRM1 is an export receptor for leucine-rich nuclear export signals. *Cell*, **90**, 1051–1060.

Fukuda, M., Asano, S., Nakamura, T., Adachi, M., Yoshida, M., Yanagida, M. *et al.* (1997) CRM1 is responsible for intracellular transport mediated by the nuclear export signal. *Nature*, **390**, 308–311.

Ganem, D. and Varmus, H.E. (1987) The molecular biology of the hepatitis B viruses. *Annu. Rev. Biochem.*, **56**, 651–693.

Gorlich, D. and Kutay, U. (1999) Transport between the cell nucleus and the cytoplasm. *Annu. Rev. Cell Dev. Biol.*, **15**, 607–660.

Gorlich, D. and Mattaj, I.W. (1996) Nucleocytoplasmic transport. *Science*, **271**, 1513–1518.

Gorlich, D., Pante, N., Kutay, U., Aebi, U. and Bischoff, F.R. (1996) Identification of different roles for RanGDP and RanGTP in nuclear protein import. *EMBO J.*, **15**, 5584–5594.

Gruter, P., Tabernero, C., von Kobbe, C., Schmitt, C., Saavedra, C., Bachi, A. *et al.* (1998) TAP, the human homologue of Mex67p, mediates CTE-dependent RNA export from the nucleus. *Mol. Cell*, **1**, 649–659.

Guzyk, B.W., Levesque, L., Prasad, S., Bor, Y.-C., Black, B.E., Pashal, B.M. *et al.* (2001) NXT1 (p15) is a crucial cellular cofactor in TAP-dependent export of intron-containing RNA in mammalian cells. *Mol. Cell. Biol.*, **21**, 2545–2554.

Hildinger, M., Abel, K.L., Ostertag, W. and Baum, C. (1999) Design of 5' untranslated sequences in retroviral vectors developed for medical use. *J. Virol.*, **73**, 4083–4089.

Hirose, Y. and Manley, J.L. (2000) RNA polymerase II and the integration of nuclear events. *Gene Dev.*, **14**, 1415–1429.

Hodge, C.A., Colot, H.V., Stafford, P. and Cole, C.N. (1999) Rat8p/Dbp5p is a shuttling transport factor that interacts with Rat7p/Nup159p and Gle1p and suppresses the mRNA export defect of xpo1-1 cells. *EMBO J.*, **18**, 5778–5788.

Hope, T.J., Huang, X.J., McDonald, D. and Parslow, T.G. (1990) Steroid-receptor fusion of the human immunodeficiency virus type 1 Rev transactivator: mapping cryptic functions of the arginine-rich motif. *Proc. Natl. Acad. Sci. USA*, **87**, 7787–7791.

Hope, T.J., Klein, N.P., Elder, M.E. and Parslow, T.G. (1992) Trans-dominant inhibition of human immunodeficiency virus type 1 Rev occurs through formation of inactive protein complexes. *J. Virol.*, **66**, 1849–1855.

Huang, J. and Liang, T.J. (1993) A novel hepatitis B virus (HBV) genetic element with Rev response element-like properties that is essential for expression of HBV gene products. *Mol. Cell. Biol.*, **13**, 7476–7486.

Huang, Y., Wimler, K.M. and Carmichael, G.G. (1999) Intronless mRNA transport elements may affect multiple steps of pre-mRNA processing. *EMBO J.*, **18**, 1642–1652.

Huang, Z.-M. and Yen, T.S.B. (1995) Role of the hepatitis B virus posttranscriptional regulatory element in export of intronless transcripts. *Mol. Cell. Biol.*, **15**, 3864–3869.

Huang, Z.M., Zang, W.Q. and Yen, T.S. (1996) Cellular proteins that bind to the hepatitis B virus posttranscriptional regulatory element. *Virology*, **217**, 573–581.

Ismail, S.I., Kingsman, S.M. and Uden, M. (2000) Split-intron retroviral vectors: enhanced expression with improved safety. *J. Virol.*, **74**, 2365–2371.

Izaurralde, E. and Adam, S. (1998) Transport of macromolecules between the nucleus and the cytoplasm. *RNA*, **4**, 351–364.

Izaurralde, E., Kutay, U., von Kobbe, C., Mattaj, I.W. and Gorlich, D. (1997a) The asymmetric distribution of the constituents of the Ran system is essential for transport into and out of the nucleus. *EMBO J.*, **16**, 6535–6547.

Izaurralde, E., Jarmolowski, A., Beisel, C., Mattaj, I. W., Dreyfuss, G. and Fischer, U. (1997b) A role for the M9 transport signal of hnRNP A1 in mRNA nuclear export. *J. Cell Biol.*, **137**, 27–35.

Izaurralde, E. and Mattaj, I.W. (1995) RNA export. *Cell*, **81**, 153–159.

Jackson, D.A., Pombo, A. and Iborra, F. (2000) The balance sheet for transcription: an analysis of nuclear RNA metabolism in mammalian cells. *FASEB J.*, **14**, 242–254.

Jarmolowski, A., Boelens, W.C., Izaurralde, E. and Mattaj, I.W. (1994) Nuclear export of different classes of RNA is mediated by specific factors. *J. Cell Biol.*, **124**, 627–635.

Kadowaki, T., Chen, S., Hitomi, M., Jacobs, E., Kumagai, C., Liang, S. *et al.* (1994) Isolation and characterization of Saccharomyces cerevisae mRNA transport-defective (mtr) mutants. *J. Cell Biol.*, **126**, 649–659.

Kang, Y., Bogerd, H.P. and Cullen, B.R. (2000) Analysis of cellular factors that mediate nuclear export of RNAs bearing the Mason-Pfizer monkey virus constitutive transport element. *J. Virol.*, **74**, 5863–5871.

Kang, Y., Bogerd, H.P., Yang, J. and Cullen, B.R. (1999) Analysis of the RNA binding specificity of the human TAP protein, a constitutive transport element-specific nuclear RNA export factor. *Virology*, **262**, 200–209.

Kang, Y. and Cullen, B.R. (1999) The human TAP protein is a nuclear mRNA export factor that contains novel RNA-binding and nucleocytoplasmic transport sequences. *Genes Dev.*, **13**, 1126–1139.

Katahira, J., Strasser, K., Podtelejnikov, A., Mann, M., Jung, J.U. and Hurt, E. (1999) The Mex67p-mediated nuclear mRNA export pathway is conserved from yeast to human. *EMBO J.*, **18**, 2593–2609.

Kataoka, N., Yong, J., Kim, V.N., Velazquez, F., Perkinson, R.A., Wang, F. *et al.* (2000) Pre-mRNA splicing imprints mRNA in the nucleus with a novel RNA-binding protein that persists in the cytoplasm. *Mol. Cell*, **6**, 673–682.

Keminer, O., Siebrasse, J.P., Zerf, K. and Peters, R. (1999) Optical recording of signal-mediated protein transport through single nuclear pore complexes. *Proc. Natl. Acad. Sci. USA*, **96**, 11842–11847.

Khamlichi, A.A., Rocca, A. and Cogne, M. (1994) The effect of intron sequences on expression levels of Ig cDNAs. *Gene*, **150**, 387–390.

Kim, V.N., Yong, J., Kataoka, N., Abel, L., Diem, M.D. and Dreyfuss, G. (2001) The Y14 protein communicates to the cytoplasm the position of exon-exon junctions. *EMBO J.*, **20**, 2062–2068.

Kjems, J., Calnan, B.J., Frankel, A.D. and Sharp, P.A. (1992) Specific binding of a basic peptide from HIV-1 Rev. *EMBO J.*, **11**, 1119–1129.

Krecic, A.M. and Swanson, M.S. (1999) hnRNP complexes: composition, structure, and function. *Curr. Opin. Cell Biol.*, **11**, 363–371.

Kutay, U., Bischoff, F.R., Kostka, S., Kraft, R. and Gorlich, D. (1997) Export of importin*α* from the nucleus is mediated by a specific nuclear transport factor. *Cell*, **90**, 1061–1071.

Le Hir, H., Izaurralde, E., Maquat, L.E. and Moore, M.J. (2000a) The spliceosome deposits multiple proteins 20–24 nucleotides upstream of mRNA exon-exon junction. *EMBO J.*, **19**, 6860–6869.

Le Hir, H., Moore, M.J. and Maquat, L.E. (2000b) Pre-mRNA splicing alters mRNP composition: evidence for stable association of proteins at exon-exon junctions. *Genes Dev.*, **14**, 1098–1108.

Li, K.J. and Garoff, H. (1998) Packaging of the intron-containing genes into retrovirus vectors by alpha virus vectors. *Proc. Natl. Acad. Sci. USA*, **95**, 3650–3654.

Liker, E., Fernandez, E., Izaurralde, E. and Conti, E. (2000) The structure of the mRNA export factor TAP reveals a *cis* arrangement of a non-canonical RNP domain and an LRR domain. *EMBO J.*, **19**, 5587–5598.

Loeb, J.E., Cordier, W.S., Harris, M.E., Weitzman, M.D. and Hope, T.J. (1999) Enhanced expression of transgenes from adeno-associated virus vectors with the woodchuck hepatitis virus posttranscriptional regulatory element: implications for gene therapy. *Hum. Gene Ther.*, **10**, 2295–2305.

Lounsbury, K.M. and Macara, I.G. (1997) Ran-binding protein1 (RanBP1) forms a ternary complex with Ran and karyopherin *β* and reduces Ran GTPase-activating protein (RanGAP) inhibition by karyopherin b. *J. Biol. Chem.*, **272**, 551–555.

Luo, M.J. and Reed, R. (1999) Splicing is required for rapid and efficient mRNA export in metazoans. *Proc. Natl. Acad. Sci. USA*, **96**, 14937–14942.

Malim, M.H., Bohnlein, S., Hauber, J. and Cullen, B.R. (1989a) Functional dissection of the HIV-1 Rev *trans*-activator – derivation of a *trans*-dominant repressor of Rev function. *Cell*, **58**, 205–214.

Malim, M.H., Hauber, J., Le, S.Y., Maizel, J.V. and Cullen, B.R. (1989b) The HIV-1 rev *trans*-activator acts through a structured target sequence to activate nuclear export of unspliced viral mRNA. *Nature*, **338**, 254–257.

Matsumoto, K., Wassarman, K.M. and Wolffe, A.P. (1998) Nuclear history of a pre-mRNA determines the translational activity of cytoplasmic mRNA. *EMBO J.*, **17**, 2107–2121.

Mattaj, J.W. and Englmeier, L. (1998) Nucleocytoplasmic transport: the soluble phase. *Annu. Rev. Biochem.*, **67**, 265–306.

Matunis, M.J., Coutavas, E. and Blobel, G. (1996) A novel ubiquitin-like modification modulates the partitioning of the RanGAP1 between cytosol and the nuclear pore complex. *J. Cell Biol.*, **135**, 1457–1470.

Mautino, M.R., Keiser, N. and Morgan, R.A. (2000) Improved titers of HIV-based lentiviral vectors using the SRV-1 constitutive transport element. *Gene Ther.*, **7**, 1421–1424.

Meyer, B.E. and Malim, M.H. (1994) The HIV-1 Rev trans-activator shuttles between the nucleus and the cytoplasm. *Genes Dev.*, **8**, 1538–1547.

Michael, W.M., Eder, P.S. and Dreyfuss, G. (1997) The K nuclear shuttling domain: a novel signal for nuclear import and nuclear export in the hnRNP K protein. *EMBO J.*, **16**, 3587–3598.

Moroianu, J., Hijikata, M., Blobel, G. and Radu, A. (1995) Mammalian karyopherin a1b and a2b heterodimers: a1 or a2 subunit binds nuclear localization signal and b subunit interacts with peptide repeat-containing nucleoporins. *Proc. Natl. Acad. Sci. USA*, **92**, 6532–6536.

Murphy, R. and Wente, S.R. (1996) An RNA-export mediator with an essential nuclear export signal. *Nature*, **383**, 357–360.

Nakielny, S. and Dreyfuss, G. (1997) Nuclear export of proteins and RNAs. *Curr. Opin. Cell Biol.*, **9**, 420–429.

Nakielny, S. and Dreyfuss, G. (1999) Transport of proteins and RNAs in and out of the nucleus. *Cell*, **99**, 677–690.

Nakielny, S., Fischer, U., Michael, W.M. and Dreyfuss, G. (1997) RNA transport. *Annu. Rev. Neurosci.*, **20**, 269–298.

Nehrbass, U. and Blobel, G. (1996) Role of the nuclear transport factor p10 in nuclear import. *Science*, **272**, 120–122.

Neugebauer, K.M. and Roth, M.B. (1997) Transcription units as RNA processing units. *Gene Dev.*, **11**, 3279–3285.

Neville, M. and Rosbash, M. (1999) The NES-Crm1p export pathway is not a major mRNA export route in Saccharomyces cerevisae. *EMBO J.*, **18**, 3746–3756.

Neville, M., Stutz, F., Lee, L., Davis, L.I. and Rosbash, M. (1997) The importin-beta family member Crm1p bridges the interaction between Rev and the nuclear pore complex during nuclear export. *Curr. Biol.*, **7**, 767–775.

Ossareh-Nazari, B., Bachelerie, F. and Dargemont, C. (1997) Evidence for a role of CRM1 in signal-mediated nuclear protein export. *Science*, **278**, 141–144.

Otero, G.C., Harris, M.E., Donello, J.E. and Hope, T.J. (1998) Leptomycin B inhibits equine infectious anemia virus Rev and feline immunodeficiency virus rev function but not the function of the hepatitis B virus posttranscriptional regulatory element. *J. Virol.*, **72**, 7593–7597.

Otero, G.C. and Hope, T.J. (1998) Splicing-independent expression of the herpes simplex virus type 1 thymidine kinase gene is mediated by three *cis*-acting RNA sub-elements. *J. Virol.*, **72**, 9889–9896.

Paine, P.L., Moore, L.C. and Horowitz, S.B. (1975) Nuclear envelope permeability. *Nature*, **254**, 109–114.

Paraskeva, E., Izaurralde, E., Bischoff, F.R., Huber, J., Kutay, U., Hartmann, E. *et al.* (1999) CRM1-mediated recycling of snurportin 1 to the cytoplasm. *J. Cell Biol.*, **145**, 255–264.

Pasquinelli, A.E., Ernst, R.K., Lund, E., Grimm, C., Zapp, M.L., Rekosh, D. *et al.* (1997a) The constitutive transport element (CTE) of Mason-Pfizer monkey virus (MPMV) accesses a cellular mRNA export pathway. *EMBO J.*, **16**, 7500–7510.

Pasquinelli, A.E., Powers, M.A., Lund, E., Forbes, D. and Dahlberg, J.E. (1997b) Inhibition of mRNA export in vertebrate cells by nuclear export signals conjugates. *Proc. Natl. Acad. Sci. USA*, **94**, 14394–14399.

Paterna, J.C., Moccetti, T., Mura, A., Feldon, J. and Bueler, H. (2000) Influence of promoter and WHV post-transcriptional regulatory element on AAV-mediated transgene expression in the rat brain. *Gene Ther.*, **7**, 1304–1311. Politz, J.C. and Pederson, T. (2000) Review: movement of mRNA from transcription site to the nuclear pores. *J. Struct. Biol.*, **129**, 252–257.

Politz, J.C. and Pederson, T. (2000) Movement of mRNA from transcription site to nuclear pores. *J. Struct. Biol.*, **129**, 252–257.

Powers, M.A., Forbes, D.J., Dahlberg, J.E. and Lund, E. (1997) The vertebrate GLFG nucleoporin, Nup98, is an essential component of multiple RNA export pathways. *J. Cell Biol.*, **136**, 241–250.

Radu, A., Blobel, G. and Moore, M.S. (1995a) Identification of a protein complex that is required for nuclear protein import and mediates docking of import substrates to distinct nucleoporins. *Proc. Natl. Acad. Sci. USA*, **92**, 1769–1773.

Radu, A., Moore, M.S. and Blobel, G. (1995b) The peptide repeat domain of nucleoporin Nup98 functions as a docking site in transport across the nuclear pore complex. *Cell*, **81**, 215–222.

Ramezani, A., Hawley, T.S. and Hawley, R.G. (2000) Lentiviral vectors for enhanced gene expression in human hematopoietic cells. *Mol. Ther.*, **2**, 458–469.

Ribbeck, K., Lipowsky, G., Kent, H.M., Stewart, M. and Gorlich, D. (1998) NTF2 mediates nuclear import of Ran. *EMBO J.*, **17**, 6587–6598.

Rout, M.P., Aittchison, J.D., Suprapto, A., Hjertaas, K., Zhao, Y. and Chait, B.T. (2000) The yeast nuclear pore complex. Composition, architecture, and transport mechanism. *J. Cell Biol.*, **148**, 635–652.

Ryan, K.J. and Wente, S.R. (2000) The nuclear pore complex: a protein machine bridging the nucleus and cytoplasm. *Curr. Opin. Cell Biol.*, **12**, 361–371.

Saavedra, C., Felber, B. and Izauralde, E. (1997) The simian retrovirus-1 constitutive transport element, unlike the HIV-1 RRE, uses factors required for cellular mRNA export. *Curr. Biol.*, **7**, 619–628.

Salmon, P., Kindler, V., Ducrey, O., Chapuis, B., Zubler, R.H. and Trono, D. (2000) High-level transgene expression in human hematopoietic progenitors and differentiated blood lineages after transduction with improved lentiviral vectors. *Blood*, **96**, 3392–3398.

Santos-Rosa, H., Moreno, H., Simos, G., Segref, A., Fahrenkrog, B., Pante, N. *et al.* (1998) Nuclear mRNA export requires complex formation between Mex67p and Mtr2p at the nuclear pores. *Mol. Cell. Biol.*, **18**, 6826–6838.

Schambach, A., Wodrich, H., Hildinger, M., Bohne, J., Krausslich, H.G. and Baum, C. (2000) Context dependence of different modules for posttranscriptional enhancement of gene expression from retroviral vectors. *Mol. Ther.*, **2**, 435–445.

Singh, O.P., Bjorkroth, B., Masich, S., Wieslander, L. and Daneholt, B. (1999) The intranuclear movement of Balbiani ring pre-messenger ribonucleoprotein particle. *Exp. Cell Res.*, **251**, 135–146.

Stade, K., Ford, C.S., Guthrie, C. and Weis, K. (1997) Exportin 1 (Crm1p) is an essential nuclear export factor. *Cell*, **90**, 1041–1050.

Stoffler, D., Fahrenkrog, B. and Aebi, U. (1999) The nuclear pore complex: from molecular architecture to functional dynamics. *Curr. Opin. Cell Biol.*, **11**, 391–401.

Strasser, K., Bassler, J. and Hurt, E. (2000) Binding of the Mex67p/Mtr2p heterodimer to FXFG, GLFG, and FG repeat nucleoporins is essential for nuclear mRNA export. *J. Cell Biol.*, **150**, 695–706.

Strasser, K. and Hurt, E. (2000) Yra1p, a conserved nuclear RNA-binding protein, interacts directly with Mex67p and is required for mRNA export. *EMBO J.*, **19**, 410–420.

Strawn, L.A., Shen, T. and Wente, S.R. (2001) The GLFG regions of Nup116p and Nup100p serve as binding sites for both Kap95p and Mex67p at the nuclear pore complex. *J. Biol. Chem.*, **276**, 6445–6452.

Stutz, F. and Rosbash, M. (1998) Nuclear RNA export. *Genes Dev.*, **12**, 3303–3319.

Stutz, F., Bachi, A., Doerks, T., Braun, I.C., Seraphin, B., Wilm, M. *et al.* (2000) REF, an evolutionary conserved family of hnRNP-like proteins, interacts with TAP/Mex67p and participates in mRNA nuclear export. *RNA*, **6**, 638–650.

Stutz, F., Izaurralde, E., Mattaj, I.W. and Rosbash, M. (1996) A role for nucleoporin FG repeat domains in export of human immunodeficiency virus type 1 Rev protein and RNA from the nucleus. *Mol. Cell. Biol.*, **16**, 7144–7150.

Tabernero, C., Zolotukhin, A.S., Valentin, A., Pavlakis, G.N. and Felber, B.K. (1996) The posttranscriptional control element of the simian retrovirus type 1 forms an extensive RNA secondary structure necessary for its function. *J. Virol.*, **70**, 5998–6011.

Weighardt, F., Biamonti, F. and Riva, S. (1996) The roles of heterogeneous nuclear ribonucleoproteins (hnRNP) in RNA metabolism. *BioEssay*, **18**, 747–756.

Weis, K. (1998) Importins and exportins: how to get in and out of the nucleus. *Trends Biochem. Sci.*, **23**, 185–189.

Wen, W., Meinkoth, J.L., Tsien, R.Y. and Taylor, S.S. (1995) Identification of a signal for rapid export of proteins from the nucleus. *Cell*, **82**, 463–473.

Wodrich, H., Schambach, A. and Krausslich, H.G. (2000) Multiple copies of the Mason-Pfizer monkey virus constitutive RNA transport element lead to enhanced HIV-1 Gag expression in a context-dependent manner. *Nucleic Acids Res.*, **28**, 901–910.

Yang, Q., Rout, M.P. and Akey, C.W. (1998) Three-dimensional architecture of the isolated yeast nuclear pore complex: functional and evolutionary implications. *Mol. Cell.*, **1**, 223–234.

Yen, T.S.B. (1993) Regulation of hepatitis B virus gene expression. *Semin. Virol.*, **4**, 33–42.

Zang, W.Q. and Yen, B. (1999) Distinct export pathway utilized by the hepatitis B virus posttranscriptional regulatory element. *Virology*, **259**, 299–304.

Zapp, M.L., Hope, T.J., Parslow, T.G. and Green, M.R. (1991) Oligomerization and RNA binding domains of the type 1 human immunodeficiency virus Rev protein: a dual function for an arginine-rich binding motif. *Proc. Natl. Acad. Sci. USA*, **88**, 7734–7738.

Zhou, Z., Luo, M.J., Straesser, K., Katahira, J., Hurt, E. and Reed, R. (2000) The protein Aly links pre-messenger-RNA splicing to nuclear export in metazoans. *Nature*, **407**, 401–405.

Zolotukhin, A.S., Valentin, A., Pavlakis, G.N. and Felber, B.K. (1994) Continuous propagation of RRE(-) and Rev(-)RRE(-) human immunodeficiency virus type 1 molecular clones containing a *cis*-acting element of simian retrovirus type 1 in human peripheral blood lymphocytes. *J. Virol.*, **68**, 7944–7952.

Zufferey, R., Donello, J.E., Trono, D. and Hope, T.J. (1999) Woodchuck hepatitis virus posttranscriptional regulatory element enhances expression of transgenes delivered by retroviral vectors. *J. Virol.*, **73**, 2886–2892.

14 Naked plasmid DNA delivery of a therapeutic protein

Holly M. Horton and Suezanne E. Parker

INTRODUCTION

Naked plasmid DNA (pDNA) has been shown to be taken up by mammalian cells, resulting in gene expression at substantial levels in certain tissues. The use of naked pDNA can avoid the costly and tedious steps necessary for the production of viral vectors or recombinant protein and therefore, may enable us to use naked pDNA as pharmaceuticals. Over the past decade, numerous preclinical studies have revealed the ability of pDNA injections to result in measurable serum levels of the expressed transgene, in addition to producing a marked therapeutic effect. pDNA gene delivery has been found to be efficacious in preclinical models of cancer, metabolic and infectious diseases. It also requires much less frequent injection compared to therapy with recombinant protein. Early clinical studies of pDNA delivery of a therapeutic protein in humans have yielded encouraging results with minimal side effects, further recommending the continued study of this type of gene delivery.

In this chapter, we will discuss the history and current status of naked pDNA delivery of a therapeutic protein. The related topic of pDNA vaccines will not be covered in this chapter and the reader is referred to several recent comprehensive reviews in this area (Lai and Bennett, 1998; Donnelly *et al.*, 1997; Horton *et al.*, 1999a). This chapter will focus on the technology of therapeutic protein delivery by injection of naked pDNA into muscle or other organs in a variety of different species.

IN VIVO TRANSFECTION OF MUSCLE USING NAKED pDNA

In 1990, a novel method of *in vivo* gene delivery was described in which the injection of pDNA into mouse muscle led to measurable, long-term levels of a reporter gene (Wolff *et al.*, 1990). Previous studies of *in vivo* gene delivery had required encapsulation of pDNA (Nicolau *et al.*, 1983) or complex formation with cationic liposomes (Felgner *et al.*, 1987) or calcium phosphate co-precipitation (Benvenisty and Reshef, 1986) or pDNA condensation with polylysine–glycoprotein carrier (Wu and Wu, 1988) for efficient uptake into tissues. The unexpected finding by Wolff *et al.* (1990) that skeletal muscle tissue injected with 'naked' DNA (not complexed with lipid or other carrier) could take up the DNA and express the transgene opened a new chapter in gene delivery. Wolff and his colleagues at Vical,

Inc. demonstrated that a single injection of naked pDNA expressing a reporter gene into the mouse quadriceps muscle could lead to localized expression in the myofibers for up to 60 days after injection. The importance of this work was that it identified a simple procedure for *in vivo* gene delivery in a tissue that was easily accessible. Furthermore, the technique did not require a viral vector for gene delivery, thereby avoiding the safety concerns of using infectious or replicating virus as a vector for gene delivery.

A later study in rhesus monkeys evaluated the ability of primate muscle to take up naked pDNA (Jiao *et al.*, 1992). A single injection of luciferase-expressing pDNA into the rectus femoris of monkeys led to luciferase expression in the muscle, which was 100-fold above background levels. Biopsy specimens revealed that both type I and II myofibers were transfected and luciferase was expressed for up to four months after the pDNA injection. The researchers compared the injection of a solution of pDNA versus the surgical implant of pDNA pellets into monkey muscle. Interestingly, higher levels of gene expression were found after the implant of pDNA pellets. Several different muscle groups were injected in the monkeys: biceps brachii, brachioradialis, rectus femoris or tibialis anterior. The different muscle types all expressed similar levels of luciferase, with somewhat higher levels of expression after the implant of pDNA pellets versus the injection of pDNA in solution. In the same study, cat muscles were also found to take up naked pDNA. Thus, muscle tissue in higher animals also has the ability to take up exogenous pDNA in the absence of lipid or other carriers.

MECHANISM OF pDNA ENTRY INTO MUSCLE TISSUE

The mechanism of pDNA entry into muscle was first evaluated by Wolff *et al.* (1992a,b) in both *in vitro* and *in vivo* studies. *In vitro* transfection of various cell lines, including muscle cells, with luciferase-encoding pDNA complexed with cationic lipid, resulted in high levels of luciferase expression, while transfection of the cell lines with naked pDNA resulted in low levels of luciferase expression. In contrast, *in vivo* intramuscular (i.m.) injection of naked pDNA resulted in high levels of gene expression, whereas i.m. injection of pDNA complexed with cationic lipid led to a 100-fold decrease in gene expression. Thus, it appears that pDNA needs to be complexed with lipid for efficient *in vitro* transfection, but transfection of muscle tissue *in vivo* is more efficient with naked pDNA. Histological analysis of muscle tissue revealed that pDNA complexed with lipid did not enter the muscle myofibers and appeared to be unable to cross the external lamina, while naked pDNA was able to enter the myofibers. Hence, *in vitro* studies of the mechanism of naked pDNA entry into muscle may not adequately reflect *in vivo* processes.

The uptake of pDNA into mouse muscle appears to be a saturable process with 25–100 µg pDNA resulting in optimal levels of gene expression (Levy *et al.*, 1996). When salmon sperm DNA was added in 40-fold excess to luciferase pDNA, reporter gene expression was completely arrested. The latter finding supports a receptor-mediated uptake mechanism for pDNA entry into muscle. In addition, co-injection of pDNA with the negatively charged polymer dextran sulfate also abolished reporter gene expression of the pDNA. The negatively charged dextran sulfate may compete with pDNA for binding sites.

The form of the injected pDNA is important. Injection of covalently closed-circular or open-circular forms of pDNA resulted in a 100-fold higher gene expression than the injection of linearized pDNA (Wolff *et al.*, 1992b). Southern blot analyses suggested that the linearized pDNA degraded more quickly than the circular forms after i.m. injection. Gold-labeled pDNA was followed to determine the distribution of the pDNA after i.m. injection in mouse muscle. As early as five minutes post-injection, gold-labeled pDNA was found in T tubules and caveolae but not in endocytic vesicles, suggesting a possible role for these structures in the pDNA uptake.

IN VIVO TRANSFECTION OF OTHER TISSUES BY NAKED pDNA

A number of studies have examined whether other tissues, in addition to muscle, are able to take up and express a transgene after pDNA injection. When the brain, liver, spleen, uterus, stomach, lung, kidney or heart of rats was injected with luciferase encoding naked pDNA only the heart tissue was found to express significant amounts of luciferase (Acsadi *et al.*, 1991a). Upon injection of 100–200 µg of pDNA into the apex of the heart, luciferase was detected in the tissue from 7–14 days post-pDNA administration. Histological analysis of the tissue revealed that the myocardial cells in the heart expressed the transgene, while other cells such as endothelial cells, fibroblasts or blood cells had no luciferase expression. The results of this study suggested that skeletal and cardiac cells may differ from other cells in their ability to take up naked pDNA. However, later studies revealed that a variety of tissues are, in fact, able to acquire and express a transgene after naked pDNA administration.

A subsequent study evaluated direct pDNA injection into the liver of rats and cats treated with dexamethasone to suppress inflammation after surgery (Hickman *et al.*, 1994). pDNA at doses of 500 µg/2 ml (rats) or 100–500 µg/3 ml (cats) were injected directly into the hepatic parenchyma. The liver tissue was assayed 48 hours later and luciferase expression was evident in both species. A dose-response was established with increasing amounts of pDNA, resulting in increasing luciferase expression. Multiple injections of pDNA led to higher expression levels than a single injection. Furthermore, injection of a fixed dose of pDNA in the two species led to higher luciferase expression in the cats. The researchers also administered pDNA encoding α-1 antitrypsin into the liver of rats and cats. Several different lobes were injected for a total pDNA dose of 1 mg in rats and 3 mg in cats. Serum levels of α-1 antitrypsin were found in rats and cats 48 hours after injection and in cats expression persisted for seven days, demonstrating that pDNA injection into the liver of several species could lead to measurable serum levels of the protein encoded by the pDNA.

DNA injection directly into mouse diaphragm has also resulted in luciferase expression and there appeared to be no damage to the diaphragm due to the DNA injections (Davis and Jasmin, 1993). In a related study, β-galactosidase (β-gal)-encoding pDNA injected into the articular space of rabbit knee joints resulted in β-gal expression in the joints (Yovandich *et al.*, 1995). In the same study, chloramphenicol acetyltransferase (CAT) encoding pDNA injected into rat knee joints also led to reporter gene expression, with peak expression 48 hours after injection and with no detectable activity 15 days later.

Injection of β-gal expression plasmids into the dermis of swine has also led to β-gal expression in the skin for up to three weeks after injection (Hengge *et al.*, 1995). At later time points, the cells expressing β-gal were found in the outer, more differentiated layers of the epidermis, suggesting that the transfected cells migrated to the outer layers as part of the normal differentiating process of the epidermis. In the same study, pDNA encoding human IL-8 was injected into swine dermis to assess whether a biologically active protein could be expressed after pDNA dermal injection. The IL-8 pDNA injection resulted in marked neutrophil accumulation in the dermis. A later study revealed that direct injection of pDNA into human skin could lead to gene expression (Hengge *et al.*, 1996). In this study, human skin grafted onto immunodeficient mice and injected with naked β-gal encoding pDNA was found to express β-gal 24 hours later.

Intracerebral injection of luciferase pDNA in mouse brain has also been demonstrated to result in a dose-dependent expression of the reporter gene in the brain (Schwartz *et al.*, 1996). The degree of reporter gene expression appeared to be lower than that demonstrated for muscle and expression declined significantly by five days post-injection.

Naked pDNA encoding luciferase has also been able to transfect rat stomach where reporter gene expression was found up to day 21 post pDNA injection (Takehara *et al.*, 1996). Histological analyses revealed that primarily smooth muscle cells and mesenchymal cells were transfected while epithelial cells had no apparent reporter gene expression.

These studies demonstrated for the first time that the injection of naked pDNA in a variety of tissues could lead to gene expression over several weeks. Most importantly, the results of these studies validated the technique of *in vivo* injection of pDNA. The next phase of pDNA-based gene therapy research involved the determination of the biological activity of the protein encoded by the pDNA when delivered by i.m. injection.

CLINICAL APPLICATIONS OF NAKED pDNA

Biological activity of naked pDNA

The use of naked pDNA to deliver a therapeutic gene was first attempted by Acsadi *et al.* (1991b) with the demonstration that pDNA encoding human dystrophin injected i.m. into mdx mice resulted in human dystrophin protein in the cytoplasm and sarcolemma of 1% of the myofibers. Although the expression levels of the transgene were very low in this study, they were important for demonstrating the principle that naked pDNA could be used to deliver a biologically active protein.

An early study by Raz *et al.* (1993) examined the biological effect of naked pDNA delivery of a cytokine gene. In this study, BALB/c mice were injected intramuscularly with 100 µg of pDNA expressing IL-2, IL-4 or TGFβ once per week for three weeks followed by three injections of keyhole limpet hemocyanin (KLH) in the same thigh. Serum was collected from the mice at various time points and tested for antibody to KLH. Mice injected intramuscularly with IL-2 pDNA or IL-4 pDNA followed by KLH had high levels of KLH-specific antibody by weeks nine–ten. In contrast, mice injected with TGFβ pDNA followed by KLH injection had significantly lower antibody levels to KLH. Co-injection of IL-2 and TGFβ pDNA resulted in very low levels of antibody to KLH, most likely due to the immunosuppressive effects of TGFβ overcoming the immunostimulatory effects of IL-2. Circulating serum levels of TGFβ (2.6 ng/ml) were found four weeks after i.m. injection of naked TGFβ pDNA. This study represents one of the first to characterize the biological efficacy of i.m. pDNA delivery of a therapeutic gene to demonstrate that cytokine delivery by pDNA can modulate the immune response to a foreign antigen, and to achieve measurable serum levels of a therapeutic protein after i.m injection of naked pDNA. Most importantly, the biological effects of the i.m. cytokine pDNA injections were evident for many weeks after the final pDNA injection, indicating a long-term effect after only a few injections of cytokine encoding pDNA.

In another study examining the biological activity of a protein delivered by naked pDNA administration, i.m. injection of naked pDNA encoding erythropoietin (Epo) was found to markedly raise the hematocrits of mice (Tripathy *et al.*, 1996). A single i.m. injection of as little as 10 μg Epo pDNA was found to raise hematocrits for 90 days. Similar to the study by Raz *et al.* (1993), this study demonstrated that long-term expression and biological activity of a therapeutic gene was possible after i.m. pDNA injection.

In a related study, the injection into rat muscle of a pDNA encoding human apolipoprotein E (apo-E2) was found to result in serum levels of the protein (Fazio *et al.*, 1994). A receptor-binding defective apo-E2 was used as the transgene to detect serum levels of the protein, which was unable to bind to the receptor. Intramuscular injection of apo-E2 pDNA resulted in serum levels of human apo-E2 for up to 45 days after pDNA injection. In a related study, single i.m. injection of 80 μg pDNA encoding apo-E3 in apo-E-deficient mice resulted in serum levels of 600 ng/ml apo-E3 for one week after pDNA injection, with measurable serum levels of apo-E3 for as long as four weeks post-injection (Rinaldi *et al.*, 2000). Remarkably, apo-E-deficient mice injected i.m. once with 80 μg apo-E3 pDNA had a significant decrease in serum cholesterol for up to 16 weeks after injection. Furthermore, a marked decrease in very low density lipoprotein (VLDL) and LDL and a corresponding increase in high density lipoprotein (HDL) was found after the pDNA therapy. Thus, pDNA delivery of apo-E3 resulted in long-term serum levels of apo-E3, as well as a long-term therapeutic effect. With further study and optimization of the treatment regimen, this type of pDNA therapy may someday be useful for the treatment of hyperlipidemic conditions in humans.

pDNA therapy of viral infection

Intramuscular pDNA therapy has also been found to be able to protect against certain viral infections in mouse models. In one study, mice were ocularly infected with HSV-1 followed by topical application of 25 μg interferon α (IFNα) pDNA at 12 hour intervals beginning at either 12, 24 and 48 hours post-infection (Noisakran and Carr, 2000). Only the mice treated with IFNα pDNA beginning at 12 hours post-infection had a significantly increased survival rate. Mice treated with IFNα pDNA at 12 hours had reduced viral load in the trigeminal ganglia. In a similar study, intravaginal delivery of IFNα pDNA 24 hours post HSV-2 infection resulted in a significantly increased survival rate (Haarle *et al.*, 2001). In contrast, treatment with 500 U recombinant IFNα protein did not enhance survival. The increase in survival was correlated with a decrease in viral transcripts and protein in vaginal tissue. If the IFNα pDNA therapy was administered 48 hours post-HSV-2 infection, however, the mice had a survival rate similar to the control pDNA-treated group. Thus, if a viral disease is identified early enough, pDNA delivery of a therapeutic protein may be beneficial in reducing viral infection.

pDNA therapy of autoimmune diseases

Naked pDNA delivery of cytokines has also been evaluated in a number of mouse models of autoimmune disease. Naked pDNA delivery of TGFβ to a murine model of systemic lupus erythematosus (SLE) led to lower serum IgG levels, decreased glomerulonephritis and increased survival (Raz *et al.*, 1995). The pDNA (100 µg) was injected i.m. at 6, 10, 14, 18 and 22 weeks. Administration of IL-2 encoding pDNA had the opposite effect, resulting in increased serum IgG, increased glomerulonephritis, and decreased survival, demonstrating that a disease course could be significantly modulated by naked pDNA therapy. The pDNA (100 µg) was injected once in every two weeks for a total of five injections. Circulating serum levels of either IL-2 or TGFβ were detected up to two weeks after the final pDNA injection into the muscle.

In a related study by Kon *et al.* (1999) streptozotocin (stz)-induced diabetes in BALB/c mice was ameliorated by i.m. injection of naked pDNA encoding rat proinsulin and furin. However, in this study the proinsulin pDNA had to be injected prior to induction of diabetes by stz. Post-stz therapy with proinsulin pDNA had no significant effect on the disease. Similar results were found by Abai *et al.* (1999), suggesting that although naked pDNA delivery of insulin may be a novel therapy for diabetes, improvements in expression, delivery or dosing may be necessary to achieve a more substantial therapeutic effect for this particular disease.

Models of autoimmune diabetes in nonobese diabetic mice (NOD) mice, insulin-dependent diabetes, and experimental allergic encephalyomyelitis (EAE) were also used to evaluate naked pDNA therapy. In the latter models, a predominant Th1 cytokine response is thought to play a role in disease symptoms and etiology. Treatment of these mouse models with a TH2 type cytokine, such as IL-10 or IL-4, has been found to shift the immune response and lessen the severity of disease. Therefore, the efficacy of pDNA delivery of a Th2 cytokine was explored in these specific models.

In a study using the NOD mouse model, i.m. injection of pDNA encoding IL-10 resulted in a significantly decreased incidence of diabetes (Nitta *et al.*, 1998). However, the IL-10 pDNA therapy was only effective when delivered to one-week old mice; delivery of the pDNA at later time points had no therapeutic effect. Furthermore, although the incidence of diabetes was reduced, there was no difference in the ultimate severity of insulitis between IL-10 pDNA and control pDNA-treated groups. Perhaps with higher-expressing pDNA vectors or optimized dosing regimens, the IL-10 pDNA therapy described in this study could be enhanced.

In a related study using the NOD model, mice were injected i.m. with pDNA encoding an IL-4/IgG fusion protein (Chang and Prud'homme, 1999). Beginning at the age of six weeks, mice were injected i.m. with 100 µg IL-4/IgG pDNA once in every three weeks for a total of five injections. The mice receiving the IL-4/IgG pDNA therapy were significantly protected from the development of diabetes. Despite the fact that serum levels of IL-4 were not detected even with an ELISA having a sensitivity of 10 pg/ml, the pDNA therapy was still remarkably effective. These results suggested that even though i.m. pDNA delivery of a therapeutic gene may result in low serum levels, the therapy can still be highly effective and may lead to much lower side-effects compared to therapy with bolus injection of recombinant protein.

The intramuscular injection of naked pDNA has also been evaluated for therapy of EAE, a mouse model of multiple sclerosis. The disease is induced in mice by s.c. injection of myelin basic protein (MBP) or proteolipid protein (PLP). In a recent study, mice were injected i.m. with pDNA encoding either IL-4/IgG or TGFβ 48 hours prior to each MBP injection (on days zero and seven) (Piccirillo and Prud'-homme, 1999). The disease severity was 70% lower in the IL-4/IgG or TGFβ-treated mice and the mean clinical scores were significantly reduced in both groups. In addition, the IL-4 and TGFβ-treated mice had significantly reduced CNS inflammation, reduced T cell proliferative responses to MBP and low levels of the Th1 cytokines IL-12 and IFNγ. Thus, the pDNA therapy appeared to shift the mice to a Th2 response, which was therapeutic and reduced the severity of the disease.

The results of the latter studies suggest that naked pDNA encoding a therapeutic gene and administered as an i.m. injection may be beneficial for the treatment of a variety of autoimmune diseases. In many of the studies, the disease course was altered significantly by the pDNA therapy and a clear biological activity of the delivered gene was demonstrated. Studies in which the biological activity of the delivered gene is low are also important for demonstrating that optimized plasmids or injection regimens may be required to achieve significant efficacy for pDNA therapy.

pDNA therapy of cancer

Tumor tissue has also been demonstrated to take up naked pDNA following direct intratumoral injection, but this ability may be dependent on tumor type and the pDNA construct. In an important study by Vile and Hart (1993), mice bearing subcutaneous (s.c.) B16F1 melanoma or Colo 26 colon carcinoma were injected intratumorally with naked β-gal pDNA or β-gal pDNA/calcium phosphate precipitates. The tumors were collected on days 2, 4, 6 and 10 after the pDNA intratumoral injection. A gradual increase in blue-staining cells was found in the transfected melanomas with 10–15% of the cells expressing β-gal by day ten. In contrast, none of the colon carcinoma tumors was positive for β-gal. One explanation for the lack of *in vivo* transfection of the colon carcinoma is that the β-gal pDNA constructs contained melanoma-specific promoters (tyrosinase and TRP promoters). This study demonstrated that using an appropriate promoter established tumors could take up and express naked pDNA.

In a similar study by Yang and Huang (1996), melanoma tumors in mice were *in vivo* transfected by the direct intratumoral administration of naked pDNA, resulting in reporter gene expression for up to ten days. In another study, Walker 256 carcinoma tumors in rats were found to express CAT after intratumoral injection of naked pDNA encoding CAT (Nomura *et al.*, 1997). More recently electroporation has been used to deliver naked pDNA to tumors (described further in the following section).

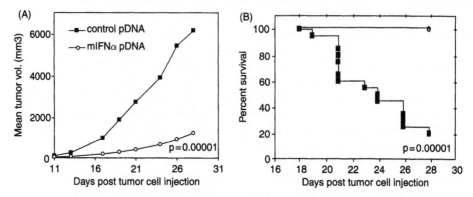

Figure 14.1 I.m. delivery of IFNα pDNA reduces the growth of s.c. B16F10 tumors and increases survival. C57BL/6 mice were injected s.c. with 10^4 B16F10 cells. Beginning four days after tumor cell injection and continuing twice per week for three weeks, mice were injected i.m. with 100 μg control or IFNα pDNA. The tumors were measured with calipers to determine tumor volume. A significant decrease in (A) s.c. B16F10 tumor growth and (B) survival was identified for the IFNα pDNA-treated mice. N = 10 mice per group. ■ = control pDNA-treated mice, ○ = IFNα pDNA-treated mice. Adapted from Horton *et al.* (1999b).

The administration of naked pDNA by i.m. injection, rather than by intratumoral injection, has also been demonstrated to have a significant antitumor effect (Figure 14.1). In the first study evaluating this type of tumor therapy, mice bearing s.c. B16F10 melanoma were injected i.m. with pDNA encoding IFNα (Horton *et al.*, 1999b). Mice receiving the i.m. IFNα pDNA therapy had a significant inhibition of primary and metastatic B16F10 tumor growth as well as a significant prolongation of survival (Horton *et al.*, 1999b). The IFNα pDNA therapy was effective when as little as 25 μg of IFNα pDNA was injected i.m. once every other week for a total of three injections. The antitumor response elicited by the IFNα pDNA therapy involved CD8+ T cells and was also able to inhibit the growth of distant metastatic tumors in the lung. The results of this study demonstrated for the first time that naked pDNA encoding a therapeutic gene could be administered at a site distal from the tumor (into the muscle) and still have a highly significant antitumor effect. Later studies suggested that i.m. injection of IFNα pDNA could significantly reduce the growth of intradermal (i.d.) Renca primary tumors also markedly reduce the establishment of lung metastases (Figure 14.2, H. Horton and C. Luke, unpublished data).

Subsequent studies by other groups also demonstrated that naked i.m. pDNA could be used to treat tumors. IL-12 pDNA injected i.m. at the time of tumor cell implant reduced melanoma metastases and the effect involved both CD8+ T cell and natural killer (NK) cells (Schultz *et al.*, 1999). In a similar study, i.m. injection of pDNA encoding the anti-angiogenic gene, endostatin, significantly reduced the growth of s.c. renal carcinoma and Lewis lung carcinoma (Blezinger *et al.*, 1999).

The results of these preclinical tumor studies revealed that distant primary and metastatic tumors may be treated by i.m. injection of a therapeutic pDNA. This type of anti-cancer therapy could be useful for the treatment of human neoplasms.

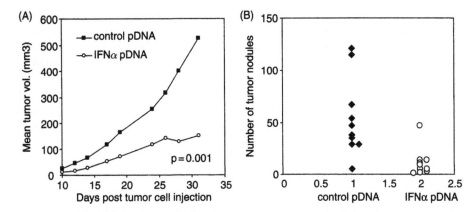

Figure 14.2 I.m. delivery of IFNα pDNA reduces the growth of primary i.d. Renca tumors and lung metastases. BALB/c mice were injected (a) i.d. or (b) i.v. with 10^5 Renca cells. Beginning four days after tumor cell injection and continuing twice per week for 2 weeks, mice were injected i.m. with 100 µg control or IFNα pDNA. The i.d. tumors were measured with calipers to determine tumor volume. Mice injected i.v. with Renca cells were euthanized on day 18, lungs were collected, fixed and lung metastases were enumerated. The IFNα pDNA therapy markedly decreased (a) i.d. Renca primary tumor growth and (b) lung metastatic nodules. N = 10 mice per group. ■ = control pDNA-treated mice, ○ = IFNα pDNA-treated mice.

One advantage of this type of therapy is that tumors in organs that are difficult to access may be treated by a simple i.m. injection. The therapy may also prevent the growth and spread of metastases.

The latter studies on pDNA delivery of a therapeutic gene to treat metabolic diseases, autoimmune diseases, viral infections or cancer suggest that naked pDNA could be used for gene delivery. The advantages of this type of therapy include the simplicity of i.m. injection, the requirement for only a limited number of i.m. injections to achieve measurable serum levels of the therapeutic protein, the maintenance of stable serum levels of the protein thereby avoiding side-effects associated with bolus protein delivery and the avoidance of the use of viral vectors which pose safety concerns and which can induce anti-vector antibodies. With improvements in pDNA design and delivery, this type of gene therapy may some-day prove useful for therapy of a variety of human diseases.

IMPROVEMENTS IN pDNA VECTORS

Vector design and vehicles

One way to enhance pDNA-based gene expression is to modify the pDNA backbone by improving promoter or enhancer sequences and removing extraneous sequences that may interfere with transgene expression. A study by Hartikka *et al.* (1996) evaluated various modifications in the regulatory elements of pDNA to construct a high expressing pDNA vector for *in vivo* gene delivery. Modifications were made in the promoter, enhancer, introns, and transcriptional terminator elements. Antibiotic resistance genes, backbone elements and viral sequences were also altered or removed. Specific modifications resulted in a pDNA that expressed 150-fold higher than pDNAs commercially available at that time. Thus, these types of alterations in regulatory elements may be important for increasing gene expression of pDNAs.

Another way to improve expression from pDNA vectors is to modify the vehicle used for pDNA injection. While early studies of i.m. pDNA therapy involved treatment of muscle with myotoxins, such as bipuvicaine, to generate muscle regeneration and facilitate pDNA uptake, more recent studies suggest that muscle damage is not required for high level pDNA expression and may, in fact, interfere with optimal gene expression (reviewed in Norman *et al.*, 2000). The use of high expression pDNAs such as those described in Hartikka *et al.* (1996) abolishes the requirement for myotoxin injection. More recently, a sodium phosphate buffer vehicle was demonstrated to increase gene expression after i.m. pDNA injection by two- to seven-fold (Hartikka *et al.*, 2000). Further improvements in the pDNA backbone, as well as in the delivery vehicles, may be required to increase *in vivo* transfection levels to the degree required for effective therapy of human disease.

Electroporation

In one of the first studies of *in vivo* delivery of pDNA using electroporation, Titomirov *et al.* (1991) demonstrated that the skin of newborn mice could take up and express a reporter gene after pDNA injection followed by the application of electric pulses. In a later study, Heller *et al.* (1996) injected the liver of rats with pDNA encoding β-gal followed by the administration of electric pulses. In the rat study, long-term expression of β-gal occurred after pDNA electroporation (up to day 21 post pDNA injection) and 30–35% of the hepatocytes were transfected.

More recently, enhancement of i.m. pDNA delivery by electroporation has also been applied to tumor therapy. C3H bearing s.c. squamous cell carcinoma (SCC) were treated by i.m. injection of 10 μg of either IL-12 pDNA or IFNα pDNA, followed by electroporation using caliper electrodes (Hanna *et al.*, 2001; Li *et al.*, 2001). The pDNA therapy was administered on days 7, 14 and 21 post-tumor cell implantation. Mice receiving the IL-12 or IFNα pDNA therapy had a significant reduction in s.c. tumor growth. In both studies i.m. pDNA therapy was more effective when combined with electroporation.

In another tumor study, C3H mice bearing s.c. hepatocellular carcinoma (HCC) were injected intratumorally with 100 μg IL-12 encoding pDNA, followed by electroporation into the tumor (Yamashita *et al.*, 2001). Remarkably a single injection of IL-12 pDNA followed by electroporation resulted in measurable serum levels of IL-12. By day five after pDNA injection, a mean of 4 pg/ml of IL-12 was detected in the serum and 2 ng/ml of IL-12 was detected as late as 28 days after pDNA injection. Furthermore, a single intratumoral injection of IL-12 pDNA followed by electroporation resulted in a significant inhibition of tumor growth as well as a reduction in the growth of a distant tumor. Tumors treated with IL-12 pDNA and electroporation were infiltrated with NK cells and CD3+ T cells and a tumor-specific CTL response was generated.

The mechanism by which electroporation enhances i.m. pDNA expression and efficacy requires further study. For muscle transfection, it has been demonstrated that electroporation appears to increase the number of muscle fibers transfected by as much as ten-fold (Dupuis *et al.*, 2000). In addition, the number of muscle nuclei containing transfected pDNA is higher after electroporation. The mechanism by which electroporation enhances transfection of tumor tissue is unclear at this time.

Although electroporation of pDNA appears to markedly enhance gene expression, there may be some degree of tissue damage induced by the electric pulses. While damage to tumor tissue may not be of great concern and may in fact be beneficial in generating an anti-tumor immune response, damage to normal muscle after i.m. pDNA electroporation should be thoroughly evaluated. Rizzuto *et al.* (1999) reported that necrotic areas with lymphocyte infiltration were sometimes detected in the electroporated muscle; however, one month later, the damage was no longer apparent. At present, there are no reports of a systematic examination of tissue damage occurring after electroporation of pDNA and presumably, further studies on this topic will be required before approval for use of this technique in human trials.

SAFETY OF NAKED pDNA

Many of the safety issues concerning naked pDNA are similar to those of conventional pharmaceutical agents, such as the inherent toxicity of the pDNA itself. However, the use of pDNA for the delivery of therapeutic proteins poses novel theoretical safety concerns. These concerns involve any toxicity associated with expression of the encoded protein, the potential for unexpected and untoward consequences as a result of the persistent expression of a therapeutic protein which could lead to autoimmune disease, the biodistribution of the pDNA, and the potential for a transformation event resulting from the integration of the pDNA into chromosomal DNA. The safety of naked pDNA has now been well documented in pre-clinical studies in animals, and more recently, in clinical trials in humans.

Preclinical safety studies

In regards to biodistribution, several preclinical studies have now documented the fate of the pDNA in animals following i.m. administration. In mice, pDNA has been reported to be detected initially in highly vascularized tissues at early time points post-administration but is retained predominately at the site of administration (Parker *et al.*, 1999, 2001; Manam *et al.*, 2000; Dupuis *et al.*, 2000) where it has been demonstrated to persist for up to 19 months post i.m. administration (Wolff *et al.*, 1992a). In rabbits, pDNA has been detected in the skin, muscle (injection site) and plasma for the first 24 hours following an i.m. injection, but was no longer detected in the skin by 28 days post-injection (Winegar *et al.*, 1996).

With regard to safety, pDNA has been found to be safe and well-tolerated in a variety of species. In mice, the repeated i.m. administration of pDNA has not been found to be associated with the induction of autoimmune disease in animals prone to developing autoimmune disease (Mor *et al.*, 1997). In mice and rabbits, the repeated i.m. or combined i.m./intradermal (i.d.) administration of pDNA-based malaria vaccines – one comprised of a pDNA encoding a single antigen (Parker *et al.*, 1999) and the second comprised of a cocktail of five pDNA's encoding malaria antigens plus one pDNA encoding granulocyte-macrophage colony-stimulating factor (GM-CSF) (Parker *et al.*, 2001) – was found to be safe and well-tolerated without any adverse toxicological effects. I.m. or i.m./i.d. administration of the pDNA vaccines had no adverse effects on clinical chemistry, hematology or histopathology, and no anti-DNA or anti-nuclear antibodies were found. Furthermore, in the case of the GM-CSF expressing pDNA, even after repeated administration, none of the toxicity associated with GM-CSF overproduction was observed (Lang, 1987), nor were antibodies to GM-CSF generated (Parker *et al.*, 2001). In non-human primates, the repeated i.m. administration of an HIV-1 encoding pDNA vaccine was also found to be safe and well-tolerated in adult, pregnant, and infant chimpanzees (Bagarazzi *et al.*, 1998).

The concern over integration of pDNA into the host chromosomal pDNA is a significant safety concern since random integration could result in the activation of a proto-oncogene. To date, in preclinical studies, there is no direct evidence that pDNA integrates into chromosomal DNA following i.m. administration (Nichols *et al.*, 1995; Martin *et al.*, 1999; Ledwith *et al.*, 2000; Manam *et al.*, 2000). It has been determined that if such an event were to occur, it would be well below the level of the natural spontaneous mutation rate and would not pose a significant safety concern (Martin *et al.*, 1999).

Clinical trials of pDNA delivery of a therapeutic protein

The first human trial of naked pDNA delivery of a therapeutic gene involved the intra-arterial injection of a naked pDNA encoding the angiogenic gene and vascular endothelial growth factor (VEGF) to treat ischemic patients (Baumgartner *et al.*, 1998). An increase in collateral blood vessel growth was demonstrated in this trial and amelioration of the ischemia was found in some of the patients. The therapy was well tolerated without any adverse side-effects. Another clinical study by the same group evaluated the direct myocardial injection of VEGF pDNA to treat myocardial ischemia (Losordo *et al.*, 1998). In this study, the therapy elicited minimal side-effects and led to reduced symptoms and improved myocardial perfusion in some patients. Several more recent clinical trials of pDNA involved Phase I/II studies of pDNA vaccines for either HIV (MacGregor *et al.*, 1998), hepatitis B virus (Roy *et al.*, 2001), or malaria (Le *et al.*, 1999). In all of the latter Phase I/II safety trials, the pDNA vaccine induced no adverse events as measured by clinical chemistry or hematology and did not induce anti-DNA antibodies.

The clinical trials of pDNA therapy in humans to date have reinforced the findings of the preclinical studies that pDNA therapy is well tolerated and induces only mild symptoms. Unlike viral vectors, pDNA does not appear to induce anti-vector antibodies, thereby allowing for repeat dosing. The favorable safety profile for pDNA administration is supportive of further evaluation of pDNA therapies for human disease.

CONCLUDING REMARKS

The pDNA delivery of a therapeutic protein has advanced significantly since the pioneering studies of Wolff *et al.* (1990, 1992a) and Acsadi *et al.* (1991a). While the early studies demonstrated naked pDNA transfection of muscle and heart, later studies revealed that other tissues, including liver, diaphragm, joints, skin, brain and stomach could also acquire naked pDNA and express the encoded transgene (Hickman *et al.*, 1994; Davis *et al.*, 1993; Yovandich *et al.*, 1995; Hengge *et al.*, 1995; Schwartz *et al.*, 1996; Takehara *et al.*, 1996). In many tissues, a single injection of a reporter gene encoding pDNA often resulted in expression of the reporter gene for several weeks. Although numerous studies have reported successful *in vivo* transfection with naked pDNA, the mechanism of pDNA uptake into the cytoplasm and entry into the nucleus still needs to be resolved. Although one study suggested that T tubules and caveolae of muscle can take up pDNA (Wolff *et al.*, 1992b), the mechanism by which this occurs requires much greater study. A thorough understanding of the mechanism of pDNA entry into cells will result in greater optimization of pDNA gene delivery.

One major challenge will be to demonstrate that pDNA administration in humans can lead to the required level of *in vivo* transfection and expression levels necessary to ameliorate disease. Improvements over the years in the pDNA backbone, including promoter modifications and removal of viral sequences, have resulted in as much as a 300-fold increase in gene expression after *in vivo* i.m. administration (Hartikka *et al.*, 1996). Changes in the vehicle used to deliver the pDNA have also markedly enhanced the expression level (Hartikka *et al.*, 2000). Further improvements in naked pDNA technology include new techniques for the administration of naked pDNA, including delivery of pDNA by electroporation. In preclinical models, lower doses of pDNA appear to be required for electroporation and this technique has been shown to be useful in treating tumor models, as well as for high level expression of a therapeutic protein after i.m. pDNA injection (Hanna *et al.*, 2001; Li *et al.*, 2001; Yamashita *et al.*, 2001). Mechanism and safety studies of electroporation, however, may be necessary before this type of pDNA delivery is applied to human disease.

The early reporter gene studies established that many tissues are susceptible to *in vivo* transfection with naked pDNA and that muscle cells in particular are able to take up and express high levels of the encoded transgene. Therefore, subsequent studies evaluated the ability of naked pDNA to treat disease. In preclinical models, naked pDNA was found to be effective for therapy of a variety of metabolic diseases, viral infections, cancers and immune-mediated diseases, such as EAE, diabetes and lupus (Raz *et al.*, 1993, 1995; Haarle *et al.*, 2001; Kon *et al.*, 1999; Abai *et al.*, 1999; Nitta *et al.*, 1998; Chang *et al.*, 1999; Piccirillo and Prud'homme, 1999). Exhaustive preclinical safety studies of naked pDNA found that pDNA injection elicited few side-effects, no autoimmune responses and no anti-DNA or anti-nuclear antibodies. In several clinical trials, pDNA delivery of a therapeutic protein has been shown to be safe and well tolerated. In humans, pDNA delivery of the angiogenic gene, VEGF, demonstrated therapeutic efficacy in patients with ischemia (Baumgartner *et al.*, 1998; Losordo *et al.*, 1998). Thus, pDNA administration appears to be safe and has demonstrated beneficial effects in preclinical models of disease, as well as in human trials. The promising results of numerous preclinical studies of naked pDNA therapy, as well as the encouraging results of several human clinical trials, lead one to expect further advances in this field with the ultimate goal of using pDNA to successfully treat human disease.

REFERENCES

Abai, A., Hobart, P. and Barnhart, K. (1999) Insulin delivery with plasmid DNA. *Hum. Gene Ther.*, **10**, 2637–2649.

Acsadi, G., Jiao, S., Jani, A., Duke, D., Williams, P., Chong, W. *et al.* (1991a) Direct gene transfer and expression into rat heart *in vivo*. *New Biol.*, **3**, 71–81.

Acsadi, G., Dickson, G., Love, D.R., Jani, A., Walsh, F.S., Gurusinghe, A. *et al.* (1991b) Human dystrophin expression in mdx mice after intramuscular injection of DNA constructs. *Nature*, **352**, 815–818.

Bagarazzi, M.L., Boyer, J.D., Ugen, K.E., Javadian, M.A., Chattergoon, M., Shah, A. *et al.* (1998) Safety and immunogenicity of Hiv-1 DNA constructs in chimpanzees. *Vaccine*, **16**, 1836–1841.

Baumgartner, I., Pieczek, A., Manor, O., Blair, R., Kearney, M., Walsh, K. *et al.* (1998) Constitutive expression of phVEGF165 after intramuscular gene transfer promotes collateral vessel development in patients with critical limb ischemia. *Circulation*, **97**, 1114–1123.

Benvenisty, N. and Reshef, L. (1986) Direct introduction of genes into rats and expression of the genes. *Proc. Natl. Acad. Sci. USA*, **83**, 9551–9555.

Blezinger, P., Wang, J., Gondo, M., Quezada, A., Mehrens, D., French, M. *et al.* (1999) Systemic inhibition of tumor growth and tumor metastases by intramuscular administration of the endostatin gene. *Nat. Biotech.*, **17**, 343–348.

Chang, Y. and Prud'homme, G.J. (1999) Intramuscular administration of expression plasmids encoding interferon-γ receptor/IgG1 or IL-4/IgG1 chimeric proteins protects from autoimmunity. *J. Gene Med.*, **1**, 415–423.

Davis, H.L. and Jasmin, B.J. (1993) Direct gene transfer into mouse diaphragm. *FEBS Lett.*, **333**, 146–150.

Donnelly, J.J., Ulmer, J.B., Shiver, J.W. and Liu, M.A. (1997) DNA vaccines. *Annu. Rev. Immunol.*, **15**, 617–648.

Dupuis, M., Denis-Mize, K., Woo, C., Goldbeck, C., Selby, M.J., Chen, M. *et al.* (2000) Distribution of DNA vaccines determines their immunogenicity after intramuscular injection in mice. *J. Immunol.*, **165**, 2850–2858.

Fazio, V.M., Fazio, S., Rinaldi, M., Catani, M.V., Zotti, S., Ciafre, S.A. *et al.* (1994) Accumulation of human apolipoprotein-E in rat plasma after *in vivo* intramuscular injection of naked pDNA. *Biochem. Biophys. Res. Commun.*, **200**, 298–305.

Felgner, P.L., Gadek, T.R., Holm, M., Roman, R., Chan, H.W., Wenz, M. *et al.* (1987) Lipofection: a highly efficient, lipid-mediated DNA-transfection procedure. *Proc. Natl. Acad. Sci. USA*, **84**, 7413–7417.

Haarle, P., Noisakran, S. and Carr, D.J. (2001) The application of a plasmid DNA encoding IFN-α1 postinfection enhances cumulative survival of herpes simplex virus type 2 vaginally infected mice. *J. Immunol.*, **166**, 1803–1812.

Hanna, E., Zhang, X., Woodlis, J., Breau, R., Suen, J. and Li, S. (2001) Intramuscular electroporation delivery of IL-12 gene for treatment of squamous cell carcinoma located at distant site. *Cancer Gene Ther.*, **8**, 151–157.

Hartikka, J., Sawdey, M., Cornefert-Jensen, F., Margalith, M., Barnhart, K., Nolasco, M. *et al.* (1996) Characterization of plasmid DNA transfer into mouse skeletal muscle: evaluation of uptake mechanism, expression and secretion of gene products into blood. *Gene Ther.*, **3**, 201–211.

Hartikka, J., Boozoukova, V., Jones, D., Mahajan, R., Wloch, M.K., Sawdey, M. *et al.* (2000) Sodium phosphate enhances plasmid DNA expression *in vivo*. *Gene Ther.*, **7**, 1171–1182.

Heller, R., Jaroszeski, M., Atkin, A., Moradpour, D., Gilbert, R., Wands, J. *et al.* (1996) *In vivo* gene electroinjection and expression in rat liver. *FEBS Lett.*, **389**, 225–228.

Hengge, U.R., Chan, E.F., Foster, R.A., Walker, P.S. and Vogel, J.C. (1995) Cytokine gene expression in epidermis with biological effects following injection of naked DNA. *Nat. Genet.*, **10**, 161–166.

Hengge, U.R., Walker, P.S. and Vogel, J.C. (1996) Expression of naked pDNA in human, pig and mouse skin. *J. Clin. Invest.*, **97**, 2911–2916.

Hickman, M.A., Malone, R.W., Lehman-Bruinsma, K., Sih, T.R., Knoell, D., Szoka, F.C. *et al.* (1994) Gene expression following direct injection of DNA into liver. *Hum. Gene Ther.*, **5**, 1477–1483.

Horton, H.M., Parker, S.E., Wloch, M.K. and Norman, J.A. (1999a) DNA vaccines for cancer therapy. *Exp. Opin. Invest. Drugs*, **8**, 2017–2026.

Horton, H.M., Anderson, D., Hernandez, P., Barnhart, K.M., Norman, J.A. and Parker, S.E. (1999b) A gene therapy for cancer using intramuscular injection of plasmid DNA encoding interferon α. *Proc. Natl. Acad. Sci. USA*, **96**, 1553–1558.

Jiao, S., Williams, P., Berg, R.K., Hodgeman, B.A., Liu, L., Repetto, G. *et al.* (1992) Direct gene transfer into nonhuman primate myofibers *in vivo*. *Hum. Gene Ther.*, **3**, 21–33.

Kon, O.L., Sivakumar, S., Teoh, K.L., Lok, S.H. and Long, Y.C. (1999) Naked plasmid-mediated gene transfer to skeletal muscle ameliorates diabetes mellitus. *J. Gene Med.*, **1**, 186–194.

Lai, W.C. and Bennett, M. (1998) DNA vaccines. *Crit. Rev. Immunol.*, **18**, 449–484.

Lang, R.A. (1987) Transgenic mice expressing a hemopoietic growth factor gene (GM-CSF) develop accumulations of macrophages, blindness, and a fatal syndrome of tissue damage. *Cell*, **20**, 675–686.

Le, T.P., Coonan, K.M., Hedstrom, R.C., Charoenvit, Y., Sedegah, M., Epstein, J.E. *et al.* (2000) Safety, tolerability and humoral immune responses after intramuscular administration of a malaria DNA vaccine to healthy adult volunteers. *Vaccine*, **18**, 1893–1901.

Ledwith, B.J., Manam, S., Troilo, P.J., Barnum, A.B., Pauley, J., Griffiths, T.G. *et al.* (2000) Plasmid DNA vaccines: investigation of integration following intramuscular injection in mice. *Intervirology*, **43**, 258–272.

Levy, M.Y., Barron, L.G., Meyer, K.B. and Szoka, F.C. (1996) Characterization of plasmid DNA transfer into mouse skeletal muscle: evaluation of uptake mechanism, expression, and secretion of gene products into blood. *Gene Ther.*, **3**, 201–211.

Li, S., Zhang, X., Xia, X., Zhou, L., Breau, R., Suen, J. and Hanna, E. (2001) Intramuscular electroporation delivery of IFN-α gene therapy for inhibition of tumor growth located at a distant site. *Gene Ther.*, **8**, 400–407.

Losordo, D.W., Vale, P.R., Symes, J.F., Dunnington, C.H., Esakof, D.D., Maysky, M. *et al.* (1998) Gene therapy for myocardial angiogenesis: initial clinical results with direct myocardial injection of phVEGF165 as sole therapy for myocardial ischemia. *Circulation*, **98**, 2800–2804.

MacGregor, R.R., Boyer, J.D., Ugen, K.E., Lacy, K.E., Gluckman, S.J., Bagarazzi, M.L. *et al.* (1998) First human trial of a DNA-based vaccine for treatment of human immuno-deficiency virus type I infection: Safety and host response. *J. Infect. Dis.*, **178**, 92–100.

Manam, S., Ledwith, B.J., Barnum, A.B., Troilo, P.J., Pauley, C.J., Harper, L.B. *et al.* (2000) Plasmid DNA vaccines: Tissue distribution and effects of DNA sequence, anjuvants and delivery methods on integration into host DNA. *Intervirology*, **43**, 273–281.

Martin, T., Parker, S.E., Hedstrom, R., Le, T., Hoffman, S.L., Norman, J. and Lew, D. (1999) Plasmid DNA malaria vaccine: The potential for genomic integration following intramuscular injection. *Hum. Gene Ther.*, **10**, 759–768.

Mor, G., Singla, M., Steinberg, A.D., Hoffman, S.L., Okuda, K. and Klinman, D.M. (1997) Do DNA vaccines induce autoimmune disease? *Hum. Gene Ther.*, **8**, 293–300.

Nichols, W.W., Ledwith, B.J., Manam, S.V. and Troilo, P.J. (1995) Potential DNA vaccine integration into host cell genome. *Ann. N. Y. Acad. Sci.*, **772**, 30–39.

Nicolau, C., Le Pape, A., Soriano, P., Fargette, F. and Juhel, M.F. (1983) *In vivo* expression of rat insulin after intravenous administration of the liposome-entrapped gene for rat insulin I. *Proc. Natl. Acad. Sci. USA*, **80**, 1068–1072.

Nitta, Y., Tashiro, F., Tokui, M., Shimada, A., Takei, I., Tabayahsi, K. and Miyazaki, J.-I. (1998) Systemic delivery of interleukin-10 by intramuscular injection of expression plasmid DNA prevents autoimmune diabetes in nonobese diabetic mice. *Hum. Gene Ther.*, **9**, 1701–1707.

Noisakran, S. and Carr, D.J.J. (2000) Therapeutic efficacy of DNA encoding IFN-α 1 against corneal HSV-1 infection. *Curr. Eye Res.*, **20**, 405–412.

Nomura, T., Nakajima, S., Kawabata, K., Yamashita, F., Takakura, Y. and Hashida, M. (1997) Intratumoral pharmacokinetics and *in vivo* gene expression of naked plasmid DNA and its cationic liposome complexes after direct gene transfer. *Cancer Res.*, **57**, 2681–2686.

Norman, J., Hartikka, J., Strauch, P. and Manthorpe, M. (2000) Adjuvants for plasmid DNA vaccines. *Methods Mol. Med.*, **29**, 185–196.

Parker, S.E., Borellini, F., Wenk, M., Hobart, P., Hoffman, S.L., Le, T. *et al.* (1999) Plasmid DNA malaria vaccine: Tissue distribution and safety studies in mice and rabbits. *Hum. Gene Ther.*, **10**, 741–758.

Parker, S.E., Monteith, D., Horton, H., Hof, R., Hernandez, P., Vilalta, A. *et al.* (2001) Safety of a GM-CSF adjuvant-plasmid DNA malaria vaccine. *Gene Ther.*, **8**, 1011–1023.

Piccirillo, C.A. and Prud'homme, G.J. (1999) Prevention of experimental allergic encephalomyelitis by intramuscular gene transfer with cytokine-encoding plasmid vectors. *Hum. Gene Ther.*, **10**, 1915–1922.

Raz, E., Watanabe, A., Baird, S.M., Eisenberg, R.A., Parr, T.B., Lotz, M. *et al.* (1993) Systemic immunological effects of cytokine genes injected into skeletal muscle. *Proc. Natl. Acad. Sci. USA*, **90**, 4523–4527.

Raz, E., Dudler, J., Lotz, M., Baird, S.M., Berry, C.C., Eisenberg, R.A. *et al.* (1995) Modulation of disease activity in murine systemic lupus erythematosus by cytokine gene delivery. *Lupus*, **4**, 266–292.

Rinaldi, M., Catapano, A.L., Parrella, P., Ciafre, S.A., Signori, E., Seripa, D. *et al.* (2000) Treatment of severe hypercholesterolemia in apolipoprotein E-deficient mice by intramuscular injection of plasmid DNA. *Gene Ther.*, **7**, 1795–1801.

Rizzuto, G., Cappelletti, M., Maione, D., Savino, R., Lazzaro, D., Ciliberto, G. *et al.* (1999) Efficient and regulated erythropoietin production by naked DNA injection and muscle electroporation. *Proc. Natl. Acad. Sci. USA*, **96**, 6417–6422.

Roy, M.J., Wu, M.S., Barr, L.J., Fuller, J.T., Tussey, L.G., Speller, S. *et al.* (2001) Induction of antigen-specific CD8+ T cells, T helper cells, and protective levels of antibody in humans by particle-mediated administration of a hepatitis B virus DNA vaccine. *Vaccine*, **19**, 764–778.

Schultz, J., Pavlovic, J., Strack, B., Nawrath, M. and Moelling, K. (1999) Long-lasting antimetastatic efficiency of interleukin 12-encoding plasmid DNA. *Hum. Gene Ther.*, **10**, 407–417.

Schwartz, B., Benoist, C., Abdallah, B., Rangara, R., Hassan, A., Scherman, D. *et al.* (1996) Gene transfer by naked DNA into adult mouse brain. *Gene Ther.*, **3**, 405–411.

Takehara, T., Hayashi, N., Yamamoto, M., Miyamoto, Y., Fusamoto, H. and Kamada, T. (1996) *In vivo* gene transfer and expression in rat stomach by submucosal injection of plasmid DNA. *Hum. Gene Ther.*, **7**, 589–593.

Titomirov, A.V., Sukharev, S. and Kistanova, E. (1991) *In vivo* electroporation and stable transformation of skin cells of newborn mice by plasmid DNA. *Biochim. Biophys. Acta.*, **1088**, 131–134.

Tripathy, S.K., Svensson, E.C., Black, H.B., Goldwasser, E., Margalith, M., Hobart, P.M. *et al.* (1996) Long-term expression of erythropoietin in the systemic circulation of mice after intramuscular injection of a plasmid DNA vector. *Proc. Natl. Acad. Sci. USA*, **93**, 10876–10880.

Vile, R.G. and Hart, I.R. (1993) *In vitro* and *in vivo* targeting of gene expression to melanoma cells. *Cancer Res.*, **53**, 962–967.

Wang, R., Doolan, D.L., Le, T.P., Hedstrom, R.C., Coonan, K.M., Charoenvit, Y. *et al.* (1998) Induction of antigen-specific cytotoxic T lymphocytes in humans by a malaria DNA vaccine. *Science*, **282**, 476–480.

Winegar, R.A., Monforte, J.A., Suing, K.D., O'Loughlin, K.G., Rudd, C.J. and Macgregor, J.T. (1996) Determination of tissue distribution of an intramuscular plasmid vaccine using PCR and in situ DNA hybridization. *Hum. Gene Ther.*, **7**, 2185–2194.

Wolff, J.A., Malone, R.W., Williams, P., Chong, W., Acsadi, G., Jani, A. *et al.* (1990) Direct gene transfer into mouse muscle *in vivo*. *Science*, **247**, 1465–1468.

Wolff, J.A., Ludkte, J.J., Williams, P. and Jani, A. (1992a) Long-term persistence of plasmid DNA and foreign gene expression in mouse muscle. *Hum. Mol. Genet.*, **1**, 363–369.

Wolff, J.A., Dowty, M.E., Jiao, S., Repetto, G., Berg, R.K., Ludtke, J.J. *et al.* (1992b) Expression of naked plasmids by cultured myotubes and entry of plasmids into T tubules and caveolae of mammalian skeletal muscle. *J. Cell Sci.*, **103**, 1249–1259.

Wu, G.Y. and Wu, C.H. (1988) Receptor-mediated gene delivery and expression *in vivo*. *J. Biol. Chem.*, **263**, 14621–14624.

Yamashita, Y., Shimada, M., Hasegawa, H., Minagawa, R., Rikimaru, T., Hamatsu, T. *et al.* (2001) Electroporation-mediated interleukin-12 gene therapy for hepatocellular carcinoma in the mice model. *Cancer Res.*, **61**, 1005–1012.

Yang, J.-P. and Huang, L. (1996) Direct gene transfer to mouse melanoma by intratumor injection of free DNA. *Gene Ther.*, **3**, 542–548.

Yovandich, J., O'Malley, B., Sikes, M. and Ledley, F.D. (1995) Gene transfer to synovial cells by intra-articular administration of plasmid DNA. *Hum. Gene Ther.*, **6**, 603–610.

15 Cationic lipid-based gene delivery

Gerardo Byk

INTRODUCTION

The human genome project has led to the emergence of numerous genes that mediate both genetic and acquired diseases (McPherson *et al.*, 2001). These dramatic advances make gene therapy an important avenue for the treatment of human genetic diseases, as well as major acquired killers like cancer and AIDS. Therefore, it is of crucial importance to have access to reliable gene transfer techniques. Unfortunately, gene transfer is still a rather inefficient process hampered by several limitations intrinsically paired to the specific gene delivery approaches. A breakthrough in gene therapy clinical trials will probably emerge from the combination and application of substantially different gene delivery techniques based on viral and synthetic vectors.

Viral vectors are the most efficient delivery system for foreign gene transfer to eukaryotic cells. In viral vectors, the genetic material is part of the genome of a replicative-defective virus. Penetration, integration and transcription in the host cell via the viral natural pathway lead to transgene expression. Although a variety of viral vectors have been developed during the last 20 years (Boulikas, 1996; Smith, 1995) and clinical trials using viral vectors are ongoing (French Anderson, 1998), their use is hampered by limitations such as the size of the foreign gene to be transferred, the risk of intrinsic viral propagation and immunogenicity (Bishop, 1987; Yang *et al.*, 1994). To circumvent the drawbacks associated with viral vectors, a variety of non-viral gene delivery systems have been developed.

Synthetic gene delivery systems will be, in principle, devoid of propagation risks, will not induce immune responses, and will not be limited in the size of the foreign gene to be expressed. However, their capacity to transfect cells permitting penetration and transcription of the foreign gene, as well as their tissue-specific targeting and transgene integration, remain to be improved. Various hybrid systems have been described, exploiting the advantages of both viral and non-viral gene delivery systems, such as adeno-Lipofection or retro-Lipofection in which infection with adenovirus (Meunier-Durmort *et al.*, 1996; Byk *et al.*, 1998d; Schleef *et al.*, 2001) or retrovirus (Themis *et al.*, 1998; Sharma *et al.*, 2000; Song *et al.*, 2000) is performed in the presence of cationic lipid vectors, where classical viral transfection is poor, resulting in improved transgene expression. Finally, another synergy between different gene transfer methodologies is exemplified by the exciting approach of plasmovirus (Noguiez-Hellin *et al.*, 1996). Plasmoviruses are plasmids capable of expressing all the viral genes required for generating infectious particles and packaging a defective genome containing a transgene. Plasmids transfected using cationic lipids transform the transduced cells into packaging cells that release infectious replication-defective retrovirus vectors (RV) containing a transgene, which will infect nearby neighbor cells. Such a vector can efficiently 'propagate' the transgene after transfection. This system is especially suited for suicide gene strategies (Mozorov *et al.*, 1997).

WHY CATIONIC LIPIDS FOR GENE DELIVERY?

Among non-viral systems, cationic lipids are the most efficient systems for gene delivery. Although their efficiency was shown to be lower than that of viral particles, they display higher transfection efficiency as compared to polymers and peptide-based systems. Their relatively higher efficiency is the result of the development of various generations of cationic lipids obtained by chemical modification of the different chemical entities in the cationic lipid, as well as the development of different formulations. Thus, along the different cationic lipid generations, the transfection efficiency *in vitro* was improved by three orders of magnitude. The high efficiency of some of these cationic lipids can be rationalized in terms of their ability to form virus-like particles. Cationic lipids possess two elements that are crucial for efficient gene delivery: a cationic headgroup to condense DNA and a lipid moiety as fusogenic group for improved penetration into the host cell. The nature of each of these elements will have a significant effect on gene transfer. For example, the presence of double-lipid chains as a fusiogenic group and the introduction of spermine as a cationic entity instead of the originally applied quaternary ammonium salts, confer a compacted state of the DNA, resulting in well defined virus-like particles arranged as multilamellar bilayers which enclose the DNA between the lipid bilayers. In various approaches, other elements were introduced into the cationic lipids. For example, fluorescent probes were included by co-formulation with fluorescently labeled DOPE or by direct labeling of cationic lipids, allowing intracellular trafficking studies of cationic lipid/DNA complexes. Alternatively, targeting molecules were introduced allowing cell or tissue-specific gene delivery. Finally, efforts were invested to modulate the stability of the self-assembling system between the cationic lipid and the DNA. In different works, chemical groups were introduced as 'modulating switches' for a controlled formation and/or disruption of the non-viral complexes to obtain improved transgene expression.

In this chapter, the synthesis and structure of commonly used cationic lipids for gene delivery and the influence of their physicochemical properties on transfection activity will be described.

STRUCTURE AND SYNTHESIS OF COMMONLY USED CATIONIC LIPIDS

Since the introduction of the transfection reagent Lipofectin™, a cationic liposome composed of 1:1 (w/w) mixture of the quaternary ammonium cationic lipid *N*[1-(2,3-dioleyloxy)propyl]-*N*, *N*, *N*-trimethylammonium chloride (DOTMA) and a colipid dioleoylphosphatidylethanolamine (DOPE) (Felgner *et al.*, 1987), an increasing number of cationic lipids have been developed. To date, cationic lipids can be grouped into seven different categories:

- Quaternary ammonium salt lipids
- Lipopolyamines
- Amidinium salts cationic lipids
- Imidazole, phosphonium, arsonium salts and miscellaneous cationic entities
- Targeted cationic lipids
- Biodegradable cationic lipids
- Non electrostatic DNA-groove binding lipids

Quaternary ammonium salt lipids

The first approach of gene delivery using cationic lipids was proposed in 1987 by Felgner *et al.* The principle was to form electrostatic complexes between the phosphate groups of the DNA and the cationic headgroups of the lipids. Quaternary ammonium salts were linked to a lipid moiety that plays the role of forming and maintaining a self-assembling system with DNA and promotes fusion with the cell membrane. The excess of positive charges in the complex facilitates the adhesion to the cell membrane. Thus, plasmid DNA (Felgner *et al.*, 1987) and RNA (Malone *et al.*, 1989) delivery was at first accomplished using Lipofectin^{TM}. The transfection efficiency was increased by 5–100 fold compared to the calcium phosphate precipitation method. In a separate study, Gershon *et al.* (1993) have shown that plasmid DNA collapses when mixed with Lipofectin^{TM}, leading to the formation of condensed structures. Nucleic acids can be encapsulated within the fused lipid bilayers in a fast and highly cooperative process, since their exposed surface is substantially smaller than that of the extended DNA molecules. This encapsulation was assessed using Kleinschmidt metal-shadowing electron microscopy assays in which cationic lipid particles appeared to localize DNA-bound spherical clusters at low cationic lipid/DNA ratios (panel A in Figure 15.1). The size of these clusters progressively increased and their structure changed to rod-shapes as the cationic lipid/DNA ratio (+/− charge) was increased (panels B, C, D, E in Figure 15.1).

The synthesis of DOTMA was performed first using D-mannitol-3,4-acetonide as a starting material (Figure 15.2). This tedious procedure was improved for the synthesis of a variety of DOTMA related cationic lipids (Bennett *et al.*, 1995). Their synthesis was accomplished using a simplified synthetic approach also suitable for the synthesis of DOTMA (Figure 15.3). This procedure allowed access to quaternary ammonium esters with less toxicity and to a variety of quaternary ammonium salts (Figure 15.4) with improved transfection efficacy.

To provide biodegradability to the cationic lipid, di-ester bonds were introduced instead of the di-ether bonds in DOTMA, resulting in biodegradable lipid 1,2-bis (oleoyloxy)-3-(trimethylammonio)propane (DOTAP), which was used to study the structure of complexes formed with DNA (Radler *et al.*, 1997; Templeton *et al.*, 1997; Zuidam *et al.*, 1999) and *in vivo* experiments (Tseng *et al.*, 1997; Templeton *et al.*, 1997; Gregoriadis *et al.*, 1997). Introduction of an alkylene alcohol in 1,2-dimyristyloxy-propyl-3-dimethyl hydroxyethyl (DMRIE), 1,2-dioleyloxypropyl-3-dimethylhydroxy-methyl ammonium bromide (DORIE) and 1,2-dioleoyl-3-dimethyl hydroxyethyl ammonium bromide (DORI) or an alkylene amine in *N*-(3-aminopropyl)-*N*,

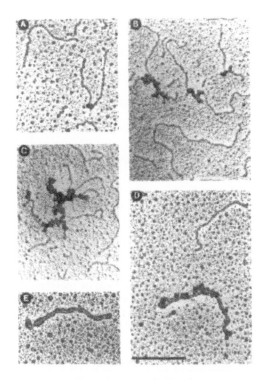

Figure 15.1 Kleinschmidt metal-shadowing electron microscopy of liposome/DNA complexes. Lipid/DNA complexes were prepared with gradually increasing amounts of DOPE/DOTMA liposomes and a constant amount of DNA (3.5 µg/mL). Liposome/DNA (+/− charge) ratios were 0.2 (A), 0.4 (B), 0.6 (C), 1 (D), and 1.5 (E). The scale bar represents 0.5 µm. This figure was reproduced with permission from Gershon *et al.* (1993).

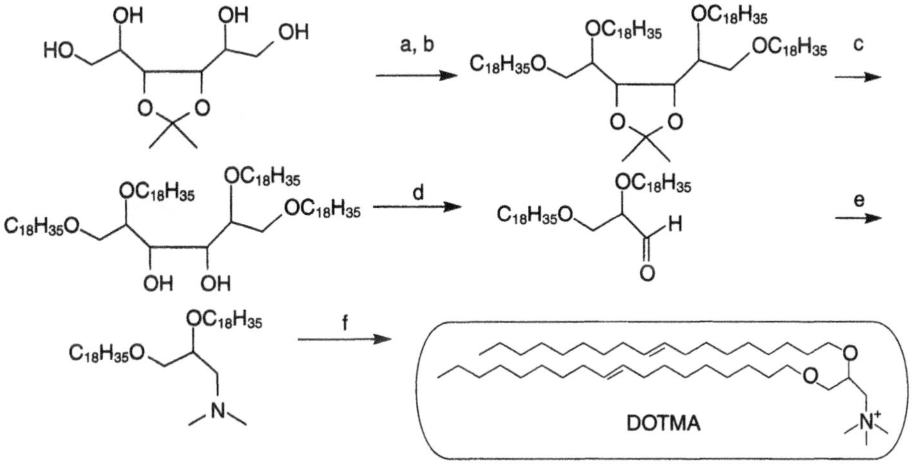

Figure 15.2 Synthesis of DOTMA and its analogs: (A) DMF/NaH/50 °C/1 hour; (B) $C_{18}H_{35}$-OTs or $C_{18}H_{35}$-Br/90 °C/2 hours; (C) 10% TFA in water/1 hour/50 °C; (D) Lead tetraacetate in chloroform/2 hours/20 °C; (E) Secondary amine in MeOH/molecular sieves/NaCNBH$_3$/40 °C/three days; and (F) CH$_3$Cl/48 hours/70 °C.

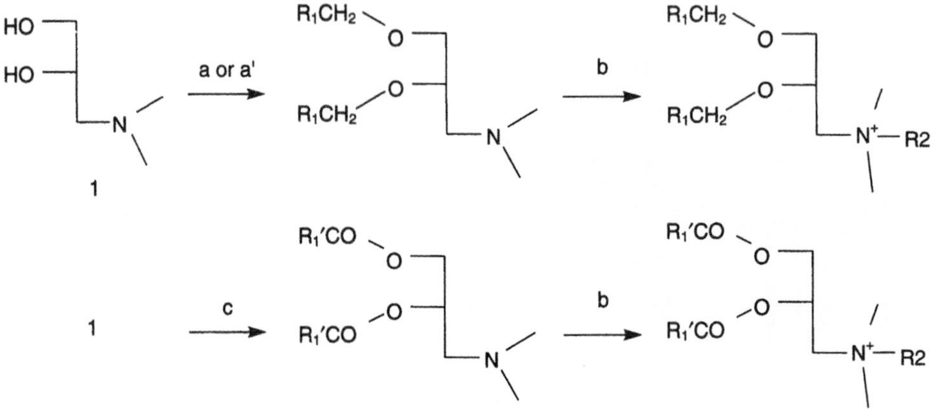

Figure 15.3 Improved synthesis of DOTMA and related quaternary ammonium lipids: a-xylene, tBuOK (3 eq), R₁-CH₂-O-toluenesulfonate (3 eq) or mesylate (3 eq), 140 °C, three hours. The following procedure was repeated three times: (a) NaH (1 eq) in DMF one hour 20 °C, R₁CH₂Br (1 eq) 20 °C one hour; (b) R₁-CH₂-Cl, 70 °C, 48 hours; (c) Et₂O, pyridine, R1'-COCl, 40 hours.

N-dimethyl-2, 3-bis(dodecyloxy)-1-propylammonium bromide (GAP-DLRIE) (Figure 15.4), brought about enhanced transfection activities (Zabner *et al.*, 1995; Ochiya *et al.*, 1999). DOTAP (Porteous *et al.*, 1997) and DMRIE (Galanis *et al.*, 1999) were used for gene delivery in clinical trials. The common feature of the quaternary ammonium salt lipids shown in Figure 15.4 is that they have to be co-formulated with a non-charged lipid such as DOPE or cholesterol for efficient transgene expression. Various authors

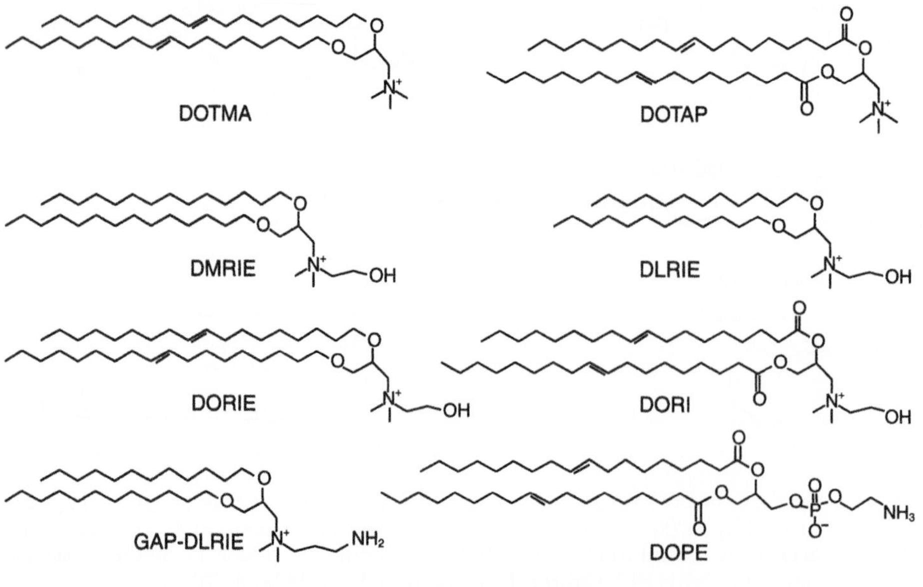

Figure 15.4 Chemical structures of quaternary ammonium salts.

proposed special formulations of DOTMA (Anwer *et al.*, 2000; Ren *et al.*, 2000) or other quaternary ammonium salt lipids (Nantz *et al.*, 1999) directly derived from DOTAP such as DODHF, DODMP or DOFEP containing cholesterol, DOPE or other co-lipids.

Extensive physicochemical characterization of various DNA/quaternary ammonium salt complexes demonstrated the formation of condensed DNA particles. Lasic *et al.* (1997b), Radler *et al.* (1997) and Koltover *et al.* (1998, 2000) demonstrated independently that quaternary ammonium salt lipids combined with neutral co-lipids lead to the formation of multilamellar bilayer vesicles. The impact of the final supramolecular state of the lipid/DNA complexes on transgene expression was elegantly illustrated for DOTAP/DNA complexes by Koltover *et al.* (1998), who showed that DOTAP:DOPC/DNA form multilamellar bilayers and do not lead to transgene expression, while DOTAP:DOPE/DNA complexes form hexagonal cylindrical structures which display significant transfection efficiency. These characteristic structures, obtained for different formulations of DOTAP, should be considered cautiously as other cationic lipid/DNA complexes with different supra-molecular structure can display high transfection efficiency, as discussed in the following sub-sections.

Lipopolyamines

Chronologically, this is the second family of cationic lipids that were employed for gene delivery. The pioneering work was presented by Behr *et al.* (1989), who had proposed to take advantage of DNA condensing property of a naturally occurring polyamine, such as spermine. Indeed, during cell division, spermine plays a central role in DNA compaction. The introduction of a carboxyl-spermine analogue into a lipopolyamine to give dioctadecyl-glycyl-carboxyspermine (DOGS) afforded self-assemblies with increased transfection efficiency compared to quaternary ammonium salts. In this case, DNA was unambiguously compacted by the lipopolyamine and, unlike their quaternary ammonium counterparts, the use of co-lipids was not necessary to obtain significant levels of transgene expression *in vitro* and *in vivo*.

DOGS is synthesized by a multi-step, convergent procedure, which includes the generation of carboxy-spermine by the addition of acrylonitrile (a in Figure 15.5) to ornithine, followed by exhaustive reduction of the intermediate nitriles using Raney-Nickel catalyst under 50 atm of hydrogen (b in Figure 15.5). The carboxy-spermine is then protected with t-butoxycarbonyl (Boc) groups (c in Figure 15.5) and coupled with glycinyl-dioctadecylamide in the presence of dicyclohexylcarbodiimide (d in Figure 15.5). Finally, DOGS is obtained after cleaving the Boc groups with trifluoroacetic acid (e in Figure 15.5).

DOGS efficiently condenses DNA and unlike quaternary ammonium salts, the use of co-lipids such as DOPE or dioleoylphosphatidylcholine (DOPC) is not needed for efficient transgene expression. Boukhnikachvili *et al.* (1997) showed that, upon complex formation with DNA, DOGS forms multilamellar bilayers similar to those obtained with DOTAP in the presence of neutral lipid. These results suggest that the presence of multilamelar bilayers in complexes is necessary for efficient transfection.

In another pioneering approach, Gao and Huang (1991) used cholesterol instead of the double fatty acid chains as lipid entity. $3\beta[N-(N', N'-\text{dimethyl-aminoethane})\text{-carbamoyl}]$cholesterol (DC-Chol) harbors a tertiary amine linked

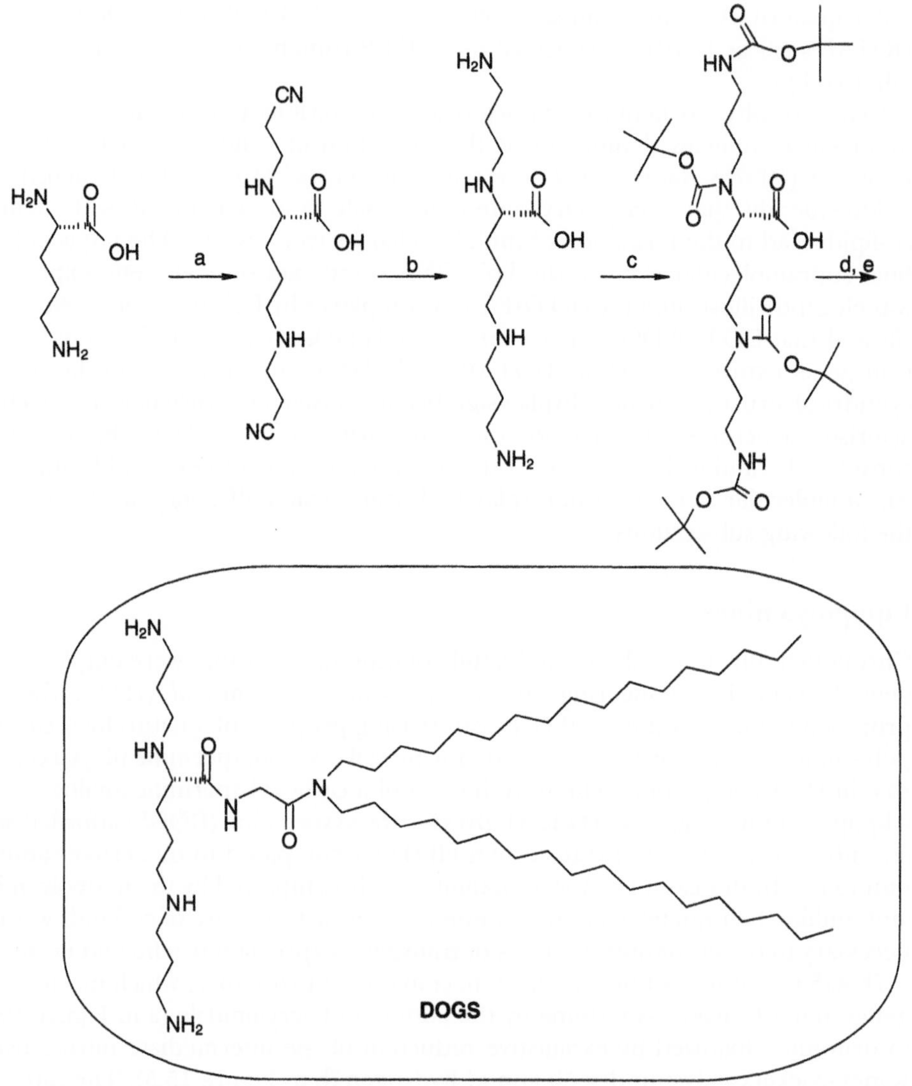

Figure 15.5 Synthesis scheme of dioctadecylamidoglycylspermine (DOGS).

to a cholesteryloxy chloroformate. This was the first lipid composed of cholesterol instead of double fatty chains. Another original aspect of this approach was the introduction of a tertiary amine as a cationic entity instead of the quaternary ammonium salt. Compared to quaternary ammonium salts, tertiary amines are weaker protein kinase C inhibitors and thus they display potentially fewer side-effects. Cholesteryl lipids are not capable of forming bilayers, however they can intercalate into bilayers formed by at least 20 mol% of DOPE. The formation of DC-Chol/ DNA complexes has been shown to be dependent on the mixing conditions, co-lipid type, charge ratio and the surrounding pH (Lasic, 1997b; Stewart

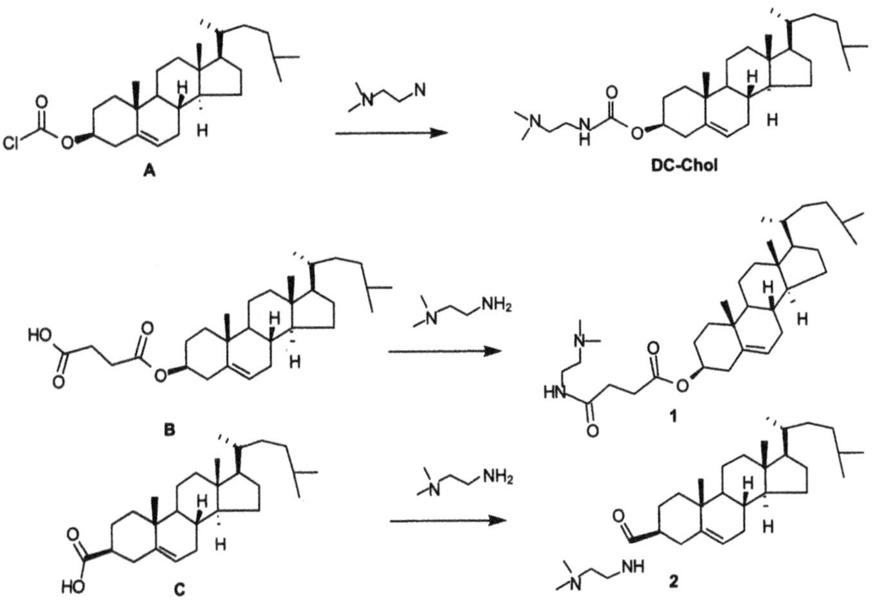

Figure 15.6 Synthesis of DC-Chol and related derivatives.

et al., 2001). DC-Chol was the first cationic lipid used in clinical trials (Caplen *et al.*, 1995; Gill *et al.*, 1997). Similarly to quaternary ammonium salt lipids, cholesteryl derivatives are mixed with a neutral co-lipid DOPE or DOPC to form liposomes for efficient transfection. Thus, the neutral co-lipids are predominant in the formation of transfecting particles and not the cholesteryl moiety, which inserts in between the fatty chains formed by DOPE in the liposomes. This assumption is supported by recent physicochemical studies performed on DC-Chol (Stewart *et al.*, 2001).

Other cholesterol derivatives include cholesteryl-3β-oxy-succinamido-ethylenedi-methylamine (product 1 in Figure 15.6) and cholesteryl-3β-carboxyamidoethylene-dimethylamine (product 2 in Figure 15.6) (Bottega and Epand, 1992). DC-Chol and its derivatives were synthesized starting from cholesteryl chloroformate. Thus, aminolysis of A, B and C with $(CH_3)_2NCH_2CH_2NH_2$ resulted in the formation of DC-Chol and derivatives 1 and 2 respectively (Figure 15.6).

Lee *et al.* (1996) determined the effect of spacer and the type and orientation of cationic headgroups on transfection efficiency. A series of linear polyamines (mainly spermine or spermidine derivatives) were linked in different manners to a hydrophobic group such as cholesteryl carbamate (product 1 in Figure 15.7), fatty alcohols (product 2 in Figure 15.7) or fatty acids (product 3 in Figure 15.7), through an amide bond between one of the amino groups of the polyamine and the hydrophobic group. Some of the cationic lipids display enhanced transfection of pulmonary-epithelium CFT1 cells *in vitro* as compared to DMRIE or DC-Chol. Moreover, it has been shown that *in vitro* transfection activity on CFT1 cells does not correlate with the *in vivo* transfection activity on BALB/c mouse lungs.

Compound 2 of Figure 15.7, which displayed the highest transfection activity on the CFT1 model, was inefficient in the BALB/c mouse lung model. However,

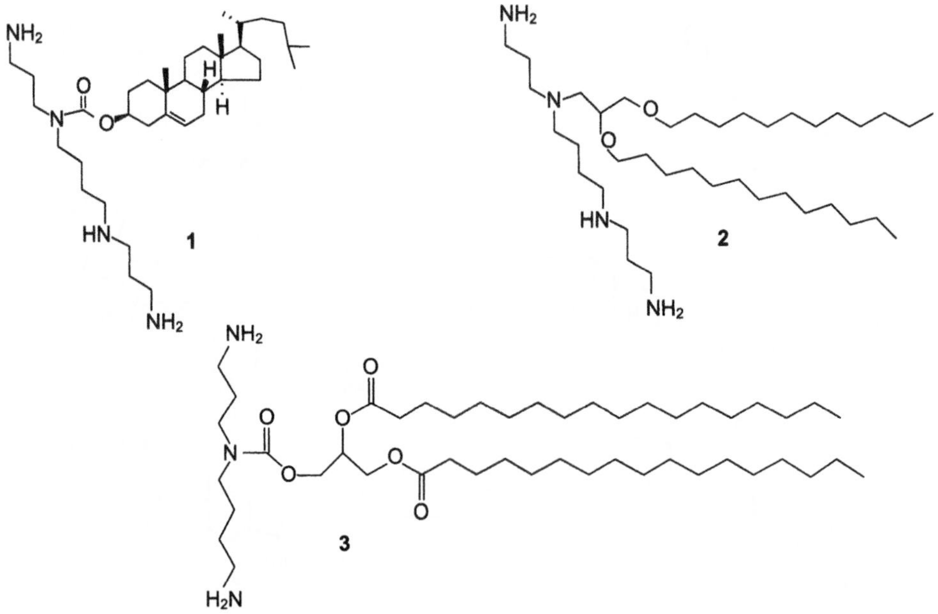

Figure 15.7 Chemical structures of polyamines.

compound 1 (Figure 15.7) with lower *in vitro* activity on CFT1 cells as compared to 2, displayed the highest level of gene expression in the BALB/c mouse lung model. In addition, it could be established that a relationship exists between the structure and geometry of the agent and the transfection activity. In the model of intranasal instillation to the lung, the T-shaped polyamines were more efficient than their linear shaped counterparts. Moreover, cholesterol derivatives displayed higher transfection activity as compared to their double chain lipid counterparts. The data suggested out that the activity of a formulation of compound 1 (in Figure 15.7) with DOPE is approximately 100 times more efficient than DC-Chol/DOPE for *in vivo* delivery of plasmid DNA encoding chloramphenicol acetyltransferase.

A systematic analysis to determine the biophysical characteristics of some cationic lipid/DNA complexes from this series was undertaken (Eastman *et al.*, 1997). Product 1 (Figure 15.7) is currently being used in clinical trials as a carrier of CFTR gene in cystic fibrosis. The synthesis of these cholesteryl derivatives is similar to that of DC-Chol: cholesteryl chloroformate is reacted with spermine or spermidine as polycation (Lee *et al.*, 1996).

In a second separate approach we proposed a novel family of lipopolyamines (Byk *et al.*, 1997a,b, 1998a,b,c). The novel approach uses, for the first time, solid phase combinatorial chemistry to obtain a variety of geometrically varied mono-functionalized polyamines. The polyamine, the spacer and the lipid moiety of the lipopolyamines were systematically modified, and the effect of these modifications on transfection efficiency was demonstrated both *in vitro* and *in vivo* (Byk *et al.*, 1998a) (Figure 15.8).

In agreement with the data published by Lee *et al.* (1996), the geometry of the cationic entity affects the transfection efficiency. Linear-shaped lipopolyamines

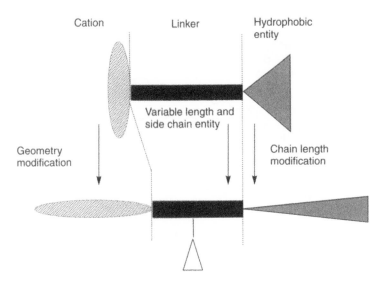

Figure 15.8 Structure–activity relationship studies of lipopolyamines.

bearing double lipid chains such as RPR-120535 were more efficient in transfection in various cell lines than T-shaped RPR-126096, globular-shaped RPR-120528 or branch-shaped RPR-120525 lipopolyamines (Figure 15.9). These lipids were synthesized using polyamine-building blocks obtained by solid phase organic synthesis (Figure 15.10). The use of a solid phase support for the synthesis of geometrically varied polyamines significantly simplifies the number of steps in the synthesis (Byk *et al.*, 1997b). Thus, taking advantage of a dilution effect obtained by linking a bromo-acetyl group to the solid support, a variety of mono-functionalized protected polyamines were obtained in a single step without isolating any inter-mediate. After cleavage from the solid support, the carboxylic function of the building blocks was reacted with the proper linkers and lipids to obtain the desired products.

Another novelty of this approach was the introduction of a new element in the lipopolyamine backbone called 'side-chain entity'. This side-chain could play various roles such as the targeting, labeling or stabilizing of lipid/DNA complexes. Using this approach, we synthesized a series of lipopolyamines bearing a variety of side-chains suitable for targeting (Figure 15.11); biotinyl (RPR-122761), arachidonyl (RPR-130605) and glycosyl (RPR-130596), for labelling; rhodaminyl (RPR121653) or guanidyl (RPR120531 and RPR121650) for the physicochemical stabilization of complexes with DNA. We demonstrated that the introduction of a linker bearing a side-chain entity is allowed for transfection both *in vitro* and *in vivo*. Additionally, the introduction of a molecular probe, such as rhodaminyl, allowed for the inves-tigation of the intracellular fate of DNA/cationic lipid complexes (Escriou *et al.*, 1998).

Extensive physicochemical studies on RPR120535, a leading product of the series, demonstrated the presence of characteristic multilamellar bilayers, particles of 200 nm, with a surprising periodicity of 80 A (Pitard *et al.*, 1997). Unlike quaternary

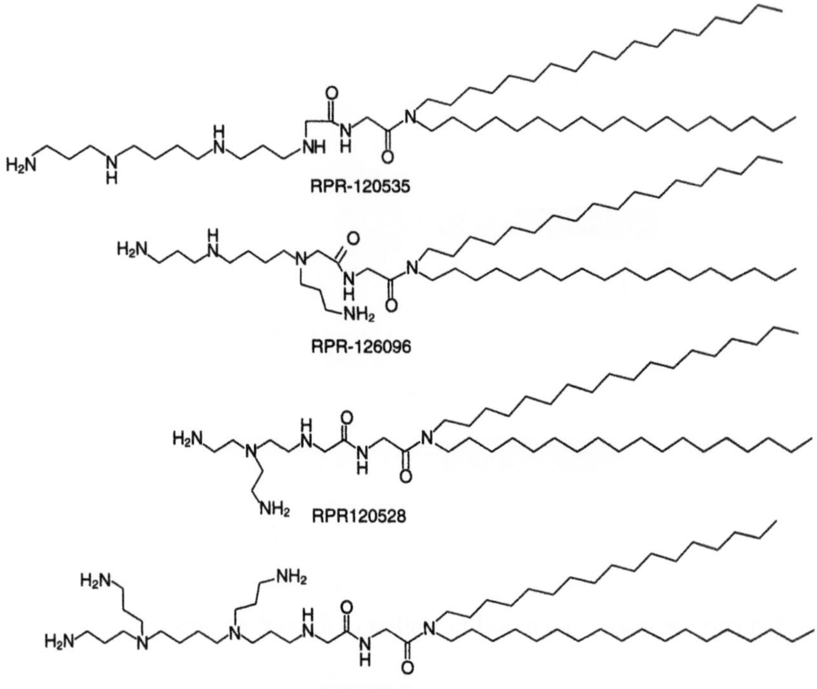

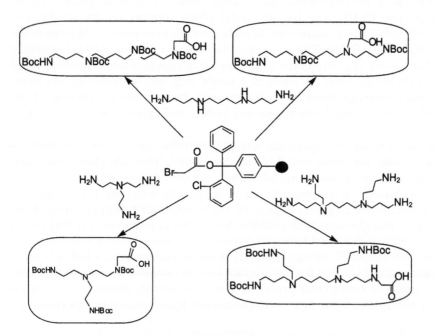

Figure 15.9 Geometrically varied lipopolyamines for structure–activity relationship studies.

RPR-120535

RPR-126096

RPR120528

RPR120525

Figure 15.10 Synthesis of geometrically varied mono-functionalized polyamine building blocks for the synthesis of geometrically varied lipopolyamines.

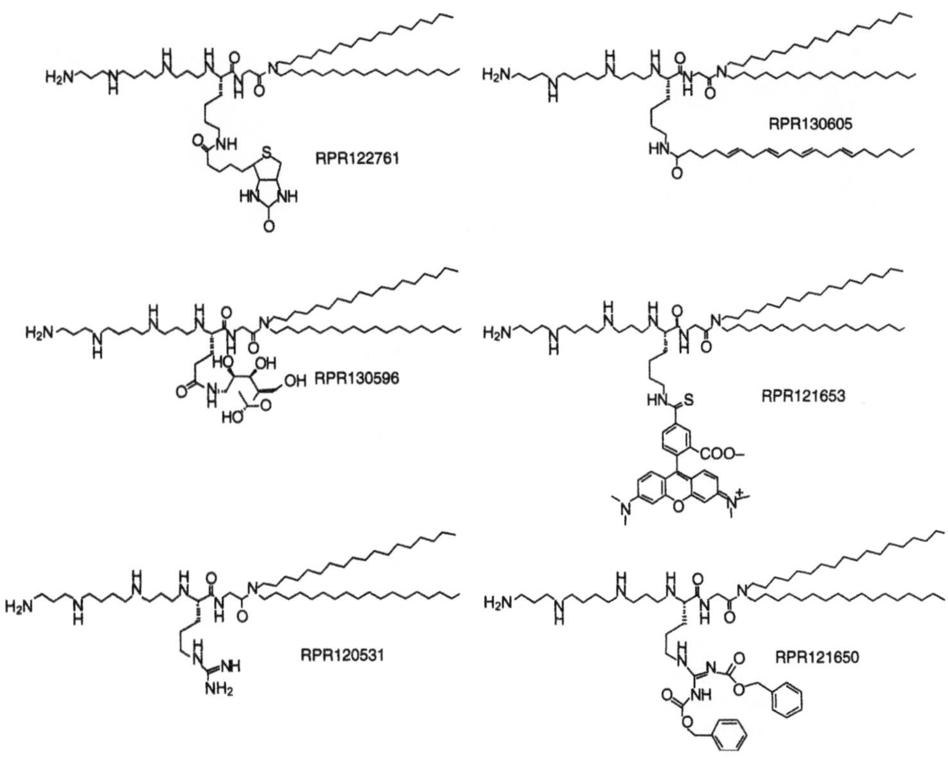

Figure 15.11 Introduction of side chain entities in lipopolyamines.

ammonium lipids, these multilamellar particles are formed in the presence or absence of any helper lipid, such as DOPE (Figure 15.12).

In a recent extensive study, the structural polymorphism of DNA/RPR120535 complexes has been studied by X-ray diffraction and cryo-electron microscopy. Monovalent salts and temperature effects have been analyzed. Depending on the treatment applied to the lipid solution prior to DNA addition, two types of structures can be obtained for identical final conditions: a classical lamellar structure and small facetted vesicles (Raspaud *et al.*, 2001).

Overall, the results obtained for the last two families suggest that the geometry of cationic lipid plays an important role in the final structure of the bilayers and thus affects the transfection efficiency. Nevertheless, this geometric effect seems to differ for different tissue models.

An interesting but different approach towards site-specific gene delivery is the use of cationic facial amphiphiles as transfection agents proposed first by Walker *et al.* (1996). The coupling of polyamines to bile acids allows the formation of a facial amphiphile able to fulfill different functions, including binding to DNA through polyamine, permeabilization of cell membrane through the hydrophobic face and target-specific gene delivery through the glycoside hydrophilic face (Figure 15.13). These amphiphile lipopolyamines can be easily synthesized by coupling a glycoside derivative of the bile acid with an appropriate polyamine (Figure 15.14).

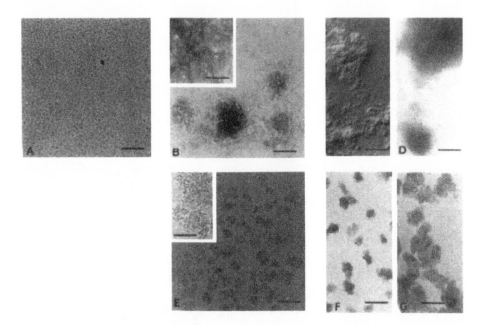

Figure 15.12 RPR120535 and RPR120535/DNA complexes from zones A, B and C, visualized by light microscopy (TEM). (A) Cryo-TEM micrographs of an aqueous solution of RPR120535 alone. (B) Electron micrograph of uranyl acetate-stained complexes from zone A (charge ratio +/−:0.3). Inset shows the same complexes at higher magnification. (C) Complexes from zone B (charge ratio +/−:1.65) observed by light microscopy. (D) Same complexes as (C) stained with uranyl acetate. (E) Cryo-TEM micrograph of RPR120535/DNA complexes from zone C (charge ratio +/−:6) Inset shows the visualization by cryo-TEM of the ordered domains in these complexes. (F) Electron micrograph of uranyl acetate stained complexes from zone C. (G) Cryo-phosphotungstate-TEM micrograph of the same complexes. In this micrograph, the complexes seem to have agrewgated because the thickest part of the vitrified film allows them to be superimposed. The scale bar represents 100 nm in A, B inset, and D-G; 500 nm in B; and 10 micron in C. Reproduced with permission from Pitard *et al.* (1997).

The ability of the series to induce beta-galactosidase transgene expression in COS-7 cells was measured and compared with Lipofectin™ (quaternary ammonium salt lipid). The transfection activity of the bile acid conjugates ranged from low (38%) in product 2c to 1000% in product 4c, as compared to Lipofectin™, which was ranked as 100%. The *in vitro* success of these unusual cationic facial amphiphiles is inspiring for the development of more efficient chemical methods based on tissue/cell targeting enabled by the polar face of the amphiphile.

Other lipopolyamines having unique properties were recently reported (Vierling *et al.*, 2001; Gaucheron *et al.*, 2001). For example, highly fluorinated derivatives of DOGS, whose transfection efficiency was significantly higher than that of DOGS in lung epithelial A549 cells with minimal cytotoxicity. In another approach, the same group proposed a new concept of lipo-polycationic telomers which, upon contact with DNA, forms a teloplex (Verderone *et al.*, 2000)

Polar face
Non polar face
DNA binding domain

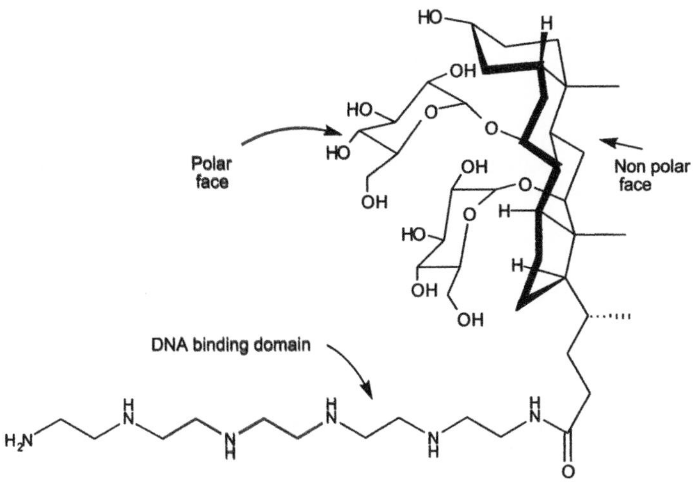

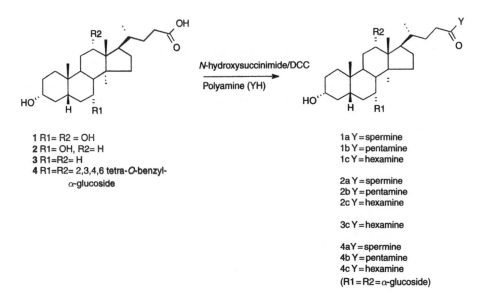

Figure 15.13 Cationic facial amphiphiles.

(Figure 15.15). The efficiency of teloplexes was assessed *in vitro* for plasmid delivery to lung epithelial A549 cells and was significantly more active than pcTG90/DOPE, a previously reported lipopolyamine from the same group (Nazih *et al.*, 1999).

Amidinium salts cationic lipids

Other nitrogen-based cationic lipids are amidinium lipid salts. This family was described by Ruysschaert *et al.* (1994) with a double lipid chain linked to an amidinium group. This product was commercialized later with the name Clonfectin.

N-hydroxysuccinimide/DCC
Polyamine (YH)
1 R1= R2 = OH
2 R1= OH, R2= H
3 R1=R2= H
4 R1=R2= 2,3,4,6 tetra-O-benzyl-α-glucoside
1a Y=spermine
1b Y=pentamine
1c Y=hexamine
2a Y=spermine
2b Y=pentamine
2c Y=hexamine
3c Y=hexamine
4aY=spermine
4b Y=pentamine
4c Y=hexamine
(R1=R2=α-glucoside)

Figure 15.14 Synthesis of cationic facial amphiphiles.

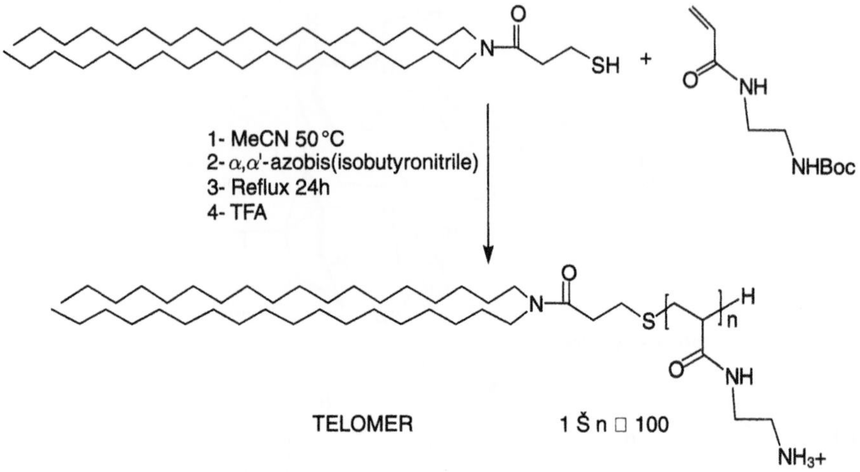

Figure 15.15 Synthesis scheme of telomer.

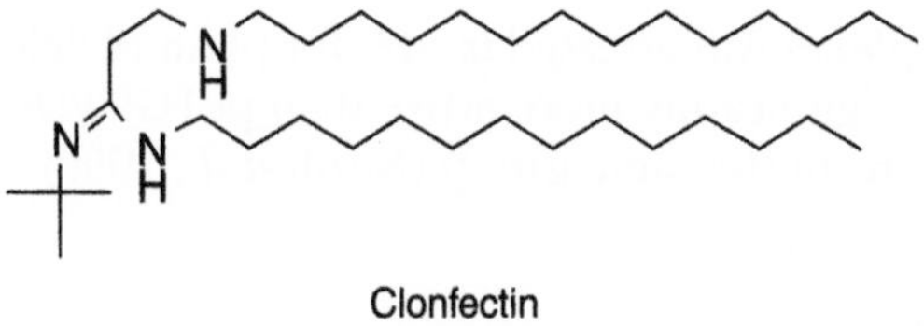

Clonfectin

Figure 15.16 Chemical structure of Clonfectin.

It is composed of two C14 lipids linked to the two arms of amino-ethyl amidine as shown in Figure 15.16.

For oligonucleotide delivery to eukaryotic cells compound GS2888 (Figure 15.17) was synthesized by Lewis *et al.* (1996). This compound can be used both in the presence and absence of serum with high reproducibility and minimal toxicity.

Various approaches based on guanidinium moieties as cationic headgroups have been explored. Some approaches introduced both polyamines and guanidinium groups. Product RPR115335 in Figure 15.18, displayed enhanced transfection

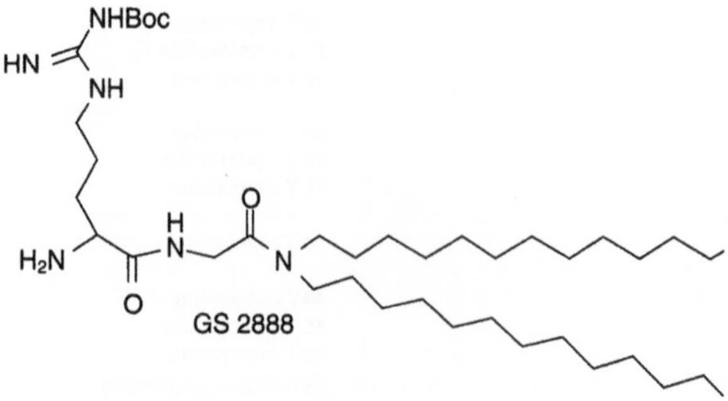

GS 2888

Figure 15.17 Chemical structure of cationic lipid GS 2888.

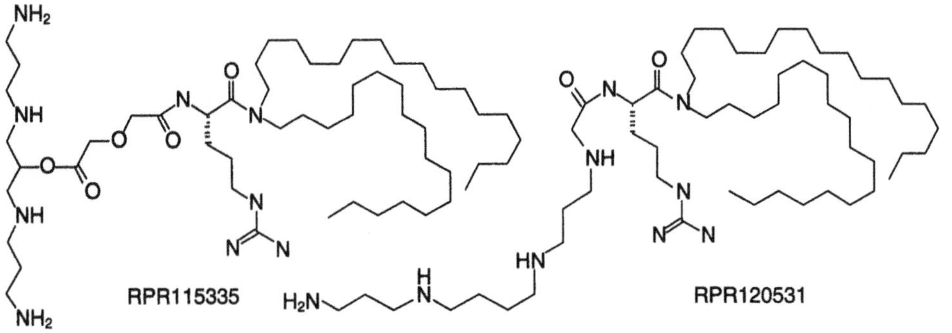

Figure 15.18 Structures of cationic lipids RPR115335 and 120531.

activity as compared to LipofectAMINE^{TM} in NIH3T3, rabbit SMC, 3LL Lewis lung and CaCO$_2$ colon carcinoma cell lines (Byk *et al.*, 1997c). RPR-120531 (Figure 15.18), displayed a high level of transgene expression even in the presence of serum (Byk *et al.*, 1997a, 1998a).

In another approach presented by Vigneron *et al.* (1996), bis-guanidinium was combined with cholesterol to give BGTC. In recent publications different *in vitro* and *in vivo* applications of this family have been demonstrated (Oudrhiri *et al.*, 1997; Densmore *et al.*, 1999; Hajri *et al.*, 2000; Gautam *et al.*, 2001). The synthesis scheme and chemical structure of BGTC are shown in Figure 15.19. In an extensive physicochemical characterization study by Pitard *et al.* (1999), the structure of complexes formed between BGTC and DNA were studied both as isolated particles (see left panel in Figure 15.20) and during gene delivery to cells (see right panel in Figure 15.20).

An extended family of poly-guanidinium lipids was obtained by exploiting a combinatorial chemistry approach (Figure 15.21). In application of the concept of 'libraries from libraries', a second generation library of mono-functionalized (polyguanidinium)-amines was synthesized and introduced into cationic lipids (Byk *et al.*, 1998b).

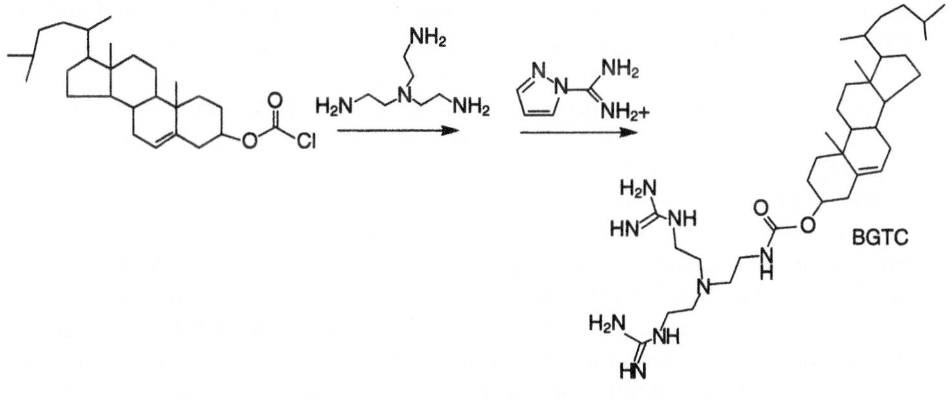

Figure 15.19 Synthesis of Bis-guanidinium lipopolyamine BGTC.

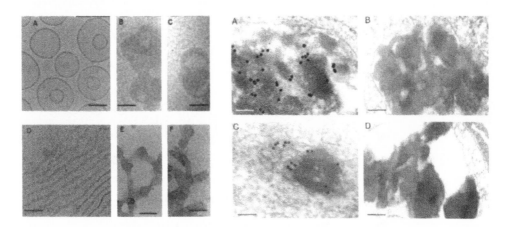

Figure 15.20 Left four panels: Cryo-TEM micrographs of BGTC/DOPE liposomes, BGTC/
DOPE–DNA lipoplexes, BGTC and BGTC–DNA lipoplexes. (A) Unreacted
BGTC/DOPE liposomes at 10 mM BGTC in 20 mM Hepes, pH 7.4. (B and C)
BGTC/DOPE–DNA lipoplexes from zone C (10 nmols BGTC/μg DNA). (D)
Lipid BGTC in aqueous solution. (E and F) Cryophosphotungstate-TEM
micrographs of BGTC–DNA lipoplexes from zone C (10 nmols BGTC/μg
DNA). The sample was mixed with phosphotungstate just before water vitri-
fication to enhance the contrast. Scale bar:100 nm. Right four panels: Electron
micrographs of HeLa cells transfected with DNA complexed with BGTC/
DOPE liposomes (A and B) or reagent BGTC (C and D). In A and C, plasmid
DNA was gold labeled before complexation with the cationic lipid. In B, C,
and D, the cells were processed for electron microscopy after one hour of
exposure to the transfection mixture, whereas they were fixed at 24 hours
after transfection in A. Scale bar:100 nm. Reproduced with permission from
Pitard *et al.* (1999).

Imidazole, phosphonium, arsonium salts and miscellaneous cationic entities

Imidazole derivatives have been developed by Solidin *et al.* (1995) and extensively studied in the laboratory of Robert Debs (Gaensler *et al.*, 1999; Meuli-
Simmen *et al.*, 1999; Liu *et al.*, 1999). The most important lipid from this family is
DOTIM. The synthesis of 1,3-dialkylated imidazolinium derivatives was accomplished through the well-known intramolecular aminolysis (Figure 15.22). In the
first step *O, O*-diacylated derivatives of bis-(2-hydroxyethyl)ethylene diamine were
prepared. Prior to acylation, the amino groups were protected with t-butoxycarbonyl groups to avoid side reactions. After the acylation, the intermediate double
ester was deprotected by treatment with 4M HCl in dioxane. The obtained
di-hydrochloride was dissolved in ethylene glycol and heated at 110 °C for 30
minutes. The imidazolinium derivatives DMTIM, DPTIM and DOTIM were
obtained with a yield of 72–78% (Solodin *et al.*, 1995). From this series the most
promising cationic lipid was DOTIM whose cholesterol and DOPE formulations
are being applied *in vivo* after systemic, intrauterine, intracerebroventricular
and intrathecal administration (Gaensler *et al.*, 1999; Meuli-Simmen *et al.*, 1999;
Liu *et al.*, 1999).

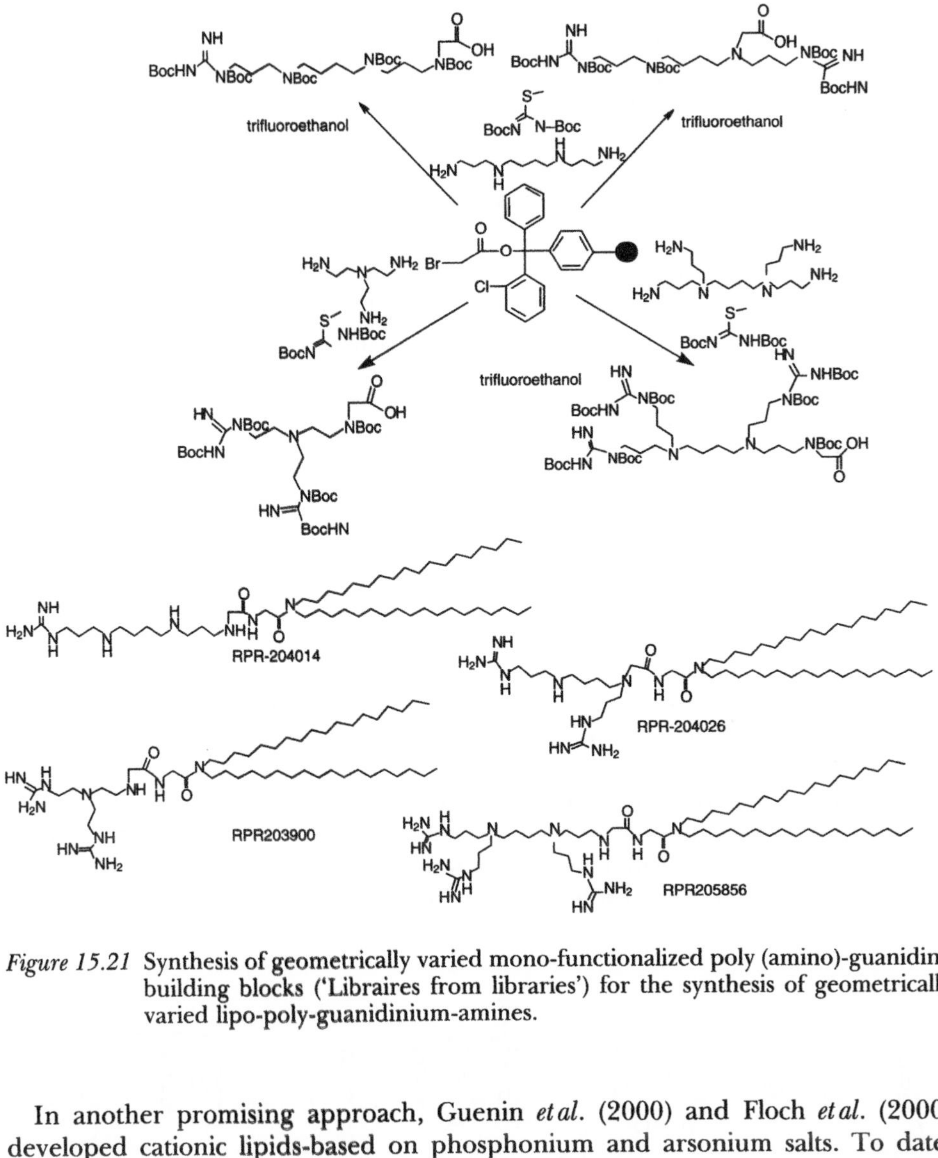

Figure 15.21 Synthesis of geometrically varied mono-functionalized poly (amino)-guanidine building blocks ('Libraires from libraries') for the synthesis of geometrically varied lipo-poly-guanidinium-amines.

In another promising approach, Guenin *et al.* (2000) and Floch *et al.* (2000) developed cationic lipids-based on phosphonium and arsonium salts. To date, these are the unique cationic lipids whose cationic entities are not based on charged nitrogens (with the exception of the work of Haces and Ciccarone described in the patent literature). The rationale of this approach is based on the prior knowledge that the replacement of the quaternary ammonium polar head in edelfosin and miltefosin (anti-neoplastic zwitterionic phospholipids) by a phosphonium or arsonium group results in maintained cytostatic activity together with decreased cellular toxicity (Steckar *et al.*, 1995). Unlike arsenic (III) compounds, arsonium salts such as arsenobetaines are not cytotoxic for humans. Since exchanging the nitrogen atom with a phosphorous or arsenic atom in quaternary ammonium salt lipids increases the volume of the cationic head, one can expect a modification of the interactions of the vector with the solvent and DNA.

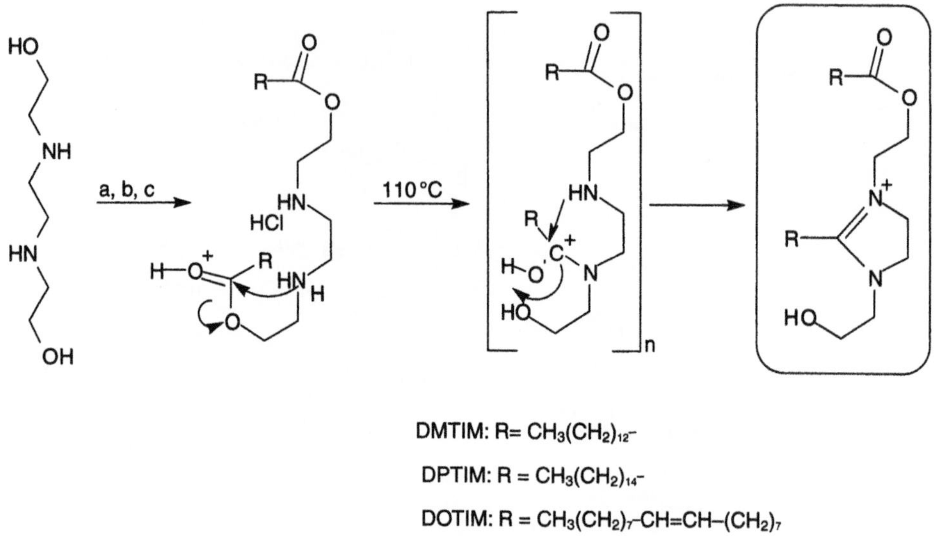

DMTIM: R= $CH_3(CH_2)_{12}-$

DPTIM: R = $CH_3(CH_2)_{14}-$

DOTIM: R = $CH_3(CH_2)_7-CH=CH-(CH_2)_7$

Figure 15.22 Synthesis of imidazole-based cationic lipids.

Two different synthetic strategies were proposed to obtain a variable linker between the phosphoester and the cationic entity. The first was based on the treatment of a fatty dialkylchlorophosphate (obtained from $POCl_3$ and two equivalents of fatty alcohol) with phosphorous and arsenic ylides, which resulted, after acidification, in the phosphonium and arsonium methylenephosphonates. Trimethylsilyl stabilized ylides were used for arsonium compounds. The silyl groups were removed at the end with methanol or water. This strategy is limited to a linker of one atom between the phosphoesters and the cation (Figure 15.23).

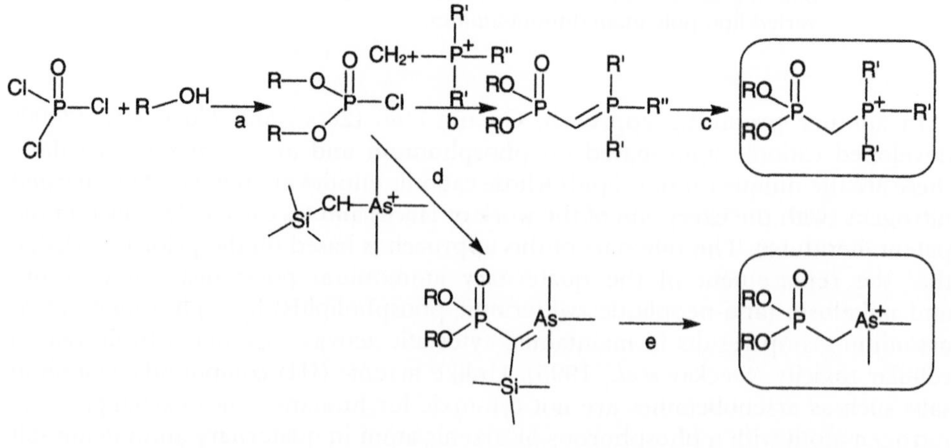

Figure 15.23 Synthesis of phosphonium and arsonium based cationic lipids: linker with single carbon.

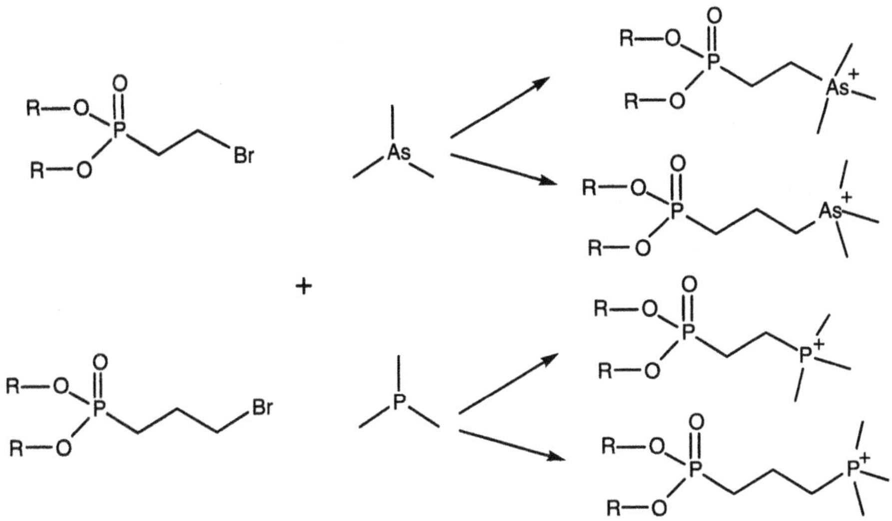

Figure 15.24 Synthesis of phosphonium and arsonium based cationic lipids: linker with various carbons.

To study the effect of this linker length on the transfection activity, a modified strategy was applied to obtain a variety of linkers (Figure 15.24). The transfection activities of the new cationic phosphonolipids were studied *in vitro* in different cell lines (HeLa, CFT1, K562) and *in vivo* using Luciferase reporter gene. It has been demonstrated that cation substitution on the polar domain of cationic phosphono-lipids from N to P or As results in a significant increase in transfection activity for both *in vitro* and *in vivo* assays and a decrease of cytotoxicity (Floch *et al.*, 2000).

Other cationic lipids combine several elements of different families, for example DOSPA, which is composed of a quaternary ammonium salt and polyamine spermine. The formulation of DOSPA with DOPE results in the well-known commercial Lipofectamine (Hawley-Nelson *et al.*, 1993). Although this lipid displayed high transfection activity, its cytotoxicity prevented its further development.

Targeted cationic lipids

Targeting strategies have been applied successfully for drug delivery to specific tissues or cells. This application was accomplished using different formulations of the drug with targeting moieties or by direct covalent conjugation of the targeting ligand with the drug. In the case of classical drugs, a higher concentration in a specific tissue promoted by the targeting ligand is directly proportional to the therapeutic effect. In many cases, promoting a longer presence of the drug in the blood stream was enough to obtain better therapeutic effects. This field advanced considerably with the emerging strategy of phage display peptide libraries, which facilitates the identification of targeting peptides for many different tissue types. Some of them were successfully conjugated to drugs, resulting in interesting therapeutic effects (Ruoslahti *et al.*, 1996; Pasqualini *et al.*, 1996).

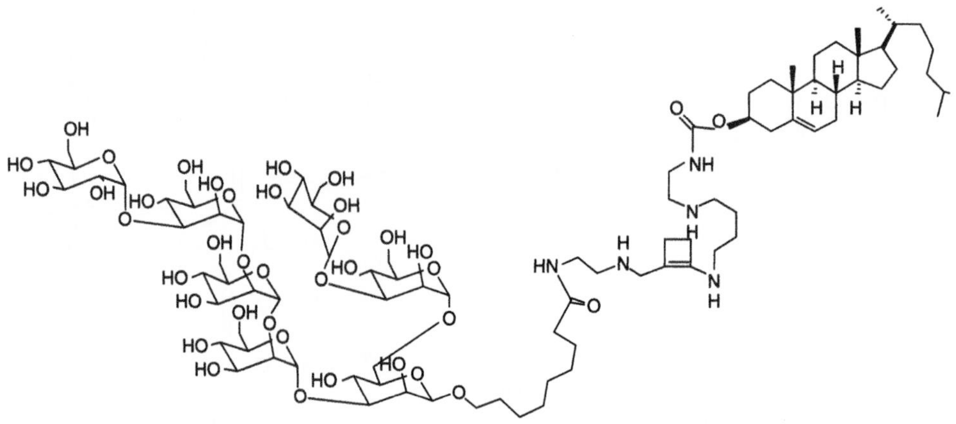

Figure 15.25 Chemical structure of mannose containing cationic cholesterol lipid.

Nevertheless, one has to be conscious that unlike for classical drugs, targeting a plasmid is not a guarantee for its penetration into the target cell and expression of the transgene. Plasmids differ from classical drugs in many aspects, such as molecular weight (more than three million Daltons against 500 Da in drugs), cell repulsive negative charges, lack of physiological stability, etc. A drug can be conjugated relatively easily through a temporary or stable covalent bond with the targeting ligand, while only a few attempts in which targeting ligands were covalently bound to plasmids did not lead to the loss of the functionality of the latter (Ciolina *et al.*, 1999; Neves *et al.*, 1999). One of the attractive ways to deliver genes to specific disease targets is to take advantage of targeting proteins found on the outer side of the viral envelope, such as pentons and penton-base. To date, there are not many targeting attempts directly applied to cationic lipids. Most of the works focus on the targeting of an additive lipid or modification of cationic polymers. Cationic facial amphiphiles are a good scaffold to support on one face a targeting ligand such as glycosides, while the other hydrophobic face remains fusiogenic for cell penetration (Walker *et al.*, 1996).

We choose to show one recent and representative example of additives that can target cationic lipid/DNA complexes after appropriate formulation (Duffels *et al.*, 2000). An oligomannose moiety isolated from the glycoprotein 63 of the parasite *Leishmania mexicana amazonensis* is an interesting ligand for active macrophage targeting of cationic lipid/DNA complexes. The oligomannose was synthesized and covalently coupled to a cholesterol-based lipid. This targeted additive was formulated with a cationic lipid and DNA for *in vivo* intraperitoneal administration (Figure 15.25).

Biodegradable cationic lipids

Many groups were concerned by cellular toxicity of cationic lipids and biodegradable elements were included in many of the presented cationic lipids (Kwok *et al.*, 2001). The stability of the formed particles with DNA is also affected by the chemical compatibility of the different functional groups present in the formulation. Recently, some scientists focused on the release of DNA from transfecting

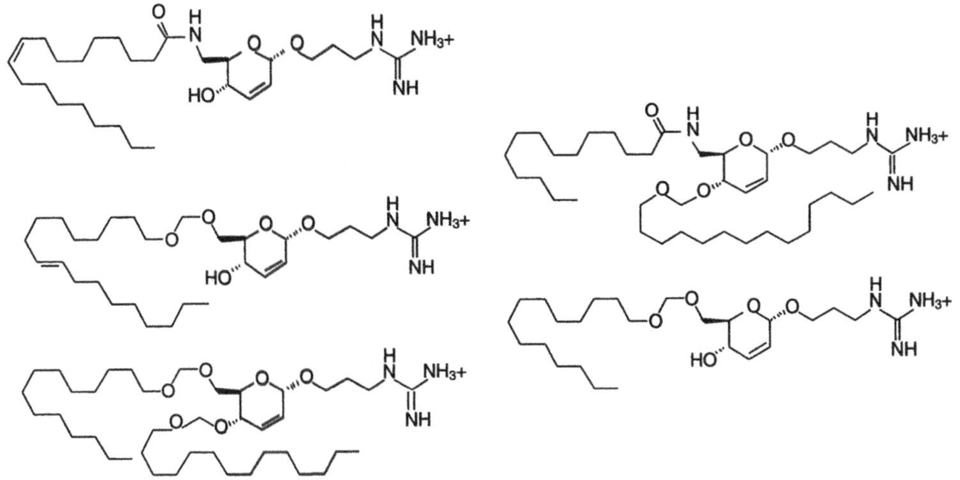

Figure 15.26 Unsaturated guanidine glycosides with acetal degradable functions.

particles after internalization into cell. The basic functions first used as biodegradable groups were carboxylic esters, which upon contact with physiological medium undergo hydrolysis mediated by surrounding esterases. The ester approach was successfully applied to various quaternary ammonium salts (see DORI in Figure 15.4), however it was not suitable for primary and secondary lipopolyamines as polyamines cross-react with the ester functions.

Recently, interesting new biodegradable cationic lipid-based on guanidinium groups have been proposed by Herscovici *et al.* (2001). These lipids contain acetal arms between the fatty chains and unsaturated glycoside as scaffold, which supports a guanidine cationic function through the anomeric acetal. The fatty chains, as well as the scaffold, are moderately sensitive to intracellular acidic pH. Thus, DNA can be released from the transfecting particles as a result of the progressive hydrolysis of the acetal functions (Figure 15.26).

The most important advances in terms of biodegradation and modulated release of DNA from cationic lipid complexes were carried out in two different groups. To facilitate the release of DNA from complexes after cell penetration, Tang and Hughes (1998) proposed to use a disulfide bond between the polar and aliphatic domains in the cationic lipid. This disulfide bond could easily be cleaved under the action of the cell environment. The obtained lipid DOSDSO had to be co-formulated with DOPE to obtain a significant transgene expression. Using appropriate negative controls, it has been shown that DOGSDSO:DOPE/DNA is five to ten times more active than DOTAP/DOPE, a known quaternary ammonium salt lipid with regular transfection activity. The authors demonstrated *in vitro* that the complexes are reduced and decomposed by the application of DTT, a strong disulfide bond reducing agent (Figure 15.27).

In an independent approach, we have designed and synthesized original cationic lipids for modulated release of DNA from cationic lipid/DNA complexes (Byk *et al.*, 1998c, 2000). Our rationale was that modulated degradation of the lipids during

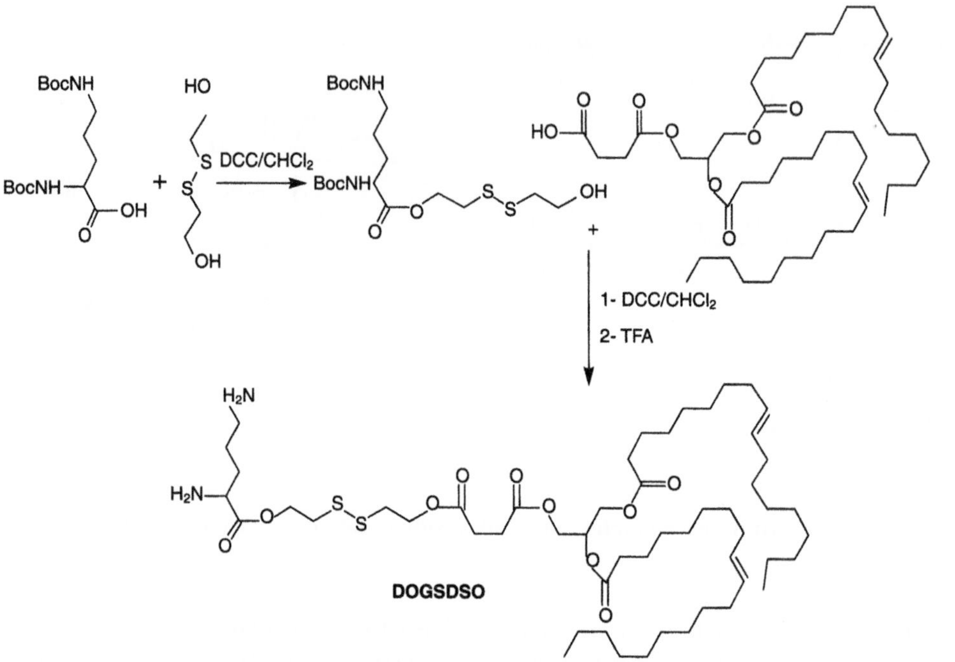

Figure 15.27 Synthesis of DOGSDSO, a biodegradable cationic lipid.

or after penetration into the cell could improve the trafficking of DNA to the nucleus, resulting in increased transgene expression. The new Reduction-Sensitive Lipopolyamines (RSL) harbor a disulfide bridge within different positions in the backbone of the lipids as a bio-sensitive function. A synthetic method was developed to obtain unsymmetrical disulfide bridged molecules with good yields and reproducibility, starting from symmetrical disulfides and thiols (Byk *et al.*, 2000). The new lipopolyamines are good candidates for *in vivo* gene delivery. To optimize the transfection efficiency in these novel series, we have carried out structure–activity relationship studies by placing the disulfide bridge at different positions in the backbone of the cationic lipid, and by systematic variation of the lipid chain length. The results indicate that the transfection level can be modulated as a function of the location of the disulfide bridge in the molecule (Figure 15.28 and 15.29).

We suggested that an early release of DNA during or after penetration into the cell, probably promoted by the reduction of a disulfide bridge placed between the polyamine and the lipid, implies a total loss of transfection efficiency. On the other hand, proper modulation of DNA release by the insertion of the disulfide bridge between one lipid chain and the rest of the molecule, brings about increased transfection efficiency as compared to the previously described non-degradable lipopolyamine analogs. Finally, physicochemical characterization studies of the complexes by Byk *et al.* (2000) and Wetzer *et al.* (2001) demonstrate that DNA release from complexes can be modulated as a function of the surrounding

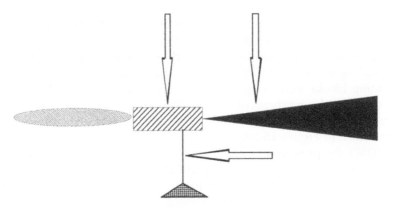

Arrows indicate the sites where disulfide
bridges can be introduced in lipopolyamines

Figure 15.28 Synthesis of reduction-sensitive lipopolyamine building blocks.

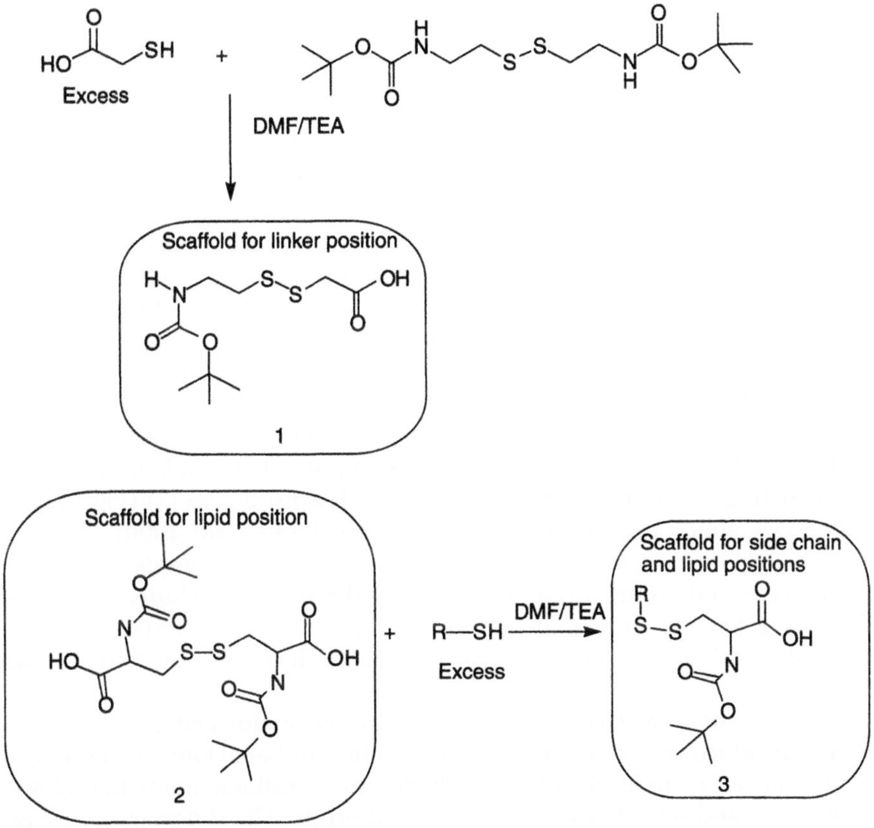

Excess
DMF/TEA
Scaffold for linker position
1
Scaffold for lipid position
2
R—SH
Excess
DMF/TEA
Scaffold for side chain
and lipid positions
3

Figure 15.29 Structure–activity relationship studies on cationic lipids.

reducing conditions of the complexes and of the localization of the disulfide bridge within the lipopolyamine. Our results suggest that RSL is a promising new approach for gene delivery. The synthesis is based in a convergent approach. In the first step building blocks 1, 2 and 3 were prepared as described in Figure 15.29. The building blocks were coupled to the corresponding lipids and carboxylspermines used for the synthesis of RPR120535 (Figure 15.9 and 15.10), by successive peptide couplings and deprotection of Boc groups. The structures of the compounds are drawn in Figure 15.30.

Unlike DOGSDSO, the present series harbor disulfide bonds in every important position of the cationic lipid. Similarly to RPR120535, these cationic lipids are not formulated with DOPE or other co-lipid(s) for optimal transfection efficiency. Based on exhaustive structure–activity relationship studies, we concluded that RPR-132688 is ten times more active than RPR120535.

Non electrostatic DNA-groove binding lipids

The possibility exists to condense DNA through proton donor and proton acceptor non-electrostatic interactions with DNA-grooves. This type of non-electrostatic complex has been developed for sequence-specific binding to DNA. Several prominent works were recently accomplished in this field (Dervan, 1997; Kielkopf *et al.*, 1998; Minehan *et al.*, 2000).

The necessity of more efficient gene delivery methods prompted the search for novel, less charged or non-cationic gene delivery systems. These non-electrostatic complexes can be advantageous for *in vitro* and *in vivo* applications, since unlike cationic lipid/DNA complexes, the novel molecules could not lead to a compacted state of DNA, and could therefore potentially lead to different kinetics of DNA release from complexes. Several compounds are able to bind to double stranded DNA along the grooves by the formation of hydrogen bonds. Groove binding typically exerts only subtle changes in DNA conformation, and DNA remains essentially in the native form. Therefore, groove-binding complexes will be essentially different from cationic lipid/DNA complexes, in which DNA is compacted within a multi-lamellar bilayer. We have set a prototype of new DNA vectors consisting of an amphiphile that is able to bind to DNA through hydrogen bond interactions based on Hoechst 33258 (1) (Figure 15.31), a well-known minor groove DNA binding agent (Soto *et al.*, 2000). Thus, alkyl derivatives of Hoechst 33258 were synthesized and their complexes with DNA were characterised using physicochemical methods, and included comparative studies using known cationic lipid/DNA complexes for gene delivery. The synthesis of dodecyl (2) and octadecyl (3) carbamate derivatives of 1 are shown in Figure 15.31.

The physicochemical characterization of complexes formed between plasmid DNA and products 2 and 3 demonstrates a different behaviour of the new lipid/DNA complexes, compared to previously described cationic lipids that classically compact DNA and retard DNA in gel electrophoresis. The different nature of the complexes, and especially the unperturbed electrophoretical mobility we have observed, propose them as potential self-assembling systems for gene delivery (Scherman *et al.*, 2001).

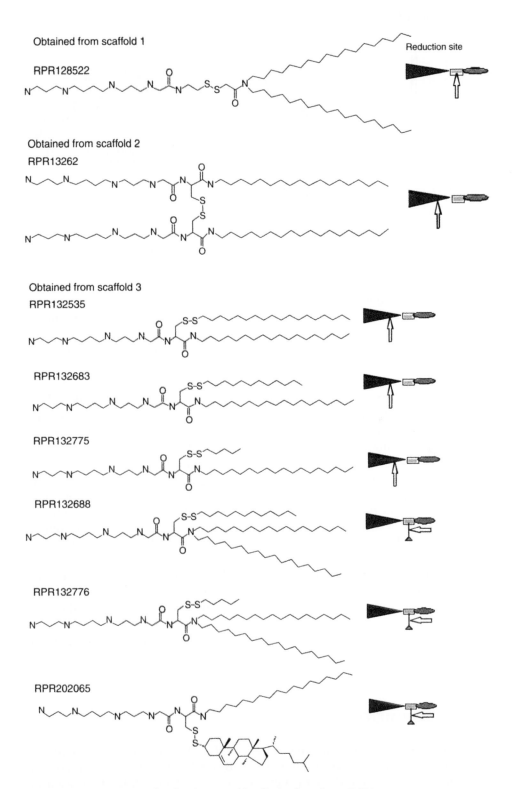

Obtained from scaffold 1

RPR128522

Obtained from scaffold 2

RPR13262

Obtained from scaffold 3

RPR132535

RPR132683

RPR132775

RPR132688

RPR132776

RPR202065

Reduction site

Figure 15.30 Structure of reduction sensitive lipopolyamines (RSL).

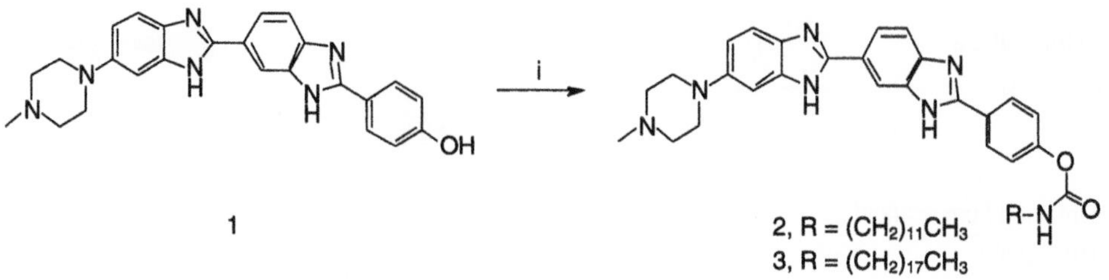

Figure 15.31 Synthesis of DNA-groove binding lipids (i) dodecyl or octadecyl isocyanate (1.5 eq), DIEA (excess), DMF, 50 °C, 18 hours, 41% yield.

CONCLUDING REMARKS

Numerous non-viral gene delivery systems have been developed in the last sixteen years. Attempts have been made to study the nature of the cationic entity, the type of lipid, the geometry of the cationic entity, the biodegradability properties of linkers, the controlled release of DNA from complexes, and targeting elements for site-specific gene delivery. A great effort has been invested in the effort to elucidate the physicochemical properties of the different cationic lipid/DNA complexes. In the near future, there is a great need to present an extensive physico-chemical characterization of complexes side by side with the synthesis of the molecules, the biodistribution of the complexes and the biological activity studies. The development of efficient site-specific gene delivery systems by taking advantage of the increasing number of tissue targeting molecules emerging from phage libraries (Pasqualini *et al.*, 1996) and other targeting ligand technologies might bring about a breakthrough in tissue-specific complex targeting. These targeting ligands, can be part of cationic lipids or co-formulated with the DNA/cationic lipid complexes. Another emerging development to take into account for *in vivo* biodistribution studies of cationic lipid/DNA complexes is the use of magnetic resonance for detecting and assessing gene transfer (Bell and Taylor-Robinson, 2000).

   Although cationic lipid/DNA complexes penetrate efficiently into the cytosol, the release of DNA from these complexes followed by its translocation to the nucleus are still a major problem in non-viral gene delivery. Understanding the mechanism of DNA release followed by translocation to the nucleus and the final expression of the transgene shall be of great concern in the near future. A breakthrough in gene therapy clinical trials will probably emerge from the combination and application of substantially different gene delivery techniques based on viral and synthetic vectors.

ACKNOWLEDGMENTS

The laboratory of Dr. Gerardo Byk is part of 'The Marcus Center for Medicinal Chemistry', his research is supported by the 'BSF USA/ Israel Binational Foundation', the 'AFIRST France/Israel program from the Israeli Ministry of Sciences', the 'Arc En Ciel France-Israel Program 1999 and 2000', 'the Israeli Academy of

Sciences (ISF)', 'TEVA Pharmaceutical Industries Ltd' and by an internal grant from Bar Ilan University.

REFERENCES

Anwer, K., Meaney, C., Kao, G., Hussain, N., Shelvin, R., Earls, R.M. *et al.* (2000) Cationic lipid-based delivery system for systemic cancer gene therapy. *Cancer Gene Ther.*, **7**, 1156–1164.

Behr, J.P., Demeneix, B., Loeffler, J.P. and Perez-Mutul, J. (1989) Efficient gene transfer into mammalian primary endocrine cells with lipopolyamine-coated DNA. *Proc. Natl. Acad. Sci. USA*, **86**, 6982–6986.

Bell, J.D. and Taylor-Robinson, S.D. (2000) Assessing gene expression *in vivo*: magnetic resonance imaging and spectroscopy. *Gene Ther.*, **7**, 1259–1264.

Bennett, M.J., Malone, R.W. and Nantz, M.H. (1995) A flexible approach to synthetic lipid ammonium salts for polynucleotide transfection. *Tetrahedron Lett.*, **36**, 2207–2210.

Bishop, J.M. (1987) The molecular genetics of cancer. *Science*, **235**, 305–311.

Blagbrough, I.S., Geall, A.J. and David, S.A. (2000) Lipopolyamines incorporating the tetraamine spermine, bound to an alkyl chain, sequester bacterial lipopolysaccharide. *Bioorg. Med. Chem. Lett.*, **10**, 1959–1962.

Bottega, R. and Epand, R.M. (1992) Inhibition of protein kinase C by cationic amphiphiles. *Biochemistry*, **31**, 9025–9030.

Boukhnikachvili, T., Aguerre-Chariol, O., Airiau, M., Lesieur, S., Ollivon, M. and Vacus, J. (1997) Structure of in-serum transfecting DNA-cationic lipid complexes. *FEBS Lett.*, **409**, 188–194.

Boulikas, T. (1996) Gene therapy to human diseases: *ex vivo* and *in vivo* studies. *Int. J. Onc.*, **9**, 1239–1251.

Byk, G., Scherman, D., Schwartz, B. and Dubertret, C. (1997a) Lipopolyamines as transfection agents and pharmaceutical uses thereof. *Patent Application*, WO961774.

Byk, G., Frederic, M. and Scherman, D. (1997b) One pot synthesis of unsymmetrically functionalized polyamines by a solid phase strategy starting from their symmetrical Polyamine-Counterparts. *Tet Lett.*, **38**, 3219–3222.

Byk, G., Dubertret, C., Schwartz, B., Frederic, M., Jaslin, G., Rangara, R. *et al.* (1997c) Novel nonviral vectors for gene delivery: synthesis and applications. *Lett. Pep. Sci.*, **4**, 263–268.

Byk, G., Dubertret, C., Escriou, V., Frederic, M., Jaslin, G., Rangara, R. *et al.* (1998a) Synthesis, activity, and structure–activity relationship studies of novel cationic lipids for DNA transfer. *J. Med. Chem.*, **41**, 224–235.

Byk, G., Soto, J., Mattler, C., Frederic, M. and Scherman, D. (1998b) Novel non-viral vectors for gene delivery: Synthesis of a second generation library of mono-functionalized poly-(guanidinium)amines. *Biotech. Bioeng.*, **61**, 81–87.

Byk, G., Dubertret, C., Pitard, B. and Scherman, D. (1998c) Transfecting compositions comprising DNA-binding, disulfide bond-containing compounds and their use in gene therapy. *Patent Application*, WO990128.

Byk, T., Haddada, H., Vainchenker, W. and Louache, F. (1998d) Lipofectamine and related cationic lipids strongly improve adenoviral infection efficiency of primitive human hematopoietic cells. *Hum. Gene Ther.*, **9**, 2493–2502.

Byk, G., Wetzer, B., Frederic, M., Dubertret, C., Pitard, B., Jaslin, G. *et al.* (2000) Reduction-sensitive lipopolyamines as a novel nonviral gene delivery system for modulated release of DNA with improved transgene expression. *J. Med. Chem.*, **43**, 4377–4387.

Caplen, N.J., Alton, E.W., Middleton, P.G., Dorin, J.R., Stevenson, B.J., Gao, X. *et al.* (1995) Liposome-mediated CFTR gene transfer to the nasal epithelium of patients with cystic fibrosis. *Nat. Med.*, **1**, 39–46.

Chesnoy, S. and Huang, L. (2000) Structure and function of lipid–DNA complexes for gene delivery. *Annu. Rev. Biomol. Struct.*, **29**, 27–47.

Ciolina, C., Byk, G., Blanche, F., Thuillier, V., Scherman, D. and Wils, P. (1999) Coupling of nuclear localization signals to plasmid DNA and specific interaction of the conjugates with importin. *Bioconjug. Chem.*, **10**, 49–55.

Densmore, C.L., Giddings, T.H., Waldrep, J.C., Kinsey, B.M. and Knight, V. (1999) Gene transfer by guanidinium-cholesterol: Dioleoylphosphatidyl-ethanolamine liposome–DNA complexes in aerosol. *J. Gene. Med.*, **1**, 251–264.

Dervan, P.B. (1997) Gene-specific transcription inhibition in vivo by designed ligands. *FASEB J.*, **11**, 2546.

Duffels, A., Green, L.G., Ley, S.V. and Miller, A.D. (2000) Synthesis of high-mannose type neoglycolipids: Active targeting of liposomes to macrophages in gene therapy. *Chem. Eur. J.*, **6**, 1416–1430.

Eastman, S.J., Siegel, C., Tousignant, J., Smith, A.E., Cheng, S.H. and Scheule, R.K. (1997) Byophysical characterization of cationic lipids for efficient gene transfer to the lung. *Hum. Gene Ther.*, **7**, 1701–1717.

Escriou, V., Ciolina, C., Lacroix, F., Byk, G., Scherman, D. and Wils, P. (1998) Cationic lipid-mediated gene transfer: effect of serum on cellular uptake and intracellular fate of lipopolyamine/DNA complexes. *Biochim. Biophys. Acta-Biomembranes*, **1368**, 276–288.

Fasbender, A., Lee, J.H., Walters, R.W., Moninger, T.O., Zabner J. and Welsh, M.J. (1997) Complexes of adenovirus with polycationic polymers and cationic lipids increase the efficiency of gene transfer *in vitro* and *in vivo*. *J. Biol. Chem.*, **272**, 6479–6489.

Felgner, P.L., Gadek, T.R., Holm, M., Roman, R., Chan, H.W., Wenz, M. *et al.* (1987) Lipofection: A highly efficient, lipid mediated DNA–transfection procedure. *Proc. Natl. Acad. Sci. USA*, **84**, 7413–7417.

Floch, V., Loisel, S., Guenin, E., Herve, A.C., Clement, J.C., Yaouanc, J.J. *et al.* (2000) Cation Substitution in cationic phosphonolipids: A new concept to improve transfection activity and decrease cellular toxicity. *J. Med. Chem.*, **43**, 4617–4628.

French Anderson, W. (1998) Human gene therapy. *Nature*, **392**, 25–30.

Gaensler, K.M.L., Tu, G.H., Bruch, S., Liggitt, D., Lipshutz, G.S., Metkus, A. *et al.* (1999) Fetal gene transfer by transuterine injection of cationic liposome–DNA complexes. *Nat. Biotech.*, **17**, 1188–1192.

Galanis, E., Hersh, E.M., Stopeck, A.T., Gonzalez, R., Burch, P., Spier, C. *et al.* (1999) Immunotherapy of advanced malignancy by direct gene transfer of an interleukin-2 DNA/DMRIE/DOPE lipid complex: phase I/II experience. *J. Clin. Oncol.*, **17**, 3313–3323.

Gao, X. and Huang, L. (1991) A novel cationic liposome reagent for efficient transfection of mammalian cells. *Biochem. Biophys. Res. Commun.*, **179**, 280–285.

Gaucheron, J., Santaella, C. and Vierling, P. (2001) Highly fluorinated lipospermines for gene transfer: Synthesis and evaluation of their *in vitro* transfection efficiency. *Bioconjug. Chem.*, **12**, 114–128.

Gautam, A., Densmore, C.L. and Waldrep, J.C. (2001) Pulmonary cytokine responses associated with PEI-DNA aerosol gene therapy. *Gene Ther.*, **8**, 254–257.

Geall, A.J. and Blagbrough, I.S. (2000) Homologation of polyamines in the rapid synthesis of lipospermine conjugates and related lipoplexes. *Tetrahedron*, **56**, 2449–2460.

Gershon, H., Ghirlando, R., Guttman, S.B. and Minsky, A. (1993) Mode of formation and structural features of DNA-cationic liposome complexes used for transfection. *Biochemistry*, **32**, 7143–7151.

Gill, D.R., Southern, K.W., Mofford, K.A., Seddon, T., Huang, L., Sorgi, F. *et al.* (1997) A placebo-controlled study of liposome-mediated gene transfer to the nasal epithelium of patients with cystic fibrosis. *Gene Ther.*, **4**, 199–209.

Gregoriadis, G., Saffie, R. and De Souza, J.B. (1997) Liposome-mediated DNA vaccination. *FEBS Lett.*, **402**, 107–110.

Guenin, E., Herve, A.C., Floch, V., Loisel, S., Yaouanc, J.J., Clement, J.C. *et al.* (2000) Cationic phosphonolipids containing quaternary phosphonium and arsonium groups for DNA transfection with good efficiency and low cellular toxicity. *Angew. Chem. Int. Edit.*, **39**, 629–631.

Hajri, A., Wack, S., Lehn, P., Vigneron, J.P. and Lehn, J.M. (2000) Efficient transfer of double suicide genes (herpes simplex virus-thymidine kinase and Escherichia coli-CD) into peritoneal disseminated pancreatic tumor cells by the cationic lipid BGTC. *Cancer Gene Ther.*, **7**, 1393–1393.

Hawley-Nelson, P., Ciccarone, V., Gebeyehu, G., Jesse, J. and Felgner, P.L. (1993) *Focus*, **15**, 73–79.

Herscovici, J., Egron, M.J., Quenot, A., Leclarcq, F., Leforestier, N., Mignet, N. *et al.* (2001) Synthesis of new cationic lipids from an unsaturated glycoside scaffold. *Org. Lett.*, **3**, 1893–1896.

International Human Genome Sequencing Consortium (2001) Initial sequencing and analysis of the human genome. *Nature*, **409**, 860–921.

Katsel, P.L. and Greenstein, R.J. (2000) Eukaryotic gene transfer with liposomes: effect of differences in lipid structure. *Biotechnol. Ann. Rev.*, **5**, 197–220.

Kielkopf, C.L., White, S., Szewczyk, J.W., Turner, J.M., Baird, E.E., Dervan, P.B. *et al.* (1998) A structural basis for recognition of A center dot T and T center dot A base pairs in the minor groove of B-DNA. *Science*, **282**, 111–115.

Koltover, I., Salditt, T., Radler, J.O. and Safinya, C.R. (1998) An inverted hexagonal phase of cationic liposome–DNA complexes related to DNA release and delivery. *Science*, **281**, 78–81.

Koltover, I., Wagner, K. and Safinya, C.R. (2000) DNA condensation in two dimensions. *Proc. Natl. Acad. Sci. USA*, **97**, 14046–14051.

Kwok, K.Y., Yang, Y.S. and Rice, K.G. (2001) Evolution of cross-linked non-viral gene delivery systems. *Curr. Opin. Mol. Ther.*, **3**, 142–146.

Lasic, D.D. (1997a) Recent developments in medical applications of liposomes: sterically stabilized liposomes in cancer therapy and gene delivery *in vivo*. *J. Controlled Release*, **48**, 203–222.

Lasic, D.D., Strey, H., Stuart, M.C.A., Podgornik, R. and Frederik, P.M. (1997b) The structure of DNA–liposome complexes. *J. Am. Chem. Soc.*, **119**, 832–833.

Lee, E.R., Marshall, J., Siegel, C.S., Jiang, C., Yew, N.S., Nichols, M.R. *et al.* (1996) Detailed analysis of structures and formulations of cationic lipids for efficient gene transfer to the lung. *Hum. Gene Ther.*, **7**, 1701–1717.

Lewis, J.G., Lin, K.Y., Kothavale, A., Flanagan, W.M., Matteucci, M.D., DePrince, R.B. *et al.* (1996) A serum-resistant cytofectin for cellular delivery of antisense oligodeoxynucleotides and plasmid DNA. *Proc. Natl. Acad. Sci. USA*, **93**, 3176–3181.

Liu, Y., Thor, A., Shtivelman, E., Cao, Y.H., Tu, G.H., Heath, T.D. *et al.* (1999) Systemic gene delivery expands the repertoire of effective antiangiogenic agents. *J. Biol. Chem.*, **274**, 13338–13344.

Malone, R.W., Felgner, P.L. and Verma, I.M. (1989) Cationic liposome-mediated RNA transfection. *Proc. Natl. Acad. Sci. USA*, **86**, 6077–6081.

Maslov, M.A., Syicheva, E.V., Morozova, N.G. and Serebrennikova, G.A. (2000) Cationic amphiphiles of both lipid and non lipid nature in gene therapy. *Russian Chem. Bull.*, **49**, 385–401.

McPherson, J.D. *et al.* (2001) A physical map of the human genome. *Nature*, **409**, 934–941.

Meuli-Simmen, C., Liu, Y., Yeo, T.T., Liggitt, D., Tu, G.H., Yang, T. *et al.* (1999) Gene expression along the cerebral-spinal axis after regional gene delivery. *Hum. Gene Ther.*, **10**, 2689–2700.

Meunier-Durmort, C., Ferry, N., Hainque, B., Delattre, J. and Forest, C. (1996) Efficient transfer of regulated genes in adipocytes and hepatoma cells by the combination of liposomes and replication-deficient adenovirus. *Eur. J. Biochem.*, **237**, 660–667.

Miller, A.D. (1998) Cationic liposomes for gene therapy. *Angew. Chem. Int. Ed.*, **37**, 1768–1785.

Miller, A.D. (2000) Progress towards third generation non-viral vectors for gene therapy. In: G. Gregoriadis and B. McCormack, B. (eds) *Targeting of Drugs*. IOS Press, London, pp. 139–145.

Minehan, T.G., Gottwald, K. and Dervan, P.B. (2000) Molecular recognition of DNA by Hoechst benzimidazoles: Exploring beyond the pyrrole-imidazole-hydroxypyrrole polyamide-pairing code. *Helv. Chim. Acta*, **83**, 2197–2213.

Morozov, V.A., Noguiez-Hellin, P., Laune, S., Tamboise, E., Salzmann, J.L. and Klatzmann, D. (1997) Plasmovirus: replication cycle of a novel nonviral/viral vector for gene transfer. *Cancer Gene Ther.*, **4**, 286–293.

Nantz, M.H., Bennett, M.J., Balasubramaniam, R.P., Aberle, A.M. and Malone, R.W. (1999) Formulations and methods for generating active cytofectin: polynucleotide transfection complexes. *US Patent*, **96**, 679971.

Nazih, A., Cordier, Y., Bischoff, R., Kolbe, H.V.J. and Heissler, D. (1999) Synthesis and stability study of the new pentammonio lipid pcTG90, a gene transfer agent. *Tet. Lett.*, **40**, 8089–8091.

Neves, C., Byk, G., Scherman, D. and Wils, P. (1999) Coupling of a targeting peptide to plasmid DNA by covalent triple helix formation. *FEBS Lett.*, **453**, 41–45.

Noguiez-Hellin, P., Robert-Le Meur, M., Salzmann, J.L. and Klatzmann, D. (1996) Plasmoviruses: Nonviral/viral vectors for gene therapy. *Proc. Natl. Acad. Sci. USA*, **93**, 4175–4180.

Ochiya, T., Takahama, Y., Baba-Toriyama, H., Tsukamoto, M., Yasuda, Y., Kikuchi, H. *et al.* (1999) Evaluation of cationic liposome suitable for gene transfer into pregnant animals. *Biochem. Biophys. Res. Commun.*, **258**, 358–365.

Oudrhiri, N., Vigneron, J.P., Peuchmaur, M., Leclerc, T., Lehn, J.M. and Lehn, P. (1997) Gene transfer by guanidinium-cholesterol cationic lipids into airway epithelial cells *in vitro* and *in vivo*. *Proc. Natl. Acad. Sci. USA*, **94**, 1651–1656.

Pasqualini, R., Koivunen, E. and Ruoslahti, E. (1996) Alpha integrins as receptors for tumor targeting by circulating ligands. *Nat. Biotech.*, **15**, 542–515.

Pitard, B., Aguerre, O., Airiau, M., Lachages, A.M., Bouknikachvilli, T., Byk, G. *et al.* (1997) Virus-sized self assembling lamellar complexes between DNA and cationic micelles promote gene transfer. *Proc. Natl. Acad. Sci. USA*, **94**, 14412–1447.

Pitard, B., Oudrhiri, N., Vigneron, J.P., Hauchecorne, M., Aguerre, O., Toury, R. *et al.* (1999) Structural characteristics of supramolecular assemblies formed by guanidinium-cholesterol reagents for gene transfection. *Proc. Natl. Acad. Sci. USA*, **96**, 2621–2626.

Porteous, D.J., Dorin, J.R., McLachlan, G., Davidson-Smith, H., David, H., Stevenson, B.J. *et al.* (1997) Evidence for safety and efficacy of DOTAP cationic liposome mediated CFTR gene transfer to the nasal epithelium of patients with cystic fibrosis. *Gene Ther.*, **4**, 210–218.

Radler, J.O., Koltover, I., Salditt, T. and Safinya, C.R. (1997) Structure of DNA-cationic liposome complexes: DNA intercalation in multilamellar membranes in distinct inter-helical packing regimes. *Science*, **275**, 810–814.

Raspaud, E., Pitard, B., Durand, D., Aguerre-Chariol, O., Pelta, J., Byk, G., Scherman, D. and Livolant, F. (2001) Polymorphism of DNA/multi-cationic lipid complexes driven by temperature and salts. *J. Phys. Chem., B*, **105**, 5291–5297.

Ren, T., Song, Y.K., Zhang, G. and Liu, D. (2000) Structural basis of DOTMA for its high intravenous transfection activity in mouse. *Gene Ther.*, **7**, 764–768.

Ruoslahti, E. (1996) RGD and other recongnition sequences for integrins. *Annu. Rev. Cell Develop. Biol.*, **12**, 697–715.

Ruysschaert, J.M., El-Ouahabi, A., Willeaume, V., Huez, G., Fuks, R., Vandenbrandem, M. *et al.* (1994) A novel cationic amphiphile for transfection of mammalian cells. *Biochem. Biophys. Res. Comm.*, **203**, 1622–1628.

Scherman, D., Bessodes, M., Pitard, B., Soto, J. and Byk, G. (2001) Oligobenzimidazole derivatives and their use as DNA transfection agents. *Patent Application*, WO 0132630.

Schleef, R.R., Olman, M.A., Miles, L.A. and Chuang, J.L. (2001) Modulating the fibrinolytic system of peripheral blood mononuclear cells with adenovirus. *Hum. Gene Ther.*, **12**, 439–445.

Sharma, S., Miyanohara, A. and Friedmann, T. (2000) Separable mechanisms of attachment and cell uptake during retrovirus infection. *J. Virol.*, **74**, 10790–10795.

Smith, A. (1995) Viral vectors in gene therapy. *Nature*, **49**, 807–838.

Solodin, I., Brown, C.S., Bruno, M.S., Chow, C.Y., Jang, E.H., Debs, R.J. *et al.* (1995) A novel series of amphiphilic imidazolinium compounds for *in-vitro* and *in vivo* gene delivery. *Biochemistry*, **34**, 13537–13544.

Song, J.J., Kim, J., Lee, H., Kim, E., Kim, J., Park, Y.S. *et al.* (2000) Enhancement of gene transfer efficiency into human cancer cells by modification of retroviral vectors and addition of chemicals. *Oncol. Rep.*, **7**, 119–124.

Soto, J., Bessodes, M., Pitard, B., Mailhe, P., Scherman, D. and Byk, G. (2000) Non-electrostatic complexes with DNA: Towards novel synthetic gene delivery systems. *Bioorg. Med. Chem. Lett.*, **10**, 911–914.

Stekar, J., Hilgard, P. and Klenner, T. (1995) Opposite effect of miltefosine on the antineoplastic activity and hematological toxicity of cyclophosphamide. *Eur. J. Cancer*, **31A(3)**, 372–374.

Stewart, L., Manvell, M., Hillery, E., Etheridge, C.J., Cooper, R.G., Stark, H. *et al.* (2001) Physico-chemical analysis of cationic liposome–DNA complexes (lipoplexes) with respect to *in vitro* and *in vivo* gene delivery efficiency. *J. Chem. Soc. Perkin Trans.*, **2**, 624–632.

Tang, F. and Hughes, J.A. (1998) Introduction of a disulfide bond into a cationic lipid enhances transgene expression of plasmid DNA. *Biochem. Biophys. Res. Comm.*, **242**, 141–145.

Templeton, N.S., Lasic, D.D., Frederik, P.M., Strey, H.H., Roberts, D.D. and Pavlakis, G.N. (1997) Improved DNA: liposome complexes for increased systemic delivery and gene expression. *Nat. Biotechnol.*, **15**, 647–652.

Themis, M., Forbes, S.J., Chan, L., Cooper, R.G., Etheridge, C.J., Miller, A.D. *et al.* (1998) Enhanced *in vitro* and *in vivo* gene delivery using cationic agent complexed retrovirus vectors. *Gene Ther.*, **5**, 1180–1186.

Tseng, W.C., Haselton, F.R. and Giorgio, T.D. (1997) Transfection by cationic liposomes using simultaneous single cell measurements of plasmid delivery and transgene expression. *J. Biol. Chem.*, **272**, 25641–25647.

Verderone, G., van Craynest, N., Boussif, O., Santaella, C., Bischoff, R., Kolbe, H.V.J. *et al.* (2000) Lipopolycationic telomers for gene transfer: Synthesis and evaluation of their *in vitro* transfection efficiency. *J. Med. Chem.*, **43**, 1367–1379.

Vierling, P., Santaella, C. and Greiner, J. (2001) Highly fluorinated amphiphiles as drug and gene carrier and delivery systems. *J. Fluorine Chem.*, **107**, 337–354.

Vigneron, J.P., Oudrhiri, N., Fauquet, M., Vergely, L., Bradley, J.C., Basseville, M. *et al.* (1996) Guanidinium-cholesterol cationic lipids: Efficient vectors for the transfection of eukaryotic cells. *Proc. Natl. Acad. Sci. USA*, **93**, 9682–9686.

Walker, S., Sofia, M. and Kakarla, R. (1996) Cationic facial amphiphiles: a promising class of transfection agents. *Proc. Natl. Acad. Sci. USA*, **93**, 1585–1590.

Wetzer, B., Byk, G., Frederic, M., Airiau, M., Blanche, F., Pitard and Scherman, D. (2001) Reducible cationic lipids for gene transfer. *Biochemical J.*, **356**, 747–756.

Yang, Y., Nunes, F.A., Berencsi, K., Furth, E.E., Gonczol, E. and Wilson, J.M. (1994) Cellular immunity to viral antigens limits E1-deleted adenoviruses for gene therapy. *Proc. Natl. Acad. Sci. USA*, **91**, 4407–4411.

Zabner, J., Fasbender, A.J., Moninger, T., Poellinger, K.A. and Welsh, M.J. (1995) Cellular and molecular barriers to gene transfer by a cationic lipid. *J. Biol. Chem.*, **270**, 18997–19007.

Zabner, J. (1997) Cationic lipids used in gene transfer. *Adv. Drug Deliv. Rev.*, **27**, 17–28.

Zuidam, N.J., Barenholz, Y. and Minsky, A. (1999) Chiral DNA packaging in DNA-cationic liposome assemblies. *FEBS Lett.*, **457**, 419–422.

16 Peptide-based gene delivery systems

Patrick Midoux and Chantal Pichon

INTRODUCTION

Gene therapy aims at introducing nucleic acids or genetic material into mammalian cells for the modulation of gene expression with the expectation of getting therapeutic benefits. To date, although viral vectors are the best vehicles to introduce genes into cells and the feasibility of this therapeutic approach has been demonstrated, clinical developments require the use of synthetic vehicles of high safety, low immunogenicity and ease of manufacture. During the last decade, efforts have been made to design peptide-based gene delivery systems that incorporate viral-like features for efficient transfection (Tomlinson and Rolland, 1996; Zauner *et al.*, 1998; Rolland, 1998; Mahato *et al.*, 1999a). By taking advantage of the DNA self-assembling with a cationic polymer to condense a plasmid DNA (pDNA), like the viral genome in the viral particles, polyplexes (DNA/cationic polymer complexes) (Felgner *et al.*, 1997) have been prospected to develop non-viral vectors. The final goal of these systems is to transform the pDNA encoding a therapeutic gene into a 'Magic Bullet', as proposed by Paul Erlich (1906), which would be suitable for the delivery of genes into the right target cells and for the translocation to the nucleus of these cells upon systemic administration.

This challenge will be achieved when the 'Magic Bullet' is able to traverse several extracellular barriers and reach the target cells. It must also pass through several intracellular barriers to reach the cell nucleus where the gene expression takes place. To traverse the extracellular barriers, it must be shielded to escape both detection by the immune system or elimination by the liver Kuppfer cells. It must get to organs or tumors upon extravasation from the vascular to the interstitial space through fenestrations or tight junctions in the endothelial layer or upon transcytosis via endothelial cells. To pass through these barriers, polyplexes require the control of DNA condensation into small particles (<100 nm). Their stabilization in physiological medium and the shielding of their positive charge is currently obtained by coupling polyethylene glycol (PEG). Such polyplexes bearing cell recognition signal (CRS) molecules will be expected to bind on to and translocate into the target cells; then pDNA can be imported into their nuclei. Although the final goal of the 'Magic Bullet' is to transfect the right target cells upon systemic administration, some gene delivery systems could be used for strategies consisting of an *ex vivo* transfection of cells, such as hematopoietic stem cells, macrophages, dendritic cells, endothelial cells, and vascular smooth muscle cells before their implantation in the body.

Peptide-based gene delivery systems are made with pDNA encoding a therapeutic gene and a peptide carrier bearing one or multiple domains with defined functions to help pDNA to cross over the above mentioned intracellular barriers (Figure 16.1), with the aim of being inside the cell nucleus. The 'ideal' system could be designed as a multi-component peptide. It would contain a domain with a DNA binding sequence (DBS) currently achieved by a sequence containing several basic amino acids allowing DNA condensation and polyplex formation. A domain exhibiting a cell recognition signal (CRS) assumes a delivery to the right target cells via receptor-mediated endocytosis. Cellular translocation of the gene requires a cytosolic translocation signal (CTS) acting to destabilize either the plasma membrane or the endosomal membrane. Once in the cytosol, pDNA unpackaging can occur; it might be a limiting or a benefit step for the pDNA import in the cell

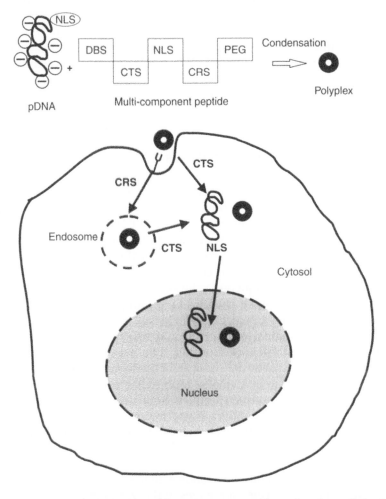

Figure 16.1 Conceptual multi-component peptide and major cellular barriers in gene transfer. DBS: DNA binding signal; CTS: cytosolic translocation signal; NLS: nuclear localization signal; CRS: cell recognition signal, and; PEG: polyethylene glycol.

nucleus. Nuclear import in the absence of cell division is mediated by a nuclear localization signal (NLS), which can be either contained in the multi-component peptide or linked to the plasmid. Once in the nucleus, gene expression requires the un-packaging of pDNA to be processed by the transcription machinery.

During the last decade, several cationic polymer-based gene delivery systems were assessed and most of them were designed using cationic polypeptides, such as polylysine (Zauner *et al.*, 1998), polyethyleneimine (Godbey *et al.*, 1999), polyamido-amine dendrimer (Haensler and Szoka, 1993), histidylated polylysine (Midoux and Monsigny, 1999) and polyallylamine (Boussif *et al.*, 1999). However, due to their high molecular weight, large degree of polymerization and high degree of poly-dispersity, cationic polymers are not well-characterized molecules in size and homogeneity. Moreover, they are cytotoxic and can induce complement activation. To circumvent these problems, low molecular weight synthetic peptides are pre-ferred because they offer the advantage of controlled synthesis and defined purity.

The objective of this chapter is to present an overview of peptide-based gene delivery systems. Some excellent reviews have been written recently on this topic, so we shall only do a summary of fusogenic peptides and then we will present our recent data. We will particularly focus on the recent progress made concerning low molecular peptide-based gene delivery systems. We will also attempt to make readers aware of the conceptual and experimental aspects of peptide-based gene delivery system design.

POLY(L-LYSINE)-BASED GENE DELIVERY SYSTEMS

Complex formation between pDNA and cationic polymers leads to a large reduction of the hydrodynamic size of the plasmid (for a review see Bloomfield, 1998). The electrostatic interactions between the negative charges of DNA (sugar-phosphate backbone groups) and the positive charges of a cationic polymer (for instance, ε-amino groups of polylysine) induce DNA condensation after the neutralization of 90% of the DNA charges. The reversible condensation process of DNA in the presence of cationic polymers in aqueous solution allows a plasmid of several thousand base pairs to turn into small particles by a complex mechanism, which is not yet well understood. Morphologically, polyplexes are toroids or spherical particles and rods under low ionic strength (<20 mM NaCl), and they form large aggregates under physiological salt concentration. The net charge of polyplexes can be characterized by ζ potential of the particles. The theoretical size of a 6.4 kb pDNA complexed with polylysine in a charge ratio of 1:1 would be 28 nm. This estimation takes into account the partial specific volume and hydration values for DNA and polylysine and assumes a spherical size for the polyplexes (see in the review by Mahato, 1999). This size is rarely achieved, however, and polyplexes exhibit a current size of 70–100 nm, suggesting that a polyplex contains several pDNA molecules.

Transmission electron micrographs have shown that many ends of DNA (up to eight) are detectable in the intermediate stages of the formation of 100 nm par-ticles between a linear pDNA and a partially gluconoylated conjugate of polylysine (unpublished results). This detection indicates that a minimum of roughly four DNA segments are included in a single toroid or a spherical aggregate. Condensation of a single pDNA molecule can be observed in very diluted solutions. However, controlled preparations of polyplexes at high pDNA concentration containing a single plasmid molecule (termed unimolecular polyplex) have been reported by Perales *et al.* (1997). This protocol to produce unimolecular polyplexes contained significant ambiguity and could not be easily reproduced under the stated conditions. Briefly, galactosylated polylysine was added over a long period (1–1.5 h) to a pDNA (1.5 mg/ml) in 0.75 M NaCl under vigorous mixing until the solution became turbid. Then, the solution was cleared by a stepwise addition of a 5 M NaCl solution. Under these conditions, homogenous particles of 12–20 nm were obtained and facilitated an efficient gene expression in rat liver. It is noticeable that the final salt concentration is largely above the physiological salt concentration. This high salt concentration indicates that the formation of unimolecular polyplex through the use of cationic polymers has not yet been achieved. Recently, new insights have been opened by the description of a controlled assembly of pDNA into small stable 23 nm and 40 nm particles by using cationic cysteine-based detergents (Blessing *et al.*, 1998; Ouyang *et al.*, 2000). The controlled formation of unimolecular polyplex will be of great interest because particles of less than 24 nm could easily be imported into the cell nucleus through the nuclear pores upon attachment of the nuclear localization signal (NLS) molecules.

ENDOSOMAL ESCAPE

Polyplexes are taken up by cells either by non-specific or receptor-mediated endocytosis when they carry a recognition signal. The recognition signal can be either proteins, such as asialoglycoproteins, transferrin, insulin, immunoglobulins, growth factors, or small ligands, such as peptides and carbohydrates. Polyplexes are internalized in intracellular vesicles from where the plasmid must escape to reach the nucleus. Although their intracellular trafficking and the mechanism allowing pDNA to reach the cell nucleus are still unknown, microscopy analysis shows that most of them route via acidic vesicular compartments (endosomes or phagosomes). The presence of pDNA in the cytosol and its location in the cell nucleus are a rare event. Therefore, the membrane of these vesicles constitutes one of the major barriers for DNA delivery in the cytosol. Cationic polymers, such as dendrimer and polyethylenimine, provide high transfection because they possess protonable amines and they can destabilize endosomal membrane (Boussif *et al.*, 1995; Tang and Szoka, 1997). In an acidic endosome, protonated polyethylen-eimine alters the osmolarity of the vesicle, leading to their swelling and their dest-abilization (Kichler *et al.*, 2001). Based on the knowledge of the endocytic pathway, chloroquine or fusogenic/permeabilizing peptides have been used as cytosolic trans-location signal (CTS) molecules in combination with polylysine- and cationic peptide-based systems to improve the transmembrane passage of pDNA or polyplexes in the cytosol upon the destabilization and/or disruption of the acid endocytic vesicles.

Chloroquine

Chloroquine drastically improves the transfection of cells when DNA/polylysine conjugates are used (Zenke *et al.*, 1990; Midoux *et al.*, 1993). So far, the mechanism of action of chloroquine has not been completely elucidated. Chloroquine is supposed to protect the internalized plasmid from intracellular degradation as a result of the neutralization of acidic compartments and the inhibition of endosome fusion with lysosomes. Furthermore, the swelling of vesicles can be induced when the concentration of chloroquine is high enough. However, there is no direct relationship between the neutralization of the acidic cell compartments and the transfection efficiency (Erbacher *et al.*, 1996a). Once taken up by the cells, chloroquine accumulates inside acidic vesicles where it can reach a concentration more than 50 mM, based on the estimated volume of the vesicular compartments. At physiological pH, 82% of chloroquine is protonated and can bind to nucleic acids. Therefore, the interaction of chloroquine with DNA appears to be of paramount importance. Indeed, we have shown in an acellular system that chloroquine induces the dissociation of pDNA/lactosylated polylysine complexes at concentrations as low as a few millimolar (Erbacher *et al.*, 1996a). Such chloroquine concentrations may dissociate polyplexes and increase the disruption of vesicles, facilitating DNA delivery into the cytosol.

Glutamic acid-rich peptides

Many amphiphilic peptides have a high affinity for lipid bilayer, but only certain sequences are able to induce membrane destabilization via either permeabilization or fusion. The most characterized fusogenic peptides were derived from viruses (for reviews see White, 1990; Kielian and Jungerwirth, 1990), but few were derived from bacteria and fungi (for reviews see Fujii *et al.*, 1993). Some fusogenic peptides exhibit membrane destabilization features in an acidic medium while others do so in both neutral and acidic media. The fusogenic and/or permeabilization features of many peptides are reliant upon their conformation, either an α-helix or a β-sheet. Peptides exhibiting an acidic pH-dependent membrane destabilization are good candidates to favor endosomal membrane destabilization, allowing cytosolic pDNA delivery. The first peptides used have been derived from the *N*-terminal segment of the HA-2 subunit of the influenza virus hemagglutinin, known to be involved in the fusion of the viral envelope with the endosomal membrane (Table 16.1). It is believed that they increase plasmid delivery into the cytosol upon membrane disruption of the acidic vesicles containing the plasmid (for a review see Wagner, 1999).

The amphiphilic anionic peptides GLFEAIAGFIENGWEGMIDGGGC and GLFEAIAEFIEGGWEGLIEGCA (E5CA) were found to increase the transfection efficiency of DNA/transferrin–polylysine complexes (Wagner *et al.*, 1992) and DNA/lactosylated–polylysine complexes (Midoux *et al.*, 1993), respectively. Then, several other amphiphilic anionic peptides listed in Table 16.1 were synthesized. The presence of naturally occurring stretch WYG in INF7 instead of GGC in INF3 makes the peptide extremely effective in lysing erythrocytes at pH 5, and therefore induces a very high gene expression in polyfection with transferrin–polylysine conjugates. Similarly, E5WYG has also been shown to be efficient in polyfection with glycosylated polylysine conjugates. In the Hemagglutinin viral fusion protein, HA-2 peptide interacts with the target membrane and initializes the fusion of viral and endosomal membranes. These trimers fuse across the two membranes to create a gated channel to release the viral particle contents (Danieli *et al.*, 1996;

Hughson, 1997). To mimic this spacial arrangement, dimerization of peptides has been performed. Dimerization of INF3 through a disulfide bond between the two C-terminal cysteines (INF3DI), or by a link between the C-terminal amino acid in the two α and ε amino groups of lysine (INF5), considerably enhances (up to 5000-fold) polyfection with transferrin–polylysine conjugates. Homodimerization of E5WYG has been also achieved via either short (G)$_2$-K or relatively long (G$\underline{A}\underline{A}$)$_2$-K arms. Depending on the dimerization arm, the effect on the transfection efficiency with glycosylated polylysine conjugates was not quite similar. With the (G)$_2$-K arm, polyfection decreased 10-fold, whereas it increased 6-fold with the (G$\underline{A}\underline{A}$)$_2$-K arm. With the latter, the amount of α-helical structure was maximal at pH 6.0, whereas it was maximal at a lower pH with the former.

Artificial peptides, such as GALA and JTS-1, and the sequence of the *N*-terminal segment of VP1 of HRV2 rhinovirus, have also been found to enhance the transfection efficiency of polylysine conjugates/DNA complexes (Table 16.1). These peptides, which contain acid residues (mainly glutamate) were shown to induce membrane fusion and permeabilization at pH lower than 6. Permeabilization and fusion activities are attributed to the protonation of the acid residues of these peptides. The protonation allows a conformational change of the peptide from random to α-helix and thereby facilitates its interaction with the membrane, leading to membrane destabilization.

These anionic peptides can be linked covalently to polylysine conjugates, but that may cause a decrease of their fusogenic features once the polyplexes are formed. For instance, we have found impairment in permeabilization of the plasma membrane upon coupling E5CA to bovine serum albumin (Midoux *et al.*, 1995).

Table 16.1 Fusogenic glutamic-acid rich peptides

Peptide sequences	Name	References
GLFGAIAGFIENGWEGMIDGWYG	HA-2	White, 1990
(X31F/68 strain)	HA-2	Murata *et al.*, 1987
GLFGAIAGFIEGGWTGMIDGWYG		
(A/PR/8/34 strain)		
GLFEAIAGFIENGWEGMIDGGGC		Wagner *et al.*, 1992
GLFEAIEGFIENGWEGMIDGGGC	INF3	Plank *et al.*, 1994
(INF3)-SS-(INF3)	INF3DI	Plank *et al.*, 1994
GLFEAIEGFIENGWEGMIDGWYG	INF7	Plank *et al.*, 1994
GLFEAIEGFIENGWEGnIDGCA	INF4	Plank *et al.*, 1994
(INF4)-SS-(INF4)	INF4DI	Plank *et al.*, 1994
GLFEAIEGFIENGWEGnIDG-K-	INF5	Plank *et al.*, 1994
GDInGEWGNEIFGEIAEFLG		
GLFEAIAEFIEGGWEGLIEGCA	E5CA	Midoux *et al.*, 1993
GLFEAIAEFIEGGWEGLIEGWYG	E5WYG	Midoux *et al.*, 1998
(E5WYGG)$_2$-KA		Kichler *et al.*, 1999
(E5WYG$\underline{A}\underline{A}$)$_2$-KA		Freulon *et al.*, 2000
WEAALAEALAEALAEHLAEALAEALEALAA	GALA	Haensler and Szoka, 1993
GLFEALLELLESLWELLLEA	JST-1	Gottschalk *et al.*, 1996
NPVENYIDEVLNEVLVVPNINSSNC	VP1	Zauner *et al.*, 1995

Note
$\underline{A}$, n and -SS- stand for β-alanine, norleucine and disulfide bond, respectively.

It is clear that the coating of DNA/polylysine complexes with anionic peptides by electrostatic interactions is easier than their covalent linkage. Quaternary complexes consisting of pDNA condensed with both a ligand-substituted and non-substituted cationic polymer, and with a fusogenic peptide ionically bound to the surface of the polyplexes, have been performed with transferrin-polylysine, polylysine and the INF family (Plank *et al.*, 1994), as well as with glycosylated polylysine, polylysine and E5WYG (Kichler *et al.*, 1999). Fusogenic peptides are strongly associated with polyplexes and thereby increase the chance of finding DNA complexes and fusogenic peptide inside the same endosomes.

Anionic peptides are almost inactive in the presence of serum because they have the disadvantage of binding to serum proteins. Amphiphilic basic peptides, such as melittin (GIGAVLKVLTTGLPALISWIKRKRQQ-*NH₂*), isolated from the venom of the European honey bee *Apis mellifera* (Dempsey, 1990) and K5, the cationic counterpart of E5 (Murata *et al.*, 1992), exhibit more efficient membrane fusion and permeabilization activities at both neutral and acidic pH than anionic peptides. However, they interact mainly with the plasma membrane and therefore are much more cytotoxic.

Histidine-rich peptides and polypeptides

Uncharged peptides, which interact neither with the plasma membrane nor with serum proteins, but become fusogenic upon protonation in an acidic medium, will be of great interest for achieving the endosomal escape of pDNA. Such peptides or polypeptides can be designed by making use of histidine. Indeed, poly-L-histidine is known to mediate both an acid-dependent fusion and leakage of negatively charged liposomes after protonation of the imidazole group of histidyl monomer of pK ~ 6.0 (Wang and Huang, 1984; Uster and Deamer, 1985). Poly-L-histidine has a better membrane fusion and leakage activity than poly-L-lysine. Fusion of negatively charged liposomes is induced at a +/− ratio (positive charges of protonated imidazoles to the negative charges of phospholipids) ≤ 0.2, whereas it occurs at a +/− ratio of 1 to 2 for poly-L-lysine. On this basis, synthesis of histidine-rich peptides and polypeptides has been achieved for the delivery of both oligonucleotides (ODN) and pDNA.

H5WYG peptide

H5WYG (GLFHAIAHFIHGGWHGLIHGWYG) peptide, the histidine counterpart of E5WYG, undergoes a dramatic conformational change between pH 7.0 and pH 6.0 that correlates with the protonation of histidines (Table 16.2).

Table 16.2 Fusogenic histidine-rich peptides

Peptide sequences	Name	References
GLFHAIAHFIHGGWHGLIHGWYG	H5WYG	Midoux *et al.*, 1998
KKALLALALHHLAHLALHLALALKKA	LAH₄	Vogt and Bechinger, 1999
LGLLLRHLRHHSNLLANI	B18	Glaser *et al.*, 1999
DSHAKRHHGYKRKFHEKHHSHRGY	Histatin5	Melino *et al.*, 1999

At neutral pH, H5WYG is weakly water-soluble and aggregates. While at pH 5.0, when all histidines are protonated, it is more soluble in water. In contrast to anionic peptides, which exhibit an α-helix structure in an acidic medium, H5WYG does not exhibit an ordered structure in acidic medium. This peptide permeabilizes cell membrane at pH 6.8 – the pH of the lumen of very early endosomes – at about one unit less acid than E5WYG, its anionic counterpart. The presence of $10\,\mu M$ H5WYG during polyfection with glycosylated polylysine drastically increases trans-fection efficiency of several human and non-human cell lines. In contrast to the anionic peptide, the effect of H5WYG is not impaired in the presence of serum (even in the medium containing 50% serum). In the presence of bafilomycin A_1, the transfection efficiency is absent because the lack of endosome acidification prevents the protonation of the imidazole groups of H5WYG and, consequently, its membrane permeabilization activity. Cytosolic and nuclear loading with fluorescein-labeled ODN can also be achieved by lowering the pH of culture medium containing both fluorescein-labeled ODN and H5WYG. Cell viability is better preserved with H5WYG than with E5WYG, which requires a more acidic pH 5.5 to permeabilize membrane.

Other peptides containing histidines listed in Table 16.2, such as those of the histatin family (antimicrobial peptides), Sea Urchin (B18) and LAH_4, strongly interact with phospholipid membranes and destabilize them. LAH_4, which does not contain other cationic residues, exhibits α-helix and is more active in an acidic medium. These peptides could be putative endosome disrupting helpers that have not yet been used for polyfection.

Histidylated polylysines (HpK)

Data obtained with H5WYG have prompted us to substitute polylysine of various degree of polymerization (dp) with histidyl residues. The resulting grafted-comb cationic polymers (HpK) (Midoux and Monsigny, 1999; Fajac *et al.*, 2000) or oligomers (HoK) (Pichon *et al.*, 2000) combine both the DNA condensation capa-city of polylysine and the membrane destabilization features of imidazole clusters on a single molecule (Figure 16.2).

Plasmid DNA mixed with a polylysine of dp 190 substituted with 109 histidyl residues form toroids with a mean diameter of 130 nm, as measured both by Quasi Elastic (dynamic) Light Scattering (QELS) and Transmission Electron Microscopy (TEM). The particles have a ζ potential of $+18\,mV$ at a theoretically $+/-$ charge ratio of 3.4 (ratio of lysyl ε-amino plus histidyl α-amino groups to pDNA phos-phates) in $10\,mM$ Hepes buffer pH 7.4 (Bello Roufai and Midoux, 2001). At physiological salt concentration, the polyplex sizes are stabilized at 100 nm and 50 nm in the presence of 10% and 50% bovine fetal serum, respectively. We have found that this stabilization is due to the absorption of several anionic serum proteins on polyplexes, which prevent hydrophobic contacts between them. In addition, the global charge of serum-stabilized polyplexes is reversed to $-25\,mV$, and, as a consequence, their non-specific binding on the cell surface is reduced. As previously described for other cationic polymers (Ogris *et al.*, 1999; Erbacher *et al.*, 1999), we found that the binding of one molecule of poly(ethylene glycol) (PEG of 5000 Da) per HpK molecule prevents aggregation of polyplexes at physiological salt concentration and reduces the ζ potential ($+6\,mV$).

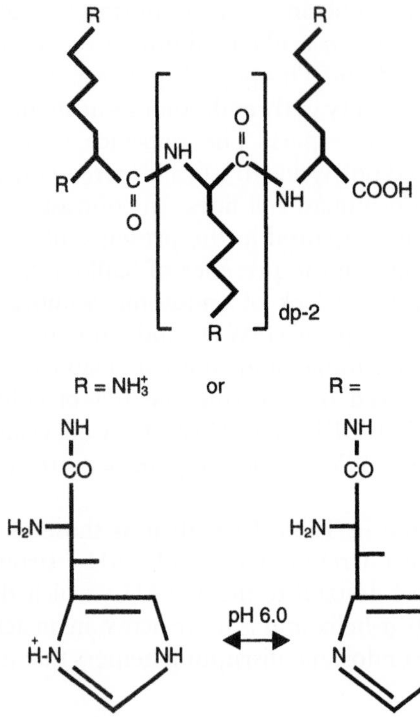

Figure 16.2 Schematic structures of histidylated polylysine (HpK: dp = 190) or histidylated oligolysine (HoK: dp = 19).

Based on Luciferase activity, we have shown that the polyfection of HepG2 cells with a pDNA encoding Luciferase gene complexed with HpK (weight ratio of 1:3) is 3–4.5 orders of magnitude higher than polyfection with pDNA complexed with pLK in the absence or presence of chloroquine or a fusogenic peptide (Midoux and Monsigny, 1999). Once inside endosomes, histidyl residues are supposed to be protonated. ζ potential of HpK polyplexes increased to 20 mV when the pH medium was lowered from pH 7.4 to pH 6.0, suggesting an increase in the number of cationic charges in the lumen of endosomes and thereby a better membrane destabilization (Bello Roufai and Midoux, 2001). With polylysine of dp 72, 36 and 19, transfection efficiency decreases drastically when histidine substitution level is more than 20% (Table 16.3). There was a significant decrease in transfection efficiency with histidylated polylysine of dp 19, probably because the number of cationic charges on the polymer was too low to stabilize condensed pDNA particles. In addition, because of the weak electrostatic interactions, polyplex solution contains a great amount of free cationic polymer, which increases the cytotoxicity. In this case, an interpeptide cross-linking via disulfide bonds are useful for stabilizing these polyplexes (Trubetskoy *et al.*, 1999; McKenzie *et al.*, 2000a). Based on our findings, a N-Ac-poly(L-histidine)-graft-poly(L-lysine) comb shaped polymer (Benns *et al.*, 2000) and a low molecular weight disulfide cross-linking peptide, Cys-His-(Lys)₆-His-Cys (McKenzie *et al.*, 2000b), have recently been described for gene delivery.

Table 16.3 Comparative evaluation of polyfection with histidylated polylysines

dp	His (%)	RLU (%)	Cytotoxicity (%)
190	35	100	24
190	45	110	21
72	23	87–96	24
72	43	0–1	12
36	22	61–100	25
36	53	0–10	4
19	25	15–26	49
19	45	9	40

Note
Polyfection was carried out with pCMVLuc (a 5 kb pDNA) on HepG2 cells for four hours at 37 °C. After 48 hours, the transfection efficiency was determined from Luciferase activity in cells measured by luminescence (RLU) and the cytotoxicity was evaluated by using the colorimetric MTT assay. dp is the polylysine degree of polymerization. The transfection efficiency is scored on a 0 to 100 scale where 0 and 100 correspond to an absence of transfection and the most effective transfection, respectively compared to the pDNA alone. His is histidyl residue.

Although histidylated polylysine of dp 19 (oligolysine, oK) is not efficient for gene transfer, highly substituted (≥80%) histidylated oligolysines (HoK) are suitable vectors for ODN delivery (Pichon *et al.*, 2000). Cells incubated with fluorescein-labeled ODN in the presence of HoK exhibit a strong fluorescence staining localized in vesicles, and also in the cytosol and the nucleus (Figure 16.3). As expected, we have found that the increase in PS-ODN delivery in the cytosol with HoK correlates with a more than 20-fold increase in the biological activity of antisense ODN. As for pDNA/HpK complexes, PEGylation prevents aggregation of HoK/ODN complexes. QELS and TEM measurements show that PEG-HoK and ODN form dense spherical particles, varying in size from 25–34 nm and a ζ potential of +17 mV which remains stable in the presence of 0.15 M NaCl, even after two weeks at 4 °C. These PEG-HoK/ODN complexes exhibit a shape and a size similar to that of complexes between PS-ODN (24-mer) and PEG-PEI (10 kDa) (Vinogradov *et al.*, 1998) and between ODN and pHPMA-b-pTMAEM block copolymers (Read *et al.*, 2000).

MEMBRANE PERMEABILIZATION

Membrane permeabilization activity of peptides is currently measured by the use of artificial membrane bilayers, such as liposomes or erythrocytes. The liposome leakage assay can be performed by using spectrofluorimetry with a concentration-dependent quenching of a dye (calcein, carboxyfluorescein) encapsulated in liposomes. Disruption of liposomes in the presence of peptide-inducing leakage will lead to an increase in the fluorescence intensity of the liposome solution. Erythrocyte lysis assay is based on the absorption of hemoglobin, which can be measured once released into the extracellular medium upon erythrocyte lysis in the presence of peptide.

Permeabilization of the plasma membranes is more relevant and can be easily performed with living cells by using flow cytometry, as previously described (Midoux *et al.*, 1995). Here, we report a flow cytometry method using stable GFP-expressing clone cells. Green Fluorescent Protein (GFP) (27 kDa), which has been

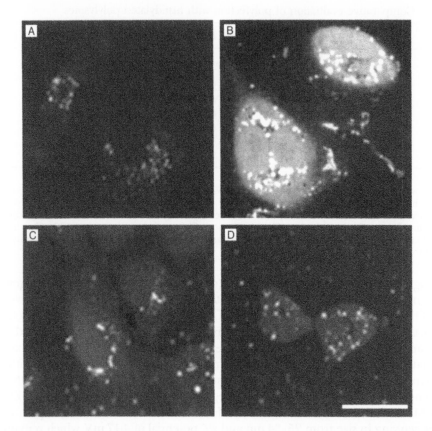

Figure 16.3 HoK induces cytosolic and nuclear delivery of ODN. A549 cells were incubated for four hours at 37 °C with fluorescein-labeled ODN (0.125 µM) either (A) in the absence of HoK, (B) in the presence of HoK, (C) AcHoK or (D) histidine-free oligolysine. Cells were fixed with 2% *p*-formaldehyde and visualized with a confocal microscope. Images were acquired by using identical settings. Scale bar = 25 µm. From Pichon *et al.*, 2000.

isolated from the jellyfish *Aequorea victoria* (Chalfie *et al.*, 1994), emits a green light at a maximum of 510 nm in the absence of added cofactors when illuminated with blue light at 488 nm. Enhanced GFP (EGFP) is a mutant emitting a brighter fluorescence, which allows a more sensitive detection. Cells transfected with plasmid encoding the GFP gene exhibit diffuse fluorescence intensity, both in the cytosol and in the cell nucleus. Because of its small size, GFP can reversibly diffuse through the nuclear pores. As shown in Figure 16.4, a clone of HeLa cells, which has integrated EGFP genes, exhibits high fluorescence intensity (Figure 16.4A). Dead cells can be evidenced upon labeling with propidium iodide (Figure 16.4B). In the presence of melittin, the green fluorescence of the cells (Figure 16.4C, upper channel) decreases rapidly (200 s) to the value of the cell autofluorescence (Figure 16.4C, lower channel). This rapid decrease indicates that EGFP leaches out of the cells upon membrane permeabilization. Indeed, the fluorescence intensity was recovered in the surpernatant upon centrifugation of the permeabilized cells.

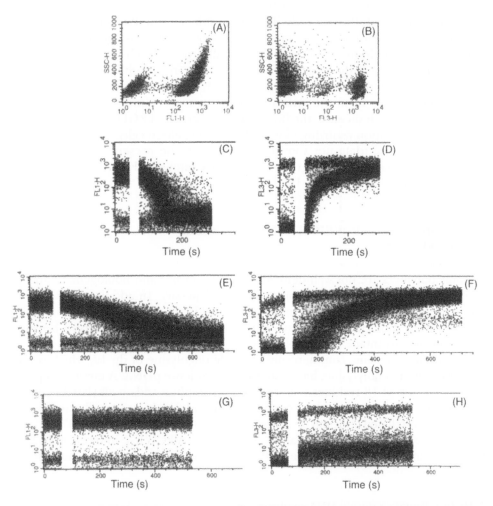

Figure 16.4 Peptide-induced membrane permeabilization. (A) Stable EGFP expressing HeLa cells exhibit a high fluorescence intensity. (B) Cells having destabilized plasma membrane are evidenced upon labeling with propidium iodide. HeLa cells (8×10^5 cells) in phosphate buffer saline, pH 7.4 were mixed with 15 nM propidium iodide and either (C and D) melittin (3.3 μM final concentration) or (G and H) H5WYG (38 μM final concentration) was added. (E and F) HeLa cells in phosphate buffer saline, pH 6.2, were mixed with 15 nM propidium iodide and H5WYG (38 μM final concentration). The cell fluorescence intensity was recorded using FACSort cytometer (Becton Dickinson) during 10 minutes both in FL1 (A, C, E and G) the green (520 nm) and in FL3 (B, D, F and H) the red (650 nm) channels immediately after the peptide addition.

Membrane destabilization can be simultaneously monitored by using propidium iodide. This non fluorescent and poorly permeant small molecule enters into the cells only upon membrane permeabilization/destabilization and becomes fluorescent upon binding to DNA in the nucleus. In the presence of melittin, cells are also rapidly (200 s) red-labeled upon peptide induced membrane permeabilization

(Figure 16.4D). It can be seen that the diffusion of propidium iodide inside the cells is correlated with the leak of EGFP. The results show that melittin induces the formation of pores in the plasma membranes allowing the passage of small molecules such as propidium iodide, as well as small proteins such as EGFP. H5WYG peptide permeabilizes the plasma membrane only in a slightly acidic medium. When the extracellular medium containing H5WYG is lowered to pH 6.2, EGFP leaches out in 400 s from the cells as propidium iodide enters the cells (Figure 16.4E and F). As with melittin, the fluorescence intensity of EGFP was recovered in the surpernatant upon centrifugation of the permeabilized cells. In the absence of H5WYG at pH 6.2 (data not shown), as well as in the presence of H5WYG at neutral pH, no decrease of the green fluorescence intensity (Figure 16.4G) and no red labeling of the cells (Figure 16.4H), are observed.

SMALL MOLECULAR WEIGHT PEPTIDE-BASED GENE DELIVERY

Cationic polymers are not well-defined molecules in size and homogeneity due to their large degree of polymerization and polydispersity. In addition they can be cytotoxic and can induce complement activation. In an effort to circumvent these problems, low molecular weight synthetic peptides should be preferred because they offer the advantage of controlled synthesis and defined purity.

Instead of polylysine, commercially available oligolysine of dp 19, which is less polydisperse than polylysine, has been used to condense pDNA. A minimal repeating lysine chain of 18 residues followed by a tryptophan and an alkylated cysteine (AlkCWK$_{18}$) has been found to condense plasmid DNA into small particles of 78 nm that mediated efficient *in vitro* transfection (Wadhwa *et al.*, 1997) (Table 16.4). Compared to a commercially available K$_{19}$, AlkCWK$_{18}$ induced a 40-fold reduction in particle size and a 1000-fold increase in transfection efficiency.

Table 16.4 Peptide inducing DNA condensation

Peptide sequences	Helper	DBS	NLS	References
AlkCWK$_{18}$	Chlo	+	−	Wadhwa *et al.*, 1997
(K$_n$)$_2$KGGC; (R$_n$)$_2$KGGC; (O$_n$)$_2$KGGC	Chlo	+	−	Plank *et al.*, 1999
YKAK$_8$WK	JTS-1	+	−	Gottschalk *et al.*, 1996
RAWARALARALRALARALRALAR (RAWA)	JTS-1	+	−	Fominaya *et al.*, 2000
(KTPKKAKKP)$_2$ (H9-2)	lipo	+	−	Schwartz *et al.*, 1999
PKKKRKV-βA-(KTPKKAKKP)$_2$ (nls-H9-2)	lipo	+	+	Schwartz *et al.*, 1999
RRRLHRIHRRQHRSCRRRKRR (Pr21)	lipo	+	−	Schwartz *et al.*, 1999
SPKRSPKRSPKR-palmitoyl	HA	+	−	Wilke *et al.*, 1996
CWK$_{17}$C	Chlo	+	−	McKenzie *et al.*, 2000a

Notes
DBS and NLS stand for DNA binding signal and nuclear localization signal, respectively. Helper indicates that the transfection is efficient in the presence of additives for the cytosolic translocation. Chlo and lipo are chloroquine and cationic lipids, respectively. JTS-1 and HA are fusogenic peptides listed in Table 1.

The more efficient pDNA condensing capacity of AlkCWK$_{18}$ was initially attributed to the presence of a tryptophan residue in the polycationic chain, which was thought to organize the condensation. However, the condensation was in fact due to the presence of a shorter chain in the commercially available K$_{19}$. Indeed, a comparison between AlkCWK$_{18}$ and a synthetic K$_{20}$ established that they both form similar particles and mediate similar transfection efficiency in cultured cells (McKenzie *et al.*, 1999). The incorporation of tryptophans into the DNA-binding moiety does not increase the DNA-compacting potency of lysine (K$_n$)$_2$KGGC, arginine (R$_n$)$_2$KGGC or ornithine (O$_n$)$_2$KGGC branched cationic peptides – where n is either 2, 3 or 4 (Table 16.4) (Plank *et al.*, 1999). Compared to polylysine, these peptides and their DNA complexes are weak activators of the complement system. No significant variations in the DNA condensation features have been observed between lysyl, arginyl and ornithyl residues and a minimum of six to eight basic amino acids are required to condense DNA and to get efficient transfection. It is worth noting that AlkCWK$_{18}$, YKAK$_8$WK and RAWA (the arginine counterpart of GALA) peptides mediate efficient transfection in the presence of either chloroquine or fusogenic peptides (Table 16.4). The anionic fusogenic JTS-1 peptide (Table 16.1) ionically bound to DNA/YKAK$_8$WK and DNA/RAWA complexes increases the transfection efficiency.

Short DNA binding sequences of natural DNA binding proteins can also be used to condense pDNA (Table 16.4). The dimeric lysine-rich peptide H9-2 of 19 residues, with the sequence KTPKKAKKP corresponding to residues 152–160 of the human histone H1, interacts with pDNA and enhances *in vitro* transfection mediated by cationic liposomes. Human protamine-derived Pr21 peptide, an arginine-rich peptide of 21 residues, displays a similar potential in transfecting cells than H9-2. The DNA binding sequence P2 (SPKRSPKRSPKR), derived from a similar tetrapeptide repeat motif (SPKR) found in Sea Urchin sperm histone H1, can also condense pDNA. The addition, of a lipid (palmitoyl) tail to the P2 sequence leads to a compound which forms ternary aggregated particles with the fusogenic peptide E5C (GLFEAIAEFIEGGWEGLIEGC) that mediate *in vitro* transfection.

Several other synthetic cationic peptides containing either lysyl or arginyl residues are also superior replacements for cationic polymers in condensing pDNA

Table 16.5 Peptide inducing DNA condensation and membrane destabilization

Peptide sequences	DBS	CTS	NLS	References
WEAKLAKALAKALAKHLAKALAKALKACEA (KALA)	+	+	–	Wyman *et al.*, 1997
Ac-LARLLARLLARLLRALLRALLRAL-*NH$_2$* (LARL)$_6$	+	+	–	Niidome *et al.*, 1999
KLLKLLLKLWKKLLKLLK (Hel 11-7)	+	+	–	Niidome *et al.*, 1999
CHKHKHHKHC; CHK$_6$HC	+	+	–	McKenzie *et al.*, 2000b
HpK; HoK	+	+	–	Midoux and Monsigny, 1999; Pichon *et al.*, 2000

Notes
DBS, CTS and NLS stand for DNA binding signal, cytosolic translocation signal and nuclear localization signal, respectively. HoK stands for histidylated oligolysine (Figure 16.2).

and mediating transfection in cultured cells (Table 16.5). KALA (the lysine counterpart of GALA), Hel 11-7 and LARL$_6$ are α-helical peptides in neutral aqueous
solution and are able to induce a membrane destabilization. These peptides exhibit
a similar organization to a hydrophilic face composed of polar or charged residues
(lysyl or arginyl) and a hydrophobic face composed of non-charged and non polar
(leucyl, alanyl) residues. The cationic hydrophilic face can bind pDNA. KALA binds
DNA, destabilizes membranes and mediates DNA transfection with an efficiency
about 100-fold greater than pDNA/polylysine complexes. Hel 11-7 and LARL$_6$
mediate transfection of COS-7 cells with an efficiency of about 10-fold less than that
obtained with lipofectin.

PEPTIDES WITH THIOL GROUPS

Generally, low molecular weight peptides mediate *in vitro* gene transfer as efficiently as their cationic polymer counterparts. However, they condense DNA with
a lower efficiency and as a consequence the resulting polyplexes have a reduced
stability in biological fluid and a less protective effect against DNA degradation.
To increase their stability, peptides with thiol groups were synthesized. Based on
the reductive features of the cytosolic compartment of the cell, a reversible cross-
linking of preformed polyplexes was achieved by forming interpeptide disulfide
bonds. These disulfide bonds can be cleaved inside the cytosol, facilitating dissociation and release of DNA from the polyplexes. This approach was first described
by Trubetskoy *et al.* (1999). Preformed DNA/polylysine complexes were cross-
linked by the addition of an heterobifunctional agent, dimethyl-3,3'-dithiobispro-
pionimidate. In addition, the cross linking of DNA complexes made with polylysine
prevented aggregation of compact particles, which occurs naturally at physiological
salt concentration. Such DNA particles were active in transfecting cells in culture.
   McKenzie and coworkers then developed a panel of cationic peptides derived
from AlkCWK$_{18}$, which contained two to five cysteine residues (McKenzie
et al., 2000a). CWK$_{17}$C, CWK$_8$CK$_8$C, CWK$_5$CK$_5$CK$_5$C and CWK$_4$CK$_3$CK$_3$CK$_4$C
peptides condense pDNA and caged plasmids are then obtained upon oxidation
by the formation of interpeptide disulfide bonds within 30 minutes at pH 7.5. The
formation of polyplexes was monitored by using the ability of the peptide to
decrease the fluorescence intensity of an intercalator dye, such as thiazole orange,
from the plasmid when polyplexes are formed. The interpeptide disulfide bond
formation displaces completely the dye from pDNA. The intracross-linking of
polyplexes was also monitored by the decrease of the fluorescence intensity of
the DNA intercalator dye SYBR Gold. Caged DNA exhibited a size of 30–50 nm,
which increased slightly to 120–170 nm upon the reduction of disulfide bridges. In
contrast to AlkCWK$_{18}$, they did not form aggregates at physiological salt concentration. Transfection of HepG2 and COS7 cells with caged DNA were 5- to 60-fold
more efficient than uncross-linked peptide DNA condensates. Amongst the tested
peptides, caged DNA with CWK$_{17}$C peptide mediated the maximal transfection efficiency. To generate an endosomolytic activity of caged DNA, histidines have been introduced in various peptides. CHK$_6$HC peptide was found
to mediate transfection in the absence of chloroquine (McKenzie *et al.*, 2000b)
(Table 16.5).

PEPTIDES FOR SITE-SPECIFIC GENE DELIVERY

A variety of receptors present on the surface of cells of interest have been prospected to achieve a specific gene delivery that avoids gene expression into undesirable cells. The coupling of ligands on cationic polymers recognized by cell surface receptors theoretically offers the possibility of targeting pDNA condensates into a given cell type and of achieving their internalization via receptor-mediated endocytosis. For instance, asialoglycoproteins, transferrin, insulin, growth factors or antibodies were evaluated to target hepatocytes, tumor cells, epithelial cells, vascular smooth muscles cells or hematopoietic stem cells. However, such protein ligands can induce an immune response and can also modify the size, charge and solubility of polyplexes. In consideration of these points, small ligands such as carbohydrates and peptides should be preferred. In fact, peptides and carbohydrates were linked to oligolysine chains of 16 or 20 residues acting as a DNA binding domain to prepare selective compounds of controlled synthesis and defined purity (Table 16.6).

Integrin targeting

Integrins are widely expressed cell surface receptors involved in cell-cell adhesion and interactions of cells with the extracellular matrix. Integrins enable the cellular uptake of structures as large as bacteria and as small as viruses. Thus, they constitute good targets for developing selective gene delivery systems.

RGD

The RGD motif exhibits a high affinity for fibronectin and vitronectin integrin receptors of several epithelial, fibroblast and endothelial cells. For this reason, it is an interesting motif for targeting genes into airway epithelial cells and especially those mutated for the CFTR gene involved in cystic fibrosis. A synthetic peptide comprising a cyclic RGD motif linked to an oligolysine of 16 residues (K_{16}–RGD) has been developed (Harbottle *et al.*, 1998). This peptide is able to condense and deliver pDNA in a specific manner to airway and intestinal epithelial cells. Transfection efficiency was improved by 30-fold in the presence of LipofectAMINE used as helper for the cytosolic delivery (Colin *et al.*, 1998). Although confocal microscopy analyses have shown that both the peptide and pDNA are localized in the cell

Table 16.6 Peptide-based gene delivery systems with selectivity

Peptide sequences	Helper	DBS	CTS	NLS	References
K_{16}-GGCRGDMFGCA (K_{16}-RGD)	lipo	+	−	+/−	Colin *et al.*, 1998
SPKRSPKRSPKR-GRGDGDV (P2-RGD)	JTS-1	+	−	−	Vaysse *et al.*, 2000
K_{16}-ICRRARGDNPDDRCT (molossin)	JST-1	+	−	−	Li *et al.*, 2000
K_{16}-CSIPPEVKFNKPFVFLI (serpin)	chlo	+	−	−	Patel *et al.*, 2001
Sugar–CWK$_{18}$	chlo	+	−	−	Collard *et al.*, 2000a

Notes
DBS, CTS and NLS stand for DNA binding signal, cytosolic translocation signal and nuclear localization signal, respectively. Chlo and lipo are chloroquine and cationic lipids, respectively. JTS-1 is a fusogenic peptide listed in Table 1.

nucleus, the translocation of pDNA in the cell nucleus remains unclear even if K_{16}-RGD containing lysine and arginine act as an NLS signal (Colin *et al.*, 2000). The DNA binding sequence (SPKRSPKRSPKR), followed by an integrin-binding motif RGD (GRGDGDV) used in ternary complexes with either E5C or JST-1 fusogenic peptides, led to the transfection of cultured cells with an efficiency of about 55% with NIH-3T3 cells (Vaysse *et al.*, 2000). A novel peptide PLAEID-GIELTY not yet tested that does not contain RGD motif has been found to bind to $\alpha_9\beta_1$-integrins highly expressed throughout the human airway epithelia and thereby would be of interest for gene delivery of cystic fibrosis (Schneider *et al.*, 1998).

Molossin

Molossin is a 15 amino acid moiety derived from the snake venom of the American pit viper *Crotuluis molossus molossus*, encompassing the RGDNP motif which has an affinity for $\alpha_5\beta_1$ and $\alpha_v\beta_3$ integrins. A 31 amino acid peptide containing molossin for cellular targeting and an oligolysine of 16 residues (K_{16}) as DNA binding moiety has been synthesized and evaluated as a receptor-mediated gene delivery system. The system was able to transfect about 30% of corneal endothelial cells of rabbit, pig and human in the presence of chloroquine (Shewring *et al.*, 1997). Associated with the fusogenic peptide of influenza, this peptide transfected 25–30% of primary cultures of vascular smooth muscle cells of man, rabbit and rat (Collins *et al.*, 2000; Li *et al.*, 2000). The molossin-based gene delivery system represents an interesting system in transplantation because the molossin peptide does not bind to vascular endothelium and pancreatic islets.

Serpins

The serpin-enzyme complex receptor (SECR) is expressed in particular on hepatocytes and macrophages. It recognizes and cleaves serine protease inhibitors (called serpins) such as α1-antitrypsin. SECR recognizes with a high affinity a critical five amino acid peptide (FVFLI) of α1-antitrypsin and induces its uptake and degradation. PAT2 peptide with an oligolysine of 16 residues (K_{16}) for DNA condensation, followed by the sequence CSIPPEVKFNKPFVFLI that contained the critical peptide for cellular targeting, has been designed (Patel *et al.*, 2001). PAT2/DNA complexes showed an efficient transfection (20–25%) of a human hepatocarcinoma cell line (HUH7 cells) in the presence of chloroquine. Transfection was ligand specific because it was blocked in the presence of the free ligand (CSIPPEVKFNKPFVFLI). This study also evidenced that the length of the space between the condensing moiety K_{16} and the ligand motif FVFLI is important for the selectivity: the peptide K_{16}-FNKPFVFLI containing only four residues was much less efficient.

Sugars

Membrane lectins that selectively recognize glycoconjugates containing complex oligosaccharide structures are expressed at the cell surface of many mammalian cells and can mediate endocytosis of glycoconjugates (for a review see Monsigny *et al.*, 1988). Galactoside-terminated glycoproteins (asialoglycoproteins) are taken up by the liver parenchymal cells via a membrane lectin recognizing galactose (Ashwell and Harford, 1982). Macrophages (Stahl *et al.*, 1984) and dendritic cells (Sallusto *et al.*, 1995; Avrameas *et al.*, 1996) express a mannose/fucose specific receptor that induces the uptake of mannosylated and fucosylated conjugates. Therefore, glycoconjugates are good candidates to design selective gene delivery systems (for a review see Monsigny *et al.*, 1994 and 1999). Mono and disaccharides have been used to prepare glycosylated polylysines (Midoux *et al.*, 1993; Erbacher *et al.*, 1996b; Kollen *et al.*, 1996; Fajac *et al.*, 1999; Allo *et al.*, 2000) and polyethylenimines (Zanta *et al.*, 1997; Erbacher *et al.*, 1999; Bettinger *et al.*, 1999; Diebold *et al.*, 1999a,b). However, complex oligosaccharides have a very high binding capacity and selectivity towards cell surface lectins as compared to mono- and disaccharides. Galactose-specific hepatocyte lectin binds triantennary oligosaccharides with Galβ-4GlcNAc moieties in a terminal non-reducing position, with an affinity 1000-fold higher than monosaccharides with a single Galβ-4GlcNAc moiety in a terminal non-reducing position (Lee *et al.*, 1983). Therefore, natural oligosaccharides isolated from biological fluids or released by enzymatic or chemical means from natural polysaccharides, glycoproteins or glycolipids are expected to be very specific and selective ligands for gene targeting. The development of efficient chemical methods will increase the use of such ligands. For instance, a method based on the transformation of the unprotected reducing end of oligosaccharides into *N*-glyco-amino acids and protection by *N*-acylation gives complex oligosaccharides, which are ready to prepare highly selective glycosylated polymers and peptides (Monsigny *et al.*, 1998).

To attach oligosaccharides onto the condensing moiety CWK$_{18}$, tyrosinamide derivatives of *N*-glycans have been synthesized (for a review see Rice, 2000). Upon transformation in *N*-iodoacetyl oligosaccharides, the sugars can be linked to CWK$_{18}$ via cysteine. A galactoside-terminated triantenary oligosaccharide (Tri-CWK$_{18}$) and an oligomannoside (Man9-CWK$_{18}$), followed by the CWK$_{18}$ peptide for pDNA condensation, have been prepared for hepatocyte and macrophage targeting (Collard *et al.*, 2000a). pDNA condensates of 110 nm and a global charge of 31 mV were obtained with the resulting glycopeptides. Unfortunately, Tri-CWK$_{18}$/DNA condensates were rapidly dissociated once injected in mouse, avoiding specific targeting to hepatocytes (Collard *et al.*, 2000b). To overcome this problem, DNA condensates were cross-linked by using glutaraldehyde, leading to particles of 50 nm with a charge of 34 mV. However, due to their high positive charge, these DNA condensates were opsonized and accumulated in the lung. When a single PEG molecule of 5000 Da was coupled to CWK$_{18}$, PEG-peptide DNA condensates exhibit a size of 80–90 nm, a reduced charge of 10 mV (versus 34 mV) and a water solubility 20-fold greater than with the non PEG-peptide. In addition, PEGylation preserves peptide DNA condensates upon freeze drying (Kwok *et al.*, 2000). Despite their low efficiency in transfecting HepG2 cells, PEGylated peptide/DNA condensates offer great advantages for *in vivo* gene delivery (Kwok *et al.*, 1999). Indeed, such modifications were found to improve the biodistribution, metabolism, cellular targeting and gene expression in mice (Collard *et al.*, 2000b). There is no doubt that caged DNA made with PEGylated CHK$_6$HC glycopeptide carrying CTS (histidyl residues) would further increase the efficiency.

PEPTIDES CONTAINING NUCLEAR LOCALIZATION SIGNAL DOMAINS

Plasmids must reach the cell nucleus for gene expression but the nuclear envelope is a highly selective barrier and the nuclear pores do not permit pDNA passage. In the absence of cell division, passive diffusion through nuclear pores occurs for molecules with a diameter of 9 nm or below (the inner diameter of a nuclear pore), such as ovalbumin (43 kDa), whereas that of serum albumin (64 kDa) does not. Larger proteins require an active transport process that involves nuclear localization signal (NLS) molecules. To date, a large number of NLS peptide sequences have been evidenced (for reviews see Nigg, 1997; Mattaj and Englmeier, 1998). Classical NLS contain one or two stretches of basic amino acid residues that are recognized by cytoplasmic carriers termed karyopherins or importins. The best known NLS is that of the large T-antigen of the SV40 virus with a minimal sequence PKKKRKV.

The addition of NLS in a non viral gene delivery system is expected to favor the nuclear import (nuclear pores allow the passage of particles of 24 nm) by using the karyopherin and importin machinery. Where should the NLS be linked, on the pDNA or on the carrier? For the latter strategy, polyplexes must not dissociate before their import in the cell nucleus. Both strategies have been prospected but with only limited success.

The assembly of NLS in peptide-based gene delivery systems has been achieved by the non-covalent binding of plasmid to either free NLS embedded with polyplexes or to NLS linked to a cationic sequence, such as $(PKKKRKV)_4\text{-}K_{20}$ (Table 16.7), $AKRARLSTSFNPVYPYEDES\text{-}K_{20}$ (Table 16.7) or H9-2 sequence (nls-H9-2) (Table 16.4). With nls-H9-2, the transfection efficiency with a formulation containing cationic lipids was quite similar to that obtained with H9-2 without NLS. Variation in the transfection efficiency using NLS could be due to differences in the intracellular trafficking of pDNA when formulated as NLS-polyplexes or NLS-lipoplexes. But the low efficiency could also result from the dissociation of the NLS from the plasmid, either in endocytic vesicles or in the cytosol before its nuclear import.

A direct attachment of the NLS sequence (CGYGPKKKRKVGG) to pDNA performed using a cyclopropapyrroloindole cross-linker was found to induce the

Table 16.7 Peptide inducing both condensation, translocation and nuclear import of DNA

Peptide sequences	DBS	CTS	NLS	References
$(PKKKRKV)_4\text{-}K_{20}$ (GenePort)	+	+/−	+	Ritter *et al.*, 1999
VAYISRGGVSTYYSDTVKGRFTRQKYNKRA-K_{19} (K_{19}-P3)	+	+	+	Avrameas *et al.*, 1998
GALFLGFLGAAGSTMGAWSQPKSKRKV (MPG)	+	+	+	Morris *et al.*, 1999
AKRARLSTSFNPVYPYEDES-K_{20}	+	+	+	Zhang *et al.*, 1999
DTWTGVEALIRILQQLLFIHFRIGCRHSRIGII QQRRTRNGASKS (Vpr52-96)	+	+	+	Kichler *et al.*, 2000
Loligomer4	+	+	+	Singh *et al.*, 1999

Notes
DBS, CTS and NLS stand for DNA binding signal, cytosolic translocation signal and nuclear localization signal, respectively.

nuclear accumulation of pDNA in digitonin-permeabilized cells (Sebestyén *et al.*, 1998). However, this conjugate did not allow the nuclear accumulation after microinjection into the cytoplasm of cultured cells. Taking into account the low diffusion of pDNA in the cytosol, this result is not surprising (Lukacs *et al.*, 2000). The cytosol of permeabilized cells is probably more fluid and therefore allows a better diffusion of the plasmid.

NLS was elegantly conjugated to specific peptide nucleic acid (PNA) and bound strongly to pDNA (Brandén *et al.*, 1999). PNA-NLS can hybridize to a plasmid containing one or more copies of the complementary DNA sequence with an affinity that is much stronger than that of a DNA–DNA hybrid. This system preserves transgene expression. In combination with polyethylenimine, the transfection was increased by only eight-fold. Nowadays, the PNA clamp technology offers the possibility of linking pDNA to any peptide sequences with a high affinity and preservation of the gene expression (Zelphati *et al.*, 1999, 2000).

In an original manner, one SV40 NLS sequence has been covalently linked to one end of a linear plasmid encoding Luciferase (Zanta *et al.*, 1999). In combination with polyethylenimine, transfection efficiency was increased 10- to 1000-fold, depending on the cell types compared to the same construction containing a non-functional mutated NLS.

Despite several attempts performed with pDNA combined with NLS, transfection efficiency has been only weakly improved. This minor improvement suggests that other strategies or other types of NLS such as sugars (Duverger *et al.*, 1995, 1996) should be explored, but also that other limiting steps have to be fully considered and optimized. Amongst them, the translocation and fate of pDNA or polyplexes in the cytosol have to be unraveled. The fact that pDNA does not diffuse in the cytosol (Lukacs *et al.*, 2000) and that a cytosolic nuclease activity has been evidenced in this compartment (Lechardeur *et al.*, 1999; Pollard *et al.*, 2001) has to be considered in new strategies for the assembling of multi-components with defined functions.

DNA UNPACKAGING

Self-assembly of pDNA in an aqueous solution induces condensation in small spherical particles, which is reversible. Although unpackaging of pDNA is expected in the nucleus for transcription, it can also occur in other compartments and can thus modify its destiny. For instance, pDNA released from polyplexes and taken up by the cells may be induced by endogenous anionic lipids, as proposed in the case of DNA/cationic lipid complexes (Xu and Szoka, 1996). We have found that polyplexes made with lactosylated polylysine are dissociated more easily by dextran sulfate than polyplexes made with histidylated polylysine (HpK). Moreover, substitution of HpK with lactosyl residues drastically reduces the stability of polyplexes. This suggests that upon dissociation, a different trafficking can occur between polymers and pDNA. Indeed, pDNA segregates rapidly within 30 minutes from either lactosylated polylysine or lactosylated histidylated polylysine into separate compartments, whereas histidylated polylysine and pDNA remain associated for a longer period. These observations are in agreement with those reported for DNA/RGD-oligolysine/LipofectAMINE complexes, which are also dissociated upon

30 minutes of uptake (Colin *et al.*, 2000). We have also noticed that the most stable polyplexes gave the best transfection efficiency. An early dissociation of polyplexes could be prevented by using caged pDNA prepared by cross-linking polymers via disulfide bonds as previously described (Trubetskoy *et al.*, 1999; McKenzie *et al.*, 2000a). But it has to be kept in mind that the stability of polyplexes could be a limiting factor for enhanced transfection by preventing pDNA release and the accessibility of the nuclear machinery.

It is still unknown if unpackaging of pDNA inside the cytoplasm is useful for efficient transfection. Several lines of evidence suggest that a decrease of the strength of electrostatic interactions between pDNA and polylysine favors pDNA dissociation from the polyplexes and enhances transfection efficiency. Indeed, reduction of the number of positive charges on polylysine after a partial substitution of the ε-amino groups with uncharged residues, such as carbohydrate moieties (Erbacher *et al.*, 1995) or polyhydroxyalcanoyl (gluconoyl) residues (Erbacher *et al.*, 1997), has been shown to facilitate *in vitro* dissociation of polyplexes and to increase the transfection efficiency. Recent data have shown that the transfection efficiency of EGF-polylysine/DNA complexes is correlated with the un-packaging of pDNA and a decrease in the stability of polyplexes according to the length of polylysine (Schaffer *et al.*, 2000). Indeed, polyplexes made with a polylysine of dp190, which are more stable than polyplexes made with polylysine of dp36, were less efficient in transfection. In addition, fluorescence microscopy analyses have shown that both pDNA and polymer are present inside the nucleus of few cells when EGF-polylysine/pDNA polyplexes are made with polylysine of dp190, indicating that polyplexes were not dissociated. Conversely, only pDNA is detected inside the cell nucleus when polyplexes are made with polylysine of dp36, indicating that polyplexes were dissociated. These data might suggest that a facilitated dissociation of polyplexes might make the plasmid more accessible to the nuclear machinery for gene expression.

An un-packaging of pDNA is expected by using disulfide-containing cationic polymers or peptides in a reductive medium such as the cytosol. This would favor the passage of pDNA bearing NLS through the nuclear pores. Indeed, it is probably excluded that in the absence of cell division pDNA condensates of 50–100 nm bearing NLS can be imported through the nuclear pores.

It has been shown that disulfide-containing cationic lipids, such as $1',2'$ dioleoyl-*sn*-glycero-$3'$-succinyl-2-hydroxyethyl disulfide ornithine conjugate (DOGSDSO) (Tang and Hughes, 1998), cholesteryl hemidithiodiglycolyl tris(aminoethyl)amine (CHDTAEA) (Tang and Hughes, 1999), as well as lipoic acid-derived amphiphiles (Balakirev *et al.*, 2000), are more efficient than their non-disulfide analogs in transfection. In the case of cationic polymers and peptides, caged DNA increases transfection efficiency both by increasing the stability of polyplexes in the extracellular medium and by the release of pDNA upon reduction of disulfide bonds in the cytosol (McKenzie, 2000a,b).

We designed disulfide-containing polylysine conjugates with amino groups interacting with phosphate DNA linked to the polymer backbone via a disulfide bond. As evidenced by agarose gel electrophoresis, polyplexes formed with this polymer are dissociated in the presence of dithiothreitol (Figure 16.5). Electron microscopy showed that polyplexes are largely de-condensed in the presence of 10 mM glutathione. Finally, we have found that the transfection of 293T7

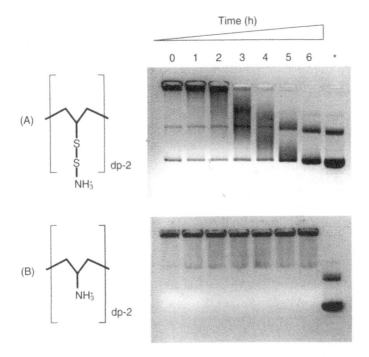

Figure 16.5 DTT releases pDNA from a disulfide-containing polylysine conjugate. pSV2luc plasmid (20 µg in 280 µl 10 mM Hepes buffer, pH 7.4) was mixed with either (A) disulfide-containing polylysine (80 µg) or (B) polylysine (40 µg) in 120 µl 10 mM Hepes buffer, pH 7.4. After 30 minutes at 20 °C, polyplexes (50 µl; 2.5 µg plasmid) were incubated at 37 °C for various times in the presence of 0.1 M DTT. Samples (20 µl) were analyzed by 0.8% agarose gel electrophoresis. *pSV2luc plasmid.

and HepG2 cells is 10- and 50-fold more efficient with the disulfide-containing polylysine conjugate than polylysine (Figure 16.6). These results indicate that disulfide-containing cationic polymers are promising DNA carriers. They could be also useful for the release of RNA and oligonucleotides in the cytosol.

PEPTIDE FROM ANTI-DNA ANTIBODIES

Anti-deoxyribonucleic acid autoantibodies from human and mice suffering from *Lupus erythematosus* can penetrate into cells and accumulate in the cell nucleus. Based on the characteristics of anti-DNA autoantibodies, VAYISRGGVSTYYS-DTVKGRFTRQKYNKRA peptide (P3), which exhibits α-helix, has been used as a vector for the intracytoplasmic and intranuclear translocation of macromolecules (Table 16.7) (Avrameas *et al.*, 1998, 1999). P3 shares similar capabilities with Antenapedia peptide (Derossi *et al.*, 1994), but in contrast P3 operates only at 37 °C by an energy dependent mechanism. P3 linked to a 19 lysine residue sequence (K_{19}-P3) forms complexes with plasmid DNA. Efficient transfection of mouse 3T3 cells and hamster lung CCL39 cells were obtained with these complexes. This transfection

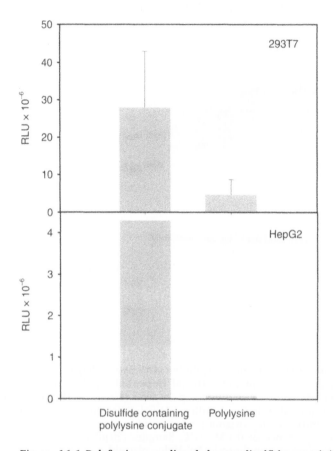

Figure 16.6 Polyfection mediated by a disulfide-containing polylysine conjugate. (A) 293-T7 cells and (B) HepG2 cells were incubated for four hours at 37 °C with pCMVluc (5 µg) complexed with either disulfide-containing polylysine (20 µg) or polylysine (15 µg) in the presence of 10% FCS and 100 µM chloroquine. The luciferase activity was measured after 48 hours culture and expressed as the relative light units (RLU) per 10^6 cells.

was not impaired by the presence of serum and did not require helper molecules such as chloroquine. These observations suggest that peptides from cell specific anti-DNA autoantibodies may represent a source of peptide-based gene delivery system with different specificities.

HIV-1 gp41

The MPG (GALFLGFLGAAGSTMGAWSQPKSKRKV) peptide that combines a fusion peptide sequence from the hydrophobic fusion protein of HIV-1 gp41 and the hydrophilic NLS sequence of SV40 large T antigen can deliver oligo-nucleotides and plasmid DNA into cells independently of the endocytic pathway (Table 16.7). Stable DNA/peptide complexes are formed via electrostatic inter-actions with the positively charged NLS sequence. It was claimed that the hydro-phobic part containing the peptide derived from the HIV-1 gp41 forms a cage around the plasmid and mediates the translocation of the complexes through the plasma membrane. In this system, no obvious data showed the involvement of the NLS sequence in the nuclear import of pDNA.

ADENOVIRAL FIBER PROTEIN-BASED PEPTIDES

Structural proteins of the adenovirus, such as fiber proteins, are synthesized in the cytoplasm and then transported to the nucleus of infected cells where the virus assembly takes place. AKRARLSTSFNPVYPYEDES peptide corresponding to the 20 N-terminal residues of adenoviral fiber protein, followed with a short polylysine of 20 lysine residues, has been synthesized (Zhang *et al.*, 1999) (Table 16.7). The peptide contains a nuclear localization signal (AKRARLSTS) and a hydrophobic domain (FNPVYPYEDES), which contains the tyrosine motif (NPVY) found in the cytoplasmic domain of the low density lipoprotein receptor involved in the endocytosis of LDL. Plasmid DNA encoding Luciferase complexed with the above peptide was able to enter the nucleus and transfect the cells. The transfection level was better than that obtained with liposomes such as DOTAP and DOSPER. The FNPVYPY motif, reminiscent of a transmembrane domain, is supposed to interact with and disturb membranes, and thus favors the cytosolic translocation of pDNA. In contrast to the HIV-1 TAT peptide and the third helix of *Antenapedia*, this peptide is not active at 4 °C. The translocation through endosomes was not clear and the internalization mediated by endocytosis pathway was not demonstrated.

Viral protein R (Vpr)

The viral protein R (Vpr) of HIV-1 plays a significant role early in the viral life cycle by facilitating the nuclear import of the preintegration complex in non-dividing cells. The C-terminal domain of Vpr (Vpr52-96), which condenses plasmid DNA, mediates DNA transfection in a variety of human and non-human cell lines (Table 16.7). The Vpr52-96 sequence (DTWTGVEALIRILQQLLFIH-FRIGCRHSRIGIIQQRRTRNGASKS) contains an α-helix domain (residues 52–78), a leucine/isoleucine rich domain (residues 60–84) and an arginine rich domain (residues 73–96) (Kichler *et al.*, 2000). Depending on the cell lines, Vpr52-96 is 10- (HeLa cells) to 500- (HepG2 cells) fold more active in transfecting cells than polylysine. Vpr52-96 was 2- to 20-fold more efficient than polyethylenimine; 26% of 293 cells expressed GFP upon transfection with Vpr52-96, which was as great (37%) as the transfection efficiency with DOTAP. The majority of complexes were found in endosomes, but the transfection efficiency was shown to be insensitive to bafilomycin A1, a specific inhibitor of the vacuolar protein pump. The authors suggest that the active fraction of Vpr52-96/pDNA complexes ending up in the nucleus either avoids the endocytic route or can be released from endosomes by a pH-independent mechanism.

Loligomers

Loligomers are branched or squid-like peptides that contain multifunctional domains presented on a tentacular scaffold. In general, lysine residues give rise to a branched peptide, which presents multiple domains that code for functions, such as cellular delivery, cell signaling, and/or cytotoxicity. Loligomer4 consists of a 5 amino acid long (KCGYA) C-terminal region and eight identical N-terminal arms linked together via two glycyl residues through a branched lysine polymer. Each N-terminal arm contains a SV40 large T antigen NLS domain (TPPKKKRKVEDP) and a lysine pentapeptide acting as a cytoplasmic translocation signal (CTS) domain, which allow it to penetrate cells and relocate to their nucleus (Singh *et al.*, 1999). Loligomer4 was synthesized by solid-phase peptide synthesis. Loligomer4 forms electrostatic complexes with pDNA via its cationic structure and the phosphate backbone of pDNA. Despite the multi-domain combination, pDNA/Loligomer4 complexes (weight ratio of 1:3) showed Luciferase expression of 3×10^7 RLU/mg protein corresponding to the transfection of 5–10% CHO cells. Transfection efficiency of Loligomer4/plasmid complexes was greater when cells were maintained as suspension instead of monolayers (Singh *et al.*, 1999).

RECOMBINANT PROTEIN-BASED GENE DELIVERY SYSTEMS

New concepts for the design of powerful multi-component peptides could be inspired by data obtained using chimeric fusion proteins that combine several domains with defined functions. This strategy was explored using the first 147 amino acids of the Yeast transcriptional activator GAL4 containing a specific DNA binding domain. This domain also contains a NLS different from that of the SV40 virus recognized by the β subunit of the importin complex instead of the α subunit. Chimeric proteins containing both a DNA-binding signal (DBS), cytoplasmic translocation signal (CTS), CRS and NLS domains are exemplified by GD5 and TEG fusion proteins (Table 16.8). GD5 combines the GAL4 DNA binding domain, the translocation domain Val^{195}-Gly^{383} of the diphteria toxin (DT) as CTS domain and a scFv fragment of antibodies directed against ErbB2, a tumor associated antigen over-expressed in many human tumors, for cellular targeting. TEG was engineered by the fusion of cDNA fragment of the tumor growth factor alpha (TGFα) for cellular targeting via the EGF receptor to sequences encoding the GAL4 DNA binding domain and the translocation domain of *pseudomonas* exotoxin A (ETA) as CTS. It is worth noting that polylysine has to be added to protein/DNA complexes to neutralize excessive pDNA charges and to facilitate pDNA condensation.

Table 16.8 Recombinant protein-based gene delivery systems

	DBS	CTS	NLS	CRS	*References*
GAL4 – DT – ErbB2scFv (GD5)	+	+	+	+	Uherek *et al.*, 1998
GAL4 – ETA – TGFα (TEG)	+	+	+	+	Fominaya *et al.*, 1998
GAL4 – PLSSIFSRIGDP-NLS (PreS2)	+	+	+	–	Hildt *et al.*, 1999
GAL4-MSH + pLK-NLS	+	–	+	+	Chan and Jans, 2001

Notes
DBS, CTS, NLS and CRS stand for DNA binding signal, cytosolic translocation signal, nuclear localization signal and cell recognition signal, respectively. MSH is α-melanocyte stimulating hormone. pLK is polylysine.

Transfection efficiency of these chimeric proteins remained low. This low transfection efficiency is probably due to the fact that GAL4 is inefficient for targeting pDNA in the nucleus. Indeed, DBS and NLS activities of GAL4 are mutually exclusive (Chan *et al.*, 1998). Recently, Chan and Jans (2001) have reported that SV40 NLS linked to polylysine, combined with a GAL4 system, increased the pDNA nuclear targeting and transfection efficiency (Table 16.8). Another example is GAL4 combined with the PreS2-domain of hepatitis B virus surface antigens (Table 16.8). PreS2 domain (41–52) exhibits a short amphipathic α-helical PLSSIFSRIGDP peptide which confers a cell permeability activity to PreS2 protein, as well as to any unrelated proteins when fused to it. PreS2 protein is translocated both at 4 and 37 °C in the cytoplasmic compartment but does not reach the cell nucleus. When linked to EGFP, the peptide 41–52 is sufficient to translocate the functional protein across the plasma membrane of cultured and primary cells (Oess and Hildt, 2000). Derived peptides with the following sequences PISSIFS-RIGDP, PISSIFSRTGDP and HISSISARTGDP sharing the amphipathic character exhibit a similar efficiency to PreS2. On this basis, a GAL4 DNA binding domain fusion protein was produced that contained the peptide 41–52 of PreS2 and a NLS. When complexed with plasmid encoding EGFP, the fusion protein allowed a very high transfection.

CONCLUDING REMARKS

Therapeutic applications of non-viral gene delivery systems are rather limited despite the latest achievements performed in the design of various systems. Multi-component peptides exhibiting several attributes for bypassing extracellular and intracellular barriers are promising for designing efficient gene delivery systems. Most of the described gene delivery systems need an endosome destabilization. Combined with peptides enabling DNA condensation and cell selectivity, various acidic pH-dependent fusogenic peptides have demonstrated their efficiency in transfecting cultured cells. Amongst them, histidine-rich peptides exhibiting membrane destabilization in a less acidic medium (close to that of the early endosome lumen), which is not impaired in the presence of serum, seem more interesting than glutamic-rich peptides. But the non-covalent or covalent assembly of fusogenic peptides with polyplexes is still not achieved for *in vivo* gene delivery. Therefore, binding of small devices enabling endosome destabilization on peptides exhibiting DNA condensation will allow DNA formulations to reach the cytoplasm more efficiently. This is the case for polylysine substituted with histidyl residues and cationic peptides containing histidines such as CHK_6HC. Despite the fact that small peptides are well-defined compounds, they form polyplexes that are unstable in extracellular medium. Intercross-linking of polyplexes via disulfide bonds is an elegant way to prevent their dissociation until they reach the cytosol.

Conceptually, DBS, CTS, NLS and CRS attributes have proven to confer their respective functions quite efficiently. However, when they were combined in a multi-component system, enhancement of the transfection efficiency was not as high as expected. This low transfection efficiency is the case of peptides listed in Table 16.7 and recombinant protein-based gene delivery systems listed in Table 16.8. This suggests that the assembly of the attributes does not meet all the requirements needed for efficient translocation of genes into the nucleus. The structure, intracellular trafficking and cytosolic stability of the polyplexes have significant influences on transfection efficiency. More knowledge about these processes will be helpful in choosing the right attributes for an efficient gene delivery system. For instance, the activity of an NLS contained in a multi-component system will depend on the formation of small polyplexes and the preservation of their stability until they reach the cell nucleus. While polycations should dissociate from plasmids in the cytosol, NLS should remain in contact with the plasmids to facilitate their translocation to the nucleus. A better knowledge on the intracellular trafficking of polyplexes, the fate of plasmid DNA in the cytosol, and a control of DNA packaging and un-packaging inside cells would enhance the levels of transgene expression. Finally, the engineering of pDNA with specific DNA sequences recognized by transcription factors that are imported in the nucleus, as well as the sequences for gene regulation, should also be explored. In addition, the biology and the host cell response of the target cells deserve more attention to the correct design of the corresponding gene delivery system. Indeed, one system, which will allow efficient transfection in epithelial cells or hepatocytes will unlikely be efficient for macrophages or dendritic cells.

ACKNOWLEDGMENTS

Our works reported in this chapter were supported by grants from Agence Nationale de Recherche contre le Sida (ANRS), Association pour la Recherche sur le Cancer (ARC), Association Française de Lutte contre la Mucoviscidose (AFLM) and European Union (EU Bio4-CT97-2216).

REFERENCES

Allo, J.-C., Midoux, P., Merten, M., Souil, E., Lipecka, J., Figarella, C. *et al.* (2000) Efficient gene transfer into human normal and cystic fibrosis tracheal gland serous cells with synthetic vectors. *Am. J. Res. Cell Mol. Biol.*, **22**, 166–175.

Ashwell, G. and Harford, J. (1982) Carbohydrate-specific receptors of the liver. *Annu. Rev. Biochem.*, **51**, 531–554.

Avrameas, A., Mc Ilroy, D., Hosmalin, A., Autran, B., Debré, P., Monsigny, M. *et al.* (1996) Expression of a mannose/fucose membrane lectin on human dendritic cells. *Eur. J. Immunol.*, **26**, 394–400.

Avrameas, A., Ternynck, T., Gasmi, L. and Buttin, G. (1999) Efficient gene delivery by a peptide derived from a monoclonal anti-DNA antibody. *Bioconjug. Chem.*, **10**, 87–93.

Avrameas, A., Ternynck, T., Nato, F., Buttin, G. and Avrameas, S. (1998) Polyreactive anti-DNA monoclonal antibodies and a derived peptide as vectors for the intracytoplasmic and intranuclear translocation of macromolecules. *Proc. Natl. Acad. Sci. USA*, **95**, 5601–5606.

Balakirev, M., Schoehn, G. and Chroboczek, J. (2000) Lipoic acid-derived amphiphiles for redox-controlled DNA delivery. *Chem. Biol.*, **7**, 813–819.

Bello-Roufai, M. and Midoux, P. (2001) Histidylated polylysine as DNA vector: elevation of the imidazole protonation and reduced cellular uptake without change in the polyfection efficiency of serum stabilized negative polyplexes. *Bioconjug. Chem.*, **12**, 92–99.

Benns, J.M., Choi, J.-S., Mahato, R.I., Park, J.-S. and Kim, S.W. (2000) pH-sensitive cationic polymer gene delivery vehicle: N-Ac-poly(l-histidine)-graft-poly(L-lysine) comb shaped polymer. *Bioconjug. Chem.*, **11**, 637–645.

Bettinger, T., Remy, J.S. and Erbacher, P. (1999) Size reduction of galactosylated PEI/DNA complexes improves lectin-mediated transfer into hepatocytes. *Bioconjug. Chem.*, **10**, 558–561.

Blessing, T., Remy, J.S. and Behr, J.P. (1998) Monomolecular collapse of plasmid DNA into stable virus-like particles. *Proc. Natl. Acad. Sci. USA*, **95**, 1427–1431.

Bloomfield, V.A. (1998) DNA condensation by multivalent cations. *Biopolymers*, **44**, 269–282.

Boussif, O., Delair, T., Brua, C., Veron, L., Pavirani, A. and Kolben, H.V.J. (1999) Synthesis of polyallylamine derivatives and their use as gene transfer vectors *in vitro*. *Bioconjug. Chem.*, **10**, 877–883.

Boussif, O., Lezoualc'h, F., Zanta, M.A., Mergny, M.D., Scherman, D., Demeinex, B. *et al.* (1995) A versatile vector for gene and oligonucleotide transfer into cells in culture and *in vivo*. *Proc. Natl. Acad. Sci. USA*, **92**, 7297–7301.

Branden, L.J., Mohamed, A.J. and Smith, C.I. (1999) A peptide nucleic acid-nuclear localization signal fusion that mediates nuclear transport of DNA. *Nat. Biotechnol.*, **17**, 784–787.

Chalfie, M., Tu, Y., Euskirchen, G., Ward, W.W. and Prasher, D.C. (1994) Green fluorescent protein as a marker for gene expression. *Science*, **263**, 802–805.

Chan, C.K., Hübner, S., Hu, W. and Jans, D.A. (1998) Mutual exclusivity of DNA binding and nuclear localization signal recognition by the yeast transcription factor GAL4: implications for nonviral DNA delivery. *Gene Ther.*, **5**, 1204–1212.

Chan, C.K. and Jans, D.A. (2001) Enhancement of MSH receptor- and GAL4-mediated gene transfer by switching the nuclear import pathway. *Gene Ther.*, **8**, 166–171.

Colin, M., Harbottle, R.P., Knight, A., Kornprobst, M., Cooper, R.G., Miller, A.D. *et al.* (1998) Liposomes enhance delivery and expression of an RGD-oligolysine gene transfer vector in human tracheal cells. *Gene Ther.*, **5**, 1488–1498.

Colin, M., Maurice, M., Truggnan, G., Kornprobst, M., Harbottle, R.P., Knight, A. *et al.* (2000) Cell delivery, intracellular trafficking and expression of an integrin-mediated gene transfer vector in tracheal epithelial cells. *Gene Ther.*, **7**, 139–152.

Collard, W.T., Evers, D.L., McKenzie, D.L. and Rice, K.G. (2000a) Synthesis of homogeneous glycopeptides and their utility as DNA condensing agents. *Carbohydrate Res.*, **323**, 176–184.

Collard, W.T., Yang, Y., Kwok, K.Y., Park, Y. and Rice, K.G. (2000b) Biodistribution, metabolism, and *in vivo* gene expression of low molecular weight glycopeptide polyethylene glycol peptide DNA co-condensates. *J. Pharm. Sci.*, **89**, 499–512.

Collins, L., Sawyer, G.J., Zhang, X.-H., Gustafsson, K. and Fabre, J.W. (2000) *In vitro* investigation of factors important for the delivery of an integrin-targeted nonviral DNA vector in organ transplantation. *Transplantation*, **69**, 1168–1176.

Danieli, T., Pelletier, Henis, Y.I. and White, J.M. (1996) Membrane fusion mediated by the influenza virus hemagglutinin requires the action of at least three hemagglutinin trimers. *J. Cell Biol.*, **133**, 559–569.

Dempsey, C.E. (1990) The actions of melittin on membranes. *Biochim. Biophys. Acta*, **1031**, 143–161.

Derossi, D., Joliot, A.H., Chassaing, G. and Prochiantz, A. (1994) The third helix of the Antennapedia homeodomain translocates through biological membranes. *J. Biol. Chem.*, **269**, 10444–10450.

Diebold, S.S., Kursa, M., Wagner, E., Cotten, M. and Zenke, M. (1999a) Mannose polyethylenimine conjugates for targeted DNA delivery into dendritic cells. *J. Biol. Chem.*, **274**, 19087–19094.

Diebold, S.S., Lehrmann, H., Kursa, M., Wagner, E., Cotten, M. and Zenke, M. (1999b) Efficient gene delivery into human dendritic cells by adenovirus polyethylenimine and mannose polyethylenimine transfection. *Hum. Gene Ther.*, **10**, 775–786.

Duverger, E., Pellerin-Mendes, C., Mayer, R., Roche, A.C. and Monsigny, M. (1995) Nuclear import of glycoconjugates is distinct from the classical NLS pathway. *J. Cell Sci.*, **108**, 1325–1332.

Duverger, E., Roche, A.C. and Monsigny, M. (1996) *N*-acetylglucosamine-dependent nuclear import of neoglycoproteins. *Glycobiology*, **6**, 381–386.

Ehrlich, P. (1906) *Collected Studies on Immunity*. John Wiley, New-York, Vol. II, pp. 442–447.

Erbacher, P., Bettinger, T., Belguise-Valladier, P., Zou, S., Coll, J.L., Behr, J.P. *et al.* (1999) Transfection and physical properties of various saccharide, poly(ethylene glycol) and antibody-derivatized polyethylenimines (PEI). *J. Gene Med.*, **1**, 210–222.

Erbacher, P., Roche, A.C., Monsigny, M. and Midoux, P. (1995) Glycosylated polylysine/DNA complexes: Gene transfer efficiency in relation with the size and the sugar substitution level of glycosylated polylysines and with the plasmid size. *Bioconjug. Chem.*, **6**, 401–410.

Erbacher, P., Roche, A.C., Monsigny, M. and Midoux, P. (1996a) Putative role of chloroquine in gene transfer into a human hepatoma cell line by DNA/lactosylated polylysine complexes. *Exp. Cell Res.*, **225**, 186–194.

Erbacher, P., Bousser, M.-T., Raimond, J., Monsigny, M., Midoux, P. and Roche, A.C. (1996b) Gene transfer by DNA/glycosylated polylysine complexes into human blood monocyte-derived macrophages. *Hum. Gene Ther.*, **7**, 721–729.

Erbacher, P., Roche, A.C., Monsigny, M. and Midoux, P. (1997) The reduction of the positive charges of polylysine by partial gluconoylation increases the transfection efficiency of polylysine/DNA complexes. *Biochim. Biophys. Acta*, **1324**, 27–36.

Fajac, I., Allo, J.-C., Souil, E., Merten, M., Pichon, C., Figarella, C. *et al.* (2000) Histidylated polylysine as a synthetic vector for gene transfer into cystic fibrosis airway surface and airway gland serous cells. *J. Gene Med.*, **2**, 368–378.

Fajac, I., Briand, P., Monsigny, M. and Midoux, P. (1999) Sugar-mediated uptake of glycosylated polylysines and gene transfer into normal and cystic fibrosis airway epithelial cells. *Hum. Gene Ther.*, **10**, 395–406.

Felgner, P.L., Barenholz, Y., Behr, J.P., Cheng, S.H., Cullis, P., Huang, L. *et al.* (1997) Nomenclature for synthetic gene delivery systems. *Hum. Gene Ther.*, **8**, 511–512.

Fominaya, J., Gasset, M., Garcia, R., Roncal, F., Albar, J.P. and Bernad, A. (2000) An optimized amphiphilic cationic peptides as an efficient non-viral gene delivery vector. *J. Gene Med.*, **2**, 455–464.

Fominaya, J., Uherek, C. and Wels, W. (1998) A chimeric fusion protein containing transforming growth factor-alpha mediates gene transfer via binding to the EGF receptor. *Gene Ther.*, **5**, 521–530.

Freulon, I., Monsigny, M., Midoux, P. and Mayer, R. (2000) Spacer length dependence on the efficiency of dimeric anionic peptides in gene transfer by glycosylated polylysine/plasmid complexes. *Biosci. Rep.*, **20**, 383–398.

Fujii, G., Selsted, M.E. and Eisenberg, D. (1993) Defensins promote fusion and lysis of negatively charged membranes. *Protein Sci.*, **2**, 1301–1312.

Glaser, R.W., Grüne, M., Wandelt, C. and Ulrich, A.S. (1999) Structure analysis of a fusogenic peptide sequence from the Sea Urchin fertilization protein binding. *Biochemistry*, **38**, 2560–2569.

Godbey, W.T., Wu, K.K. and Mikos, A.G. (1999) Poly(ethylenimine) and its role in gene delivery. *J. Control. Release*, **60**, 149–160.

Gottschalk, S., Sparrow, J.T., Hauer, J., Mims, M.P., Leland, F.E., Woo, S.L.C. *et al.* (1996) A novel DNA-peptide complex for efficient gene transfer and expression in mammalian cells. *Gene Ther.*, **3**, 448–457.

Haensler, J. and Szoka, F.C. (1993) Polyamidoamine cascade polymers mediate efficient transfection of cells in culture. *Bioconjug. Chem.*, **4**, 372–379.

Harbottle, R.P., Cooper, R.G., Hart, S.L., Ladhoff, A., McKay, T., Knight, A.M. *et al.* (1998) An RGD-oligolysine peptide: a prototype construct for integrin-mediated gene delivery. *Hum. Gene Ther.*, **9**, 1037–1047.

Hildt, E., Oess, S. and Wollersheim, M. (1999) Cell permeable GAL4-DNA binding domain as an efficient tool in gene transfer. *J. Gene Med.*, **1** (Suppl. 6), 31.

Hughson, F.M. (1997) Enveloped viruses: a common mode of membrane fusion? *Curr. Biol.*, **7**, R565–R569.

Kichler, A., Freulon, I., Boutin, V., Mayer, R., Monsigny, M. and Midoux, P. (1999) Glycofection in the presence of anionic fusogenic peptides: a study of the parameters affecting the peptide-mediated enhancement of the transfection efficiency. *J. Gene Med.*, **1**, 134–143.

Kichler, A., Leborgne, C., Coeytaux, E. and Danos, O. (2001) Polyethylenimine-mediated gene delivery: a mechanistic study. *J. Gene Med.*, **3**, 135–144.

Kichler, A., Pages, J.C., Leborgne, C., Druillennec, S., Lenoir, C., Coulaud, D. *et al.* (2000) Efficient DNA transfection mediated by the C-terminal domain of human immuno-deficiency virus type 1 viral protein R. *J. Virol.*, **74**, 5424–5431.

Kielian, M. and Jungerwirth, S. (1990) Mechanisms of enveloped virus entry into cells. *Mol. Biol. Med.*, **7**, 17–31.

Kollen, W.J.W., Midoux, P., Erbacher, P., Yip, A., Roche, A.C., Monsigny, M. *et al.* (1996) Gluconoylated and glycosylated polylysines as vectors for gene transfer into cystic fibrosis airway epithelial cells. *Hum. Gene Ther.*, **7**, 1577–1586.

Kwok, K.Y., Adami, R.C., Hester, K.C., Park, Y., Thomas, S. and Rice, K.G. (2000) Strategies for maintaining the particle size of peptide DNA condensates following freeze-drying. *Int. J. Pharm.*, **203**, 81–88.

Kwok, K.Y., McKenzie, D.L., Evers, D.L. and Rice, K.G. (1999) Formulation of highly soluble poly(ethyle glycol)-peptide DNA condensates. *J. Pharm. Sci.*, **88**, 996–1003.

Lechardeur, D., Sohn, K.J., Haardt, M., Joshi, P.B., Monck, M., Graham, R.W. *et al.* (1999) Metabolic instability of plasmid DNA in the cytosol: a potential barrier to gene transfer. *Gene Ther.*, **6**, 482–497.

Lee, Y.C., Townsend, R.R., Hardy, M.R., Lonngren, J., Arnap, J., Haraldsson, M. *et al.* (1983) Binding of synthetic oligosaccharides to the hepatic Gal/GalNAc lectin. Dependence one fine structural features. *J. Biol. Chem.*, **258**, 199–202.

Li, J.-M., Collins, L., Zhang, X.-H., Gustafsson, K. and Fabre, J.W. (2000) Efficient gene delivery to vascular smooth muscle cells using a nontoxic, synthetic peptide vector system targeted to membrane integrins: a first step toward the gene therapy of chronic rejection. *Transplantation*, **70**, 1616–1624.

Lukacs, G.L., Haggie, P., Seksek, O., Lechardeur, D., Freedman, N. and Verkman, A.S. (2000) Size-dependent DNA mobility in cytoplasm and nucleus. *J. Biol. Chem.*, **275**, 1625–1629.

Mahato, R.I., Monera, O.D., Smith, L.C. and Rolland, A. (1999) Peptide-based gene delivery. *Curr. Opn. Mol. Ther.*, **1**, 226–243.

Mahato, R.I. (1999) Non-viral peptide-based approaches to gene delivery. *J. Drug Target.*, **7**, 249–268.

Mattaj, I.W. and Englmeier, L. (1998) Nucleocytoplasmic transport: the soluble phase. *Annu. Rev. Biochem.*, **123**, 265–306.

McKenzie, D.L., Collard, W.T. and Rice, K.G. (1999) Comparative gene transfer efficiency of low molecular weight polylysine DNA-condensing peptides. *J. Pept. Res.*, **54**, 311–318.

McKenzie, D.L., Kwok, K.Y. and Rice, K.G. (2000a) A potent new class of reductively activated peptide gene delivery agents. *J. Biol. Chem.*, **275**, 9970–9977.

McKenzie, D.L., Smiley, E., Kwok, K.Y. and Rice, K.G. (2000b) Low molecular weight disulfide cross-linking peptides as nonviral gene delivery carriers. *Bioconjug. Chem.*, **11**, 901–909.

Melino, S., Rufini, S., Sette, M., Morero, R., Grottesi, A., Paci, M. *et al.* (1999) Zn^{2+} ions selectively induce antimicrobial salivary peptide Histatin-5 to fuse negatively charged vesicles. Identification and characterization of a zinc-binding motif present in the functional domain. *Biochemistry*, **38**, 9626–9633.

Midoux, P., Kichler, A., Boutin, V., Maurizot, J.C. and Monsigny, M. (1998) Membrane permeabilization and efficient gene transfer by a peptide containing several histidines. *Bioconjug. Chem.*, **9**, 260–267.

Midoux, P., Mayer, R. and Monsigny, M. (1995) Membrane permeabilization by alpha-helical peptides: a flow cytometry study. *Biochim. Biophys. Acta*, **1239**, 249–256.

Midoux, P., Mendes, C., Legrand, A., Raimond, J., Mayer, R., Monsigny, M. *et al.* (1993) Specific gene transfer mediated by lactosylated poly-L-lysine into hepatoma cells. *Nucleic Acids Res.*, **21**, 871–878.

Midoux, P. and Monsigny, M. (1999) Efficient gene transfer by histidylated polylysine/pDNA complexes. *Bioconjug. Chem.*, **10**, 406–411.

Monsigny, M., Midoux, P., Mayer, R. and Roche, A.C. (1999) Glycotargeting: influence of the sugar moiety on both the uptake and the intracellular trafficking of nucleic acid carried by glycosylated polymers. *Biosci. Rep.*, **19**, 125–132.

Monsigny, M., Quétard, C., Bourgerie, S., Delay, D., Pichon, C., Midoux, P. *et al.* (1998) Glycotargeting: the preparation of glyco-amino acids and derivatives from unprotected reducing sugars. *Biochimie*, **80**, 99–108.

Monsigny, M., Roche, A.C., Kieda, C., Midoux, P. and Obrenovitch, A. (1988) Characterization and biological implications of membrane lectins in tumor, lymphoid and myeloid cells. *Biochimie*, **70**, 1633–1649.

Monsigny, M., Roche, A.C., Midoux, P. and Mayer, R. (1994) Glycoconjugates as carriers for specific delivery of therapeutic drugs and genes. *Adv. Drug Deliv. Rev.*, **14**, 1–24.

Morris, M.C., Chaloin, L., Méry, J., Heitz, F. and Divita, G. (1999) A novel potent strategy for gene delivery using a single peptide vector as a carrier. *Nucleic Acids Res.*, **27**, 3510–3517.

Murata, M., Sugahara, Y., Takahashi, S. and Ohnishi, S. (1987) pH-dependent membrane fusion activity of a synthetic twenty amino acid peptide with the same sequence as that of the hydrophobic segment of Influenza virus hemagglutinin. *J. Biochem.*, **102**, 957–962.

Murata, M., Takahashi, S., Kagiwada, S., Suzuki, A. and Ohnishi, S. (1992) pH-dependent membrane fusion and vesiculation of phospholipid large unilamellar vesicles induced by amphiphilic anionic and cationic peptides. *Biochemistry*, **31**, 1986–1992.

Nigg, E.A. (1997) Nucleocytoplasmic transport: signals, mechanisms and regulation. *Nature*, **386**, 779–787.

Niidome, T., Takaji, K., Urakawa, M., Ohmori, N., Wada, A., Hirayama, T. *et al.* (1999) Chain length of cationic alpha-helical peptide sufficient for gene delivery into cells. *Bioconjug. Chem.*, **10**, 773–780.

Oess, S. and Hildt, E. (2000) Novel cell permeable motif derived from the PreS2-domain hepatitis-B virus surface antigens. *Gene Ther.*, **7**, 750–758.

Ogris, M., Brunner, S., Schuller, S., Kircheis, R. and Wagner, E. (1999) PEGylated DNA/transferrin-PEI complexes: reduced interaction with blood components, extended circulation in blood and potential for systemic gene delivery. *Gene Ther.*, **6**, 595–605.

Ouyang, M., Remy, J.S. and Szoka, F.C. (2000) Controlled template-assisted assembly of plasmid DNA into nanometric particles with high DNA concentration. *Bioconjug. Chem.*, **11**, 104–112.

Patel, S., Zhang, X.-H., Collins, L. and Fabre, J.W. (2001) A small synthetic peptide for gene delivery via the serpin-enzyme complex receptor. *J. Gene Med.*, **3**, 271–279.

Perales, J.C., Grossmann, G.A., Molas, M., Liu, G., Ferkol, T., Harpst, J. *et al.* (1997) Biochemical and functional characterization of DNA complexes capable of targeting genes to hepatocytes via the asialoglycoprotein receptor. *J. Biol. Chem.*, **272**, 7398–7407.

Pichon, C., Bello-Roufai, M., Monsigny, M. and Midoux, P. (2000) Histidylated oligolysines increase the transmembrane passage and the biological activity of antisense oligonucleotides. *Nucleic Acids Res.*, **28**, 504–512.

Plank, C., Oberhauser, B., Mechtler, K., Koch, C. and Wagner, E. (1994) The influence of endosome-disruptive peptides on gene transfer using synthetic virus-like gene transfer systems. *J. Biol. Chem.*, **269**, 12918–12924.

Plank, C., Tang, M.X., Wolfe, A.R. and Szoka, F.C. (1999) Branched cationic peptides for gene delivery: role of type and number of cationic residues in formation and *in vitro* activity of DNA polyplexes. *Hum. Gene Ther.*, **10**, 319–332.

Pollard, H., Toumaniantz, G., Amos, J.L., Avet-Loiseau, H., Guihard, G., Behr, J.P. *et al.* (2001) Ca^{2+}-sensitive cytosolic nucleases prevent efficient delivery to the nucleus if injected plasmids. *J. Gene Med.*, **3**, 153–164.

Read, M.L., Dash, P.R., Clark, A., Howard, K.A., Oupicky, D., Toncheva, V. *et al.* (2000) Physicochemical and biological characterization of an antisense oligonucleotide targeted against the bcl-2 mRNA complexed with cationic-hydrophilic copolymers. *Eur. J. Pharm. Sci.*, **10**, 169–177.

Rice, K.G. (2000) Derivatization strategies for preparing *N*-glycan probes. *Anal. Biochem.*, **283**, 10–16.

Ritter, W., Plank, C. and Rosenecker, J. (1999) *In vitro* gene delivery with a new non viral vector: Geneport. *J. Gene Med.*, **1** (Suppl. 6), 34.

Rolland, A.P. (1998) From genes to gene medicines: recent advances in nonviral gene delivery. *Crit. Rev. Ther. Drug Carrier Syst.*, **15**, 143–198.

Sallusto, F., Cella, M., Danieli, C. and Lanzavecchia, A. (1995) Dendritic cells use macropinocytosis and the mannose receptor to concentrate macromolecules in the major histocompatibility complex class II compartment: downregulation by cytokines and bacterial products. *J. Exp. Med.*, **182**, 389–400.

Schaffer, D.V., Fidelman, N.A., Dan, N. and Lauffenburger, D.A. (2000) Vector unpacking as a potential barrier for receptor-mediated polyplex gene delivery. *Biotechnol. Bioeng.*, **67**, 598–606.

Schneider, H., Harbottle, R.P., Yokosaki, Y., Kunde, J., Sheppard, D. and Coutelle, C. (1998) A novel peptide, PLAEIDGIELTY, for the targeting of $\alpha 9\beta 1$-integrins. *FEBS Letters*, **249**, 269–273.

Schwartz, B., Ivanov, M.-A., Pitard, B., Escriou, V., Rangara, R., Byk, G. *et al.* (1999) Synthetic DNA-compacting peptides derived from human sequence enhance cationic lipid-mediated gene transfer *in vitro* and *in vivo*. *Gene Ther.*, **6**, 282–292.

Sebestyen, M.G., Ludtke, J.J., Bassik, M.C., Zhang, G., Budker, V., Lukhtanov, E.A. *et al.* (1998) DNA vector chemistry: the covalent attachment of signal peptides to plasmid DNA. *Nat. Biotech.*, **16**, 80–85.

Shewring, L., Collins, L., Lightman, S.L., Hart, S., Gustafsson, K. and Fabre, J.W. (1997) A non viral system for efficient gene transfer to corneal endothelial cells via membrane integrins. *Transplantation*, **64**, 763–769.

Singh, D., Bisland, S.K., Kawamura, K. and Gariépy, J. (1999) Peptide-based intracellular shuttle able to facilitate gene transfer in mammalian cells. *Bioconjug. Chem.*, **10**, 745–754.

Stahl, P.D., Wileman, T.E., Diment, S. and Shepherd, V.L. (1984) Mannose-specific oligosaccharide recognition by mononuclear phagocytes. *Biol. Cell*, **51**, 215–218.

Tang, F. and Hughes, J.A. (1998) Introduction of a disulfide bond into a cationic lipid enhances transgene expression of plasmid DNA. *Biochem. Biophys. Res. Commun.*, **242**, 141–145.

Tang, F. and Hughes, J.A. (1999) Use of dithiodiglycolic acid as a tether for cationic lipids decreases the cytotoxicity and increases transgene expression of plasmid DNA *in vitro*. *Bioconjug. Chem.*, **10**, 791–796.

Tang, M.X. and Szoka, F.C. (1997) The influence of polymer structure on the interactions of cationic polymers with DNA and morphology of the resulting complexes. *Gene Ther.*, **4**, 823–832.

Tomlinson, E. and Rolland, A.P. (1996) Controlled gene therapy pharmaceutics of non-viral gene delivery systems. *J. Control. Release*, **39**, 357–372.

Trubetskoy, V.S., Loomis, A., Slattum, P.M., Hagstrom, J.E., Budker, V.G. and Wolff, J.A. (1999) Caged DNA does not aggregate in high ionic strength solutions. *Bioconjugate Chem.*, **10**, 624–628.

Uherek, C., Fominaya, J. and Wels, W. (1998) A modular DNA carrier protein based on the structure of Diphtheria Toxin mediates target cell-specific gene delivery. *J. Biol. Chem.*, **273**, 8835–8841.

Uster, P.S. and Deamer, D.W. (1985) pH-dependent fusion of liposomes using titratable polycations. *Biochemistry*, **24**, 1–8.

Vaysse, L., Burgelin, I., Merlio, J.P. and Arveiler, B. (2000) Improved transfection using epithelial cell line-selected ligands and fusogenic peptides. *Biochim. Biophys. Acta*, **1475**, 369–376.

Vinogradov, S.V., Bronich, T.K. and Kabanov, A.V. (1998) Self-assembly of Polyamine-Poly(ethylene glycol) copolymers with phosphorothioate oligonucleotides. *Bioconjug. Chem.*, **9**, 805–812.

Vogt, T.C.B. and Bechinger, B. (1999) The interactions of Histidine-containing amphipatic helical peptide antibiotics with lipid bilayers. *J. Biol. Chem.*, **274**, 29115–29121.

Wadhwa, M.S., Collard, W.T., Adami, R.C., McKenzie, D.L. and Rice, K.G. (1997) Peptide-mediated gene delivery: influence of peptide structure on gene expression. *Bioconjug. Chem.*, **8**, 81–88.

Wagner, E. (1999) Application of membrane-active peptides for nonviral gene delivery. *Adv. Drug Deliv. Rev.*, **38**, 279–289.

Wagner, E., Plank, C., Zatloukal, K., Cotten, M. and Birnstiel, M.L. (1992) Influenza virus hemagglutinin HA-2 N-terminal fusogenic peptides augment gene transfer by transferrin-polylysine–DNA complexes: toward a synthetic virus-like gene-transfer vehicle. *Proc. Natl. Acad. Sci. USA*, **89**, 7934–7938.

Wang, C.-Y. and Huang, L. (1984) Polyhistidine mediates an acid-dependent fusion of negatively charged liposomes. *Biochemistry*, **23**, 4409–4416.

White, J.M. (1990) Viral and cellular membrane fusion proteins. *Annu. Rev. Physiol.*, **52**, 675–697.

Wilke, M., Fortunati, E., Van den Broek, M., Hoogeveen, A.T. and Scholte, B.J. (1996) Efficacy of a peptide-based gene delivery system depends on mitotic activity. *Gene Ther.*, **3**, 1133–1142.

Wyman, T.B., Nicol, F., Zelphati, O., Scaria, P.V., Plank, C. and Szoka, F.C. (1997) Design, synthesis, and characterization of a cationic peptide that binds to nucleic acids and permeabilizes bilayers. *Biochemistry*, **36**, 3008–3017.

Xu, Y. and Szoka, F.C. (1996) Mechanism of DNA release from cationic liposome/DNA complexes used in cell transfection. *Biochemistry*, **35**, 5616–5623.

Zanta, M.-A., Boussif, O., Adib, A. and Behr, J.P. (1997) *In vitro* gene delivery to hepatocytes with galactosylated polyethylenimine. *Bioconjug. Chem.*, **8**, 839–844.

Zanta, M.A., Belguise-Valladier, P. and Behr, J.P. (1999) Gene delivery: a single nuclear localization signal peptide is sufficient to carry DNA to the cell nucleus. *Proc. Natl. Acad. Sci. USA*, **96**, 91–96.

Zauner, W., Blaas, D., Kuechler, E. and Wagner, E. (1995) Rhinovirus-mediated endosomal release of transfection complexes. *J. Virol.*, **69**, 1085–1092.

Zauner, W., Ogris, M. and Wagner, E. (1998) Polylysine-based transfection systems utilizing receptor-mediated delivery. *Adv. Drug Deliv. Rev.*, **30**, 97–113.

Zelphati, O., Liang, X., Hobart, P. and Felgner, P.L. (1999) Gene chemistry: functionally and conformationally intact fluorescent plasmids. *Hum. Gene Ther.*, **10**, 15–24.

Zelphati, O., Liang, X., Nguyen, C., Barlow, S., Sheng, S., Shao, Z. *et al.* (2000) PNA-dependent gene chemistry: stable coupling of peptides and oligonucleotides to plasmid DNA. *Biotechniques*, **28**, 304–310.

Zenke, M., Steinlein, P., Wagner, E., Cotten, M., Beug, H. and Birnstiel, M.L. (1990) Receptor-mediated endocytosis of transferrin-polycation conjugates: an efficient way to introduce DNA into hematopoietic cells. *Proc. Natl. Acad. Sci. USA*, **87**, 3655–3659.

Zhang, F., Andreassen, P., Fender, P., Geissler, E., Hernandez, J.H. and Chroboczek, J. (1999) A transfecting peptide derived from adenovirus fiber protein. *Gene Ther.*, **6**, 171–181.

17 Cationic and non-condensing polymer-based gene delivery

Heidi L. Holtorf and Antonios G. Mikos

INTRODUCTION

The course of action of exogenous gene delivery to a mammalian cell proceeds through the following general pathway: formation of small DNA containing particles, uptake of the particles into the cell, entrance of the particles into the cytoplasm, transport of intact DNA to the nucleus and finally expression of delivered gene. The delivery process may be thwarted at any one of these many steps, resulting in reduced overall transfection efficiency. Viruses have evolved the machinery to proceed through each of these phases with ease, allowing their DNA to reach the nucleus and be expressed in high quantities. This unique property has led many researchers to reverse engineer these viruses to produce highly efficient gene transfer vectors without the associated harmful effects. However, these vectors are limited by an immune response, a limited capacity to carry DNA, and a short shelf-life. In an attempt to overcome these issues, an alternate approach to gene delivery was devised using entirely synthetic carriers. One such family of synthetic carriers utilizes polycationic polymers to condense DNA via electrostatic interactions, thus facilitating its cellular uptake. Another approach utilizes neutral amphiphilic polymers that bind to DNA via hydrogen bonding but do not condense it. Currently, the major drawback of these gene delivery systems is the much lower transfection efficiencies than those observed in viral systems. Thus, a majority of research in this area is devoted to increasing transfection efficiency while simultaneously gaining a better understanding of how both polycationic and non-condensing polymers help mediate gene delivery.

Three families of polymers have been used to study transfection mechanisms: polyamines, polyamides, and polyvinyl type polymers. The transfection efficiencies achievable with these systems vary widely, so an in-depth analysis of each polymer family and subsequent comparison of what affects gene delivery will be discussed in this chapter. In addition to high transfection efficiency, it is important for the polymeric systems to be relatively nontoxic to cells *in vitro* and not to elicit an immune response *in vivo*. Thus, the effect of transfection parameters on cytotoxicity and immunogenicity will also be examined.

DNA CONDENSATION

One of the most important criteria of transfection with polycationic polymers is the ability of the polymer to condense plasmid DNA. Naked DNA can be taken up by cells and expressed, however not at sufficiently high levels, presumably due to degradation at one or multiple points in the transfection process. In solution, DNA assumes a highly extended, solvated structure due to the high density of negative charge along its backbone; making the backbone easily accessible to nucleases present in extracellular fluid, endolysosomes and cytosol. In the presence of poly-cationic polymers, DNA will condense into a compact structure of folded loops, forming spherical, cylindrical or toroidal shaped particles with diameters of 50–100 nm (Arscott *et al.*, 1990; Chattoraj *et al.*, 1978; Dunlap *et al.*, 1997; Haynes *et al.*, 1970; Marquet *et al.*, 1987; Plum *et al.*, 1990). The transfection efficiency of DNA increases tremendously when it is condensed into these small particles by a polycation because the polymer reduces the electrostatic repulsion between DNA and cells by neutralizing the negative charge on the DNA while also creating a physical barrier to degradative enzymes. In general, a polycationic polymer's ability to form small, compact structures with DNA is a necessity for its success as a gene delivery carrier.

The ability of a polycation to condense DNA may be largely dependant on the structure of the polycation. Wolfert *et al.* (1999) studied the effect of distance of cationic charge from the backbone (i.e., length of side-chain), order of charged amine (primary, tertiary, or quaternary), charge spacing along the polymer backbone (i.e., charge density), and polymer molecular weight on particle formation using polymers based on a methacrylate backbone. Shorter side-chains caused DNA to condense into smaller particles, and the order of charge and charge density had little or no effect on the size of polymer/DNA complexes while the effect of molecular weight was varied. When there was an effect of polymer molecular weight on DNA condensation, one of two trends was observed: there was either continually increasing compaction with increasing molecular weight or increasing compaction with increasing molecular weight until a maximum level was reached followed by decreasing compaction at higher molecular weights. Interestingly, there was not a direct relationship observed between size of complexes and transfection efficiency. While it was necessary for DNA to condense into a small, tightly packed structure, there was a negative effect on transfection efficiency with the most highly compact particles. The overall effect of physical parameters was higher transfection efficiency with longer side chains, primary or tertiary amines, and higher charge density, while transfection efficiency tended to either increase with higher molecular weight polymers or reach a maximum at an intermediate value of molecular weight.

Once DNA has been condensed by a polycation, it is important for these complexes to retain a certain level of stability in salt solutions to allow sufficient time for cellular uptake of the particles. Izumrudov *et al.* (1999) studied the stability of a variety of polymers including polyvinylpyridines, linear polyamines, branched polyamines, polymethacrylates, and polyamides in salt solutions at a variety of pHs. They observed that polymers with predominantly primary amines produced the most stable polymer/DNA complexes followed by tertiary then quaternary amines, while higher molecular weight polymers resulted in more stable complexes for all amine types. Thus, it may be possible to specifically control complex stability by adjusting the relative amount of each amine type in the polymer.

CELLULAR TRAFFICKING

In general, when naked DNA is taken up by a cell via endocytosis it follows a general pathway. The DNA binds to the cell surface receptors and a pit starts to form in the membrane. Eventually, this pit forms a vesicle that pinches off from the cell membrane and begins traveling toward the interior of the cell. This newly formed endosome undergoes gradual acidification to pH of about 5.5 when it merges with a lysosome; at which time a majority of the DNA is degraded by pH dependent nucleases. A very small number of DNA molecules escape from the acidic vesicles into the cytoplasm where they are transported to the nucleus and then transcribed by host cell machinery. The purpose of using a polymeric carrier is to increase the amount of DNA taken up by the cell and to prevent digestion of DNA as it progresses through the cell trafficking machinery. While it is generally believed that DNA/polymer complexes follow the same cellular processing pathway as naked DNA, there is recent evidence by Godbey *et al.* (2000a) that certain polycationic vectors may take a slightly different path, in particular by escaping into the cytosol prior to endosome acidification. Thus, an understanding of how these vectors achieve their goals is essential to the development of novel carriers.

POLYLYSINE

One of the first polycations used as a gene delivery vehicle was poly(L-lysine) (PLL), a polyamide of the amino acid lysine containing a primary amino nitrogen in each repeating unit (Figure 17.1). A detailed evaluation of PLL as a gene carrier is outside the scope of this chapter, however a brief discussion here is warranted. PLL was first described as a gene carrier in 1973 by Li *et al.* and since then it has been widely studied as a gene carrier. PLL is able to mediate higher levels of cell transfection than when DNA is used alone, however its efficiency is greatly increased by the addition of an endosomolytic agent such as chloroquine (Cotten *et al.*, 1990). While this strategy works *in vitro*, there are limitations on the use of chloroquine *in vivo*. To overcome this shortcoming, a host of PLL derivatives have been synthesized, including polymers with covalently linked targeting ligands, membrane disrupting peptides, or lipophilic molecules. In addition, graft copolymers of PLL and hydrophilic polymers have been synthesized to reduce the nonspecific interaction of the polymer/DNA complexes with blood components. These polymer modification strategies were later applied to different polymer groups, such as those discussed below. In general, PLL is not a very efficient vector and the chain length heterogeneity of commercially available PLL is so great as to preclude its use in generating consistent transfections. Thus, the following polymers were developed to improve upon existing systems utilizing PLL.

POLYETHYLENIMINE

Polyethylenimine (PEI) was chosen as a candidate for gene delivery because of its unique structure. It is a highly branched polymer of ethylamine containing

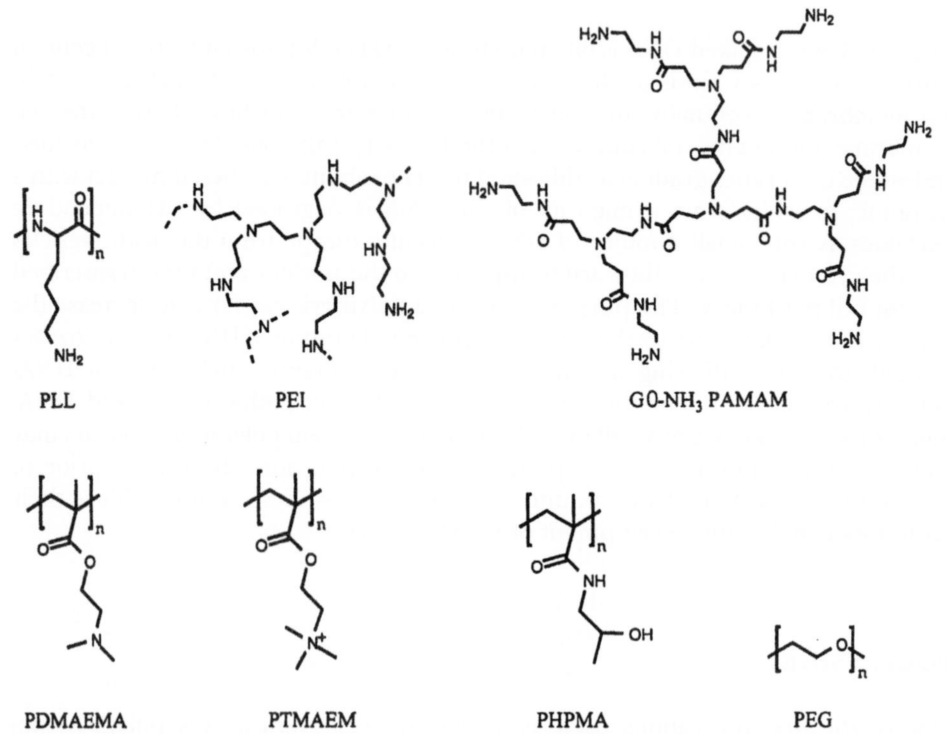

Figure 17.1 Chemical structures of polycationic polymers used as gene delivery vectors.

primary, secondary and tertiary amines at a corresponding ratio of 1:2:1 (Suh *et al.*, 1994) (Figure 17.1). Every third atom in the polymer is an amino nitrogen, giving it the highest possible cationic charge density of any molecule. Only a portion of its amine groups are positively charged at physiological pH, allowing it to complex with DNA and condense it while remaining amine groups retain the ability to become charged at lower pH's (Suh *et al.*, 1994). The ability of PEI to condense DNA and protect it from degradation by nuclease has been evaluated by several groups. Godbey *et al.* (2000a) exposed PEI/plasmid DNA complexes to DNase I and DNase II in solution and found that DNA remained intact even after 24 hours of incubation at high enzyme concentrations, whereas free DNA was completely digested in three minutes at much lower concentrations. Marschall *et al.* (1999) condensed 2.3 Mb yeast artificial chromosome (YAC) with PEI and subsequently transfected cells via lipofection. The YAC remained intact in 100% of positively transfected cells when PEI was used to condense the DNA, while 0% of DNA was intact when NaCl was used as the condensing molecule. Thus, PEI is able to protect even large pieces of DNA from degradation by nucleases.

PEI was first described as a possible gene delivery vehicle by Boussif *et al.* (1995) and has been extensively studied since then to optimize its transfection efficiency both *in vitro* and *in vivo*. The ratio of PEI nitrogens to DNA phosphates, frequently called the charge ratio, is an important transfection parameter (Boussif *et al.*, 1995).

At low charge ratios, there is not enough cationic charge to neutralize the negative charge on the DNA, resulting in incompletely condensed particles with large diameters and subsequent low cellular uptake. At high charge ratios, there is excess cationic polymer, causing a noticeable increase in cytotoxicity. An optimum ratio lies between these two extremes where there is high gene expression with comparatively low toxicity. Optimal *in vitro* charge ratios have been reported from 5 to 13.5 (Boussif *et al.*, 1995; Kichler *et al.*, 2001; Godbey *et al.*, 1999b; Poulain *et al.*, 2000). The variability in these numbers is more than likely an artifact of variation in the physical properties (degree of branching, molecular weight and polydispersity) of PEI or cell type used for transfection.

Other parameters likely to influence transfection include pH and salt concentration of the compaction medium, amount of DNA, cell type, and polymer molecular weight and polydispersity. Forming the complexes at lower pH does not have a significant effect on transfection efficiency (Godbey *et al.*, 1999a); lower salt concentrations and greater amounts of DNA resulted in higher efficiencies (Boussif *et al.*, 1995). When transfection was optimized among these three parameters, there was still a wide variance of luciferase expression across the eight different cell types tested. This wide variance is not surprising since different cell types process material in different manners, however the specific cause of increased gene expression in some cell types is not yet known. Godbey *et al.* (1999a) observed an increase in transfection efficiency with increasing molecular weight of PEI from nominal molecular weight of 600 up to 70,000. Figure 17.2 demonstrates the variation of transfection efficiency with molecular weight of PEI. Relatively high transfection was obtained with molecular weights of 10,000 and 70,000 while molecular weights of 1,800 and lower resulted in negligible or no transfection. The initial pH of PEI did not affect transfection. More polydisperse polymers also tended to give higher transfection efficiencies, and when small molecular weight

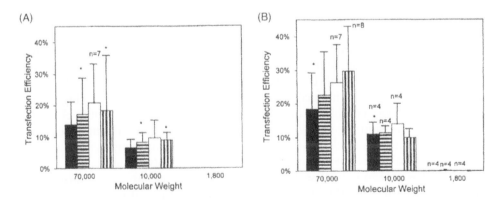

Figure 17.2 Percentages of positive cells for GFP expression using PEI of various molecular weights and starting pH values. Molecular weights of 1,200 and 600 were tested but are not shown because they yielded zero transfection. The number of replications was $n = 6$ unless otherwise stated; error bars indicate one standard deviation. An asterisk (*) over an error bar indicates the molecular weights 70,000 and 10,000 were not significantly different for the given time at the given pH. Two time points were tested: (A) 24 hour post-transfection; (B) 48 hour post-transfection. pHs: ■ = 5.0; ≡ = 6.0; □ = 7.0; ▥ = 8.0. (Reproduced with permission from Godbey *et al.*, 1999a).

PEI molecules were added to complexes preformed with high molecular weight PEI, transfection efficiency was enhanced greatly (Godbey *et al.*, 1999b).

As stated earlier, the transfection efficiency of PLL is enhanced by the addition of chloroquine to the media. Comparable transfection efficiency is achievable with PEI alone and the addition of chloroquine does not result in any enhancement of gene transfer. This observation led Boussif *et al.* (1995) to hypothesize that PEI acts in a similar manner as chloroquine to aid DNA escape from the lysosomes. This idea, known as the proton–sponge hypothesis, is based on the fact that the highly branched PEI contains tertiary amines that are still protonable at physiological pH. Polymer/DNA complex containing endosomes begin to acidify as they move toward the cell interior due to ATP driven proton pumps. Large volumes of positively charged protons enter the endosome, protonating previously uncharged amino nitrogens on the PEI. The increase in positive charge in the endosome results in an inflow of negative ions such as Cl^- to relieve the electrical gradient. The increasing concentration of ions inside the endosome results in swelling due to osmosis and eventual bursting of the endosomes, thus releasing the DNA containing complexes into the cytosol. Recent work by Kichler *et al.* (2001) supports this hypothesis. They investigated the effect of proton pump inhibitors on the transfection efficiency of PEI and found that transfection efficiency decreased up to 70-fold in the presence of the proton pump inhibitor bafilomycin A1. However, recent work by Godbey *et al.* (2000a) challenges the proton – sponge hypothesis. They observed that lysosome pH remained constant over a five hour time period (the amount of time required for gene delivery to the cell nucleus), as well as an absence of endosome–lysosome fusion. These observations suggest that PEI/DNA complexes escape from endosomes prior to acidification. Figures 17.3 and 17.4 show transfection of cells with either PEI or PLL. The polymers were fluorescently labeled with a green fluorophore while lysosomes were identified using a red fluorophore, a yellow color indicates overlap of polymer and lysosome.

After the complexes are released in the cytosol, they must be transported to the nucleus and cross the nuclear membrane. At some point in the transfection cascade, the DNA must be released from the PEI to allow expression of the gene and this may occur before or after transport across the nuclear membrane. Godbey *et al.* (1999c) showed that both DNA and PEI are delivered to the nucleus, however it remains unclear how the molecules get there, as the complexes are too big to pass through nuclear pore complexes in their native state. Pollard *et al.* (1998) observed comparable expression kinetics when naked DNA and PEI/DNA complexes were microinjected into the nucleus, suggesting that the rate-limiting step in nuclear transport is crossing the membrane rather than vector unpacking.

While PEI is able to condense DNA and effectively mediate gene transfer into mammalian cells, it is not the ideal carrier, as rather significant levels of cell death have been observed with PEI transfection. Fischer *et al.* (1999) found that low molecular weight (LMW) PEI was less toxic to cells than high molecular weight (HMW) PEI. The HMW-PEI showed less than 20% cell survival after one hour of exposure to 0.1 mg/mL of the polymer. Godbey *et al.* (2000b) saw similar cell death for free PEI, while the effect was lessened when PEI was complexed with DNA, resulting in 50% survival rates. When the cells were visualized by phase contrast microscopy, the live cells exhibited a highly altered morphology, they were rounded rather than spread and smaller than normal cells. Godbey *et al.* (2001)

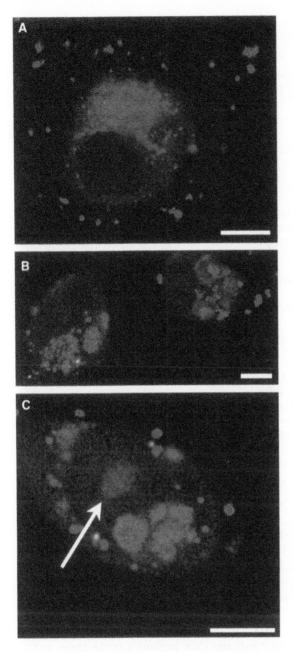

Figure 17.3 Tracking of labeled PEI/DNA complexes (green) in cells with labeled lysosomes (red). Each bar indicates 10 μm. Times post-transfection are as follows: (A) two hours – clumps of PEI/DNA complexes are present on the plasma membrane, and lysosomes are scattered throughout the cytoplasm; (B) three hours – PEI/DNA complexes are located in endocytotic vesicles and are somewhat surrounded by lysosomes. There is no overlap of PEI and lysosomal probes; (C) five hours – PEI/DNA complexes have entered the nucleus (shown by arrow) while cytoplasmic vesicles containing PEI/DNA complexes still have not fused with lysosomes. (Reproduced with permission from Godbey *et al.*, 2000a). (*see Color Plate 12*)

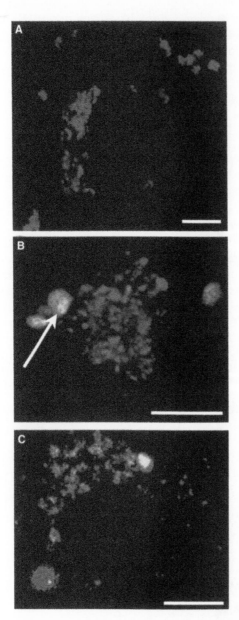

Figure 17.4 Tracking of labeled PLL/DNA complexes (green) in cells with labeled lysosomes (red). Yellow color indicates close proximity of the green and red fluorophores and therefore complex/lysosome interaction. Each bar indicates 10 μm. Times post-transfection are as follows: (A) two hours – as with PEI, PLL/DNA complexes aggregate in clumps on cell exteriors. Note, however, that the PLL/DNA clumps are larger and less spherical (compare to Figure 17.3); (B) four hours – after the PLL/DNA complexes enter the cytoplasm, they are seen to meet up with lysosomes. These endolysosomes are visible as yellow and are denoted by arrows; (C) five hours – the large endolysosomes are quickly dissipated as the PLL/DNA complexes are degraded. (Reproduced with permission from Godbey *et al.*, 2000a). (*see Color Plate 13*)

saw another toxic effect of PEI/DNA complexes on endothelial cell function. In addition to increased cell death, there were increased levels of some endogenous proteins, even when the delivered gene contained no promoter. This increased level is significant in that some cell toxicity assays are based on total amount of cell protein in solution. If protein levels are enhanced due to the exogenous DNA, then one could have a certain level of cell death that would be masked by the increased protein levels in positively transfected cells.

Although *in vitro* gene delivery is important, the goal of most gene therapy projects is to develop a system that could be delivered directly to a patient and targeted to a specific tissue without exhibiting toxicity or eliciting an immune response. One major problem with cationic carriers for systemic delivery *in vivo* is activation of the complement system. Plank *et al.* (1996) determined the effect of several cationic polymers used for gene delivery on complement activation, finding that all positively charged polymers activated complement, however the effect was reduced when polymers were complexed with DNA. This reduction was dependent on the charge ratio of the complexes, with less complement activation as the ratio approached neutrality. Unfortunately, these complexes are also less soluble in water and tend to aggregate, causing other problems, such as increased clearance by the liver and spleen (Pouton and Seymour, 1998). Simultaneous reduction of complement activation and increased complex solubility can be achieved by coating the complexes with uncharged hydrophilic polymers such as poly(ethylene oxide) (PEO), poly(propylene oxide) (PPO) or Pluronics (triblock copolymers of PEO-*b*-PPO-*b*-PEO) (Nguyen *et al.*, 2000). Complexes formed with these polymers grafted to PEI had zeta potentials close to neutrality. PEI grafted to Pluronic formed particles with positive zeta potentials when complexed with DNA and could attain transfection efficiency as high as that of free PEI.

Other criteria for the systemic delivery of genes *in vivo* include the ability to target the DNA to a specific tissue and to remain in blood circulation for an extended period of time. To target a molecule to a specific tissue, it is necessary to both eliminate nonspecific interaction of polymer/DNA complexes with cells and facilitate uptake in the desired cell type. One approach to lowering random interactions is the attachment of hydrophilic polymers to the surface of the complexes. Indeed, Nguyen *et al.* (2000) showed that certain PEI–PEO conjugates are unable to spontaneously transfect cells. A variety of molecules, including transferrin (Wightman *et al.*, 1999), avidin (Wojda and Miller, 2000), mannose (Diebold *et al.*, 1999) and galactose (Zanta *et al.*, 1997) have been attached to PEI/DNA conjugates for the purpose of targeted gene delivery. In each case, these targeting systems were tested *in vitro* and transfection efficiencies of targeted complexes were the same or higher than PEI/DNA complexes alone for cells expressing the appropriate receptor. Ogris *et al.* (1999) examined the *in vitro* transfection of cells with DNA/transferrin-PEI/PEG complexes and found that the addition of PEG to DNA/transferrin–PEI complexes had no effect on the overall transfection efficiency, while *in vivo* studies performed by the same group showed reduced nonspecific tissue uptake when PEG was added to transferrin modified PEI/DNA complexes.

Delivery of genes via the airway offers an alternative to systemic gene delivery when the lungs are the target tissue. The major barrier in aerosol delivery of genes to the lung is stabilizing the transfection complexes to the aerosolization process as well as to pulmonary surfactants. The process of nebulization causes plasmids to degrade, lowering their transfection efficiency (Eastman *et al.*, 1998). Additionally, the transfection of liposome/plasmid complexes is inhibited by pulmonary surfactants (Tsan *et al.*, 1997). Polycationic polymers offer a good alternative gene delivery system, as polymer/DNA complexes were shown to remain intact during nebulization and resulted in high pulmonary transfection with less starting material (Densmore *et al.*, 2000).

POLYAMIDOAMINES

Polyamidoamine (PAMAM) dendrimers are synthesized via the stepwise addition of methacrylate and ethylenediamine (EDA) to a core molecule, typically ammonia or tris(2-aminoethyl)amine (TAEA) (Tomalia *et al.*, 1985, 1990). Ethylamine adds to methacrylate forming an amide linkage with a terminal amine. This amine serves as a branching point for the next cycle of synthesis or generation, so the polymer structure is built up in spherical shells around the core molecule. A generation zero dendrimer includes the core molecule and its associated branches after one round of methacrylate/ethylenediamine addition (Figure 17.1). Two branches form from each terminal amine group of the dendrimer, resulting in a two-fold increase in the number of available primary amino groups on the surface of the molecule with each successive generation, creating increasingly high surface charge density. The molecule can continue to grow until the outer layer of amine groups touch each other, forming a closed nanoparticle and creating steric hindrance from the addition of another generation (Esfand and Tomalia, 2001). The biggest advantage of this dendrimeric structure is that the degree of branching is strictly controlled (polydispersity less than 1.10) and likewise, the surface charge of the molecules. This allows for the study of charge and molecular weight effects on transfection efficiency in a more precise manner than for the highly polydispersed branched polyethylenimine.

PAMAM dendrimers can condense DNA into small toroidal particles without altering the structure of the DNA (Bielinska *et al.*, 1997). These complexes were shown to form via electrostatic interactions, by the observation that DNA binding affinity is directly proportional to the number of charged surface amines. When dendrimer was complexed with DNA at excess positive charge, the polymer protected DNA from nuclease digestion and prevented DNA transcription in a cell free model system, showing that PAMAM dendrimers are able to provide a physical barrier to DNA against cellular components.

The first use of polyamidoamine dendrimers as DNA delivery molecules was by Haensler and Szoka (1993). They reported high levels of transfection in a variety of cell types *in vitro* with low toxicity. The level of transfection was dependent on the dendrimer terminal amine to DNA phosphate ratio as well as the size (generation) of the dendrimer. Maximum transfection levels were found to occur with generation six ammonia core (G6-NH$_3$) dendrimers at a charge ratio of six amines: one phosphate. However, they were unable to repeat the experiment with newly synthesized, highly purified dendrimers, leading them to believe that the original batch of PAMAM had degraded somewhat at the time of transfection (Tang *et al.*, 1996).

To test this hypothesis, Tang *et al.* (1996) synthesized several generations of PAMAM dendrimers and partially degraded them by solvolysis aided by heat. They synthesized generation five and six dendrimers based on a TAEA core (G5-TAEA and G6-TAEA), resulting in molecules with three-fold core symmetry, similar to the previously studied G6-NH$_3$ dendrimers, and generation six and eight dendrimers based on an EDA core (G6-EDA and G8-EDA), resulting in molecules with four-fold core symmetry. The newly synthesized intact dendrimers exhibited 100-fold lower β-galactosidase activity and 1000-fold lower luciferase activity than the previously tested G6-NH$_3$ core dendrimers. Heating of the newly synthesized dendrimers in the presence of a solvolytic solvent, such as water, 1-butanol, 2-butanol, or 2-ethoxyethanol, resulted in increased transfection efficiencies with increased heating time up to a maximum, with efficiency then trailing off. Maximal transfection coincided with minimal polymer/DNA complex diameter for generation six dendrimers. While individual complex size did not differ much with heating time, there was a significant amount of complex aggregation at low heating times. The optimal transfection efficiency was noted when there was minimal interparticle aggregation and individual polymer/DNA complexes were evenly dispersed throughout the transfection mixture. Kukowska *et al.* (1996) observed less complex aggregation and greater transfection efficiency of dendrimers when DEAE-dextran was added to the transfection medium. Luciferase expression comparable to that of lipofection was obtained with G7-EDA/DEAE-dextran dendrimer mediated transfection. Thus, transfection efficiency can be improved overall by reducing particle aggregation.

Size exclusion chromatography of heat-treated dendrimers revealed a bimodal distribution of molecular weights. Upon fractionation of the mixture, it was discovered that the highest molecular weight fragments mediated the majority of transfection, while the smallest fragments mediated the lowest level of transfection, although the intact mixture was still the most efficient mediator of transfection. Tang *et al.* (1996) called these high molecular weight fragments 'fractured' dendrimers and hypothesized that they were composed of the original dendrimer core with a large percentage of its branches cleaved off. This type of structure would yield a highly charged polymer molecule with much greater flexibility than the intact dendrimer. The flexibility parameter assumes that the degraded polymer occupies the same volume as the intact dendrimer, and is determined by normalizing the volume of a sphere to molecular weight of the degraded dendrimer. When the flexibility parameters of each dendrimer formulation were compared, maximal transfection efficiency of all formulations occurred at a flexibility parameter of approximately 7.5, indicating that a certain amount of flexibility in the polymer backbone is necessary to mediate high levels of transfection. To further illustrate this point, viscosity measurements were taken for both intact and fractured dendrimers at different pH levels. Viscosity of a polymer solution is directly related to the size of the polymer molecule, so a highly extended polymer will have a greater diameter and a corresponding greater viscosity than a very compacted polymer. While the intact dendrimers retained the same viscosity at pH 7.2 and 10.5, the fractured dendrimers showed a three-fold increase in viscosity at pH 7.2 over both intact dendrimer and fractured dendrimer at pH 10.5.

This increase has two-fold implications. First, it implies that the fractured dendrimer is more flexible than the intact dendrimer and second, that the fractured dendrimer may expand due to an increase in positive charge at lower pH, a quantity that was described as essential for PEI mediated transfection. Indeed, when branched PEI was subjected to the same set of experiments, the same three-fold increase in viscosity was observed, lending support to the idea that PAMAM dendrimers act as proton sponges. Evidence of lysosomal buffering capability of PAMAM dendrimers was shown by Kukowska-Latallo *et al.* (1996) when they observed that the efficiency of G5-EDA dendrimers was enhanced by the addition of chloro-quine, while the same molecule could not enhance transfection of G10-EDA dendri-mers, which contain 40-fold more surface amine groups for proton absorption.

Bielinska *et al.* (1996) studied the effectiveness of PAMAM dendrimers in delivering a 27 base antisense oligonucleotide to cells permanently expressing Luciferase. Using G7-EDA dendrimers at a 10:1 surface amine: phosphate charge ratio to transfect cells expressing the luciferase gene, baseline luciferase expression was reduced by 30–40%, indicating that it may be easier to deliver small oligo-nucleotides than large plasmids using intact PAMAM dendrimers. They also assessed cytotoxicity of G7-EDA dendrimers and saw no significant cell death compared to controls, while both lipofectamine and diethylaminoethyl (DEAE)-dextran showed high levels of cytotoxicity.

The toxicity of generation 3, 5 and 7 NH_3 core dendrimers was tested *in vitro* and *in vivo* by Roberts *et al.* (1996). There was a concentration and generation dependent toxicity *in vitro*, with higher concentrations and generations being more toxic, while no immunogenicity was observed *in vivo*. However, *in vitro* toxicity was measured at levels well above those seen during a typical transfection and at the lowest concentration of particles tested (100 nM) the dendrimers exhibited relatively low levels of toxicity. In general, there was no significant cytotoxicity of PAMAM dendrimers observed by any group.

Qin *et al.* (1998) demonstrated the efficiency of polyamidoamine dendrimers on the *in vivo* transfection of murine cardiac grafts. The grafts were injected with polymer/DNA complexes and β-galactosidase activity was detected up to 28 days post-injection. Similarly, when the grafts were injected with G5-EDA/DNA complexes containing the gene for IL-10, an interleukin that has been shown to down regulate the immune system and thus reduces the possibility of host rejection of a transplant, the hearts survived over twice as long as controls, indicating sufficient delivery and expression of the gene to reduce the activity of the recipi-ent's immune system.

Hudde *et al.* (1999) demonstrated the efficiency of activated (fractured) dendri-mers for *ex vivo* delivery of genes to corneal endothelium. Transfection efficiency was dependent on the charge ratio and the amount of DNA delivered to the cells. Maximum transfection was observed at 18:1 weight ratio of polymer:DNA and total DNA amount of 2 µg/cell well, at which point 6–10% of cells were expressing the reporter gene β-galactosidase. In addition, corneas were transfected with dendrimer/DNA complexes containing the TNFR-Ig gene, which reduced the risk of recipient rejection and found continued expression of the factor up to nine days post-transfection.

While the dendrimer architecture is the most popular form of polyamidoamine polymers for gene delivery, linear polyamidoamines have also been evaluated for their effectiveness as gene transfer agents to assess the importance of polymer structure on transfection ability and cytotoxicity. Hill *et al.* (1999) synthesized a series of polyamidoamines with various functionalities in the backbone that may influence transfection ability. These variables include amine type (piperazine or methyl amine), distance of charged moieties from each other along the backbone and overall polymer molecular weight. Increasing molecular weight or charge density resulted in increasing cytotoxicity, while methylamine groups tended to be more toxic than piperazine groups. However, the most toxic polyamidoamine structures were also the only formulations able to mediate a detectable level of transfection level of luciferase, leading to speculation that the same parameter that mediates cytotoxicity also mediates an essential step in transfection. Examination of the physical properties of linear polyamidoamine/DNA complexes showed more positive zeta potentials and smaller hydrodynamic radii, with methylamines and higher charge density (Jones *et al.*, 2000). In general, important chemical properties seem to be high charge density and amine type, while important physical properties are positive zeta potentials and small complex size.

POLYAMINOMETHACRYLATES

A variety of amino methacrylate polymers have been studied for their potential as gene delivery vehicles. The first polymer of this sort to be characterized was poly(2-(dimethylamino)ethyl methacrylate) (PDMAEMA) (Figure 17.1), which is synthesized by free radical polymerization of 2-(dimethylamino)ethyl methacrylate in water using ammonium peroxydisulphate as an initiator. The result is a high molecular weight linear polymer with a large polydispersity that is able to condense DNA and provide a physical barrier to nuclease digestion, similar to polyethylenimine (Arigita *et al.*, 1999). Cherng *et al.* (1996) characterized the physical parameters of PDMAEMA/DNA particles via zeta potential and dynamic light scattering, finding that at a polymer/DNA weight ratio of one and higher, the particles had positive zeta potentials and at weight ratios of two and higher the average particle diameter was 150 nm. While particle size remained constant at a variety of ratios, the polydispersity of particles reached a minimum at the ratio corresponding to the highest transfection efficiency. The particle size of PDMAEMA/plasmid complexes is also dependent on the pH, ionic strength and viscosity of the solution in which the complexes are formed, with the smallest particles being formed at low pH, low ionic strength and low viscosity (Cherng *et al.*, 1999b).

Cherng *et al.* (1996) were the first to describe the transfection capabilities and toxicity of PDMAEMA. They showed that PDMAEMA promoted cellular uptake and expression of exogenous DNA and the resulting transfection levels were dependent on the polymer/DNA weight ratio, as well as the total number of complexes. While transfection efficiency peaked at midrange weight ratios and particle concentrations, cell viability continually decreased with increasing levels of each parameter. This low level of cell survival was attributed to high levels of polymer, as naked PDMAEMA was shown to be cytotoxic, while its effect was lessened by complexing it with DNA. Transfection efficiency was also found to depend on DNA topology if the order was supercoiled > open-circular > linear, suggesting that in therapeutic applications it may be beneficial to use plasmid DNA rather than linear (Cherng *et al.*, 1999a).

Van de Wetering *et al*. (1999a) studied the effects of various structural properties on the transfection efficiency of amino methacrylate polymers. They found that while changing the length of the side-chain, the type of side-chain linkage, or the degree of the charged amine had no affect on the complex size or zeta potential, these parameters did have an effect on transfection efficiency with the following trends increasing the side chain-length and changing the acrylate bond to an acrylamide bond decreased efficiency and changing the tertiary amine to a quaternary amine virtually eliminated transfection. The difference in transfection could have been due to differences in the strength of polymer/DNA interactions and corresponding complex stability. Molecular modeling experiments showed that polymers with side-chains containing one extra methylene group bound to DNA more strongly, which probably stabilized the complexes, resulting in lower transfection due to reduced polymer/DNA uncoupling. A similar increase in polymer/DNA binding strength resulted from replacing the acrylate bond in the monomer with an acrylamide bond. Substituting a permanently charged quaternary amine for the sometimes charged tertiary amine did not alter the stability of the complexes but did eliminate the ability of the polymer to absorb protons, and thus eliminating the ability of complexes to escape from endosomal compartments.

In the previous experiments, β-galactosidase was used as a reporter, but Van de Wetering *et al*. (1998) later found that the transfection efficiency determined using β-galactosidase reporter was altered by the amount of time the coloring assay was allowed to run. This observation led them to use the green fluorescent protein as their reporter gene instead, and they found that transfection efficiency was three times higher than previously thought, or about 7% total. They also studied the effect of molecular weight on efficiency, finding that higher molecular weight PDMAEMA was more efficient at transfecting cells. To gain a better understanding of the chemical properties of these polymers that are important in mediating cell transfection, they copolymerized DMAEMA with monomers of varying degrees of hydrophobicity. *N*-vinyl pyrrolidone (NVP) was chosen as a hydrophilic monomer, methyl methacrylate (MMA) as a hydrophobic monomer and ethoxytriethylene glycol methacrylate (triEGMA) as an intermediately hydrophilic/hydrophobic monomer. Copolymers of NVP and DMAEMA gave higher transfection efficiencies and lower cytotoxicity than the DMAEMA homopolymer, while copolymers formulated with the other two monomers had either a detrimental or no effect on either property, indicating that monomer hydrophilicity is an important transfection parameter.

One important requirement of non-viral gene delivery devices is that they possess a long shelf life; this would be one of the biggest advantages of using polymeric carriers over viral carriers, as they are not easy to store for long periods of time. With this in mind, Cherng *et al*. (1997) examined the potential of freeze-dried PDMAEMA/plasmid complexes to transfect cells. When PDMAEMA/plasmid complexes were formed in $> 2\%$ sucrose solution, they could be freeze-dried and reconstituted in water without loss of transfection efficiency. They later showed (Cherng *et al*., 1999c) that PDMAEMA/plasmid complexes were stable in aqueous solution for ten months when stored under refrigeration, but their transfection ability was reduced when stored at $40\,^{\circ}\mathrm{C}$ for the same length of time. Freeze-dried samples retained their transfection ability for the ten month period, even when stored at $40\,^{\circ}\mathrm{C}$, indicating that the freeze-drying process stabilizes polymer/plasmid complexes and is a viable means of long term storage.

As for polyethylenimines and polyamidoamines, PDMAEMA has been assessed for its transfection ability *in vivo*. Van de Wetering *et al.* (1999b) examined the efficiency of PDMAEMA *in vivo* and found that while ovarian carcinoma cells were able to be transfected *in vitro* and *ex vivo* at efficiencies up to 10%, they were not transfected *in vivo*. Components present in body fluids that are not present in the *in vitro* model may be responsible for the disappearance of transfection activity. This idea is supported by evidence that the presence of hyaluronic acid, one of many fluid components, greatly reduced *in vitro* transfection efficiency.

Wolfert *et al.* (1996) examined the transfection and cytotoxicity of poly (*N*-2-hydroxypropyl methacrylamide)-*b*-poly(trimethylaminoethyl methacrylate) (PHPMA-PTMAEM), an amino methacrylate polymer with quaternary amine groups connected to an uncharged hydrophilic polymer of similar structure (Figure 17.1). It has been proposed that this neutral hydrophilic block will coat the surface of the complex and shield the surface charge to reduce nonspecific interaction of the complexes with fluid components *in vivo*. For these experiments, chloroquine was added as a lysosomotropic agent to enhance transfection efficiency and it was found that while cytotoxicity of the copolymer did not differ much from the homopolymer, the transfection efficiency was enhanced by the addition of the PHPMA block.

The addition of PHPMA block to PTMAEM improves the solubility of charge neutralized complexes by reducing the hydrophobicity of the complexes (Oupicky *et al.*, 1998). The reduction in hydrophobicity also reduces complex aggregation in a manner dependent on the relative amount of *N*-2-hydroxypropylmethacrylamide (HPMA). At high levels of this hydrophilic block, complexes existed as single particles in solution. In conjunction with reduced particle aggregation, higher HPMA levels also increased complex stability in salt solutions, an indication that these copolymers will be better transfection agents *in vivo* due to the large amount of ions present in physiological solutions. To further test the stability of these complexes, Oupicky *et al.* (1999) examined the ability of the anionic protein albumin to exchange the bound DNA from the polymer, as well as its effect on particle size. Albumin was chosen as the polyanion because it is the most common negatively charged protein in blood plasma, and though it did form a ternary complex with the PHPMA-PTMAEM/DNA particles, resulting in slightly larger particles, it was unable to release DNA from the polymer. A more rigorous exchange experiment was performed using the synthetic polyanion poly(styrene-sulfonate) (PSS), a polymer with a much higher negative charge density than albumin. It was shown that this highly charged polymer was unable to exchange DNA from the cationic polymer in the absence of salt, and did so only very slowly in high concentration of salt. Thus, the major concern with anionic blood components is an increase in particle size and possible enhancement of particle aggregation, rather than premature DNA release from hydrophilic cationic block copolymers. An *in vivo* biodistribution study of the PHPMA-*b*-PTMAEM complexes revealed that a majority of them were cleared from the bloodstream by the liver within 30 minutes of intravenous injection. This high level of liver clearance is unlikely to be due to the size of ternary albumin/polymer/DNA complexes; rather, they are being marked for clearance by plasma proteins. This led Oupicky *et al.* (1999) to conclude that there were exposed hydrophobic sites on the surface of the complexes. These exposed sites may have been due to a large portion of the HPMA chains being trapped in the interior of the DNA complexes, leaving the surface incompletely coated with hydrophilic polymer.

NON-CONDENSING POLYMERS

An alternative to the condensing polycationic polymers discussed above is a neutral polymer that will bind to but not condense DNA, while still affording it an adequate level of protection. These polymers are amphiphilic molecules with a hydrophobic backbone and hydrophilic-side chains that are either hydrogen bond donors or acceptors that stabilize DNA through hydrogen bonding, rather than charge neutralization. Two polymers have been identified and studied as non-condensing polymers, poly(vinyl pyrrolidone) (PVP) as a hydrogen bond accepting polymer and poly(vinyl alcohol) (PVA) as a hydrogen bond donating polymer (Figure 17.5).

The side-chains of PVP form hydrogen bonds with nucleotide bases in the major groove of the DNA double helix, while the hydrophobic backbone is exposed to the exterior of the molecule, providing the plasmid with a hydrophobic coating (Mumper *et al.*, 1998). When DNA is coated with PVP, it is afforded some protection against nuclease degradation over uncoated DNA (Mumper *et al.*, 1996). The hydrophobic coating also has an effect on the zeta potential of DNA; it increases with increasing levels of PVP, but even at 40:1 weight ratio of PVP to DNA the plasmids retained a substantial negative surface charge (Mumper *et al.*, 1998). PVP and PVA are both uncharged molecules and observation of DNA/polymer conjugates by electron microscopy and laser light scattering gave no evidence of plasmid condensation into small particles, indicating that the PVP coats the surface of the plasmid while allowing it to retain an extended flexible structure. When a portion of vinyl pyrrolidone monomers was substituted for vinyl acetate, which is less able to form hydrogen bonds, the transfection efficiency decreased with increasing vinyl acetate substitution, indicating that hydrogen bonding is indeed the main cause of PVP/DNA interaction (Mumper and Rolland, 1998).

The effect of pH and salt concentration on gene expression was also determined, with higher expression observed when plasmid/PVP conjugates were formed in solutions of pH ≤ 3.75 and high salt concentrations. PVP has been shown to deliver plasmids coding for IL-12 to tumor cells, resulting in increased gene expression over naked plasmid (Mendiratta *et al.*, 1999). Comparative *in vivo* transfections of rat tibialis muscle with PVP and PVA showed that at optimal weight ratios and doses, both exhibited higher transfection than plasmid injected with

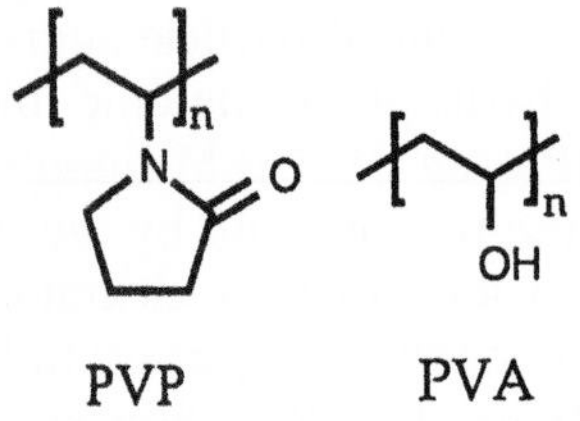

PVP   PVA

Figure 17.5 Chemical structures of non-condensing polymers used as gene delivery vectors.

saline, with PVA exhibiting higher gene expression than PVP (Mumper *et al.*, 1996). Although physical characterization similar to that performed on PVP was not performed on PVA, it is believed that this molecule operates in a similar fashion to PVP. The difference in transfection can be attributed to differences in hydrogen bonding of the side-chains to DNA bases.

CONCLUDING REMARKS

To develop novel gene carriers, it is important to identify the essential parameters of successful delivery with currently available systems. The above cationic polymer systems all showed similar dependence on transfection efficiency to a variety of physical and chemical parameters. When these polymers condense DNA into small particles, they are able to mediate much higher levels of transfection than naked DNA. However, the overall transfection efficiency can be further enhanced in the following ways: optimization of the charge ratio; using intermediate side chain lengths; using primary or tertiary amines; increasing the positive charge density; increasing side chain flexibility; increasing polymer polydispersity; increasing polymer molecular weight; increasing the proton absorbing capability; increasing the amount of DNA; lowering complex aggregation; lowering salt concentrations; attaching targeting molecules, and; adding a hydrophilic block. Table 17.1 summarizes the important parameters affecting gene transfer. While it is necessary for polymers to condense DNA into small structures, there is a negative effect on transfection efficiency when these complexes are extremely compact and highly stable. At this extreme, dissociation of the DNA from the polymer becomes a problem and limits the transfection efficiency. Examination of a dendrimer structure has also led to the conclusion that a certain level of backbone flexibility is necessary to mediate high levels of transfection.

Two of the polymer structures exhibit significant toxicities while the other does not. PEI and amino methacrylate polymers both exhibited a great degree of cytotoxicity, while polyamidoamines did not. The most striking difference between these two groups is the degradability of their backbones; polyethylenimine and poly(aminomethacrylate) (PAM) are not degradable while polyamidoamines have been shown to break down over long periods of time *in vitro*. The toxicity of PEI and PAM increases with higher charge ratios, higher polymer molecular weight, higher charge density, and greater complex concentration, while it decreases with

Table 17.1 Factors affecting transfection efficiencies of different cationic polymers

- N/P ratios
- Salt concentrations
- DNA concentration
- Molecular weight of polymer
- Polydispersity
- Aggregation
- Side-chain length
- Number of primary, secondary and tertiary amines
- Hydrophilic components/block

Table 17.2   Guidelines for design of nontoxic polycationic polymers for gene delivery

Polymer type	Parameter	Reference
Polyethylenimine	low molecular weight hydrophilic block	Fischer *et al.* (1999) Nguyen *et al.* (2000)
Polyamidoamine	degradability low molecular weight low charge density	Roberts *et al.* (1996); Hill *et al.* (1999) Hill *et al.* (1999)
Polymethacrylates	low molecular weight low [particles]	Cherng *et al.* (1996) Cherng *et al.* (1996)

the addition of hydrophilic blocks. The introduction of hydrophilic segments or blocks was shown to drastically reduce complement activation *in vivo* by reducing surface charge and hydrophobicity. Table 17.2 summarizes the parameters necessary for the design of a polycationic polymer with low cytotoxicity.

The design of a new polymer system should take into consideration all of the parameters identified to increase transfection efficiency and those that decrease cytotoxicity and immune response.

REFERENCES

Arigita, C., Zuidam, N.J., Crommelin, D.J.A. and Hennink, W.E. (1999) Association and dissociation characteristics of polymer/DNA complexes used for gene delivery. *Pharm. Res.*, **16**, 1534–1541.

Arscott, P.G., Li, A.Z. and Bloomfield, V.A. (1990) Condensation of DNA by trivalent cations. 1. Effects of DNA length and topology on the size and shape of condensed particles. *Biopolymers*, **30**, 619–630.

Bielinska, A., Kukowska-Latallo, J.F., Johnson, J., Tomalia, D.A. and Baker, Jr., J.R. (1996) Regulation of *in vitro* gene expression using antisense oligonucleotides or antisense expression plasmids transfected using starburst PAMAM dendrimers. *Nucleic Acids Res.*, **24**, 2176–2182.

Bielinska, A.U., Kukowska-Latallo, J.F. and Baker, Jr., J.R. (1997) The interaction of plasmid DNA with polyamidoamine dendrimers: mechanism of complex formation and analysis of alterations induced in nuclease sensitivity and transcriptional activity of the complexed DNA. *Biochim. Biophys. Acta.*, **1353**, 180–190.

Boussif, O., Lezoualc'h, F., Zanta, M.A., Mergny, M.D., Scherman, D., Demeneix, B. and Behr, J.P. (1995) A versatile vector for gene and oligonucleotide delivery into cells in culture and *in vivo*: Polyethylenimine. *Proc. Natl. Acad. Sci. USA*, **92**, 7297–7301.

Chattoraj, D.K., Gosule, L.C. and Schellman, A. (1978) DNA condensation with polyamines. II. Electron microscopic studies. *J. Mol. Biol.*, **121**, 327–337.

Cherng, J.-Y., Van de Wetering, P., Talsma, H., Crommelin, D.J.A. and Hennink, W.E. (1996) Effect of size and serum proteins on transfection efficiency of poly((2-dimethyl-amino)ethyl methacrylate)-plasmid nanoparticles. *Pharm. Res.*, **13**, 1038–1042.

Cherng, J.Y., Van de Wetering, P., Talsma, H., Crommelin, D.J.A. and Hennink, W.E. (1997) Freeze-drying of poly((2-dimethylamino)ethyl methacrylate)-based gene delivery systems. *Pharm. Res.*, **14**, 1838–1841.

Cherng, J.-Y., Schuurmans-Nieuwenbroek, N.M.E., Jiskoot, W., Talsma, H., Zuidam, N.J., Hennink, W.E. and Crommelin, D.J.A. (1999a) Effect of DNA topology on the transfection efficiency of poly((2-dimethylamino)ethyl methacrylate)-plasmid complexes. *J. Control. Release*, **60**, 343–353.

Cherng, J.-Y., Talsma, H., Verrijk, R., Crommelin, D.J.A. and Hennink, W.E. (1999b) The effect of forumulation parameters on the size of poly((2-dimethylamino)ethyl methacrylate)-plasmid complexes. *Eur. J. Pharm. Biopharm.*, **47**, 215–224.

Cherng, J.-Y., Talsma, H., Crommelin, D.J.A. and Hennink, W.E. (1999c) Long term stability of poly((2-dimethylamino)ethyl methacrylate)-based gene delivery systems. *Pharm. Res.*, **16**, 1417–1423.

Cotten, M., Laengle-Rouault, F. and Kirlappos, H. (1990) Transferrin-polycation-mediated introduction of DNA into human leukemic cells: stimulation by agents that affect the survival of transfected DNA or modulate transferrin receptor levels. *Proc. Natl. Acad. Sci. USA*, **87**, 4033–4037.

Densmore, C.L., Orson, F.M., Xu, B., Kinsey, B.M., Waldrep, J.C., Hua, P. *et al.* (2000) Aerosol delivery of robust polyethyleneimine–DNA complexes for gene therapy and genetic immunization. *Mol. Ther.*, **1**, 180–188.

Diebold, S.S., Kursa, M., Wagner, E., Cotten, M. and Zenke, M. (1999) Mannose polyethylenimine conjugates for targeted DNA delivery into dendritic cells. *J. Biol. Chem.*, **274**, 19087–19094.

Dunlop, D.D., Maggi, A., Soria, M.R. and Monaco, L. (1997) Nanoscopic structure of DNA condensed for gene delivery. *Nucleic Acids Res.*, **25**, 3095–3101.

Eastman, S.J., Tousignant, J.D., Lukason, M.J., Chu, Q., Cheng, S.H. and Scheule, R.K. (1998) Aerosolization of cationic lipid:pDNA complexes: *In vitro* optimization of nebulizer parameters for human clinical studies. *Hum. Gene Ther.*, **9**, 43–52.

Esfand, R. and Tomalia, D.A. (2001) Poly(amidoamine) (PAMAM) dendrimers: from biomimicry to drug delivery and biomedical applications. *Drug Discovery Today*, **6**, 427–436.

Fisher, D., Bieber, T., Li, Y., Elsasser, H.P. and Kissel, T. (1999) A novel non-viral vector for DNA delivery based on low molecular weight, branched polyethylenimine: effect of molecular weight on transfection efficiency and cytotoxicity. *Pharm. Res.*, **51**, 321–328.

Godbey, W.T., Barry, M.A., Saggau, P., Wu, K.K. and Mikos, A.G. (2000a) Poly(ethylenimine)-mediated transfection: A new paradigm for gene delivery. *J. Biomed. Mater. Res.*, **51**, 321–328.

Godbey, W.T., Wu, K.K. and Mikos, A.G. (1999a) Size matters: Molecular weight affects the efficiency of poly(ethylenimine) as a gene delivery vehicle. *J. Biomed. Mater. Res.*, **45**, 268–275.

Godbey, W.T., Wu, K.K., Hirasaki, G.J. and Mikos, A.G. (1999b) Improved packing of poly(ethylenimine)/DNA complexes increases transfection efficiency. *Gene Ther.*, **6**, 1380–1388.

Godbey, W.T., Wu, K.K. and Mikos, A.G. (1999c) Tracking the intracellular path of poly(ethylenimine)/DNA complexes for gene delivery. *Proc. Natl. Acad. Sci. USA*, **96**, 5177–5181.

Godbey, W.T. and Mikos, A.G. (2000b) Non-viral gene delivery. In: K.D. Park, I.C. Kwon, N. Yui, S.Y. Jeong and K. Park (eds) *Biomaterials and Drug Delivery toward New Millenium.* Han Rim Won Publishing Company, Seoul, pp. 223–236.

Godbey, W.T., Wu, K.K. and Mikos, A.G. (2001) Poly(ethylenimine)-mediated gene delivery affects endothelial cell function and viability. *Biomaterials*, **22**, 471–480.

Haensler, J. and Szoka, Jr., F.C. (1993) Polyamidoamine cascade polymers mediate efficient transfection of cells in culture. *Bioconjug. Chem.*, **4**, 372–379.

Haynes, M., Garrett, R.A. and Gratzer, W.B. (1970) Structure of nucleic acid-poly base complexes. *Biochemistry*, **9**, 4410–4416.

Hill, I.R.C., Garnett, M.C., Bignotti, F. and Davis, S.S. (1999) *In vitro* cytotoxicity of poly(amidoamine)s: relevance to DNA delivery. *Biochim. Biophys. Acta.*, **1427**, 161–174.

Hudde, T., Rayner, S.A., Comer, R.M., Weber, M., Isaacs, J.D., Waldmann, H., Larkin, D.F.P. and George, A.J.T. (1999) Activated polyamidoamine dendrimers, a non-viral vector for gene transfer to the corneal endothelium. *Gene Ther.*, **6**, 939–943.

Izumrudov, V.A., Zhiryakova, M.V. and Kudaibergenov, S.E. (1999) Controllable stability of DNA-containing polyelectrolyte complexes in water-salt solutions. *Biopolymers*, **52**, 94–108.

Jones, N.A., Hill, I.R.C., Stolnik, S., Bignotti, F., Davis, S.S. and Garnett, M.C. (2000) Polymer chemical structure is a key determinant of physicochemical and colloidal properites of polymer–DNA complexes for gene delivery. *Biochim. Biophys. Acta.*, **1517**, 1–18.

Kichler, A., Leborgne, C., Coeytaux, E. and Danos, O. (2001) Polyethylenimine-mediated gene delivery: a mechanistic study. *J. Gene Med.*, **3**, 135–144.

Kukowska-Latallo, J.F., Bielinska, A.U., Johnson, J., Spindler, R., Tomalia, D.A. and Baker, Jr., J.R. (1996) Efficient transfer of genetic material into mammalian cells using Starburst polyamidoamine dendrimers. *Proc. Natl. Acad. Sci. USA*, **93**, 4897–4902.

Li, H.J., Chang, C. and Weiskopf, M. (1973) Helix-coil transition in nucleoprotein-chromatin structure. *Biochemistry*, **12**, 1763–1772.

Marquet, R., Wyart, A. and Houssier, C. (1987) Influence of DNA length on spermine-induced condensation. Importance of the bending and stiffening of DNA. *Biochim. Biophys. Acta.*, **909**, 165–172.

Marschall, P., Malik, N. and Larin, Z. (1999) Transfer of YACs up to 2.3 Mb intact into human cells with polyethylenimine. *Gene Ther.*, **6**, 1634–1637.

Mendiratta, S.K., Quezada, A., Matar, M., Wang, J., Hebel, H.L., Long, S., Nordstrom, J.L. and Pericle, F. (1999) Intratumoral delivery of IL-12 gene by polyvinyl polymeric vector system to murine renal and colon carcinoma results in potent antitumor immunity. *Gene Ther.*, **6**, 833–839.

Mumper, R.J., Duguid, J.G., Anwer, K., Barron, M.K., Nitta, H. and Rolland, A.P. (1996) Polyvinyl derivatives as novel interactive polymers for controlled gene delivery to muscle. *Pharm. Res.*, **13**, 701–709.

Mumper, R.J. and Rolland, A.P. (1998) Plasmid delivery to muscle: Recent advances in polymer delivery systems. *Adv. Drug Deliv. Rev.*, **30**, 151–172.

Mumper, R.J., Wang, J., Klakamp, S.L., Nitta, H., Anwer, K., Tagliaferri, F. and Rolland, A.P. (1998) Protective interactive non-condensing (PINC) polymers for enhanced plasmid distribution and expression in rat skeletal muscle. *J. Control. Release*, **52**, 191–203.

Nguyen, H.-K., Lemieux, P., Vinogradov, S.V., Gebhart, C.L., Guérin, N., Paradis, G. *et al.* (2000) Evaluation of polyether-polyethyleneimine graft copolymers as gene transfer agents. *Gene Ther.*, **7**, 126–138.

Ogris, M., Brunner, S., Schüller, S., Kircheis, R. and Wagner, E. (1999) PEGylated DNA/transferrin-PEI complexes: reduced interaction with blood components, extended circulation in blood and potential for systemic gene delivery. *Gene Ther.*, **6**, 595–605.

Oupicky, D., Konák, C. and Ulbrich, K. (1998) DNA complexes with block and graft copolymers of *N*-(2-hydroxypropyl)methacrylamide and 2-(trimethylammonio)ethyl methacrylate. *J. Biomater. Sci. Polym. Ed.*, **10**, 573–590.

Oupicky, D., Konák, C., Dash, P.R., Seymour, L.W. and Ulbrich, K. (1999) Effect of albumin and polyanion on the structure of DNA complexes with polycation containing hydrophilic nonionic block. *Bioconjug. Chem.*, **10**, 764–772.

Plank, C., Mechtler, K., Szoka, F.C. and Wagner, E. (1996) Activation of the complement system by synthetic DNA complexes: a potential barrier for intravenous gene delivery. *Hum. Gene Ther.*, **7**, 1437–1446.

Plum, G.E., Arscott, P.G. and Bloomfield, V.A. (1990) Condensation of DNA by trivalent cations. 2. Effects of cation structure. *Biopolymers*, **30**, 631–643.

Pollard, H., Remy, J.S., Loussouarn, G., Demolombe, S., Behr, J.P. and Escande, D. (1998) Polyethylenimine but not cationic lipids promotes transgene delivery to the nucleus in mammalian cells. *J. Biol. Chem.*, **273**, 7507–7511.

Poulain, L., Ziller, C., Muller, C.D., Erbacher, P., Bettinger, T., Rodier, J.-F. and Behr, J.-P. (2000) Ovarian carcinoma cells are effectively transfected by polyethylenimine (PEI) derivatives. *Cancer Gene Ther.*, **7**, 644–652.

Pouton, C.W. and Seymour, L.W. (1998) Key issues in non-viral gene delivery. *Adv. Drug Deliv. Rev.*, **34**, 3–19.

Qin, L., Rahud, D.R., Ding, Y., Bielinska, A.U., Kukowska-Latallo, J.F., Baker, Jr., J.R. and Bromberg, J.S. (1998) Efficient transfer of genes into murine cardiac grafts by starburst polyamidoamine dendrimers. *Hum. Gene Ther.*, **9**, 553–560.

Roberts, J.C., Bhalgat, M.K. and Zera, R.T. (1996) Preliminary biological evaluation of polyamidoamine (PAMAM) Starburst dendrimers. *J. Biomed. Mater. Res.*, **30**, 53–65.

Suh, J., Paik, H. and Hwang, B.K. (1994) Ionization of poly(ethylenimine) and poly(allylamine) at various pH's. *Bioorg. Chem.*, **22**, 318–327.

Tang, M.X., Redemann, C.T. and Szoka, F.C. (1996) *In vitro* gene delivery by degraded polyamidoamine dendrimers. *Bioconjug. Chem.*, **7**, 703–714.

Tomalia, D.A., Baker, H., DeWald, J., Kallos, G., Martin, S., Toeck, J., Ryder, J. and Smith, P. (1985) A new class of polymers: Starburst-dendritic macromolecules. *Polymer J.*, **17**, 117–132.

Tomalia, D.A., Naylor, A.M. and Goddard, W.A. (1990) Starburst dendrimers: Molecular-level control of size, shape, surface chemistry, topology, and flexibility from atoms to macroscopic matter. *Angew. Chem. Int. Ed. Eng.*, **29**, 138–175.

Tsan, M.-F., Tsan, G.L. and White, J.E. (1997) Surfactant inhibits cationic liposome-mediated gene transfer. *Hum. Gene Ther.*, **8**, 817–825.

Van de Wetering, P., Cherng, J.-Y., Talsma, D.J.A. and Hennink, W.E. (1998) 2-(dimethylamino)ethyl methacrylate based (co)polymers as gene transfer agents. *J. Control. Release*, **53**, 145–153.

Van de Wetering, P., Moret, E.E., Schuurmans-Nieuwenbroek, N.M.E., Van Steenbergen, M.J. and Hennink, W.E. (1999a) Structure-activity relationships of water-soluble cationic methacrylate/methacrylamide polymers for nonviral gene delivery. *Bioconjug. Chem.*, **10**, 589–597.

Van de Wetering, P., Schuurmans-Nieuwenbroek, N.M.E., Hennink, W.E. and Storm, G. (1999b) Comparative transfection studies of human ovarian carcinoma cells *in vitro, ex vivo* and *in vivo* with poly(2-(dimethylamino)ethyl methacrylate)-based polyplexes. *J. Gene Med.*, **1**, 156–165.

Wightman, L., Patzelt, E., Wagner, E. and Kircheis, R. (1999) Development of transferrin-polycation/DNA based vectors for gene delivery to melanoma cells. *J. Drug Target.*, **7**, 293–303.

Wojda, U. and Miller, J.L. (2000) Targeted transfer of polyethylenimine-avidin-DNA bioconjugates to hematopoietic cells using biotinylated monoclonal antibodies. *J. Pharm. Sci.*, **89**, 674–681.

Wolfert, M.A., Schacht, E.H., Toncheva, V., Ulbrich, K., Nazarova, O. and Seymour, L.W. (1996) Characterization of vectors for gene therapy formed by self-assembly of DNA with synthetic block co-polymers. *Hum. Gene Ther.*, **7**, 2123–2133.

Wolfert, M.A., Dash, P.R., Nazarova, O., Oupicky, D., Seymour, L.W., Smart, S., Strohalm, J. and Ulbrich, K. (1999) Polyelctrolyte vectors for gene delivery: Influence of cationic polymer on biophysical properties of complexes formed with DNA. *Bioconjug. Chem.*, **10**, 993–1004.

Zanta, M.A., Boussif, O., Adib, A. and Behr, J.P. (1997) *In vitro* gene delivery to hepatocytes with galactosylated polyethylenimine. *Bioconjug. Chem.*, **8**, 839–844.

18 Device-mediated gene delivery

Alexander L. Rakhmilevich and
Georg Widera

INTRODUCTION

The introduction of DNA (or RNA) into cells of a patient for the treatment of inherited and acquired diseases has received much interest in the scientific and clinical community over the past few years. Diseases caused by a single gene mutation, such as cystic fibrosis or hemophilia, could be attenuated by long term expression of the correct form of the gene. Immunostimulatory genes might be of help to the immune system in fighting infectious diseases and cancer (Dachs *et al.*, 1997). DNA vectors encoding antigens of a pathogen or tumor might provide preventive or therapeutic use in DNA vaccines. *Ex vivo* gene therapy encompasses the removal of cells from a patient to modify these cells *in vitro* with the therapeutic gene. The manipulated cells are then returned back to the patient. *In vivo* gene therapy, on the other hand, involves the direct introduction of the gene of choice into tissues of the patient. The most persistent challenge for gene therapy, whether *ex vivo* or *in vivo*, is still the delivery of sufficient DNA molecules to specific target cells to achieve desired expression of the encoded gene (Knoell and Yiu, 1998). Several modes of DNA transfer into target cells are currently being pursued.

Viral vectors are the most widely used tools for gene transfer *in vivo* and *ex vivo*. However, viral vectors cause serious side effects and complications. Alternatives to viral systems for gene therapy are under development and some have also reached the clinical setting (Rolland, 1998; Vogel, 2000). Plasmid DNA encoding the gene of interest can be introduced into target tissues and are taken up by the cells. As the stability and uptake of 'naked' plasmid DNA in tissue is very low, chemical and mechanical means are used to increase efficacy. Liposomal formulations are used to coat DNA to protect it from degradation and to enhance binding and uptake by the cells. Even with these improvements to stability and uptake by formulation, however, gene delivery via needle injection remains relatively ineffective and extremely large amounts of DNA have to be used.

To increase the efficacy of non-viral gene delivery, new DNA delivery technologies have been developed. In this chapter, we describe several common device-mediated DNA delivery technologies, such as particle-mediated gene transfer (PMGT), electroporation and jet devices (Figure 18.1). Specific applications of these technologies to gene therapy of cancer and DNA vaccination are emphasized.

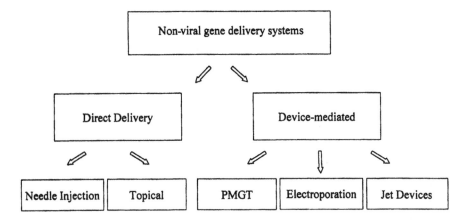

Figure 18.1 Types of non-viral gene delivery systems.

Particle-mediated gene transfer (PMGT)

The PMGT technology, popularly known as the 'gene gun' method, was originally developed for the transformation of plants (McCabe *et al.*, 1988; Christou *et al.*, 1990). High-voltage electric discharge used for these studies was later replaced by helium pulse-operating devices for mammalian gene transfer. PMGT provides a physical means of delivering biologically active molecules, including DNA, RNA, and proteins intracellularly. Because of its physical nature, this method displays properties distinct from those characteristics of chemical and biological gene transfer agents, and has been shown to be advantageous in certain cases (Heiser, 1994). During the past decade, PMGT technology has been shown to be effective for the transfection of various mammalian somatic tissues, including skin, liver, pancreas, muscle, spleen, and heart *in vivo* (Yang *et al.*, 1990; Williams *et al.*, 1991; Cheng *et al.*, 1993; Nishizaki *et al.*, 2000), brain, mammary, and leukocyte primary cultures or tissue explants *ex vivo* (Jiao *et al.*, 1993; Thompson *et al.*, 1993; Burkholder *et al.*, 1993), and a wide range of cell lines *in vitro* (Yang *et al.*, 1990; Thompson *et al.*, 1993; Burkholder *et al.*, 1993; Ye *et al.*, 1998). A major advantage of PMGT is its applicability to cells *in vivo*, an advantage primarily discussed in this review.

PMGT principles

The principles and techniques of PMGT have been described by us in detail elsewhere (Rakhmilevich and Yang, 2000). To achieve PMGT, microscopic gold particles are coated with the gene of interest and accelerated by a motive force (helium shock wave) to sufficient velocities to penetrate the target cells, resulting in intracellular delivery of the DNA molecules. To achieve PMGT, a hand-held transfection device is used (formally, an *Accell* gene delivery device, currently known as a helium-pulse Dermal PowderJect-XR device, PowderJect Vaccines, Inc., Madison, WI, or a commercially available device from Bio-Rad). Using DNA/gold particles loaded within a small teflon tube as a cartridge, the

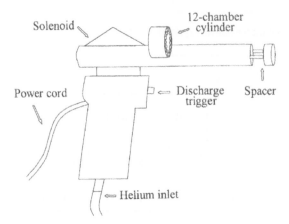

Figure 18.2 Schematic presentation of a hand-held PMGT device.

experimental hand-held helium pulse transfection device can hold 12 cartridges in a revolving cylinder (Figure 18.2). Each gene transfer can be performed in less than five seconds, thus making PMGT a highly efficient method for repeated, multiple gene deliveries. For a clinical application, a device carrying a disposable, sterile, single cartridge per transfection is currently used (Mahvi *et al.*, 1997). The amount of DNA required for PMGT is relatively low; for example, nanogram amounts of DNA per cm^2 of target area have been shown to be effective for DNA vaccine applications (Eisenbraun *et al.*, 1993). This amount corresponds to 10–500 plasmid molecules per particle, on average, assuming a uniform distribution of DNA on the particles. In other studies, the amount of 5000 copies of cDNA delivered per cell was found to be optimal for commonly used reporter genes (Yang *et al.*, 1990; Cheng *et al.*, 1993). Most current PMGT devices use macrocarriers for accelerating DNA-coated particles. Recently, a new gene transfection device that uses a hammering bullet instead of a macrocarrier has been developed and effectively used for transfecting murine liver tissues *in vivo* (Kuriyama *et al.*, 2000).

Some functional parameters that can be modified to optimize PMGT into skin include the following: physical acceleration rate for particle penetration; shape form and size of particles; particle loading rate per target surface area; and DNA loading rate per particle. For transfecting appropriately treated skin tissues, a pressure of 300–500 psi for the helium pulse device (Yang *et al.*, 1997) has been found to confer high levels of transgene expression in mouse skin. Particles made from dense materials, including gold, tungsten, iridium, and platinum are all capable of effectively delivering DNA via the PMGT. However, gold particles are most commonly chosen for two reasons: elemental gold is chemically inert with no cytotoxic effects, and, owing to its common use in the electronics industry, uniform sized gold particles are commercially available. A wide range of gold particle sizes has been evaluated for gene transfer via PMGT. These include 0.95-, 1–3-, 5–7- and 15-µm diameter gold particles. Generally, for cell transfection *in vitro*, smaller sizes of gold particles (0.95–1 µm) are recommended. For mammalian skin tissues, the 2–3-µm gold particles are recommended (Yang *et al.*, 1990; Cheng *et al.*, 1993;

Yang *et al.*, 1997). Some gold particles are available in different forms (e.g., as round particles, crystals, or even aggregates). For gene transfer into skin epidermal cells, crystal and spherical gold particles were found to be similarly useful in gene delivery.

Advantages of PMGT

One of the major advantages of the PMGT method is its capacity for intracellular delivery of high copy numbers of DNA *in vivo*. More than 5,000 copies of 5–10 kb plasmid DNA can be effectively coated onto a single 1–3-μm gold particle with a Ca^{2+}/ spermidine formulation in precipitated form. Approximately 1–2 gold particles (1–3 μm) per cell can be delivered via random distribution into the epidermis containing stratified epithelial cells. This feature of PMGT allows for the use of very small doses of a DNA plasmid for effective immunization *in vivo*. For example, in comparison with the naked DNA injection via syringe, which usually requires from 50 μg to 100 μg DNA per injection (Schreurs *et al.*, 1998; Bellone *et al.*, 2000), PMGT-mediated delivery of 1–3 μg DNA can achieve strong immunization (Biragyn *et al.*, 1999; Chen *et al.*, 2000). Moreover, we have recently shown that the effective dose of antigen DNA can be further reduced to 62.5 ng when combined with the DNA for an adjuvant such as granulocyte macrophage-colony stimulating factor (GM-CSF) (Rakhmilevich *et al.*, 2001). In a recent comparative study, PMGT was more effective than intradermal (i.d.) needle injection in vaccinating mice against malaria, even though 50 times less DNA was administered via PMGT (Weiss *et al.*, 2000).

Another important advantage of PMGT is the much reduced restriction on the size of the DNA vectors. Plasmid DNA, genomic DNA (~23 kb), and reporter genes cloned in lambda phage genomic libraries (~44 kb) can all be effectively delivered into mammalian cells by PMGT (Yang and Ziegelhoffer, 1994). Furthermore, RNA molecules can be similarly delivered as DNA vectors via the PMGT (Qiu *et al.*, 1996). In addition, PMGT offers new opportunities for transferring multiple genes into a single cell or neighboring cells. To transfer several genes into a single cell (assuming that the transfection rate is one gold particle per cell), the plasmids of interest are mixed together prior to precipitating onto gold particles, so that each gold particle is coated with all the tested plasmids. To transfer genes into the neighboring cells, each plasmid is precipitated onto separate gold particles, which are mixed together for coating onto the 'bullets'. Co-transfection of multiple genes on different plasmids has been shown to be efficiently achieved by using the PMGT method (Albertini *et al.*, 1996; Chen *et al.*, 2000). Using a cytokine gene therapy approach, we have recently shown that simultaneous delivery by PMGT of three plasmids encoding IL-12, pro-IL-18, and IFN-1β-converting enzyme (ICE), respectively, resulted in synergistic immunological and antitumor effects (Oshikawa *et al.*, 1999). In a gene vaccination approach, we have shown that co-delivery of two plasmid DNAs, one coding for a tumor-associated antigen (gp100) and another coding for a cytokine (GM-CSF), resulted in augmented protection of mice against poorly immunogenic B16 tumors (Rakhmilevich *et al.*, 2001).

Other significant advantages of PMGT include versatility, safety, low immunogenicity and time-efficiency. By using PMGT, it is possible to transfect different cell types irrespective of their lineage, state of division or differentiation. Because of the ability to transfect resting cells, PMGT is considered to be a safe alternative to the virus-mediated gene delivery, as most viruses require cell proliferation to achieve successful transfection. In addition, PMGT is much less immunogenic than virus-mediated gene transfer, which makes possible repeated gene transfections. PMGT is also a more time-efficient means to generate a tumor vaccine, compared with the virus-mediated gene delivery; thus, PMGT is capable of transfecting tumors within several hours after being removed from a patient (Mahvi *et al.*, 1996). PMGT is also a time-efficient and simple way for *in vivo* gene delivery, as it takes only several seconds to perform an effective skin transfection.

Disadvantages of PMGT

The current disadvantages of PMGT *in vivo* include the limited transfection efficiency for certain tissues, the relatively short duration of transgene expression, and the limited depth of tissue that can be accessed. Because of these features, *in vivo* tumor therapy via PMGT may be less effective than that using adenoviral gene delivery (Wright *et al.*, 1999). Although transient transfection efficiencies from 5–15% can frequently be obtained *in vivo*, and efficiencies approaching 3–50% are possible *in vitro*, efficiencies for stable (i.e., integrative) gene transfer *in vivo* are apparently low, and have not been clearly established in various transfected somatic tissues.

In skin immunization studies, it was found that approximately 90% of the transgenic antigen expression was lost within a week following PMGT, a loss consistent with the sloughing of the epidermal target site (Boyle and Robinson, 2000). Long-term gene expression may be potentially achieved through a combination of PMGT and replicating or actively integrating vector systems, but for the present it appears that the technique is most suitable in applications where short- to medium-term transgene expression is sufficient or desirable, such as DNA vaccine and cytokine gene therapy applications.

For genetic vaccine administration and cytokine gene therapy *in vivo*, PMGT is mostly used on the skin area, where the gold bead delivery is limited to the epidermis (Rakhmilevich *et al.*, 1996). Surgical procedures are required for the delivery of DNA via PMGT into the tumors located either deep in the skin (Sun *et al.*, 1995) or in the visceral organs (Weber *et al.*, 1999). Also, the PMGT method at present cannot deliver genes systemically to cell fractions scattered in large, three-dimensional tissues, like liver or brain, as can certain other gene transfer systems when administered through the circulatory system (He *et al.*, 2000).

IN VIVO APPLICATIONS OF PMGT APPROACH

Among the applications of PMGT technology, transfection of the skin tissues of live animals has resulted in the most interesting findings. High levels of transgene expression and/or induction of immune response have been first demonstrated by *in vivo* PMGT of skin epidermal tissues in rodents (Tang *et al.*, 1992; Cheng *et al.*, 1993). These results were highly reproducible in various animal models including turkeys (Vanrompay *et al.*, 1999), rabbits (Han *et al.*, 1999), dogs (Hogge *et al.*, 1998), pigs (Macklin *et al.*, 1998), horses (Lunn *et al.*, 1999), cattle (Oliveira *et al.*,

2000), and rhesus monkeys (Fuller *et al.*, 1997). Safe and effective skin transfection by PMGT has been recently demonstrated in humans (Tacket *et al.*, 1999). Moreover, induction of antigen-specific T cells and protective levels of antibody in humans by particle-mediated administration of a hepatitis B virus DNA vaccine has been recently reported (Roy *et al.*, 2000). Efficient delivery and expression of transgenes in skin tissues have been extended to several reporter genes (Yang *et al.*, 1990; Yang and Ziegelhoffer, 1994), candidate tumor antigen genes (Irvine *et al.*, 1996; Ciernik *et al.*, 1996; Conry *et al.*, 1996; Ross *et al.*, 1997), cytokine genes (Sun *et al.*, 1995; Rakhmilevich *et al.*, 1997), viral antigen genes (Fuller *et al.*, 1997; Feltquate *et al.*, 1997; Fomsgaard *et al.*, 1999), bacterial antigen genes (Fensterle *et al.*, 1999), and minigenes (Iwasaki *et al.*, 1999), demonstrating the wide ranging applicability of this gene transfer strategy. PMGT into skin tissues has been used for developing genetic immunization approaches (Fuller *et al.*, 1997; Irvine *et al.*, 1996; Ciernik *et al.*, 1996; Conry *et al.*, 1996; Feltquate *et al.*, 1997), gene therapy of subcutaneous tumors (Sun *et al.*, 1995; Rakhmilevich *et al.*, 1996; Rakhmilevich *et al.*, 1997), wound healing (Andree *et al.*, 1994), delivery of RNA as transgenes or immunogens (Qiu *et al.*, 1996), analysis of transcriptional promoters and other regulatory sequences in gene expression vectors (Cheng *et al.*, 1993; Rajagopalan *et al.*, 1995), and also for studying different cell types in transgene expression and migration following DNA immunization (Condon *et al.*, 1996; Iwasaki *et al.*, 1997). When PMGT employs different promoters, gene expression can be restricted to certain cell types, tissues and skin layers (Lin *et al.*, 2001). It appears that, depending on the model used, PMGT can be more effective (Han *et al.*, 2000), or less effective (Tanghe *et al.*, 2000) than intramuscular DNA immunization. In most cases, however, PMGT has been shown to be more effective (Weiss *et al.*, 2000) and reproducible (Yoshida *et al.*, 2000) than needle DNA immunization.

PMGT APPROACH FOR CANCER THERAPY

PMGT has been used to generate tumor vaccines by genetically-modifying tumor cells *in vitro* or *ex vivo*, primarily with cytokine genes. In addition, having many advantages as a simple and efficacious *in vivo* gene delivery method, PMGT into skin has been successfully applied to cancer research as a means of DNA vaccination or cytokine gene therapy (Rakhmilevich and Yang, 2000).

Generation of tumor vaccines *in vitro* and *ex vivo*

The potential advantage of cancer immunotherapy is the ability of the immune system to selectively recognize and attack tumor cells throughout the body. Many human cancers express tumor-associated antigens (TAA) that can be recognized by the immune system (Pardoll, 1998). Immunization using whole tumor cell vaccine, TAA peptides, or TAA genes is a promising therapeutic strategy for cancers (Roth and Cristiano, 1997). However, vaccination with tumor cells alone, without adjuvants, rarely achieved a substantial anti-tumor effect due to insufficient antigen presentation or co-stimulation (Pardoll, 1998).

The hope for clinical cancer immunotherapy was raised by the exciting findings that some 'nonimmunogenic' tumors may be genetically modified to allow them to induce immune responses which can be detected following certain experimental approaches (Pardoll, 1998; Roth and Cristiano, 1997). PMGT has been successfully used to transfect tumor cells with co-stimulatory genes (Albertini *et al.*, 1996; McCarthy *et al.*, 2000) or cytokine genes (Figure 18.3A). The transfection of weak immunogenic tumor cells with GM-CSF expression plasmids, followed by vaccination, resulted in the generation of an immune response that was able to control growth of parental tumors in several mouse tumor models (Mahvi *et al.*, 1996; Shi *et al.*, 1999). Whereas viral methods of gene delivery require the establishing of tumor cell cultures from patient's samples, PMGT was found to be an effective means for transfecting tumors within several hours after removal from a patient (Mahvi *et al.*, 1996). Based on these findings, the first clinical study using PMGT was conducted as the method of *ex vivo* transfection of tumor cells with GM-CSF expression plasmids (Mahvi *et al.*, 1997). Another group of investigators has confirmed the efficacy of PMGT for transfecting human tumors, in that primary renal carcinoma cell lines, obtained from patient tumor tissues, were found to produce high levels of GM-CSF following transfection with GM-CSF DNA using PMGT (Seigne *et al.*, 1999). Transfection of tumor cell vaccine with GM-CSF cDNA *ex vivo* via PMGT was found to result in more effective tumor protection than transfecting the skin above the cutaneous tumor vaccine with GM-CSF cDNA (Shi *et al.*, 1999). Similar to cytokine genes, the particle-mediated delivery of cDNA for the co-stimulatory molecules, such as B7-1, into human cells enhanced the antigenicity of gene-modified cells (McCarthy *et al.*, 2000). A separate approach of transfecting dendritic cells with TAA genes via PMGT for the induction of immune response has been recently described (Tüting and Albers, 2000).

DNA vaccination *in vivo*

DNA immunization, a novel method for inducing protective immune responses, was recently introduced into the scientific community (Tang *et al.*, 1992) and has proven to be very effective in animal models (Donnelly *et al.*, 1997). DNA immunization entails the direct *in vivo* administration of plasmid-based DNA vectors that encode specific antigens. Due to the immunogenicity and safety features of DNA vaccines, considerable efforts are being made to develop this new vaccination modality, which would lead to the safety and efficacy trials in humans (MacGregor *et al.*, 1998; Wang *et al.*, 1998; Tacket *et al.*, 1999). For tumor studies, this approach involves the delivery into the skin (or other tissues in rare cases) of genes encoding TAA in an attempt to induce antitumor immune responses.

Two methods of administration for the vaccine DNA are commonly used: the most widely used is the direct DNA injection into muscle (Wolf *et al.*, 1990) or skin (Raz *et al.*, 1994) by needle and syringe. This method is effective in inducing immune responses in small animals, such as mice, but it requires the administration of relatively large amounts of DNA (50 to 100 µg per mouse). To obtain immune responses in larger animals, such as rabbits, non-human primates, and humans, very large amounts of DNA have to be injected (Wang *et al.*, 1998). It remains to be seen whether this requirement for large doses of vaccine DNA turns out to be practical for safety and commercial reasons in human applications.

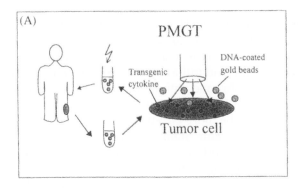

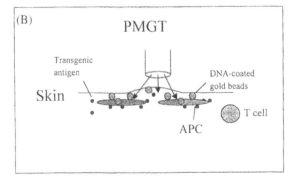

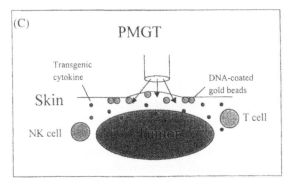

Figure 18.3 Approaches for cancer gene therapy using PMGT. (A) Generation of tumor vaccines *ex vivo*. After the tumor is removed from a patient and the single cell suspension is obtained, tumor cells are transfected via PMGT with a certain cytokine gene such as GM-CSF (Mahvi *et al.*, 1996), or with another immunomodulatory gene. The cells are then lethally irradiated and injected back into the patient as an intradermal vaccine. (B) DNA vaccination *in vivo*. The skin is transfected with the genes encoding a tumor-associated antigen, with or without adjuvant genes such as GM-CSF. Cutaneous dendritic cells can be directly transfected (Condon *et al.*, 1996) and present the transgenic tumor antigen to T cells, primarily in draining lymph nodes, resulting in induction of immune response against the tumor. (C) Cytokine gene therapy *in vivo*. The skin overlaying a subcutaneous or intradermal tumor is transfected via PMGT with the genes encoding cytokines such as IL-12 (Rakhmilevich *et al.*, 1996). The transfected epidermal cells produce the transgenic cytokine, which activates T cells, NK cells and other immune cells in the vicinity of the tumor.

The second method of administering vaccine DNA is the use of the PMGT (Figure 18.3B). Using PMGT, successful vaccinations against tumors have been achieved with the plasmid DNA encoding β-galactosidase (Irvine *et al.*, 1996; Ross *et al.*, 1997) or ovalbumin (Ross *et al.*, 1997), and mutant p53 oncoprotein (Ciernik *et al.*, 1996; Tüting *et al.*, 1999), carcinoembrionic antigen (Conry *et al.*, 1996), or human papillomavirus E7 antigen (Chen *et al.*, 1999). In the study of Ross *et al.* (1997), vaccination by PMGT was found to be more effective than vaccination with a peptide, even when combined with an adjuvant. Similarly, vaccination with DNA constructs encoding fusions of chemokines with TAA generated superior tumor protection, as compared with the protein vaccines (Biragyn *et al.*, 1999). In several comparative studies, PMGT was found to require 10–12 times less DNA than intramuscular (i.m.) injections in order to achieve a comparable level of immunization (Bennett *et al.*, 1999; Degano *et al.*, 1999).

In an attempt to elucidate the mechanism of induction of immune response by PMGT into the skin, the trafficking of cutaneous dendritic cells carrying the DNA/gold beads to draining lymph nodes has been elegantly demonstrated (Condon *et al.*, 1996). These cutaneous dendritic cells directly transfected with DNA-encoded antigen via PMGT have been shown to play a predominant role in antigen presentation to CD8$^+$T cells (Porgador *et al.*, 1998). These results suggest that the enhanced antigen presentation by bone marrow-derived dendritic cells to T lymphocytes is responsible for induction of the antitumor immunity in cutaneous gene immunization experiments (Condon *et al.*, 1996). The PMGT method for a co-delivery of adjuvant genes with TAA genes has been successfully used to further augment antigen presentation and to induce enhanced antitumor immunity in mouse models. These results were achieved by the co-delivery of plasmids encoding such cytokines as IL-12 (Tüting *et al.*, 1999; Tan *et al.*, 1999), IFN-γ (Charo *et al.*, 1999) and GM-CSF (Conry *et al.*, 1996; Charo *et al.*, 1999). We have recently established a model of gene vaccination against melanoma using PMGT for gp100 gene delivery in the skin of mice. The results show that co-administration of human gp100 and murine GM-CSF expression plasmids resulted in a much greater vaccination effect than the delivery of the gp100 cDNA vaccine alone. Moreover, this DNA combination was effective in a treatment protocol, resulting in the suppression of tumor growth and the extended survival of mice bearing established B16 melanoma that genetically expressed human gp100 (Rakhmilevich *et al.*, 2001). Similar to cytokine genes, genes encoding for heat-shock protein 70 (Chen *et al.*, 2000) or chemokines (Biragyn *et al.*, 1999) provided substantial adjuvant effect when combined with the TAA genes and delivered into the skin of mice by PMGT.

Cytokine gene therapy

Another approach using PMGT involves the treatment of already established subcutaneous tumors with cytokine genes (Figure 18.3C). We have reported a powerful, T cell-mediated tumor regression following skin transfection with the IL-12 gene in several mouse tumor models (Rakhmilevich *et al.*, 1996). Moreover, the localized IL-12 gene delivery into the skin overlaying the immunogenic tumor has resulted in a systemic effect against visceral metastases (Rakhmilevich *et al.*, 1996) and a distant solid tumor (Rakhmilevich *et al.*, 1997). Histological analysis showed that IL-12 transgene expression was readily detectable in the epidermis, although the DNA-coated gold beads did not reach the implanted tumor (Rakhmilevich *et al.*, 1996). This gene therapy approach using PMGT was also shown to be applicable and effective not only against cutaneous tumors, but also against tumors in visceral organs such as liver (Weber *et al.*, 1999). The important feature of this IL-12 gene therapy approach is the apparent lack of toxicity, in contrast to relatively toxic recombinant IL-12 protein administration (Rakhmilevich *et al.*, 1999).

In contrast to immunogenic tumors, IL-12 gene therapy of poorly immunogenic tumors via PMGT may elicit different antitumor mechanisms. Thus, IL-12 gene transfer into the skin surrounding and overlaying a poorly immunogenic 4T1 mammary adenocarcinoma has resulted in a significant reduction of spontaneous lung metastases, while having no significant effect on the growth of the primary intradermal tumor (Rakhmilevich *et al.*, 2000). In contrast to the antitumor effect of IL-12 gene therapy described above, this anti-metastatic effect was not mediated by T cells, but involved NK cells and IFN-γ. Our subsequent study using the spontaneous LLC-F5 metastasis model showed that particle-mediated IL-12 gene delivery can confer anti-metastatic activities via a combination of several mechanisms involving CD8$^+$T cells, NK cells, IFN-γ, and antiangiogenesis (Oshikawa *et al.*, 2001).

While several cytokine genes were tested in a therapeutic strategy by the PMGT (Sun *et al.*, 1995), IL-12 expression plasmid DNA was shown to be the most effective cytokine gene among six other cytokine genes tested (Rakhmilevich *et al.*, 1997). However, co-delivery of multiple genes into one cell may result in an additive or synergistic antitumor effect. Thus, co-delivery of pro-IL-18 DNA and ICE DNA with IL-12 DNA into the skin of TS/A adenocarcinoma-bearing mice substantially potentiated the antitumor and anti-metastatic activity of IL-12 gene therapy (Oshikawa *et al.*, 1999).

Depending on the mechanism of action, certain cytokine genes may be more effective in some gene therapy approaches than others. Thus, the GM-CSF gene, although shown to have a limited activity against established cutaneous tumors following PMGT *in vivo* (Rakhmilevich *et al.*, 1997; Tanigawa *et al.*, 2000), was much more effective as an adjuvant in the *ex vivo* tumor vaccine approach (Shi *et al.*, 1999), or in the DNA vaccination approach (Rakhmilevich *et al.*, 2001).

ELECTROPORATION-MEDIATED GENE DELIVERY

Electroporation is widely used *in vitro* to effectively introduce DNA into eukaryotic cells and bacteria. Application of short electrical pulses to the target cells opens pores in the cell membrane, facilitating an effective DNA uptake (Neumann *et al.*, 1982; Potter, 1988). It has only recently been found that applying an electric field to targeted tissues *in vivo* significantly increases DNA uptake and thus gene expression (Nishi *et al.*, 1996). Electroporation-augmented DNA transfer *in vivo* offers a number of advantages over viral vectors, as DNA can be introduced into all tissues or cells accessible to the applicator electrodes (Figure 18.4). The procedure is easy and takes a very short time to perform (Muramatsu *et al.*, 1998). As no immunogenicity to the vector is generated, repeated administration of DNA is

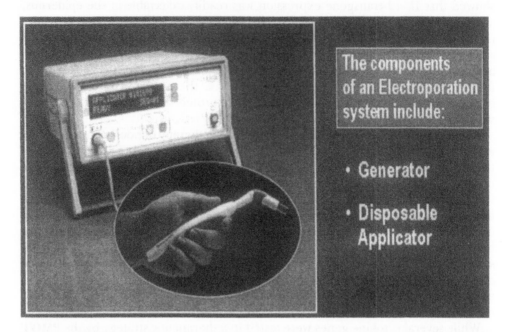

Figure 18.4 Pulse generator and applicator electrode for *in vivo* electroporation. The applicator electrode shown here consists of six needles and is used for intra-tumoral and intra-muscular applications in large animals. Two needle applicator electrodes for use in rodent muscles are commercially available.

possible, and DNA of any size can be administered. A case for using electroporation in gene therapy has been made by Matthews *et al*. (1995).

Electroporation for *ex vivo* gene therapy

Three clinical studies are currently under way employing electroporation augmented gene transfer into target cells *in vitro* and returning the manipulated cells into the patient: two involve gene transfer to ameliorate bleeding disorders, the third involves cancer immunotherapy (Keating *et al*., 1998; Keating *et al*., in press; Fakhari, personal communication). For the last study, a preclinical efficacy of electroporation as a transfection device was established in the rat glioma model (Fakhari *et al*., 1996).

Electroporation for *in vivo* gene therapy

The usefulness and positive effect of *in vivo* electroporation on gene expression has been described for a variety of genes, animal models, and tissues (Muramatsu *et al*., 1998). Titomirov *et al*. (1991) described the stable transformation of skin cells of newborn mice by plasmid DNA as early as 1991. Mouse testis (Muramatsu *et al*., 1997), hen oviduct (Ochiai *et al*., 1998), and murine spermatogenic cells (Yamazaki *et al*., 1998) are among tissues of the reproductive tract successfully transfected by *in vivo* electroporation. Rat bladder (Harimoto *et al*., 1998) and rat liver (Heller *et al.*, 1996) have been targeted. Also, cardiac tissue (chick heart) has successfully been used for electroporation-augmented gene transfer (Harrison *et al.*, 1998). Increase in the levels and duration of gene expression has been shown for reporter genes, but also for genes of interest for therapeutic applications, such as herpes simplex virus-thymidine kinase (HSV-TK), in brain tumor (Nishi *et al.*, 1996) and subcutaneous solid tumors (Goto, 2000). *In vivo* electroporation enhanced DNA and protein uptake in a murine melanoma model (Rols *et al.*, 1998).

One of the most promising tissues for gene transfer in a clinical setting is the muscle. Gene transfer into the muscle can be used for treatment and correction of muscle disorders, such as Duchenne's muscular dystrophy, for systemic secretion of therapeutic proteins, and for vaccination purposes. *In vivo* electroporation increases gene expression by 100- to 1000-fold compared to the needle injection of plasmid DNA (Ahira and Miyazaki, 1998; Mir *et al.*, 1998). Many more muscle fibers are transfected, and the variability of gene expression between individual animals is greatly decreased. Among clinically relevant genes expressed are IL-5 (Ahira and Miyazaki, 1998), fibroblast growth factor-1 (Mir *et al.*, 1999), and erythropoietin (EPO) (Kreiss *et al.*, 1999). *In vivo* electroporation of muscle tissue can be accomplished by a few monopolar electroporation pulses, using low voltage (electric field of up to 200 V/cm) and long pulse duration conditions, as demonstrated by Ahira and Miyazaki (1998) and Mir *et al.* (1998, 1999). In addition to these conditions, trains of low voltage, high frequency bipolar pulses have been used to increase gene expression in muscle by Mathiesen (1999), showing that the electroporation stimuli can be delivered in different ways to the fibers to achieve similar increases in expression. *In vivo* electroporation does differ, however, from conditions used *in vitro*, where normally high voltage and short pulse duration conditions are used.

Most studies reporting enhancement of gene expression after electroporation were done in mouse muscle, but similar increases were found in larger animals, such as rabbits and non-human primates (Mir *et al.*, 1999). As *in vivo* electroporation after i.m. injection dramatically increases gene expression, decreases variability of expression levels between individual animals, provides long lasting expression, and allows modulation of gene expression levels by varying the amount of DNA applied or varying the electroporation conditions, this method of gene delivery may be the most promising for use in a clinical setting.

Use of electroporation for DNA vaccination

As opposed to the DNA vaccination via PMGT, where DNA is introduced directly into cells by gold particles, the extracellularly-delivered DNA after needle and syringe injection has to overcome the physical barrier of the cell membrane via a passive and rather ineffective process. This very inefficient DNA uptake is most likely the reason for the large quantities of DNA needed to induce immune responses *in vivo*, especially in larger animals and human. Increased gene expression *in vivo* can be achieved by electroporation in various tissues after DNA transfer, as described above. This process is of great interest for gene therapy applications, where the use of non-viral vectors is desired because of safety and ease of production, but is hampered by the relatively lower level of gene expression and duration, compared to the best viral systems available today. We have recently demonstrated that *in vivo* electroporation could also increase the efficiency of DNA vaccination after i.m. injection (Widera *et al.*, 2000). Using a weak immunogenic hepatitis B surface antigen DNA vaccine and a potent HIV gag DNA vaccine, we have shown that *in vivo* electroporation improves DNA immunization efficacy in three ways: the immune response is observed earlier than without electroporation, the magnitude of the resulting response is increased, and far less DNA can be used to reproducibly induce an immune response. In addition to mice, immune responses were enhanced by electroporation in guinea pigs and rabbits (Widera *et al.*, 2000). Therefore, *in vivo* electroporation may prove useful at increasing effectiveness of DNA vaccines, which is of special significance for the application in large animals and potentially in humans.

JET DEVICE-MEDIATED NUCLEIC ACID DELIVERY

Of all non-viral gene delivery systems, the direct injection by needle and syringe into muscle or skin (or other tissues) is still the most widely used. The biggest drawback for needle and syringe as a delivery system when applied to gene delivery is the low efficacy achieved in larger animals and humans. The needle-free injection (jet injection) of vaccines by aerosol jet was introduced for military use almost 50 years ago, and today a variety of injectors for the injection of vaccines, proteins, or drugs are available that utilize gas pressure or spring tension to generate the aerosol jet. For example, the Biojector system (Bioject Inc., Portland, OR), one of the most studied jet devices, delivers solutions into the skin or muscle via a very thin stream generated by high pressure CO_2. Jet injection has been validated as a safe and efficacious method for delivering protein vaccines to muscle. When compared to injection by needle and syringe, the Biojector-mediated delivery of the Hepatitis B DNA vaccine resulted in a nearly four-fold greater antibody production (Davis *et al.*, 1994). In a similar comparative study, the jet-injector application of the Hepatitis A vaccine has been shown to yield a higher proportion of seroconversion (Williams *et al.*, 2000). When jet-injection of a recombinant vaccinia virus carcinoembryonic antigen (CEA) vaccine into the skin of cancer patients was compared to injection by needle and syringe, both methods proved to be equally efficient (Conry *et al.*, 1999). However, the accommodation of larger injection volumes, enhanced standardization between clinicians, and the avoidance of needles that could transmit the vaccine or blood-borne pathogens to health care workers were compelling arguments for continuing trials using the jet-injector administration technique (Conry *et al.*, 1999).

The use of needle-free jet devices for the delivery of nucleic acids has been described for various disease models, and has been found to generally enhance DNA uptake in various tissues and to increase DNA vaccine efficacy. Jet injection has been found to be an efficient method to induce papillomas in rabbits by inoculation with cottontail rabbit papillomavirus DNA (Brandsma *et al.*, 1991). Jet injection has been used to introduce DNA through the skin surface, effectively transfecting skin, muscle, fat and mammary tumor tissue (Furth *et al.*, 1992).

Especially in the application of DNA vaccination, jet injection has been found to increase efficacy when compared to the injection of DNA by needle and syringe. This has first been described for the classical i.m. route in rabbits (Davis *et al.*, 1994) and monkeys (Gramzinski *et al.*, 1998). However, with the development of specialized instruments, jet injection is also used successfully to deliver DNA vaccines to skin (Haensler *et al.*, 1999; Amara *et al.*, 2001). Comparing jet delivery to skin with i.m. delivery by needle of an influenza hemaglutinin DNA vaccine in mice and monkeys, both routes of immunization were found to be equally efficient in inducing ELISA antibody titers and hemaglutinin inhibition titers (Haensler *et al.*, 1999). When i.m. delivery of a DNA vaccine against pseudorabies in pigs by needle and syringe or jet device was compared to delivery to skin by needle, however, the skin route was found to induce better protection from challenge than i.m. inoculation (VanRooij *et al.*, 1998). The choice of route and method of delivery of a DNA vaccine will have to be determined in a relevant animal model, and will depend on the immune response necessary to achieve the desired protective or therapeutic effect.

CONCLUDING REMARKS

There are a variety of methods available to improve efficacy of DNA uptake in a non-viral manner, many of which are described in this book. A combination of mechanical and chemical means has been shown to have a synergistic effect on improving DNA vaccine efficacy. Formulation of DNA with polyvinylpyrrolidone (PVP) and delivery of this complex by using a needle-free injection device was found to elicit higher antibody titers in dogs and pigs against delivered hGH DNA then could be achieved by delivery of formulated DNA by needle or jet device delivery of naked DNA. This synergistic effect was observed for i.m. and i.d. DNA delivery (Anwer *et al.*, 1999). As non-viral gene therapy approaches are becoming more important, and as more DNA vaccines, using multiple antigens, are approaching experimentation in larger animals, a combination of several delivery systems, direct and device-mediated, might prove to be advantageous.

ACKNOWLEDGMENTS

This work was supported by the UWCCC pilot grant (A.L.R.) and the Midwest Athletes Against Childhood Cancer (MACC) Fund Grant (A.L.R.).

REFERENCES

Ahira, H. and Miyazaki, J. (1998) Gene transfer into muscle by electroporation. *Nat. Biotechnol.*, **16**, 867–870.

Albertini, M.R., Emler, C.A., Schell, K., Tans, K.J., King, D.M. and Sheehy, M.J. (1996) Dual expression of human leukocyte antigen molecules and the B7-1 co-stimulatory molecule (CD80) on human melanoma cells after particle-mediated gene transfer. *Cancer Gene Ther.*, **3**, 192–201.

Amara, R.R., Villinger, F., Altman, J.D., Lydy, S.L., O'Neil, S.P., Staprans, S.I. *et al.* (2001) Control of a mucosal challenge and prevention of AIDS by a multiprotein DNA/MVA vaccine. *Science*, **292**, 69–74.

Andree, C., Swain, W.F., Page, C.P., Macklin, M.D., Slama, J., Hatzis, D. and Eriksson, E. (1994) *In vivo* transfer and expression of an EGF gene accelerates wound repair. *Proc. Natl. Acad. Sci. USA*, **91**, 12188–12192.

Anwer, K., Earle, K.A., Shi, M., Wang, J., Mumper, R.J., Proctor, B. *et al.* (1999) Synergistic effect of formulated plasmid and needle-free injection for genetic vaccines. *Pharm. Res.*, **16**, 889–895.

Bellone, M., Cantarella, D., Castiglioni, P., Crosti, M.C., Ronchetti, A., Moro, M. *et al.* (2000) Relevance of the tumor antigen in the validation of three vaccination strategies for melanoma. *J. Immunol.*, **165**, 2651–2656.

Bennett, A.M., Phillpotts, R.J., Perkins, S.D., Jacobs, S.C. and Williamson, E.D. (1999) Gene gun mediated vaccination is superior to manual delivery for immunization with DNA vaccines expressing protective antigens from Yersinia pestis or Venezuelan Equine Encephalitis virus. *Vaccine*, **18**, 588–596.

Biragyn, A., Tani, K., Grimm, M.C., Weeks, S. and Kwak, L.W. (1999) Genetic fusion of chemokines to a self tumor antigen induces protective, T-cell dependent antitumor immunity. *Nat. Biotechnol.*, **17**, 253–258.

Boyle, C.M. and Robinson, H.L. (2000) Basic mechanisms of DNA-raised antibody responses to intramuscular and gene gun immunizations. *DNA Cell Biol.*, **19**, 157–165.

Brandsma, J.L., Yang, Z.H., Barthold, S.W. and Johnson, E.A. (1991) Use of a rapid, efficient inoculation method to induce papillomas by cottontail rabbit papillomavirus DNA shows that the E7 gene is required. *Proc. Natl. Acad. Sci. USA*, **88**, 4816–4820.

Burkholder, J.K., Decker, J. and Yang, N.-S. (1993) Transgene expression in lymphocyte and macrophage primary cultures after particle bombardment. *J. Immunol. Methods*, **165**, 149–156.

Charo, J., Ciupitu, A.M., Le Chevalier De Preville, A., Trivedi, P., Klein, G., Hinkula, J. and Kiessling, R. (1999) A long-term memory obtained by genetic immunization results in full protection from a mammary adenocarcinoma expressing an EBV gene. *J. Immunol.*, **163**, 5913–5919.

Chen, C.H., Ji, H., Suh, K.W., Choti, M.A., Pardoll, D.M. and Wu, T.C. (1999) Gene gun-mediated DNA vaccination induces antitumor immunity against human papillomavirus type 16 E7-expressing murine tumor metastases in the liver and lungs. *Gene Ther.*, **6**, 1972–1981.

Chen, C.H., Wang, T.L., Hung, C.F., Yang, Y., Young, R.A., Pardoll, D.M. and Wu, T.C. (2000) Enhancement of DNA vaccine potency by linkage of antigen gene to an HSP70 gene. *Cancer Res.*, **60**, 1035–1042.

Cheng, L., Ziegelhoffer, P. and Yang, N.-S. (1993) *In vivo* promoter activity and transgenic expression in mammalian somatic tissues evaluated by using particle bombardment. *Proc. Natl. Acad. Sci. USA*, **90**, 4455–4459.

Christou, P., McCabe, D., Martinell, B. and Swain, W. (1990) Soybean genetic engineering-commercial production of transgenic plants. *Trends Biotechnol.*, **8**, 145–151.

Ciernik, F., Berzofsky, J.A. and Carbone, D.P. (1996) Induction of cytotoxic T lymphocytes and antitumor immunity with DNA vaccines expressing single T cell epitopes. *J. Immunol.*, **156**, 2369–2375.

Condon, C., Watkins, S.C., Celluzzi, C.M., Thompson, K. and Falo, L.D. (1996) DNA-based immunization by *in vivo* transfection of dendritic cells. *Nat. Med.*, **2**, 1122–1128.

Conry, R.M., Widera, G., LoBuglio, A.F., Fuller, J.T., Moore, S.E., Barlow, D.L. *et al.* (1996) Selected strategies to augment polynucleotide immunization. *Gene Ther.*, **3**, 67–74.

Conry, R.M., Khazaeli, M.B., Saleh, M.N., Allen, K.O., Barlow, D.L., Moore, S.E. *et al.* (1999) Phase I trial of a recombinant vaccinia virus encoding carcinoembryonic antigen in metastatic adenocarcinoma: comparison of intradermal versus subcutaneous administration. *Clin. Cancer Res.*, **5**, 2330–2337.

Dachs, G.U., Dougherty, G.J., Stratford, I.J. and Chaplin, D.J. (1997) Targeting gene therapy to cancer: a review. *Oncol. Res.*, **9**, 313–325.

Davis, H.L., Michel, M.L., Mancini, M., Schleef, M. and Whalen, R.G. (1994) Direct gene transfer in skeletal muscle: plasmid DNA-based immunization against the hepatitis B virus surface antigen. *Vaccine*, **12**, 1503–1509.

Degano, P., Schneider, J., Hannan, C.M., Gilbert, S.C. and Hill, A.V. (1999) Gene gun intradermal DNA immunization followed by boosting with modified vaccinia virus Ankara: enhanced CD8$^+$ T cell immunogenicity and protective efficacy in the influenza and malaria models. *Vaccine*, **18**, 623–632.

Donnelly, J.J., Ulmer, J.B., Shiver, J.W. and Liu, M.A. (1997) DNA vaccines. *Annu. Rev. Immunol.*, **15**, 617–648.

Eisenbraun, M.D., Fuller, D.H. and Haynes, J.R. (1993) Examination parameters affecting the elicitation of humoral immune responses by particle bombardment mediated genetic immunization. *DNA Cell Biol.*, **12**, 791–797.

Fakhrai, H., Dorigo, O., Shawler, D.L., Lin, H., Mercola, D., Black, K.L. *et al.* (1996) Eradication of established intracranial rat glioma by TGF antisense gene therapy. *Proc. Natl. Acad. Sci. USA*, **93**, 2909–2914.

Feltquate, D.M., Heaney, S., Webster, R.G. and Robinson, H.L. (1997) Different T helper cell types and antibody isotypes generated by saline and gene gun DNA immunization. *J. Immunol.*, **158**, 2278–2284.

Fensterle, J., Grode, L., Hess, J. and Kaufmann, S.H. (1999) Effective DNA vaccination against listeriosis by prime/boost inoculation with the gene gun. *J. Immunol.*, **163**, 4510–4518.

Fomsgaard, A., Nielsen, H.V., Kirkby, N., Bryder, K., Corbet, S., Nielsen, C., Hinkula, J. and Buus, S. (1999) Induction of cytotoxic T-cell responses by gene gun DNA vaccination with minigenes encoding influenza A virus HA and NP CTL-epitopes. *Vaccine*, **18**, 681–691.

Fuller, D.H., Corb, M.M., Barnett, S., Steimer, K. and Haynes, J.R. (1997) Enhancement of immunodeficiency virus-specific immune responses in DNA- immunized rhesus macaques. *Vaccine*, **15**, 924–926.

Furth, P.A., Shamay, A., Wall, R.J. and Henninghaused, L. (1992) Gene transfer into somatic tissues by jet injection. *Anal. Biochem.*, **205**, 365–368.

Goto, T., Nishi, T., Tamura, T., Dev, S.B., Takeshima, H., Kochi, M., Yoshizato, K., Kuratsu, J., Sakata, T., Hofmann, G.A. and Ushio, Y. (2000) Highly efficient electro-gene therapy of solid tumor by using an expression plasmid for the herpes simplex virus thymidine kinase gene. *Proc. Natl. Acad. Sci. USA*, **97**, 354–359.

Gramzinski, R.A., Millan, C.L., Obaldia, N., Hoffman, S.L. and Davis, H.L. (1998) Immune response to a hepatitis B DNA vaccine in Aotus monkeys: a comparison of vaccine formulation, route, and method of administration. *Mol. Med.*, **4**, 109–118.

Haensler, J., Verdelet, C., Sanchez, V., Girerd-Chambaz, Y., Bonnin, A., Trannoy, E., Krishnan, S. and Meulien, P. (1999) Intradermal DNA immunization by using jet-injectors in mice and monkeys. *Vaccine*, **17**, 628–638.

Han, R., Cladel, N.M., Reed, C.A., Peng, X. and Christensen, N.D. (1999) Protection of rabbits from viral challenge by gene gun-based intracutaneous vaccination with a combination of cottontail rabbit papillomavirus E1, E2, E6, and E7 genes. *J. Virol.*, **73**, 7039–7043.

Han, R., Reed, C.A., Cladel, N.M. and Christensen, N.D. (2000) Immunization of rabbits with cottontail rabbit papillomavirus E1 and E2 genes: protective immunity induced by gene gun-mediated intracutaneous delivery but not by intramuscular injection. *Vaccine*, **18**, 2937–2944.

Harimoto, K., Sugimura, K., Lee, C.R., Kuratsukuri, K. and Kishimoto, T. (1998) *In vivo* gene transfer methods in the bladder without viral vectors. *Br. J. Urol.*, **81**, 870–874.

Harrison, R.L., Byrne, B.J. and Tung, L. (1998) Electroporation-mediated gene transfer in cardiac tissue. *FEBS Lett.*, **435**, 1–5.

He, Y., Pimenov, A.A., Nayak, J.V., Plowey, J., Falo, L.D. and Huang, L. (2000) Intravenous injection of naked DNA encoding secreted flt3 ligand dramatically increases the number of dendritic cells and natural killer cells *in vivo*. *Hum. Gene Ther.*, **11**, 547–554.

Heiser, W.C. (1994) Gene transfer into mammalian cells by particle bombardment. *Anal. Biochem.*, **217**, 185–196.

Heller, R., Jaroszeski, M., Atkin, A., Moradpour, D., Gilbert, R., Wands, J. and Nicolau, C. (1996) *In vivo* gene electroinjection and expression in rat liver. *FEBS Lett.*, **389**, 225–228.

Hogge, G.S., Burkholder, J., Culp, J., Dubielzig, R.R., Albertini, M.R., Keller, E.T. *et al.* (1998) Development of human granulocyte macrophage-colony stimulating factor transfected tumor cell vaccines for the treatment of spontaneous canine cancer. *Hum. Gene Ther.*, **9**, 1851–1861.

Irvine, K.R., Rao, J.B., Rosenberg, S.A. and Restifo, N.P. (1996) Cytokine enhancement of DNA immunization leads to effective treatment of established pulmonary metastases. *J. Immunol.*, **156**, 238–245.

Iwasaki, A., Torres, C.A.T., Ohashi, P.S., Robinson, H.L. and Barber, B.H. (1997) The dominant role of bone marrow-derived cells in CTL induction following plasmid DNA immunization at different sites. *J. Immunol.*, **159**, 11–14.

Iwasaki, A., Dela Cruz, C.S., Young, A.R. and Barber, B.H. (1999) Epitope-specific cytotoxic T lymphocyte induction by minigene DNA immunization. *Vaccine*, **17**, 2081–2088.

Jiao, S., Cheng, L., Wolff, J. and Yang, N.-S. (1993) Particle bombardment-mediated gene transfer and expression in rat brain tissues. *Bio/Technology*, **11**, 497–502.

Keating, A., Berkham, L. and Filshie, R.A. (1998) Phase I study of the translation of genetically marked autologous bone marrow stromal cells. *Hum. Gene Ther.*, **9**, 591–600.

Knoell, D.L. and Yiu, I.M. (1998) Human gene therapy for hereditary diseases: a review of trials. *Am. J. Health Syst. Pharm.*, **55**, 899–904.

Kreiss, P., Bettan, M., Crouzer, J. and Scherman, D. (1999) Erythropoietin secretion and physiological effect in mouse after intramuscular plasmid DNA electrotransfer. *J. Gene Med.*, **1**, 245–250.

Kuriyama, S., Mitoro, A., Tsujinoue, H., Nakatani, T., Yoshiji, H., Tsujimoto, T. *et al.* (2000) Particle-mediated gene transfer into murine livers using a newly developed gene gun. *Gene Ther.*, **7**, 1132–1136.

Lin, M.T.S., Wang, F., Uitto, J. and Yoon, K. (2001) Differential expression of tissue-specific promoters by gene gun. *Br. J. Dermatol.*, **144**, 34–39.

Lunn, D.P., Soboll, G., Schram, B.R., Quass, J., McGregor, M.W., Drape, R.J. *et al.* (1999) Antibody responses to DNA vaccination of horses using the influenza virus hemagglutinin gene. *Vaccine*, **17**, 2245–2258.

MacGregor, R.R., Boyer, J.D., Ugen, K.E., Lacy, K.E., Gluckman, S.J., Bagarazzi, M.L. *et al.* (1998) First human trial of a DNA-based vaccine for treatment of human immunodeficiency virus type 1 infection: safety and host response. *J. Infect. Dis.*, **178**, 92–100.

Macklin, M.D., Mccabe, D., Mcgregor, M.W., Neumann, V., Meyer, T., Callan, R. *et al.* (1998) Immunization of pigs with a particle-mediated DNA vaccine to influenza a virus protects against challenge with homologous virus. *J. Virol.*, **72**, 1491–1496.

Mahvi, D.M., Burkholder, J.K., Turner, J., Culp, J., Malter, J.S., Sondel, P.M. and Yang, N.S. (1996) Particle-mediated gene transfer of granulocyte macrophage-colony stimulating factor cDNA to tumor cells – implications for a clinically relevant tumor vaccine. *Hum. Gene Ther.*, **7**, 1535–1543.

Mahvi, D.M., Sondel, P.M., Yang, N.S., Albertini, M.R., Schiller, J.H., Hank, J. *et al.* (1997) Phase I/IB study of immunization with autologous tumor cells transfected with the GM-CSF gene by particle-mediated transfer in patients with melanoma or sarcoma. *Hum. Gene Ther.*, **8**, 875–888.

Mathiesen, I. (1999) Electropermeabilization of skeletal muscle enhances gene transfer *in vivo*. *Gene Ther.*, **6**, 508–514.

Matthews, K.E., Dev, S.B., Toneguzzo, F. and Keating, A. (1995) Electroporation for gene therapy. In: J.A. Nickoloff (ed.) *Methods in Molecular Biology*, pp. 273–280.

McCabe, D., Swain, W., Martinell, B. and Christou, P. (1988) Stable transformation of soybean (glycine max) by particle acceleration. *Bio/Technology*, **6**, 923–926.

McCarthy, D.O., Glowacki, N., Schell, K., Emler, C.A. and Albertini, M.R. (2000) Antigenicity of human melanoma cells transfected to express the B7-1 co-stimulatory molecule (CD80) varies with the level of B7-1 expression. *Cancer Immunol. Immunother.*, **49**, 85–93.

Mir, L.M., Bureau, M.F., Rangara, R., Schwartz, B. and Scherman, D. (1998) Long-term, high level *in vivo* gene expression after electric pulse-mediated gene transfer into skeletal muscle. *C. R. Acad. Sci. III*, **321**, 893–899.

Mir, L.M., Bureau, M.F., Gehl, J., Rangara, R., Rouy, D., Caillaud, J.M. *et al.* (1999) High efficiency gene transfer into skeletal muscle by electric pulses. *Proc. Natl. Acad. Sci. USA*, **96**, 4262–4267.

Muramatsu, T., Shibata, O., Ryoki, S., Ohmori, Y. and Okumura, J. (1997) Foreign gene expression in the mouse testis by localized in vivo gene transfer. *Biochem. Biophys. Res. Commun.*, **233**, 45–49.

Muramatsu, T., Nakamura, A. and Park, H.M. (1998) *In vivo* electroporation: A powerful and convenient means of non-viral gene transfer to tissues of living animals. *Intl. J. Mol. Med.*, **1**, 55–62.

Neumann, E., Schaefer-Ridder, M., Wang, Y. and Hofschneider, P.H. (1982) Gene transfer into mouse lymphoma cells by electroporation in high electric fields. *EMBO J.*, **1**, 841–845.

Nishi, T., Yoshizato, K., Yamashiro, S., Takeshima, H., Sato, K., Hamada, K. *et al.* (1996) High efficiency *in vivo* gene transfer using intra arterial plasmid DNA injection following *in vivo* electroporation. *Cancer Res.*, **56**, 1050–1055.

Nishizaki, K., Mazda, O., Dohi, Y., Kawata, T., Mizuguchi, K., Kitamura, S. and Taniguchi, S. (2000) *In vivo* gene gun-mediated transduction into rat heart with Epstein-Barr virus-based episomal vectors. *Ann. Thoracic Surg.*, **70**, 1332–1337.

Ochiai, H., Park, H.M., Nakamura, A., Sasaki, R., Okumura, J.I. and Muramatsu, T. (1998) Synthesis of human erythropoietin *in vivo* in the oviduct of laying hens by localized *in vivo* gene transfer using electroporation. *Poult. Sci.*, **77**, 299–302.

Oliveira, S.C., Harms, J.S., Rosinha, G.M., Rodarte, R.S., Rech, E.L. and Splitter, G.A. (2000) Biolistic-mediated gene transfer using the bovine herpesvirus-1 glycoprotein D is an effective delivery system to induce neutralizing antibodies in its natural host. *J. Immunol. Methods*, **245**, 109–118.

Oshikawa, K., Shi, F., Rakhmilevich, A.L., Sondel, P.M., Mahvi, D.M. and Yang, N.-S. (1999) Synergistic inhibition of tumor growth in a murine mammary adenocarcinoma model by combinational gene therapy using interleukin-12, pro-interleukin-18 and IL-1β-converting enzyme cDNA. *Proc. Natl. Acad. Sci. USA*, **96**, 13351–13356.

Oshikawa, K., Rakhmilevich, A.L., Shi, F., Sondel, P.M., Yang, N.-S. and Mahvi, D.M. (2001) Particle-mediated IL-12 gene transfer into the skin distant from tumor site elicits anti-metastatic effect equivalent to local gene transfer. *Hum. Gene Ther.*, **12**, 149–160.

Pardoll, D.M. (1998) Cancer vaccines. *Nat. Med.*, **4**, 525–531.

Porgador, A., Irvine, K.R., Iwasaki, A., Barber, B.H., Restifo, N.P. and Germain, R.N. (1998) Predominant role for directly transfected dendritic cells in antigen presentation to CD8+ T cells after gene gun immunization. *J. Exp. Med.*, **188**, 1075–1082.

Potter, H. (1988) Electroporation in biology: methods, applications, and instrumentation. *Anal. Biochem.*, **174**, 361–373.

Qiu, P., Ziegelhoffer, P., Sun, J. and Yang, N.-S. (1996) Gene gun delivery of mRNA in situ results in efficient transgene expression and immunization. *Gene Ther.*, **3**, 262–268.

Rajagopalan, L.E., Burkholder, J.K., Turner, J., Culp, J., Yang, N.-S. and Malter, J.S. (1995) Targeted mutagenesis of GM-CSF cDNA increases transgenic mRNA stability and protein expression in normal cells. *Blood*, **86**, 2551–2558.

Rakhmilevich, A.L., Turner, J., Ford, M.J., McCabe, D., Sun, W.H., Sondel, P.M., Grota, K. and Yang, N.-S. (1996) Gene gun-mediated skin transfection with interleukin 12 gene results in regression of established primary and metastatic murine tumors. *Proc. Natl. Acad. Sci. USA*, **93**, 6291–6296.

Rakhmilevich, A.L., Janssen, K., Turner, J., Culp, J. and Yang, N.-S. (1997) Cytokine gene therapy of cancer using gene gun technology: Superior antitumor activity of IL-12. *Hum. Gene Ther.*, **8**, 1303–1311.

Rakhmilevich, A.L., Timmins, J.G., Janssen, K., Pohlmann, E.L., Sheehy, M.J. and Yang, N.-S. (1999) Gene gun-mediated IL-12 gene therapy induces antitumor effects in the absence of toxicity: a direct comparison with systemic IL-12 protein therapy. *J. Immunother.*, **22**, 135–144.

Rakhmilevich, A.L. and Yang, N.-S. (2000) *In vivo* particle-mediated gene transfer for cancer therapy. In: W. Walther and U. Stein (eds) *Methods in Molecular Medicine, Vol. 35: Gene Therapy: Methods and Protocols*. Humana Press, Inc., Totowa, NJ, 331–344.

Rakhmilevich, A.L., Janssen, K., Hao, Z., Sondel, P.M. and Yang, N.-S. (2000) Interleukin 12 gene therapy of a weakly immunogenic mouse mammary carcinoma results in reduction of spontaneous lung metastases via a T cell-independent mechanism. *Cancer Gene Ther.*, **7**, 826–838.

Rakhmilevich, A.L., Imboden, M., Hao, Z., Macklin, M.D., Roberts, T., Wright, K.M. *et al.* (2001) Effective particle-mediated vaccination against mouse melanoma by co-administration of plasmid DNA encoding gp100 and granulocyte-macrophage colony-stimulating factor. *Clin. Cancer Res.*, **7**, 952–961.

Raz, E., Carson, D.A., Parker, S.E., Parr, T.B., Abai, A.M., Aichinger, G. *et al.* (1994) Intradermal gene immunization: the possible role of DNA uptake in the induction of cellular immunity to viruses. *Proc. Natl. Acad. Sci. USA*, **91**, 9519–9523.

Rolland, A.P. (1998) From genes to gene medicines: recent advances in nonviral gene delivery. *Crit. Rev. Ther. Drug Carrier Syst.*, **15**, 143–198.

Rols, M.P., Delteil, C., Golzio, M., Dumond, P., Cros, S. and Teissie, J. (1998) *In vivo* electrically mediated protein and gene transfer in murine melanoma. *Nat. Biotechnol.*, **16**, 168–171.

Roth, J.A. and Cristiano, R.J. (1997) Gene therapy for cancer: what have we done and where are we going? *J. Natl. Cancer Inst.*, **89**, 21–39.

Ross, H.M., Weber, L.W., Wang, S., Piskun, G., Dyall, R., Song, P. *et al.* (1997) Priming for T-cell-mediated rejection of established tumors by cutaneous DNA immunization. *Clin. Cancer Res.*, **3**, 2191–2196.

Roy, M.J., Wu, M.S., Barr, L.J., Fuller, J.T., Tussey, L.G., Speller, S. *et al.* (2000) Induction of antigen-specific CD8$^+$T cells, T helper cells, and protective levels of antibody in humans by particle-mediated administration of a hepatitis B virus DNA vaccine. *Vaccine*, **19**, 764–778.

Schreurs, M.W., de Boer, A.J., Figdor, C.G. and Adema, G.J. (1998) Genetic vaccination against the melanocyte lineage-specific antigen gp100 induces cytotoxic T lymphocyte-mediated tumor protection. *Cancer Res.*, **58**, 2509–2514.

Shi, F.-S., Weber, S., Gan, J., Rakhmilevich, A.L. and Mahvi, D.M. (1999) GM-CSF secreted by cDNA transfected tumor cells induces a more potent antitumor response than exogenous GM-CSF . *Cancer Gene Ther.*, **6**, 81–88.

Seigne, J., Turner, J., Diaz, J., Hackney, J., Pow-Sang, J., Helal, M., Lockhart, J. and Yu, H. (1999) A feasibility study of gene gun mediated immunotherapy for renal cell carcinoma. *J. Urol.*, **162**, 1259–1263.

Sun, W.H., Burkholder, J.K., Sun, J., Culp., J., Turner, J., Lu, X.G. *et al.* (1995) *In vivo* cytokine gene transfer by gene gun suppresses tumor growth in mice. *Proc. Natl. Acad. Sci. USA*, **92**, 2889–2893.

Tacket, C.O., Roy, M.J., Widera, G., Swain, W.F., Broome, S. and Edelman, R. (1999) Phase 1 safety and immune response studies of a DNA vaccine encoding hepatitis B surface antigen delivered by a gene delivery device. *Vaccine*, **17**, 2826–2829.

Tan, J., Yang, N.S., Turner, J.G., Niu, G.L., Maassab, H.F., Sun, J. *et al.* (1999) Interleukin-12 cDNA skin transfection potentiates human papillomavirus E6 DNA vaccine-induced antitumor immune response. *Cancer Gene Ther.*, **6**, 331–339.

Tang, D.C., DeVit, M. and Johnston, S.A. (1992) Genetic immunization is a simple method for eliciting an immune response. *Nature*, **356**, 152–154.

Tanghe, A., Denis, O., Lambrecht, B., Motte, V., van den Berg, T. and Huygen, K. (2000) Tuberculosis DNA vaccine encoding Ag85A is immunogenic and protective when administered by intramuscular needle injection but not by epidermal gene gun bombardment. *Infect Immun.*, **68**, 3854–3860.

Tanigawa, K., Yu, H., Sun, R., Nickoloff, B.J. and Chang, A.E. (2000) Gene gun application in the generation of effector T cells for adoptive immunotherapy. *Cancer Immunol. Immunother.*, **48**, 635–643.

Thompson, T.A., Gould, M.N., Burkholder, J.K. and Yang, N.-S. (1993) Transient promoter activity in primary rat mammary epithelial cells evaluated using particle bombardment gene transfer. *In vitro Cell Dev. Biol.*, **29A**, 165–170.

Titomirov, A.V., Sukharev, S. and Kistanova, E. (1991) *In vivo* electroporation and stable transformation of skin cells of newborn mice by plasmid DNA. *Biochim. Biophys. Acta.*, **1088**, 131–134.

Tüting, T., Gambotto, A., Robbins, P.D., Storkus, W.J. and DeLeo, A.B. (1999) Co-delivery of T helper 1-biasing cytokine genes enhances the efficacy of gene gun immunization of mice: studies with the model tumor antigen beta-galactosidase and the BALB/c Meth A p53 tumor-specific antigen. *Gene Ther.*, **6**, 629–636.

Tüting, T. and Albers, A. (2000) Particle-mediated gene transfer into dendritic cells – a novel strategy for the induction of immune responses against tumor antigens. In: W. Walther and U. Stein (eds) *Methods in Molecular Medicine, Vol. 35: Gene Therapy: Methods and Protocols*. Humana Press, Inc., Totowa, NJ, pp. 27–47.

Vanrompay, D., Cox, E., Vandenbussche, F., Volckaert, G. and Goddeeris, B. (1999) Protection of turkeys against Chlamydia psittaci challenge by gene gun-based DNA immunizations. *Vaccine*, **17**, 2628–2635.

VanRooij, E.M., Haagmans, B.L., de Visser, Y.E., de Bruin, M.G., Boersma, W. and Bianchi, A.T. (1998) Effect of vaccination route and composition of DNA vaccine on the induction of protective immunity against pseudorabies infection in pigs. *Vet. Immunol. Immunopathol.*, **66**, 113–126.

Vogel, J.C. (2000) Nonviral skin gene therapy. *Hum. Gene Ther.*, **11**, 2253–2259.

Wang, R., Doolan, D.L., Le, T.P., Hedstrom, R.C., Coonan, K.M., Charoenvit, Y. *et al.* (1998) Induction of antigen-specific cytotoxic T lymphocytes in humans by a malaria DNA vaccine. *Science*, **282**, 476–480.

Weber, S.M., Shi, F., Heise, C., Warner, T. and Mahvi, D.M. (1999) Interleukin-12 gene transfer results in CD8-dependent regression of murine CT26 liver tumors. *Ann. Surg. Oncol.*, **6**, 186–194.

Weiss, R., Leitner, W.W., Scheiblhofer, S., Chen, D., Bernhaupt, A., Mostbock, S., Thalhamer, J. and Lyon, J.A. (2000) Genetic vaccination against malaria infection by intradermal and epidermal injections of a plasmid containing the gene encoding the Plasmodium berghei circumsporozoite protein. *Infect. Immun.*, **68**, 5914–5919.

Widera, G., Austin, M., Rabussay, D., Goldbeck, C., Barnett, S.W., Chen, M.C. *et al.* (2000) Increased DNA vaccine delivery and immunogenicity by electroporation *in vivo*. *J. Immunol.*, **164**, 4635–4640.

Williams, R.S., Johnston, S.A., Riedy, M., DeVit, M.J., McElligot, S.G. and Sanford, J.C. (1991) Introduction of foreign genes into tissues of living mice by DNA-coated microprojectiles. *Proc. Natl. Acad. Sci. USA*, **88**, 2726–2730.

Williams, J., Fox-Leyva, L., Christensen, C., Fisher, D., Schlicting, E., Snowball, M. *et al.* (2000) Hepatitis A vaccine administration: comparison between jet-injector and needle injection. *Vaccine*, **18**, 1939–1943.

Wolff, J.A., Malone, R.W., Williams, P., Chong, W., Acsadi, G., Jani, A. and Felgner, P.L. (1990) Direct gene transfer into mouse muscle *in vivo*. *Science*, **247**, 1465–1468.

Wright, P., Braun, R., Babiuk, L., Littel-van den Hurk, S.D., Moyana, T., Zheng, C. *et al.* (1999) Adenovirus-mediated TNF-alpha gene transfer induces significant tumor regression in mice. *Cancer Biother. Radiopharm.*, **14**, 49–57.

Yamazaki, Y., Fujimoto, H., Ando, H., Ohyama, T., Hirota, Y. and Noce, T. (1998) *In vivo* gene transfer to mouse spermatogenic cells by deoxyribonucleic acid injection into seminiferous tubules and subsequent electroporation. *Biol. Reprod.*, **59**, 1439–1444.

Yang, N.-S., Burkholder, J., Roberts, B., Martinell, B. and McCabe, D. (1990) *In vivo* and *in vitro* gene transfer to mammalian somatic cells by particle bombardment. *Proc. Natl. Acad. Sci. USA*, **87**, 9568–9572.

Yang, N.-S. and Ziegelhoffer, P. (1994) The particle bombardment system for mammalian gene transfer. In: N.-S. Yang and P. Christou (eds) *Particle Bombardment Technology for Gene Transfer*. Oxford University Press, New York, pp. 117–141.

Yang, N.-S., Burkholder, J., McCabe, D., Neumann, V. and Fuller, D. (1997) Particle-mediated gene delivery *in vivo* and *in vitro*. *Curr. Protocols Hum. Genet.*, 12.6.1–12.6.14.

Ye, Z.Q., Qiu, P., Burkholder, J.K., Turner, J., Culp, J., Roberts, T., Shahidi, N.T. and Yang, N.S. (1998) Cytokine transgene expression and promoter usage in primary CD34[+] cells using particle-mediated gene delivery. *Hum. Gene Ther.*, **9**, 2197–2205.

Yoshida, A., Nagata, T., Uchijima, M., Higashi, T. and Koide, Y. (2000) Advantage of gene gun-mediated over intramuscular inoculation of plasmid DNA vaccine in reproducible induction of specific immune responses. *Vaccine*, **18**, 1725–1729.

19 Basic pharmacokinetics of oligonucleotides and genes

Makiya Nishikawa, Yoshinobu Takakura,
Fumiyoshi Yamashita and
Mitsuru Hashida

INTRODUCTION

The ultimate goal of gene therapy is to cure inheritable and acquired diseases in a straightforward manner by correcting abnormalities in genes. Various protocols have been employed to express gene product including the addition of the wild-type gene, correcting mutation in the gene, or suppressing undesirable gene products by blocking mRNA with complementary antisense oligonucleotide. Like conventional drugs and biologically active protein drugs, the administration of plasmid DNA (pDNA) and oligonucleotide (both are called 'gene drugs') directly to patients represents an ideal methodology for the treatment of a variety of diseases. Following *in vivo* administration, however, they encounter many hurdles that must be overcome for a successful therapy.

Biodistribution of a drug, which is administered externally as a free form or with a delivery system, is determined by its interaction with the body, based on the physicochemical and biological properties of the drug and the anatomical and physiological properties of the body. Therefore, drug targeting can be achieved by altering the properties of a drug with the drug delivery system (Senior, 1987; Takakura and Hashida, 1996; Nishikawa *et al.*, 1996), or by altering the properties of tissues, such as the osmotic opening of the blood-brain barrier (Robinson and Rapoport, 1987). Changing the route of administration, for example, using intraarterial injection to the target tissue instead of intravenous injection, is also a promising approach for improving the targeting efficiency of a drug (Hunt *et al.*, 1986). Similar strategies can be applied to a gene drug to deliver it to specific target tissues/cells. However, contrary to most conventional or protein drugs, pDNA and oligonucleotide should find a way to the intracellular space within the nucleus or cytoplasm where they have a chance to work.

Since Wolff *et al.* (1990) reported gene expression in skeletal muscle by a simple intramuscular injection of naked pDNA, it has widely been accepted that nucleic acids injected directly into muscle enter the cells. However, the way in which nucleic acids finally find a way to the nucleus after their cellular entry needs to be elucidated. Even for systemic administration, naked pDNA can produce a high level of transgene product when it is rapidly injected into the systemic circulation with a large-volume of solution (Zhang *et al.*, 1999; Liu *et al.*, 1999). However, a conventional intravenous injection of pDNA results in undetectable gene expression in major tissues (Kawabata *et al.*, 1995). Tissue and intracellular distribution of a gene drug would explain such differences as the level of transgene product in the final output. To improve the distribution of gene drug after *in vivo* administration, various synthetic gene carriers, such as cationic lipids, polymers and peptides, have been developed. Gene drug, a negatively charged molecule, forms an electrostatic complex with cationic carriers and, within the body, such a complex interacts with various components and shows a complicated biodistribution profile.

Clear understanding of the biodistribution of pDNA and oligonucleotides, as well as their complex with delivery systems is a prerequisite to making a strategy for developing an *in vivo* gene transfer or modulation method. Pharmacokinetics translates the biodistribution properties of a gene drug into quantitative parameters, which can be compared with parameters obtained in a different condition, or with physiological parameters, such as blood flow and the rate of fluid-phase endocytosis. This chapter focuses on the pharmacokinetic evaluation of pDNA and oligonucleotides, in both free and complexed forms, administered systemically or locally.

WHOLE BODY PHARMACOKINETICS AFTER SYSTEMIC ADMINISTRATION

After systemic administration, a drug is generally delivered to tissues in the body through blood circulation. Therefore, the concentration of drug in plasma defines the rate of tissue uptake.

In vivo fate of drugs with large molecular weight such as a gene drug can be pharmacokinetically analyzed on the basis of a physiological pharmacokinetic model, as shown in Figure 19.1. Tissue uptake of a drug consists of an uptake

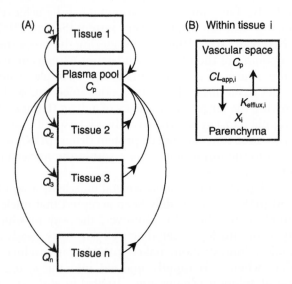

Figure 19.1 Physiological pharmacokinetic model for evaluating *in vivo* disposition of a macromolecular drug. (A) A multi-compartment model in which every tissue compartment is connected with the plasma pool by blood flow. (B) Tissue uptake of a drug from vascular space to tissue parenchyma.

from the plasma and an efflux from the tissue. When the tissue uptake rate is assumed to be independent on its concentration in the plasma and the efflux process follows the first-order rate kinetics, the change in its amount in a tissue with time can be described as follows:

$$\frac{dX_i}{dt} = CL_{app,i}C_p - k_{efflux,i}X_i \tag{1}$$

where X_i(µg) represents an amount of the drug in tissue i after administration, C_p (µg/mL) is its concentration in plasma, $CL_{app,i}$ (mL/h) expresses an apparent tissue uptake clearance from plasma to tissue i, and $k_{efflux,i}$ (h^{-1}) represents an efflux rate from tissue i. In some cases, the efflux process from tissues can be negligible, which makes it easier to analyze the distribution properties of a drug. When biodistribution of a drug is traced by the counting of radioactivity, the use of residualizing radiolabel will fit to this simplification (Ali *et al.*, 1988; Deshpande *et al.*, 1990). Polymers that are hardly metabolized after cellular uptake also remain within tissues by which they are taken up, and this feature allows for the omission of efflux processes from tissues in the pharmacokinetic analysis. However, it is not the case for gene drugs such as pDNA and oligonucleotide; they are easily degraded after cellular uptake and, in most cases, radioactivity derived from radiolabeled gene drugs is released from the cells. Even though the efflux of the tracing material occurs, the efflux from tissues should be ignored within short early periods following administration. When the efflux from tissues can be ignored, Eq (1) is simplified to:

$$\frac{dX_i}{dt} = CL_{app,i}C_p \tag{2}$$

Integration of Eq (2) from time 0 to t_1 gives:

$$CL_{app,i} = \frac{X_{i,t_1}}{\int_0^{t_1} C_p dt} = \frac{X_{i,t_1}}{AUC_{p,0-t_1}} \tag{3}$$

where $AUC_{p,0-t_1}$ (µg h/mL) is an area under the plasma concentration-time curve of a drug from time 0 to t_1. Its elimination profile from the plasma could be expressed as a function of one or more exponentials in many cases when AUC_p values at any time point can be calculated by fitting an equation to experimental data using a pharmacokinetic analysis program such as MULTI (Yamaoka *et al.*, 1981). According to Eq (3), $CL_{app,i}$ is obtained as the slope when the amount in a tissue (X_i) is plotted against AUC_p.

Tissue uptake clearance is a useful parameter to characterize the *in vivo* distribution properties of a drug since it is independent of the drug concentration in plasma. However, when the tissue uptake process depends on the drug concentration in plasma and follows non-linear kinetics, the calculated $CL_{app,i}$ represents an average value of its time-dependent clearance for the overall experimental period (Nishikawa *et al.*, 1992).

$CL_{app,i}$ is a hybrid parameter of the plasma flow rate (Q, mL/h) to a tissue and intrinsic uptake clearance ($CL_{int,i}$, mL/h) of the tissue and also expressed as:

$$CL_{app,i} = \frac{Q\,CL_{int,i}}{Q + CL_{int,i}} \tag{4}$$

When $CL_{int,i}$ is much larger than Q, $CL_{app,i}$ comes close to Q and this value (plasma flow rate to a tissue) is the upper limit of $CL_{app,i}$ whatever specific and rapid uptake mechanism is involved in the tissue uptake.

Total body clearance (CL_{total}, mL/h) of a drug can be calculated using AUC_p for infinite time ($AUC_{p,\infty}$) and an administered dose (D) as follows:

$$CL_{total} = \frac{D}{AUC_{p,\infty}} \tag{5}$$

Since CL_{total} is the sum of tissue uptake clearances and urinary excretion clearance, CL_{total} is also expressed as:

$$CL_{total} = CL_{app,liver} + CL_{app,kidney} + \cdots + CL_{urine} \tag{6}$$

$$= CL_{target} + CL_{non\text{-}target} \tag{7}$$

where CL_{target} denotes the uptake clearance of target tissue and $CL_{non\text{-}target}$ represents the sum of clearances except for CL_{target}. In the case of a gene drug, its degradation within systemic circulation is also a factor determining its efficacy. After administration, the fraction of a drug delivered to a target (F_{target}) can be calculated using CL_{target}, $CL_{non\text{-}target}$ and the degradation clearance of a drug within systemic circulation (CL_{deg}, mL/h) as follows:

$$F_{target} = \frac{CL_{target}}{CL_{total} + CL_{deg}} = \frac{CL_{target}}{CL_{target} + CL_{non\text{-}target} + CL_{deg}} \tag{8}$$

Therefore, the potential of targeted delivery of a gene drug can be quantitatively explained by the parameters of CL_{target}, $CL_{non\text{-}target}$ and CL_{deg}. Eq (8) clearly indicates that an approach increasing CL_{target} and/or reducing $CL_{non\text{-}target}$ or CL_{deg} of a gene drug is suitable for achieving an efficient gene transfer (or gene suppression) at target site. Figure 19.2A shows F_{target} as a function of CL_{target} when the sum of $CL_{non\text{-}target}$ and CL_{deg} is held constant at either 0.1, 1 or 10 mL/h. An increase in CL_{target} from 0.01 to 0.1 mL/h significantly enlarges F_{target} only when the sum of $CL_{non\text{-}target}$ and CL_{deg} is smaller than 1 mL/h. Figure 19.2B indicates that the reduction of $CL_{non\text{-}target}$ or CL_{deg} increases F_{target} of a gene drug when CL_{target} equals to 0.1 mL/h. These simulation studies clearly show a reasonable strategy for targeted delivery of a gene drug. If an inefficient delivery of a gene drug to a target is due to its rapid uptake by non-target tissues or extensive degradation in the systemic circulation, the drug should be protected from those unfavorable processes with a vector system. When a gene drug circulates in plasma for a long time (i.e., having small CL_{total}), the use of a ligand specifically recognized by the target, for example, galactose for hepatocytes, will increase the amount of drug delivered to the target.

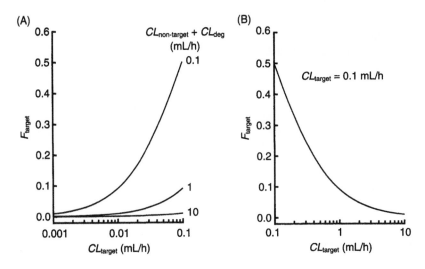

Figure 19.2 Effect of target (CL_{target}), non-target ($CL_{non-target}$) and degradation (CL_{deg}) clearances on a fraction of drug delivered to the target tissue (F_{target}) after systemic administration. The curves represent F_{target} simulated using Eq (8): (A) $CL_{non-target} + CL_{deg}$ is set at 0.1, 1 or 10 mL/h; (B) CL_{target} is fixed at 0.1 mL/h.

Figure 19.3 summarizes two major clearances governing the biodistribution of most macromolecular drugs – the hepatic uptake clearance and the urinary excretion clearance-of model compounds with diverse physicochemical characteristics following intravenous injection in mice. These plots clearly indicate that the biodistribution of macromolecules including pDNA and oligonucleotide is largely governed by their physicochemical properties such as molecular size and electrical charge.

Naked gene drug

pDNA

Systemic administration that does not require local, regional administration or surgical procedures is a desirable method for *in vivo* gene transfer. However, this route is one of the toughest ways for a gene drug to reach the target and express its function at the site because of a rapid removal by the liver and degradation.

The pharmacokinetics of naked pDNA in mice was examined using ^{32}P-labeled pDNA (Kawabata *et al.*, 1995). When naked ^{32}P-pDNA in 100 µL of saline solution was injected into mice at a dose of 1 mg/kg (about 25 µg/mouse), radioactivity was rapidly eliminated from plasma due to an extensive uptake by the liver, while it was not susceptible to glomerular filtration. In a different set of experiments, a rapid degradation by nucleases in serum was also observed. At this condition naked pDNA resulted in no gene expression in major organs (Mahato *et al.*, 1995a), possibly due to low DNA dose and its rapid degradation by nucleases. A pharmacokinetic analysis of the biodistribution of naked ^{32}P-pDNA showed that its hepatic uptake clearance (80 mL/h) is very close to the hepatic plasma flow rate of mice

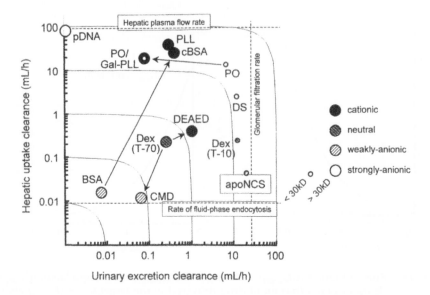

Figure 19.3 Apparent hepatic uptake clearance and urinary excretion clearance of
model compounds in mice after intravenous injection. Strongly-anionic;
pDNA (MW 2,850 kD), PO (20-mer phosphodiester oligonucleotide), DS
(dextran sulfate, MW 8 kD). Weakly-anionic; apoNCS (apoprotein of neo-
carzinostatin, MW 12 kD), CMD (carboxymethyl-dextran derived from
dextran T-70, average MW 70 kD), BSA (bovine serum albumin, MW
67 kD). Neutral; Dex(T-10) and Dex(T-70) (dextran T-10 and dextran
T-70, average MW 10 and 70 kD, respectively). Cationic; DEAED (diethyl-
aminoethyl-dextran derived from dextran T-70, average MW 70 kD),
cBSA (cationized BSA, MW 70 kD), PLL (poly-L-lysine, average MW
40 kD). Ligand-complexed; PO/Gal-PLL (PO complexed with galactosylated PLL). Original data were published in following papers: pDNA,
Kawabata *et al.* (1995); PO and PO/Gal-PLL, Mahato *et al.* (1997); DS,
Takakura *et al.* (1994); apoNCS, CMD, BSA, Dex(T-10), Dex(T-70),
DEAED, Takakura *et al.* (1990); cBSA, Fujita *et al.* (1995).

(85 mL/h for 25 g mouse) (Figure 19.3). Degradation clearance was also estimated
from the stability data of pDNA in blood after intravenous injection to be 8.3 mL/h,
about one-tenth of its hepatic uptake clearance. Thus, the pharmacokinetic analysis
of the biodistribution of naked pDNA clearly shows that the rapid hepatic uptake,
not its degradation in serum, is a major barrier for delivering pDNA to tissues,
except for the liver.

On a point of gene expression following systemic administration of naked
pDNA, Liu *et al.* (1999) and Zhang *et al.* (1999) reported that a rapid injection of
a large volume of naked pDNA solution (for example, 5 μg pDNA in 1.6 mL saline
solution for a 20 g mouse, which is almost equivalent to the total blood volume of
the animal) into mice via the tail vein could induce an efficient gene transfer in
internal organs, including the lung, spleen, heart, kidney and liver, with the highest level observed in the liver. Mechanisms for gene transfer by this approach have
not been fully understood. However, it is proposed that the injected pDNA solution accumulates in the inferior vena cava, flows back to tissues directly linked to

this vascular system, including the liver. The hydrostatic pressure forces pDNA into the liver cells before being mixed with blood (Liu *et al.*, 1999). On the other hand, a receptor-mediated process is also hypothesized for the *in vivo* uptake of naked pDNA by hepatocytes (Budker *et al.*, 2000). The gene expression level obtained by this approach is much better than those with other approaches using naked pDNA or nonviral vectors.

Such huge differences in gene expression by naked pDNA between a normal (small volume, slow) injection and a large volume injection at a high velocity would in part be explained by differences in the pharmacokinetic profile of the injected pDNA. Kobayashi *et al.* (2001) studied the biodistribution of naked ^{32}P-pDNA in mice following normal or large volume injection. In both cases, radioactivity accumulated largely in the liver. However, the hepatic uptake of ^{32}P-pDNA following normal injection was saturable and was inhibited by pDNA itself, calf thymus DNA, polyinosinic acid (poly I), and chondroitin sulfate. On the other hand, the uptake following the large volume injection was not inhibited by the administration of poly I, dextran sulfate, and heparin. In addition, proteins such as bovine serum albumin (BSA), which is hardly taken up by tissues, including the liver, in a normal condition, are also taken up, by the liver by this large volume injection. These findings suggest that the uptake of pDNA following the large volume injection is a nonspecific process, while its uptake following the conventional injection would be mediated by scavenger receptor-like mechanism(s) (Kawabata *et al.*, 1995; Takakura *et al.*, 1999).

Oligonucleotides

Compared with pDNA, oligonucleotides are very small in size, and they can be susceptible to glomerular filtration after systemic administration. Contrary to the invariable properties of pDNA, the physicochemical properties of oligonucleotides, such as the molecular weight, hydrophilicity/hydrophobicity and electrical charge, vary depending on the nature of the linkage between nucleotides. Such variations are reflected in the pharmacokinetic profile of oligonucleotides.

Due to the small size (smaller than 10 kD in most cases), oligonucleotide can be easily filtered at the kidney. In addition, its property of plasma protein binding will greatly alter the biodistribution of oligonucleotides. Compared with natural phosphodiester oligonucleotide, the phosphorothioate one has a much higher affinity with serum proteins, including albumin. A 10-mer phosphodiester oligonucleotide showed little binding with bovine serum albumin (BSA) in buffer solution and, when administered into the perfused rat kidney, it was efficiently excreted into urine (Sawai *et al.*, 1995). On the other hand, its phosphorothioate showed a high binding ability to BSA, resulting in reduced filtration at the kidney.

When injected intravenously in mice, a 10-mer phosphordiester oligonucleotide modified with ^{3}H-biotin at the *5'*-end and with methoxyethylamine at the *3'*-end was very quickly metabolized within the body; more than 90% of radioactivity in plasma was degradation product at two minutes after injection (Miyao *et al.*, 1995). Mahato *et al.* (1997) examined the biodistribution of ^{35}S-labeled 20-mer phosphordiester and phosphorothioate oligonucleotides following systemic injection in mice. Both types of oligonucleotides were eliminated rapidly from the circulation, but the tissue distribution was different. A pharmacokinetic analysis based on the clearance concept showed the phosphordiester oligonucleotide had relatively large uptake clearances for all internal organs tested and large urinary excretion clearance, while the phosphorothioate possessed small urinary clearance, reflecting its high ability of plasma protein binding.

Due to the stability and resistance to endonuclease and exonuclease degradation (Uhlmann and Peyman, 1990), phosphorothioate linkage becomes the first choice of antisense oligonucleotides. Intense accumulation of phosphorothioate oligonucleotides in the liver and kidney is a universal distribution characteristic observed in many studies (Agrawal *et al.*, 1991, 1995; Sands *et al.*, 1994; Phillips *et al.*, 1997; Peng *et al.*, 2001), irrespective of the length of oligonucleotide between 20 and 25-mer. Recently, Peng *et al.* (2001) analyzed the biodistribution of ISIS 1082, a 21-mer phosphorothioate oligonucleotide in rat, based on a physiologically based pharmacokinetic model. They also used a model, similar to the model shown in Figure 19.1, in which all tissues were represented by a two-compartment model, comprising a blood compartment and an extravascular tissue compartment, with a permeability barrier at the capillary wall membrane. They found that the equilibrium tissue/plasma partition coefficient (Kp) of oligonucleotides exceeds one for all internal tissues, despite its relatively large size (about 6 kD). This Kp could be due to the high ability of phosphorothioate oligonucleotides for binding to tissue matrix. However, they could not find any correlation between the estimated permeability-surface area product in a tissue and its corresponding Kp value. This lack of correlation might be explained by the fact that permeability is a dynamic parameter, whereas Kp reflects a value at steady state.

Nonviral vector complex

The addition of cationic liposomes or polymers to a gene drug decreases its negative charge and facilitates its interaction with the cell membrane, so various vectors have been developed and used for *in vivo* delivery of a gene drug. One major group of these vectors consists of cationic lipids or liposomes. After systemic injection, cationic lipid/pDNA complex resulted in gene expression in vascular endothelial cells (Zhu *et al.*, 1993; Liu *et al.*, 1997), especially the cells in the lung, the first tissue a pDNA complex encounters following injection.

We examined the biodistribution of cationic liposomes/pDNA complex following intravenous injection in mice and pharmacokinetically analyzed the data based on the clearance concept (Mahato *et al.*, 1995a, 1997). These analyses showed that the pharmacokinetics of ^{32}P-pDNA complexes depend on their mixing (charge) ratio, the type of cationic and helper lipids (Mahato *et al.*, 1998). When analyzed using radioactivity counting following the injection of the complex prepared with ^{32}P-pDNA, the tissue uptake clearance per g tissue (mL/h/g tissue) was large for the lung, liver and spleen, though gene expression was not correlated with this uptake characteristic; no gene expression was detected in the liver in any formulation (Mahato *et al.*, 1995b).

The preferential gene transfer in the lung following intravenous injection of cationic lipid/pDNA complex would result from complicated events occurring in the body. Positively charged liposomes/pDNA complexes bind to serum components, such as albumin, heparin, lipoprotein, or specific opsonins. This interaction is dependent on the net charge density and surface morphology of lipid/pDNA complexes (Mahato *et al.*, 1998). The biodistribution of pDNA after intravenous injection was dependent on the charge ratio of cationic liposomes/pDNA; the amount in the lung decreased by ten-fold, but that in the liver increased when the charge ratio decreased from 3:1 to 0.5:1 (+/−) (Mahato *et al.*, 1998). Sakurai *et al.* (2001) studied the tissue distribution of cationic liposomes/pDNA complexes in mice following intravenous injection, with or without preincubation of the complexes with serum or red blood cells (RBC). When a formulation contains dioleoylphosphatidylethanolamine (DOPE) as a helper lipid, cationic liposomes/pDNA complexes pre-incubated with RBC resulted in embolization in the lung, whereas a formulation with cholesterol instead of DOPE did not. Cationic liposomes/pDNA complexes induced fusion and aggregation of erythrocytes *in vitro* when DOPE was added as a helper lipid (Sakurai *et al.*, 2001). These differences in the interaction characteristics of pDNA complexes with blood components partially explain the differences in the biodistribution following intravenous injection of various complex formulations (Mahato *et al.*, 1998).

Cationic polymer is also frequently examined to increase the potential of a gene drug. Large molecular weight cationic polymers can condense pDNA more efficiently than cationic liposomes. They include: poly-L-lysine (PLL), poly-L-ornithine, polyethyleneimine (PEI), chitosan, starburst dendrimer and various novel synthetic polymers. These polymers can enhance the cellular uptake of pDNA by nonspecific adsorptive endocytosis.

Biodistribution of cationic polymer/pDNA complexes is more easily controlled than that of cationic lipid/pDNA complexes, therefore, active targeting to a specific population of cells in the body has been attempted since 1988 (Wu and Wu, 1988). Polymers such as PLL and PEI have been covalently modified with targeting ligand, which include asialoglycoproteins (Wu and Wu, 1988), carbohydrates (Perales *et al.*, 1994), transferrin (Kircheis *et al.*, 1999), and antibody (Li *et al.*, 2000). However, the pharmacokinetics of cationic polymer/pDNA complexes used in these studies was hardly examined. We determined the biodistribution profiles of galactosylated PLL (Gal-PLL)/pDNA complexes following intravenous injection in mice (Nishikawa *et al.*, 1998). As mentioned above, naked pDNA is rapidly taken up by the liver. Cell fractionation and confocal imaging of fluorescein-labeled pDNA following intravenous injection in mice has shown that pDNA is mainly taken up by sinusoidal cells such as Kupffer cells and endothelial cells (Kawabata *et al.*, 1995; Kobayashi *et al.*, 2001). Since the uptake by these cells seems to be mediated by the strong negative charge of pDNA (Takagi *et al.*, 1998b; Takakura *et al.*, 1999) and its clearance is very large (about 80 mL/h, Figure 19.3), it is important to mask the negative charge of pDNA for controlling its biodistribution. The pharmacokinetics of the DNA complexes are determined by not only a ligand but also by the overall physicochemical characteristics of the complexes (as summarized in Figures 19.2 and 19.3). After the intravenous injection of Gal-PLL/^{32}P-pDNA complexes, the hepatic uptake clearance was much greater than any of the other tissue uptake clearances. However, the physicochemical properties of Gal-PLL used for the complexation greatly affected the pharmacokinetics of the pDNA complex. Figure 19.4 shows the total body and hepatic uptake clearances of

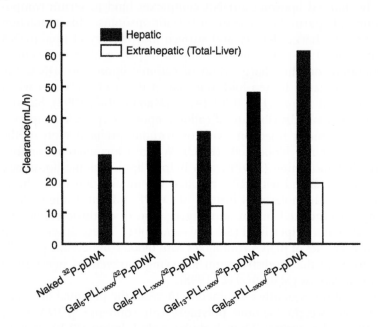

Figure 19.4 Hepatic and extrahepatic clearances of ^{32}P-pDNA and its complexes with varying Gal-PLL following intravenous injection in mice. The hepatic clearance was calculated by dividing the amount of radioactivity in the liver at an appropriate time point by the AUC up to the same time. Extrahepatic clearance represents the difference in the total-body and hepatic clearances. The numbers in the subscript represent the number of galactose (Gal-) and the molecular weight of PLL.

various Gal-PLL/^{32}P-pDNA complexes. The clearance values demonstrate that the complexes with larger Gal-PLL (13 or 29 kD in the molecular weight of PLL) have larger hepatic (target) clearance than ones with small Gal-PLL (1.8 kD), which failed to deliver efficiently pDNA to hepatocytes, probably due to the complex dissociation before reaching the target.

The figure also shows the importance of the number of galactose residues on PLL for the pDNA delivery using Gal-PLL (compare the results of complexes with Gal_5-PLL_{13000} and Gal_{13}-PLL_{13000}), as clearly demonstrated in the studies of galactosylated or mannosylated proteins (Nishikawa *et al.*, 1995; Opanasopit *et al.*, 2001). Gene expression following intravenous injection corresponded to these pharmacokinetic profiles of Gal-PLL/pDNA complexes (Nishikawa *et al.*, 1998). The pDNA complexes with cationic carriers would be internalized by cells via endocytosis, resulting in lysosomal degradation. This intracellular pathway greatly limits the efficiency of gene transfer by this approach. In addition to the control of *in vivo* pharmacokinetics by using carrier molecules like Gal-PLL, the control of intracellular sorting of pDNA can be a good approach to increase gene transfer at the target. Wagner *et al.* (1992) demonstrated the increased gene expression in cultured cells by the addition of fusogenic peptides, derived from influenza virus hemmaglutinin subunit HA-2, to pDNA complexes. We attached fusogenic peptide to a hepatocyte-targetable polymer and obtained an improved gene expression in the liver, indicating that the peptide also works in whole animals to, at least partially, avoid the intracellular degradation (Nishikawa *et al.*, 2000).

Similar to pDNA, the pharmacokinetics of oligonucleotides can be controlled by using delivery systems. Mahato *et al.* (1997) studied the pharmacokinetic characteristics of antisense oligonucleotides complexed with Gal-PLL or manno-sylated PLL (Man-PLL), whose mannose residues can be recognized by mannose receptors on macrophages and liver sinusoidal endothelial cells (Shlesinger *et al.*, 1978). Complex formation of phosphodiester or phosphorothioate oligonucle-otides with either of these modified PLL greatly reduced the urinary excretion clearance by increasing the effective size of the oligonucleotide, about 100–160 nm in diameter when measured by laser light scattering (Mahato *et al.*, 1997). Increased hepatic uptake clearances were obtained by the complex formation with Gal- or Man-PLL, but the delivery efficiency was not so outstanding for oligonucleotides as observed in pDNA delivery. Such differences suggest that the molecular weight of both components of gene drugs/cationic carrier complexes determine the stability of the complex, which is a major determinant of its pharmacokinetics.

LOCAL PHARMACOKINETICS

Isolated perfused tissue is a good system with which to analyze the pharmaco-kinetic events occurring in a specific tissue of interest following administration into the artery or by direct injection into the tissues. When isolated from the other parts of the body and perfused without recirculation (single-pass, one-loop system), the tissue can be pharmacokinetically treated as a physiological one-organ model. In this model, the circulatory system is observed as a black box under linear dispos-ition conditions and the disposition function of a drug is reflected in the output response to an input. The output response is obtained by way of the time course of the outflow concentration and can usually be regarded as a statistical distribution curve, similar to that observed in chromatography. Statistical moment analysis was applied to a single-pass local perfusion system (Kakutani *et al.*, 1985). These phar-macokinetic approaches have been applied to analyze the disposition characteris-tics of various drugs in the liver (Nishida *et al.*, 1989, 1990, 1991a, 1991b, 1992; Takakura *et al.*, 1996; Yoshida *et al.*, 1996; Takagi *et al.*, 1998b; Ogawara *et al.*, 1998, 1999), kidney (Mihara *et al.*, 1993a, 1993b, 1994; Sawai *et al.*, 1995, 1996; Takagi *et al.*, 1997) and tumor (Ohkouchi *et al.*, 1990; Imoto *et al.*, 1992; Saikawa *et al.*, 1996; Nomura *et al.*, 1997, 1998a, 1998b; Nakajima *et al.*, 2000). Here, we sum-marize the pharmacokinetics of gene drugs in these isolated tissues.

Isolated perfused liver

In the isolated perfused liver experiments, buffers containing no erythrocytes or serum proteins are used to examine the direct interaction of a gene drug with tissues and to avoid the interaction of a gene drug with blood components and possible contamination of nucleases.

Bolus injection

The statistical moment parameters for the outflow pattern of a bolusly administered drug from the portal vein are defined as follows:

$$AUC = \int_0^\infty C dt \tag{9}$$

$$\bar{t} = \int_0^\infty \frac{tC}{AUC} dt \tag{10}$$

where t (sec) is the time and C (% of dose/mL) is the concentration of compound. AUC (% of dose sec/mL) and $t(bar)$ (sec) denote the area under the concentration-time curve and mean transit time of the drug through the liver, respectively. The moments defined by Eq (9) and (10) can be calculated by numerical integration using a linear trapezoidal formula and extrapolation to infinite time based on a monoexponential equation. The $t(bar)$ values are corrected for the lag time of the catheter.

The hepatic disposition parameters of a drug, representing reversible and irreversible processes, are calculated using the following equations:

$$F = AUC \cdot Q \tag{11}$$

$$V = \frac{Q \cdot \bar{t}}{F} \tag{12}$$

$$E = 1 - F \tag{13}$$

$$t_{cor} = \frac{\bar{t}}{F} \tag{14}$$

$$k_{el} = \frac{E}{\bar{t}} \tag{15}$$

$$CL_{int} = k_{el} \cdot V \tag{16}$$

where V (mL) is the apparent retention volume, which reflects reversible interaction of drug with the tissue; t_{cor} (sec) is the corrected mean transit time, E (%) is the extraction ratio, k_{el} (min^{-1}) is the first order irreversible elimination rate constant, CL_{int} (mL/min/g tissue) is the intrinsic clearance, and Q (mL/min) is the perfusion rate. These parameters can be divided into three groups: parameters representing reversible interaction (V, t_{cor}), irreversible uptake (E, F, k_{el}), and both (CL_{int}) (Nishida *et al.*, 1990).

The pharmacokinetic analysis of the outflow dilution curve of the concentration of radioactivity following bolus injection of ^{32}P-pDNA and [32]S-oligonucleotides with different linkages translates the distribution data to the quantitative parameters (Table 19.1). The extraction (E) of gene drugs in the perfused liver was relatively high for ^{32}P-pDNA (46% at 1.33 µg/liver), ^{32}P-PS$_3$ (33% at 3 µg/liver) and ^{32}P-PS (36% at 3 µg/liver), but low for ^{32}P-PO (15% at 3 µg/liver). These results correspond to the *in vivo* distribution data following systemic administration into mice (Kawabata *et al.*, 1995; Miyao *et al.*, 1995). If a drug does not reversibly

Table 19.1 Moments and disposition parameters of ^{32}P-pDNA and ^{32}P-oligonucleotides in the single-pass rat liver perfusion system

Compound	Moment parameters			Disposition parameters				
	Dose (µg/liver)	AUC (% dose sec/mL)	t(bar) (sec)	V (mL/g tissue)	t_{cor} (min)	E (%)	k_{el} (min^{-1})	CL_{int} (mL/min/g tissue)
^{32}P-pDNA[a]	1.33	252 ± 17	12.6 ± 1.5	0.598 ± 0.09	0.313 ± 0.05	45.6 ± 0.3	21.7 ± 0.1	1.29 ± 0.12
	13.3	365 ± 14	10.3 ± 1.0	0.314 ± 0.08	0.179 ± 0.03	20.1 ± 0.8	1.17 ± 0.09	0.354 ± 0.10
^{32}P-PO[b]	3	402 ± 19	16.6 ± 1.5	0.691 ± 0.09	0.333 ± 0.02	15.3 ± 1.8	0.434 ± 0.17	0.214 ± 0.08
^{32}P-PS$_3$[b]	0.3	264 ± 27	20.8 ± 2.0	0.796 ± 0.02	0.408 ± 0.03	45.4 ± 8.5	1.45 ± 0.19	1.15 ± 0.85
	3	320 ± 12	17.2 ± 8.8	0.746 ± 0.40	0.314 ± 0.03	33.2 ± 3.1	0.857 ± 0.56	0.786 ± 0.61
	30	446 ± 6	12.5 ± 0.7	0.315 ± 0.01	0.214 ± 0.01	3.00 ± 0.84	0.162 ± 0.10	0.051 ± 0.03
^{32}P-PS[b]	3	289 ± 5	41.7 ± 2.4	1.55 ± 0.14	1.08 ± 0.09	35.8 ± 0.9	0.516 ± 0.04	0.798 ± 0.01
^{51}Cr-RBC[c]	–	471	8.89	0.209	0.148	0	–	0
^{131}I-HSA[c]	–	486	9.33	0.252	0.156	0	–	0

Notes
PO, PS$_3$, PS, 20-mer antisense oligonucleotide complementary to the human c-*myc* mRNA with different internucleotide linkages; PO, phosphodiester; PS$_3$, three phosphorothioate linkages on both ends; PS, phosphorothioate. RBC, red blood cells; HSA, human serum albumin. a Yoshida *et al.*, 1996; b Takakura *et al.*, 1996; c Nishida *et al.*, 1989.

interact with the tissue, its V value is close to the volume of the blood vessels within the liver. Compared with ^{131}I-human serum albumin (HSA), a vascular reference substrate that distributes the sinusoidal and Disse spaces in the liver, all gene drugs listed in Table 19.1 had larger V value, indicating their reversible interaction with the tissue. During the 60 minute perfusion, radioactivity could be detected in the outflow when ^{32}P-PS was bolusly administered into the liver (Takakura *et al.*, 1996), showing a very slow dissociation of the ^{32}P-PS oligonucleotide attached onto the surface of liver cells. The reversible (V) and irreversible (E) parameters of these gene drugs decreased with an increasing dose, indicating that both interactions are saturable processes.

Constant infusion

Contrary to the bolus input experiment that is particularly useful for examining the initial stages of hepatic uptake of drugs, constant infusion gives direct information on the uptake behavior of drugs at steady state. In particular, slow processes can be clearly characterized by this approach. Furthermore, the binding and internalization processes can be distinguished from each other (Nishida *et al.*, 1992). When a drug is constantly supplied to the liver, a fraction would be steadily extracted by the tissue, and the extraction ratio at steady state (E_{ss}) for the drug is calculated as follows:

$$E_{ss} = \frac{C_{in,ss} - C_{out,ss}}{C_{in,ss}} \tag{17}$$

where $C_{in,ss}$ and $C_{out,ss}$ are the concentration of the drug in the perfusate before and after passing through the liver under steady state condition. Then (at steady state), the hepatic clearance (CL_h, mL/min) of the drug is expressed as:

$$CL_h = E_{ss} \cdot Q \tag{18}$$

where Q (mL/min) is the perfusion rate.

To obtain the binding and internalization parameters of a drug, a physiological one-organ model is employed as shown in Figure 19.5 (Nishida *et al.*, 1992). In this model, the sinusoidal compartment, consisting of the vascular and Disse spaces, is assumed to be under, a well stirred condition, and the concentration is assumed to be similar to that in the outflow (C_s, corresponding to $C_{out,ss}$ in Eq 17; C_b equals to $C_{in,ss}$). The binding compartment is characterized by a maximum binding amount (X_∞) and a binding constant (K) and rapid equilibration is assumed to occur between the sinusoidal and binding compartments. V_s represents the sum of the volumes of the sinusoid and Disse spaces (assumed to be 0.180 mL/g liver). Assuming the internalization process follows a first-order rate kinetics, the internalization rate of a drug (dX/dt) is expressed as a product of a binding amount X and its rate constant (k_{int}). Then, in the sinusoidal and binding compartments, a mass-balance equation is defined as follows:

$$V_s \left(\frac{dC_s}{dt} \right) + \left(\frac{dX}{dt} \right) = QC_b - QC_s - k_{int}X \tag{19}$$

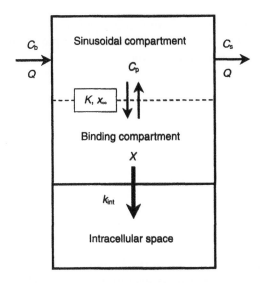

Figure 19.5 Physiological pharmacokinetic model for hepatic uptake of drug constantly infused in the isolated rat liver perfusion system. Q, flow rate (mL/min); C_b, inflow concentration (µg/mL); C_s, sinusoidal concentration (µg/mL); V_s, sinusoidal volume (mL); X, binding constant (µg); X_∞, maximum binding amount (µg); K, binding constant (mL/µg); k_{int}, internalization rate constant (min^{-1}).

Assuming the binding of a drug to the cell surface is consistent with the Langmuir equation, the following expression holds:

$$X = \frac{X_\infty K C_s}{1 + K C_s} \tag{20}$$

Differentiated with respect to t (time), Eq 20 is changed to

$$\frac{dX}{dt} = \frac{X_\infty K}{(1 + K C_s)^2}\left(\frac{dC_s}{dt}\right) \tag{21}$$

To substitute Eq (19) with Eq (21) gives the following equation:

$$\left(V_s + \frac{X_\infty K}{(1 + K C_s)^2}\right)\left(\frac{dC_s}{dt}\right) = QC_b - QC_s - \left(\frac{k_{int} X_\infty K C_s}{1 + K C_s}\right) \tag{22}$$

When the constant infusion experiments are performed at various inflow concentrations of a drug, the differential equations are numerically solved (Nishida *et al.*, 1992; Ogawara *et al.*, 1998, 1999).

When ^{32}P-pDNA was constantly infused in the isolated perfused rat liver, however, its uptake by the perfused liver did not reach a steady state during the experimental period of 60 minutes (Yoshida *et al.*, 1996). Therefore, a precise analysis of the binding and internalization characteristics could not be performed.

Isolated perfused kidney

The same statistical analytical method used for the liver can be applied to examine the disposition characteristics of a drug in the kidney. The following parameters are important to understand the renal disposition of drug:

$$AUC = \int_0^\infty Cdt \tag{23}$$

$$MTT_{kid} = \int_0^\infty \frac{tC}{AUC} dt \tag{24}$$

$$F_u = \int_0^\infty \left(\frac{dX_u}{dt}\right) dt \tag{25}$$

$$MTT_u = \frac{\int_0^\infty t\left(\frac{dX_u}{dt}\right) dt}{F_u} \tag{26}$$

where MTT_{kid} (sec) is the mean transit time of drug in the kidney; F_u denotes the urinary recovery (excretion) ratio; dX_u/dt is the urinary excretion rate, and MTT_u is the urinary mean excretion time. Then the distribution volume at steady state (V_d) is calculated from these moment parameters as follows:

$$F_0 = AUC \cdot Q \tag{27}$$

$$V_d = \frac{Q \cdot MTT_{kid}}{F_0} \tag{28}$$

where F_0 is the venous outflow recovery ratio. By adjusting the renal arterial pressure (from 70–80 to 55 mmHg) and tying off the ureters, one can have a 'nonfiltering' kidney, in which the glomerular filtration does not occur. This technique is useful to distinguish events occurring in the capillary side of the kidney from those in the luminal side.

Reference substances are required to understand the pharmacokinetic characteristics of a gene drug in the perfused kidney. Serum albumin can be used as a marker that is hardly filtered at the kidney and rarely taken up by the tissue through the passage. Inulin is a well-known marker of glomerular filtration rate. These references have unique pharmacokinetic parameters when subjected to the pharmacokinetic analysis in the isolated perfused rat kidney (Table 19.2). Oligo-nucleotides with different internucleotide linkages are found to have significant reversible interaction with the kidney (because they have larger MTT_{kid} and V_d, parameters representing reversible interaction, than those reference substances) (Sawai *et al.*, 1995, 1996).

Tissue-isolated perfused tumor

The pharmacokinetics of a gene drug within tumor tissue is a very important issue because cancer becomes one of the major targets for gene therapy, and various protocols are now under clinical trials (Roth and Cristiano, 1997). For *in vivo* gene delivery protocols, a gene drug, free or complexed with vector, is sometimes

Table 19.2 Moments and distribution volume of ^{32}P-pDNA and ^{32}P-oligonucleotides in the single-pass rat kidney perfusion system

Compound	Dose (μg/kidney)	AUC (% dose sec/mL)	MTT_{kid} (sec)	V_d (mL)
^{32}P-PO[a]	0.42	376 ± 4	1.45 ± 0.07	0.462 ± 0.013
^{32}P-PS$_3$[a]	0.42	335 ± 1	1.51 ± 0.12	0.491 ± 0.011
^{32}P-PS[a]	0.42	319 ± 23	2.54 ± 0.14	0.716 ± 0.022
^{14}C-Inulin[b]	–	352 ± 49	1.42 ± 0.10	0.449 ± 0.021
^{111}In-BSA[b]	–	302 ± 12	0.900 ± 0.014	0.240 ± 0.001

Notes
PO, PS$_3$, PS, 20-mer antisense oligonucleotide complementary to the human *c-myc* mRNA with different internucleotide linkages; PO, phosphodiester; PS$_3$, three phosphorothioate linkages on both ends; PS, phosphorothioate; BSA, bovine serum albumin. a Sawai *et al.*, 1996; b Mihara *et al.*, 1993a.

injected directly into tumor tissues (Kitajima *et al.*, 1992; Ratajczak *et al.*, 1992; Plautz *et al.*, 1993; Sun *et al.*, 1995; Wei *et al.*, 1995; Toloza *et al.*, 1996; Dow *et al.*, 1998; Nemunaitis *et al.*, 1999) because the direct administration circumvents vascular and interstitial barriers in the systemic delivery of a gene drug to the tumor. Injected intratumorally, a gene drug would distribute within the tissue, and fractions reaching to the blood vessel would be cleared by blood flow, so the profiles of the drug in the outflow include information on their disposition characteristics within the tumor tissue (Saikawa *et al.*, 1996). Quantitative evaluation of its disposition within the tumor tissues is important to assess and predict the efficiency of *in vivo* cancer gene therapy. A tissue-isolated tumor is a good experimental system to investigate the intratumoral disposition of pharmaceuticals, because (i) experimental conditions are easily controlled, (ii) its disposition features in the tumor tissue can be obtained independently from those in other normal tissues, and (iii) disposition characteristics can be quantitatively analyzed by a pharmacokinetic approach.

Since Gullino and Grantham reported in 1961 the use of a tissue-isolated tumor in studying exchanges of fluids between host and tumor, their model has been used in estimating physiological properties of tumors, such as blood flow, interstitial pressure, and energy metabolism, and in evaluating the effect of interstitial pressure on the distribution of macromolecules. In their model, blocks of Walker 256 carcinoma are inoculated in the adipose tissue around the ovary and enclosed in a plastic bag to separate it from other tissues. After an adequate period, the tumor, isolated from other tissues, can be perfused after being cannulated with tubes into the aorta and vena cava. To ensure independent perfusion for the isolated tumor, all blood vessels supplying other tissues (left renal artery and vein, right renal vein, inferior vena cava, and aorta) should be ligated. After administration of a drug, the outflowing perfusate is collected at appropriate time intervals for analysis. Figure 19.6 shows a scheme of the experimental system of the tissue-isolated tumor of Walker 256 carcinosarcoma.

Some physiological parameters of this tissue-isolated tumor vary among preparations. Necrosis can be apparently observed near the center of the tissue with the increase in the size of the tumor (Warren, 1970; Leunig *et al.*, 1992; Fox *et al.*, 1993). Therefore, the blood supply to the tissue is highly heterogeneous and, in this case, the tumor tissue can be divided into a well perfused (viable) region and

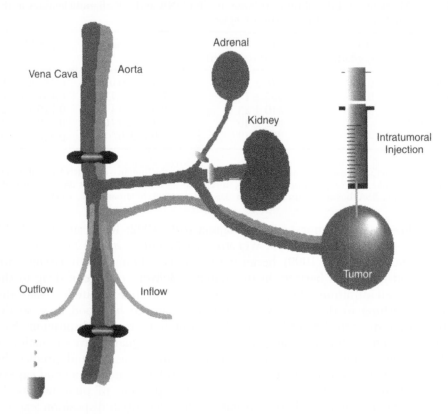

Figure 19.6 Schematic presentation of perfusion system of the tissue-isolated tumor preparation.

a poorly perfused (necrotic and/or hypoxic) region. Fluid regularly oozes out from the tumor surface (Butler *et al.*, 1975), but the fluid leakage is highly unique, for each tumor preparation and its rate hardly correlates with the size of the tumor (Saikawa *et al.*, 1996). Therefore, the tumor tissue can be divided into two regions, viable and necrotic regions. Large tumors possess widespread necrotic regions that are poorly perfused with blood. On the other hand, viable regions are enriched with vasculature. Based on these results and anatomical characteristics of tumor tissues, a pharmacokinetic model to evaluate the intratumoral behavior of a drug after intratumoral injection is developed (Figure 19.7). In the model, the tumor tissue is assumed to be composed of two compartments, well perfused and poorly perfused regions. A drug in the well perfused region is assumed to be cleared from the vascular side quickly and in the poorly perfused region it is assumed to be transferred to the well perfused region or leak out. The poorly perfused region is assumed to have little blood supply and also to contain some necrotic tissue. The well perfused region, in contrast, is assumed to consist of vascular space and its surrounding space, which is in equilibrium to the vascular space. Based on these assumptions, the following equations are derived to describe the change in the drug amount in these two regions with time:

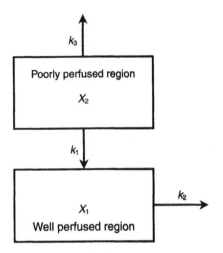

Figure 19.7 Pharmacokinetic model for analyzing drug disposition following direct intratumoral injection. k_1, rate constant of transfer from poorly perfused region to well perfused region; k_2, venous appearance rate constant; k_3, rate constant of leakage from the surface; X_1 and X_2, drug amounts in well perfused and poorly perfused regions, respectively.

$$\frac{dX_1}{dt} = k_1X_2 - k_2X_1 \tag{29}$$

$$\frac{dX_2}{dt} = -(k_1 + k_3)X_2 \tag{30}$$

where X_1 and X_2 are drug amounts in well and poorly perfused regions, respectively; k_1 is the rate constant of transfer from poorly perfused regions to well perfused regions; k_2 is the venous appearance rate constant; and k_3 is the rate constant of leakage from the surface. The integration of Eq (29) and (30) gives

$$J = Ae^{-\alpha t} + Be^{-\beta t} \tag{31}$$

$$A = k_2X_0\frac{k_1 + (1 - R)(k_3 - k_2)}{k_1 + k_3 - k_2} \tag{32}$$

$$B = -\frac{k_1k_2RX_0}{k_1 + k_3 - k_2} \tag{33}$$

$$\alpha = k_2 \tag{34}$$

$$\beta = k_1 + k_3 \tag{35}$$

where J (% of dose/min) is the appearance rate in venous outflow, which is equal to k_2X_1; X_0 is the injected dose; and R is the dosing ratio into the poorly perfused region. To estimate the pharmacokinetic parameters, k_1, k_2, k_3 and R, the venous outflow pattern is fitted to Eq (31).

This pharmacokinetic model has been applied to analyze the intratumoral disposition characteristics of lipidic drug carriers (Nomura *et al.*, 1998a), macromolecular prodrugs of MMC (Nomura *et al.*, 1998b), and naked pDNA (Nomura *et al.*, 1997). Some parameters obtained based on the model vary among tumor preparations, depending on their sizes (Saikawa *et al.*, 1996). Therefore, in order to use the pharmacokinetic model for evaluating the intratumoral behavior of a drug, the sizes of the tumor preparations should be controlled. Figure 19.8 summarizes the pharmacokinetic parameters, k_1 and k_2, representing the transfer rate within the tissue and the venous appearance rate, respectively, of ^{32}P-pDNA and other test compounds. Extensive differences in the physicochemical properties of test compounds, i.e., from low-molecular weight drugs like mitomycin C (MMC, MW 334) to particulate lipidic carriers like fat emulsions (mean diameter of 250 nm), slightly affected k_1, but greatly influenced k_2, indicating that the rate of transfer from the poorly perfused compartment to the well perfused compartment is the determining factor that controls the intratumoral behavior of a drug following its direct injection. In Figure 19.8, cationic liposome shows the smallest k_1 value, and cationic MMC-dextran conjugate (MMC-Dcat) has a larger k_1 than anionic conjugate (MMC-Dan); these results indicate that the electrical interaction of a cationic drug with the anionic surface of the tissue prolongs the drug's retention in the tumor. Furthermore, pDNA-cationic liposome complex injected in the tumor was

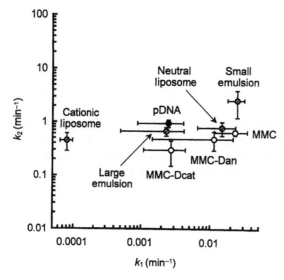

Figure 19.8 Pharmacokinetic parameters, k_1 and k_2, following direct intratumoral injection of drugs in tissue-isolated tumor. k_1 is the rate constant of transfer of drug from poorly perfused region to well perfusion region, and k_2 is the venous appearance rate constant of drug. MMC, mitomycin C; MMC-Dan, MMC conjugate with anionic dextran (T-70); MMC-Dcat, MMC conjugate with cationic dextran (T-70); Large Emulsion, egg phosphatidylcholine (PC)/soybean oil emulsion with diameter of 250 nm; Small Emulsion, egg PC/soybean oil emulsion with diameter of 86 nm; Neutral Liposome, egg PC/dioleoylphosphatidylethanolamine (DOPE) liposome with diameter of 120 nm; Cationic Liposome, Liposome, egg PC/DOPE/ dimethyldioctadecylammonium liposome with diameter of 125 nm.

hardly recovered in the outflow (Nomura *et al.*, 1997). In such cases, the pharmacokinetic analysis cannot be performed because the analysis uses the venous appearance rate of drug.

CONCLUDING REMARKS

It is important to develop vector and/or transfection methods that enable us to achieve gene expression *in vivo* that is high in its efficiency and long in its duration. Understanding the elimination pathway, rate and extent of gene drugs such as pDNA and antisense oligonucleotides is a prerequisite to designing a good approaches for improving their efficacy. Pharmacokinetic analysis will give us information on the events occurring in the body following drug administration, therefore, it is a powerful tool for developing a strategy to fight the inefficient results of gene therapy trials thus far.

REFERENCES

Agrawal, S., Temsamani, J. and Tang, J.Y. (1991) Pharmacokinetics, biodistribution, and stability of oligodeoxynucleotide phosphorothioates in mice. *Proc. Natl. Acad. Sci. USA*, **88**, 7595–7579.

Agrawal, S., Temsamani, J., Galbraith, W. and Tang, J. (1995) Pharmacokinetics of antisense oligonucleotides. *Clin. Pharmacokinet.*, **28**, 7–16.

Ali, S.A., Eary, J.F., Warren, S.D., Badger, C.C. and Krohn, K.A. (1988) Synthesis and radioiodination of tyramine cellobiose for labeling monoclonal antibodies. *Nucl. Med. Biol.*, **15**, 557–561.

Budker, V., Budker, T., Zhang, G., Subbotin, V., Loomis, A. and Wolff, J.A. (2000) Hypothesis: naked plasmid DNA is taken up by cells *in vivo* by a receptor-mediated process. *J. Gene Med.*, **2**, 76–88.

Butler, T.P., Grantham, F.H. and Gullino, P.M. (1975) Bulk transfer of fluid in the interstitial compartment of mammary tumours. *Cancer Res.*, **35**, 3084–3088.

Deshpande, S.V., Subramanian, R., McCall, M.J., DeNardo, S.J., DeNardo, G.L. and Meares, C.F. (1990) Metabolism of indium chelates attached to monoclonal antibody: minimal transchelation of indium from benzyl-EDTA chelate *in vivo*. *J. Nucl. Med.*, **31**, 218–224.

Dow, S.W., Elmslie, R.E., Willson, A.P., Roche, L., Gorman, C. and Potter, T.A. (1998) *In vivo* tumor transfection with superantigen plus cytokine genes induces tumor regression and prolongs survival in dogs with malignant melanoma. *J. Clin. Invest.*, **101**, 2406–2414.

Fox, S.B., Gatter, K.C., Bicknell, R., Going, J.J., Stanton, P., Cooke, T.G. and Harris, A.L. (1993) Relationship of endothelial cell proliferation to tumor vascularity in human breast cancer. *Cancer Res.*, **53**, 4161–4163.

Fujita, T., Takakura, Y., Sezaki, H. and Hashida, M. (1995) Control of disposition characteristics of proteins by direct cationization in mice. *Pharm. Sci.*, **1**, 371–375.

Gullino, P.M. and Grantham, F.H. (1961) Studies on the exchanges of fluids between host and tumor. I. A method for growing 'tissue-isolated' tumors in laboratory animals. *J. Natl. Cancer Inst.*, **27**, 679–689.

Hunt, C.A., MacGregor, R.D. and Siegel, R.A. (1986) Engineering targeted *in vivo* drug delivery. I. The physiological and physicochemical principles governing opportunities and limitations. *Pharm. Res.*, **3**, 333–344.

Imoto, H., Sakamura, Y., Ohkouchi, K., Atsumi, R., Takakura, Y., Sezaki, H. and Hashida, M. (1992) Disposition characteristics of macromolecules in the perfused tissue-isolated tumor preparation. *Cancer Res.*, **52**, 4396–4401.

Kakutani, T., Yamaoka, K., Hashida, M. and Sezaki, H. (1985) A new method for assessment of drug disposition in muscle: application of statistical moment theory to local perfusion systems. *J. Pharmacokin. Biopharm.*, **13**, 609–631.

Kawabata, K., Takakura, Y. and Hashida, M. (1995) The fate of plasmid DNA after intravenous injection in mice: involvement of scavenger receptors in its hepatic uptake. *Pharm. Res.*, **12**, 825–830.

Kircheis, R., Schuller, S., Brunner, S., Ogris, M., Heider, K.H., Zauner, W. and Wagner, E. (1999) Polycation-based DNA complexes for tumor-targeted gene delivery *in vivo*. *J. Gene Med.*, **1**, 111–120.

Kitajima, I., Shinohara, T., Minor, T., Bibbs, L., Bilakovics, J. and Nerenberg, M. (1992) Human T-cell leukemia virus type 1 tax transformation is associated with increased uptake of oligodeoxynucleotides *in vitro* and *in vivo*. *J. Biol. Chem.*, **267**, 25881–25888.

Kobayashi, N., Kuramoto, T., Yamaoka, K., Hashida, M. and Takakura, Y. (2001) Hepatic uptake and gene expression mechanisms following intravenous administration of plasmid DNA by conventional and hydrodynamics-based procedures. *J. Pharmacol. Exp. Ther.*, **297**, 1–8.

Leunig, M., Yuan, F., Menger, M.D., Boucher, Y., Goetz, A.E., Messmer, K. and Jain, R.K. (1992) Angiogenesis, microvascular architecture, microhemodynamics, and interstitial fluid pressure during early growth of human adenocarcinoma LS174T in SCID mice. *Cancer Res.*, **52**, 6553–6560.

Li, S., Tan, Y., Viroonchatapan, E., Pitt, B.R. and Huang, L. (2000) Targeted gene delivery to pulmonary endothelium by anti-PECAM antibody. *Am. J. Physiol.*, **278**, L504–L511.

Liu, Y., Mounkes, L.C., Liggitt, H.D., Brown, C.S., Solodin, I., Heath, T.D. and Debs, R.J. (1997) Factors influencing the efficiency of cationic liposome-mediated intravenous gene delivery. *Nat. Biotech.*, **15**, 167–173.

Liu, F., Song, Y.K. and Liu, D. (1999) Hydrodynamics-based transfection in animals by systemic administration of plasmid DNA. *Gene Ther.*, **6**, 1258–1266.

Mahato, R.I., Kawabata, K., Takakura, Y. and Hashida, M. (1995a) *In vivo* disposition characteristics of plasmid DNA complexed with cationic liposomes. *J. Drug Target.*, **3**, 149–157.

Mahato, R.I., Kawabata, K., Nomura, T., Takakura, Y. and Hashida, M. (1995b) Physicochemical and pharmacokinetic characteristics of plasmid DNA/cationic liposome complexes. *J. Pharm. Sci.*, **84**, 1267–1271.

Mahato, R.I., Takemura, S., Akamatsu, K., Nishikawa, M., Takakura, Y. and Hashida, M. (1997) Physicochemical and disposition characteristics of antisense oligonucleotides complexed with glycosylated poly(L-lysine). *Biochem. Pharmacol.*, **53**, 887–895.

Mahato, R.I., Anwer, K., Tagliaferri, F., Meaney, C., Leonard, P., Wadhwa, M.S., Logan, M., French, M. and Rolland, A. (1998) Biodistribution and gene expression of lipid/plasmid complexes after systemic administration. *Hum. Gene Ther.*, **9**, 2083–2099.

Mihara, K., Mori, M., Hojo, T., Takakura, Y., Sezaki, H., Hashida, M. (1993a) Disposition characteristics of model macromolecules in the perfused rat kidney. *Biol. Pharm. Bull.*, **16**, 158–162.

Mihara, K., Hojo, T., Fujikawa, M., Takakura, Y., Sezaki, H. and Hashida, M. (1993b) Disposition characteristics of protein drugs in the perfused rat kidney. *Pharm. Res.*, **10**, 823–827.

Mihara, K., Sawai, K., Takakura, Y. and Hashida, M. (1994) Manipulation of renal disposition of human recombinant superoxide dismutase by chemical modification. *Biol. Pharm. Bull.*, **17**, 296–301.

Miyao, T., Takakura, Y., Akiyama, T., Yoneda, F., Sezaki, H. and Hashida, M. (1995) Stability and pharmacokinetic characteristics of oligonucleotides modified at terminal linkages in mice. *Antisense Res. Develop.*, **5**, 115–121.

Nakajima, S., Koshino, Y., Nomura, T., Yamashita, F., Agrawal, S., Takakura, Y. and Hashida, M. (2000) Intratumoral pharmacokinetics of oligonucleotides in a tissue-isolated tumor perfusion system. *Antisense Nucleic Acid Drug Develop.*, **10**, 105–110.

Nemunaitis, J., Fong, T., Burrows, F., Bruce, J., Peters, G., Ognoskie, N., Meyer, W., Wynne, D., Kerr, R., Pippen, J., Oldham, F. and Ando, D. (1999) Phase I trial of interferon gamma retroviral vector administered intratumorally with multiple courses in patients with metastatic melanoma. *Hum. Gene Ther.*, **10**, 1289–1298.

Nishida, K., Tonegawa, C., Kakutani, T., Hashida, M. and Sezaki, H. (1989) Statistical moment analysis of hepatobiliary transport of phenol red in the perfused rat liver. *Pharm. Res.*, **6**, 140–146.

Nishida, K., Tonegawa, C., Nakane, S., Takakura, Y., Hashida, M. and Sezaki, H. (1990) Effect of electric charge on the hepatic uptake of macromolecules in the rat liver. *Int. J. Pharm.*, **65**, 7–17.

Nishida, K., Eguchi, Y., Takino, T., Takakura, Y., Hashida, M. and Sezaki, H. (1991a) Hepatic disposition characteristics of 111In-labeled lactosaminated bovine serum albumin in rats. *Pharm. Res.*, **8**, 1253–1257.

Nishida, K., Mihara, K., Takino, T., Nakane, S., Takakura, Y., Hashida, M. and Sezaki, H. (1991b) Hepatic disposition characteristics of electrically charged macromolecules in rat *in vivo* and in the perfused liver. *Pharm. Res.*, **8**, 437–444.

Nishida, K., Takino, T., Eguchi, Y., Yamashita, F., Hashida, M. and Sezaki, H. (1992) Pharmacokinetic analysis of uptake process of lactosaminated albumin in rat liver constant infusion experiments. *Int. J. Pharm.*, **80**, 101–108.

Nishikawa, M., Ohtsubo, Y., Ohno, J., Fujita, T., Koyama, Y., Yamashita, F., Hashida, M. and Sezaki, H. (1992) Pharmacokinetics of receptor-mediated hepatic uptake of glycosylated albumin in mice. *Int. J. Pharm.*, **85**, 75–85.

Nishikawa, M., Miyazaki, C., Yamashita, F., Takakura, Y. and Hashida, M. (1995) Galactosylated proteins are recognized by the liver according to the surface density of galactose moieties. *Am. J. Physiol.*, **268**, G849–G856.

Nishikawa, M., Takakura, Y. and Hashida, M. (1996) Pharmacokinetic evaluation of polymeric carriers. *Adv. Drug Deliv. Rev.*, **21**, 135–155.

Nishikawa, M., Takemura, S., Takakura, Y. and Hashida, M. (1998) Targeted delivery of plasmid DNA to hepatocytes *in vivo*: optimization of the pharmacokinetics of plasmid DNA/galactosylated poly(L-lysine) complexes by controlling their physicochemical properties. *J. Pharmacol. Exp. Ther.*, **287**, 408–415.

Nishikawa, M., Yamauchi, M., Morimoto, K., Ishida, E., Takakura, Y. and Hashida, M. (2000) Hepatocyte-targeted *in vivo* gene expression by intravenous injection of plasmid DNA complexed with synthetic multi-functional gene delivery system. *Gene Ther.*, **7**, 548–555.

Nomura, T., Nakajima, S., Kawabata, K., Yamashita, F., Takakura, Y. and Hashida, M. (1997) Intratumoral pharmacokinetics and *in vivo* gene expression of naked plasmid DNA and its cationic liposome complexes after direct gene transfer. *Cancer Res.*, **57**, 2681–2686.

Nomura, T., Koreeda, N., Yamashita, F., Takakura, Y. and Hashida, M. (1998a) Effect of particle size and charge on the disposition of lipid carriers after intratumoral injection into tissue-isolated tumors. *Pharm. Res.*, **15**, 128–132.

Nomura, T., Saikawa, A., Morita, S., Sakaeda (ne Kakutani), T., Yamashita, F., Honda, K., Takakura, Y. and Hashida, M. (1998b) Pharmacokinetic characteristics and therapeutic effects of mitomycin C-dextran conjugates after intratumoural injection. *J. Control Release*, **52**, 239–252.

Ogawara, K., Nishikawa, M., Takakura, Y. and Hashida, M. (1998) Pharmacokinetic analysis of hepatic uptake of galactosylated bovine serum albumin in a perfused rat liver. *J. Control Release*, **50**, 309–317.

Ogawara, K., Hasegawa, S., Nishikawa, M., Takakura, Y. and Hashida, M. (1999) Pharmacokinetic evaluation of mannosylated bovine serum albumin as a liver cell-specific carrier: quantitative comparison with other hepatotropic ligands. *J. Drug Target.*, **6**, 349–360.

Ohkouchi, K., Imoto, H., Takakura, Y., Hashida, M. and Sezaki, H. (1990) Disposition of anticancer drugs after bolus arterial administration in a tissue-isolated tumor perfusion system. *Cancer Res.*, **50**, 1640–1644.

Opanasopit, P., Shiraishi, K., Nishikawa, M., Yamashita, F., Takakura, Y. and Hashida, M. (2001) *In vivo* recognition of mannosylated proteins by hepatic mannose receptors and mannan-binding protein. *Am. J. Physiol.*, in press.

Peng, B., Andrews, J., Nestorov, I., Brennan, B., Nicklin, P. and Rowland, M. (2001) Tissue distribution and physiologically based pharmacokinetics of antisense phosphorothioate oligonucleotide ISIS 1082 in rat. *Antisense Nucleic Acid Drug Develop.*, **11**, 15–27.

Perales, J.C., Ferkol, T., Beegen, H., Ratnoff, O.D. and Hanson, R.W. (1994) Gene transfer *in vivo*: sustained expression and regulation of genes introduced into the liver by receptor-mediated uptake. *Proc. Natl. Acad. Sci. USA*, **91**, 4086–4090.

Phillips, J.A., Craig, S.J., Bayley, D., Christian, R.A., Geary, R. and Nicklin, P.L. (1997) Pharmacokinetics, metabolism, and elimination of a 20-mer phosphorothioate oligodeoxy-nucleotide (CGP 69846A) after intravenous and subcutaneous administration. *Biochem. Pharmacol.*, **54**, 657–668.

Plautz, G.E., Yang, Z., Wu, B., Gao, X., Huang, L. and Nabel, G.J. (1993) Immunotherapy of malignancy by *in vivo* gene transfer into tumors. *Proc. Natl. Acad. Sci. USA*, **90**, 4645–4649.

Ratajczak, M.Z., Kant, J.A., Luger, S.M., Hijiya, N., Zhang, J., Zon, A. and Gewirtz, A.M. (1992) *In vivo* treatment of human leukemia in a scid mouse model with c-myb antisense oligonucleotides. *Proc. Natl. Acad. Sci. USA*, **89**, 11823–11827.

Robinson, P.J. and Rapoport, S.I. (1987) Size selectivity of blood-brain barrier permeability at various times after osmotic opening. *Am. J. Physiol.*, **253**, R459–R466.

Roth, J.A. and Cristiano, R.J. (1997) Gene therapy for cancer: what have we done and where are we going? *J. Natl. Cancer Inst.*, **89**, 21–39.

Saikawa, A., Nomura, T., Yamashita, F., Takakura, Y., Sezaki, H. and Hashida, M. (1996) Pharmacokinetic analysis of drug disposition after intratumoral injection in a tissue-isolated tumor perfusion system. *Pharm. Res.*, **13**, 1438–1444.

Sakurai, F., Nishioka, T., Saito, H., Baba, T., Okuda, A., Matsumoto, O., Taga, T., Yamashita, F., Takakura, Y. and Hashida, M. (2001) Interaction between DNA-cationic liposome complexes and erythrocytes in an important factor in systemic gene transfer via the intravenous route in mice: the role of the neutral helper lipid. *Gene Ther.*, **8**, 677–686.

Sands, H., Gorey-Feret, L.J., Cocuzza, A.J., Hobbs, F.W., Chidester, D. and Trainor, G.L. (1994) Biodistribution and metabolism of internally ^{3}H-labeled oligonucleotides. I. Comparison of a phosphodiester and a phosphorothioate. *Mol. Pharmacol.*, **45**, 932–943.

Sawai, K., Miyao, T., Takakura, Y. and Hashida, M. (1995) Renal disposition characteristics of oligonucleotides modified at terminal linkages in the perfused rat kidney. *Antisense Res. Develop.*, **5**, 279–287.

Sawai, K., Mahato, R.I., Oka, Y., Takakura, Y. and Hashida, M. (1996) Disposition of oligonucleotides in isolated perfused rat kidney: involvement of scavenger receptors in their renal uptake. *J. Pharmacol. Exp. Ther.*, **279**, 284–290.

Senior, J.H. (1987) Fate and behavior of liposomes *in vivo*: a review of controlling factors. *Crit. Rev. Ther. Drug Carrier Syst.*, **3**, 123–193.

Shlesinger, P.H., Doebber, T.W., Mandell, B.F., White, R., DeSchryver, C., Rodman, J.S., Miller, M.J. and Stahl, P.D. (1978) Plasma clearance of glycoproteins with terminal mannose and *N*-acetylglucosamine by liver non-parenchymal cells. Study with beta-glucuronidase, *N*-acetyl-beta-*D*-glucosamine, ribonuclease B and agalacto-orosomucoid. *Biochem. J.*, **176**, 103–108.

Sun, W.H., Burkholder, J.K., Sun, J., Culp, J., Turner, J., Lu, X.G., Pugh, T.D., Ershler, W.B. and Yang, N.S. (1995) *In vivo* cytokine gene transfer by gene gun reduces tumor growth in mice. *Proc. Natl. Acad. Sci. USA*, **92**, 2889–2893.

Takagi, A., Yabe, Y., Oka, Y., Sawai, K., Takakura, Y. and Hashida, M. (1997) Renal disposition of recombinant human interleukin-11 in the isolated perfused rat kidney. *Pharm. Res.*, **14**, 86–90.

Takagi, A., Yabe, Y., Yoshida, M., Takakura, Y. and Hashida, M. (1998a) Hepatic disposition characteristics of recombinant human interleukin-11 (rhIL-11) in the perfused rat liver. *Biol. Pharm. Bull.*, **21**, 1364–1366.

Takagi, T., Hashiguchi, M., Mahato, R.I., Tokuda, H., Takakura, Y. and Hashida, M. (1998b) Involvement of specific mechanism in plasmid DNA uptake by mouse peritoneal macrophages. *Biochem. Biophys. Res. Commun.*, **245**, 729–733.

Takakura, Y., Fujita, T., Hashida, M. and Sezaki, H. (1990) Disposition characteristics of macromolecules in tumor-bearing mice. *Pharm. Res.*, **7**, 339–346.

Takakura, Y., Fujita, T., Furitsu, H., Nishikawa, M., Sezaki, H. and Hashida, M. (1994) Pharmacokinetics of succinylated proteins and dextran sulfate in mice: implications for hepatic targeting of protein drugs by direct succinylation via scavenger receptors. *Int. J. Pharm.*, **105**, 19–29.

Takakura, Y. and Hashida, M. (1996) Macromolecular carrier systems for targeted drug delivery: pharmacokinetic considerations on biodistribution. *Pharm. Res.*, **13**, 820–831.

Takakura, Y., Mahato, R.I., Yoshida, M., Kanamaru, T. and Hashida, M. (1996) Uptake characteristics of oligonucleotides in the isolated rat liver perfusion system. *Antisense Nucleic Acid Drug Develop.*, **6**, 177–183.

Takakura, Y., Takagi, T., Hashiguchi, M., Nishikawa, M., Yamashita, F., Doi, T. *et al.* (1999) Characterization of plasmid DNA binding and uptake by peritoneal macrophages from class A scavenger receptor knockout mice. *Pharm. Res.*, **16**, 503–508.

Toloza, E.M., Hunt, K., Swisher, S., McBride, W., Lau, R., Pang, S., Rhoades, K., Drake, T., Belldegrun, A., Glaspy, J. and Economou, J.S. (1996) *In vivo* cancer gene therapy with a recombinant interleukin-2 adenovirus vector. *Cancer Gene Ther.*, **3**, 11–17.

Uhlmann, E. and Peyman, A. (1990) Antisense oligonucleotides. A new therapeutic principle. *Chem. Rev.*, **90**, 543–584.

Wagner, E., Plank, C., Zatloukal, K., Cotten, M. and Birnstiel, M.L. (1992) Influenza virus hemagglutinin HA-2 N-terminal fusogenic peptides augment gene transfer by transferrin-polylysine-DNA complexes: toward a synthetic virus-like gene-transfer vehicle. *Proc. Natl. Acad. Sci. USA*, **89**, 7934–7938.

Warren, B.A. (1970) The ultrastructure of the microcirculation at the advancing edge of Walker 256 carcinoma. *Microvasc. Res.*, **2**, 443–453.

Wei, M.X., Tamiya, T., Hurford, Jr., R.K., Boviatsis, E.J., Tepper, R.I. and Chiocca, E.A. (1995) Enhancement of interleukin-4-mediated tumor regression in athymic mice by *in situ* retroviral gene transfer. *Gene Ther.*, **6**, 437–443.

Wolff, J.A., Malone, R.W., Williams, P., Chong, W., Acsadi, G., Jani, A. and Felgner, P.L. (1990) Direct gene transfer into mouse muscle *in vivo*. *Science*, **247**, 1465–1468.

Wu, G.Y. and Wu, C.H. (1988) Receptor-mediated gene delivery and expression *in vivo*. *J. Biol. Chem.*, **263**, 14621–14624.

Yamaoka, K., Tanigawara, Y., Nakagawa, T. and Uno, T. (1981) A pharmacokinetic analysis program (MULTI) for microcomputer. *J. Pharmaco-Dyn.*, **4**, 879–885.

Yoshida, M., Mahato, R.I., Kawabata, K., Takakura, Y. and Hashida, M. (1996) Disposition characteristics of plasmid DNA in the single-pass rat liver perfusion system. *Pharm. Res.*, **13**, 599–603.

Zhang, G., Budker, V. and Wolff, J.A. (1999) High levels of foreign gene expression in hepatocytes after tail vein injections of naked plasmid DNA. *Hum. Gene Ther.*, **10**, 1735–1737.

Zhu, N., Liggitt, D., Liu, Y. and Debs, R. (1993) Systemic gene expression after intravenous DNA delivery into adult mice. *Science*, **261**, 209–211.

20 Interstitial transport of macromolecules: implication for nucleic acid delivery in solid tumors

Sarah McGuire, David Zaharoff and Fan Yuan

INTRODUCTION

Gene delivery in solid tumors has become an important concern to the advances of molecular medicine. One of the major problems in both systemic and local delivery of genes is the interstitial resistance to transport of nucleic acids and their carriers (Jain, 1997). The problem is attributed to several unique characteristics at molecular, cellular, and tissue levels, which include: (a) low convective transport due to uniformly elevated interstitial fluid pressure (IFP) and the lack of functional lymphatics; (b) outward gradient of IFP in tumor periphery, causing convective transport of extravasated genes from interior to surrounding tissues; (c) large diffusion distance in some regions of the interstitium; (d) binding of drugs and genes to both the plasma membrane of cells and the extracellular matrix, and; (e) degradation of nucleic acids in the interstitial space. These factors may significantly hinder the interstitial penetration of genes, limit the accessibility of therapeutic agents to intracellular targets, and thus reduce the efficacy of molecular medicines.

Despite its clinical importance, the quantitative analysis of interstitial transport of genes has been neglected in most studies attempting to improve the efficacy of gene medicines. Thus, few data can be reviewed in this chapter. However, there exists a wealth of information on the transport of nucleic acids in solutions and polymeric gels, as well as across cell membranes (de Gennes, 1999; Han *et al.*, 1999), and a large number of studies have been performed on interstitial transport of macromolecules other than nucleic acids in solid tumors (Jain, 1997). To this end, we will separately review the interstitial transport of macromolecules in solid tumors and the transport of nucleic acids in solutions and polymeric gels. We hope that these data will provide some indirect information on the interstitial transport of nucleic acids and stimulate research interests in this area.

INTERSTITIAL TRANSPORT OF MACROMOLECULES IN SOLID TUMORS

Macromolecules and nanoparticles such as antibodies, liposomes, and genes are being used with more regularity in cancer treatment. However, two critical questions remain to be answered. One is how to uniformly deliver large therapeutic agents throughout a tumor at a clinically adequate dose. Another is how to selectively deliver these agents to solid tumors with minimal accumulation in normal tissues. To address the selectivity issue, antibodies, immunoliposomes, and retro-viral vectors that target tumor-associated antigens (Weiner, 1999) or extracellular matrix (Hall *et al.*, 2000) have been exploited. The antibody approach has shown promising results in treating leukemia and lymphoma (Feuring-Buske *et al.*, 2000; Foon, 2000; Kreitman *et al.*, 2000), but is less effective in solid tumors. This reduced effectivity in solid tumors is partly because delivery of large molecules in tumor tissues is difficult (Jain, 1997). The delivery problem is related to (i) hetero-geneous blood flow and vasculature (Jain, 1997; Juweid *et al.*, 1992; Milenic *et al.*, 1991; Yuan, 1998), and (ii) the interstitial resistance to drug transport, as mentioned above (Jain, 1987, 1997). Local delivery using drug-loaded polymeric devices may avoid the blood supply problem, but it is still hampered by interstitial barriers (Dang *et al.*, 1994; Fung and Saltzman, 1997; Shea *et al.*, 1999). These barriers make diffusion impractical for interstitial delivery of macromolecules. Alternatively, intratumoral infusion is a promising technique for the local delivery of macromolecules (Boucher *et al.*, 1998; Dillehay, 1997; Laske *et al.*, 1997; McGuire and Yuan, 2001; Nishikawa and Hashida, 1999; Nomura *et al.*, 1997, 1998; Order *et al.*, 1996; Zhang *et al.*, 2000). This technique relies on convection driven by an infusion-induced pressure gradient in tumors. The infusion tech-nique bypasses the problems associated with tumor vasculature and slow diffusion of macromolecules, but it has not been fully optimized (Boucher *et al.*, 1998; McGuire and Yuan, 2001; Zhang *et al.*, 2000). In addition, both controlled release devices and intratumoral infusion are limited to the local delivery of therapeutic agents. They are less effective in treating micrometastases in the body.

Given the complexity in molecular transport in tissues, understanding mech-anisms of convection, diffusion, and binding in the interstitial space regardless of administration techniques may provide the means to overcome transport barriers for more uniform and adequate delivery of large therapeutic agents in solid tumors.

Convection

The velocity of interstitial fluid in solid tumors is often lower than the resolution of experimental techniques, which is $\sim$0.1 µm/sec, except in some special tumor models. For example, Chary and Jain (1989) have examined interstitial fluid velocity in granulation tissues and VX2 mammary carcinoma grown in rabbit ear chambers, using the fluorescence recovery after photobleaching (FRAP) technique. The average velocities in both tissues are about 0.6 µm/sec.

IFP is elevated and uniform throughout a solid tumor, but decreases sharply at the tumor periphery. The sharp decrease improves convection across the micro-vessel wall in that region and results in drug transport from the tumor to sur-rounding normal tissues. Based on a tissue isolated tumor model, Butler *et al.* (1975) have shown that the rate of fluid oozing out of a tumor is 0.14–0.22 ml/hr-g tissue. The outward convection is one of the major mechanisms for macromolecule and nanoparticle accumulation in the periphery of solid tumors. It may be bene-ficial for tumor diagnosis when contrast agents are delivered, but drug delivery to peripheral tissues has minor effects on tumor treatment.

Most studies on convective transport in solid tumors are related to intratumoral infusion of therapeutic agents (Boucher *et al.*, 1998; Dillehay, 1997; McGuire and

Yuan, 2001; Zhang *et al.*, 2000). The infusion establishes a pressure gradient that drives fluid flow from the infusion needle tip to surrounding tissues. Convective transport has been quantified by the distribution volume of therapeutic agents. It is a function of time, infusion pressure, and flow rate (Bobo *et al.*, 1994; Chen *et al.*, 1999; Kroll *et al.*, 1996; McGuire and Yuan, 2001). The ratio of distribution volume (V_d) versus infused volume (V_i) is independent of infusion conditions in rigid and porous materials; it is equal to the retardation coefficient, as will be discussed later. However, the volume ratio in solid tumors depends on the infusion pressure, as has been shown in an *ex vivo* study of intratumoral infusion of Evans blue-labeled albumin in a rat fibrosarcoma (Figure 20.1A) (McGuire and Yuan, 2001). In that study, the median V_d/V_i is 2.99 at the pressure of 50 cmH$_2$O, and is reduced to 1.79 at 163 cmH$_2$O. The decrease in V_d/V_i is presumably due to changes in tissue structures. In addition, V_d/V_i varies with tumors, and the coefficient of variation at 50 cmH$_2$O is 0.13 and is increased to 0.32 at 94 cmH$_2$O and 0.46 at 163 cmH$_2$O. The increase in the coefficient of variation with pressure indicates that changes in tissue structures are haphazard. The volume ratio depends on the infusion rate as well (Figure 20.1B) (McGuire and Yuan, 2001). The dependence is statistically significant.

Intratumoral infusion has shown promising results in treating brain tumor patients (Laske *et al.*, 1997), partly due to the existence of the blood brain barrier (BBB).

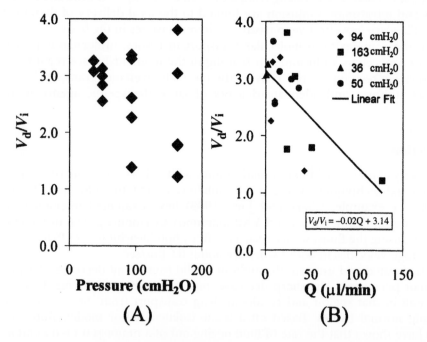

Figure 20.1 Distribution volume of Evans blue-labeled albumin in a rat fibrosarcoma as a function of (A) perfusion pressure or (B) perfusion rate. The ratio of distribution volume (V_d)/infused volume (V_i) was quantified at the infusion pressures of 36, 50, 94, and 163 in cmH$_2$O, respectively. Symbols represent data from individual experiments; $N = 2$ for pressure of 36 cmH$_2$O and $N = 5$ for other pressures. The line in (B) was obtained through linear curve-fitting of the data. Reproduced with permission (McGuire and Yuan, 2001).

The BBB limits transport of drugs and tumor cells across the microvessel wall in both directions. The limitation on cell transport significantly reduces micrometastases of brain tumors in distant organs, which cannot be treated with the local infusion technique. The limitation on drug transport makes local infusion more efficient than systemic approaches. Furthermore, the BBB reduces absorption of infused drugs into blood circulation and thus lowers systemic toxicity of drugs.

The infusion technique has also been applied to drug delivery in brain tissues (Bobo *et al.*, 1994; Laske *et al.*, 1997; Lieberman *et al.*, 1995; Morrison *et al.*, 1994). Bobo *et al.* (1994) infused solutes into cat brain with a constant flow rate. These authors found an inverse relationship between the distribution volume and molecular weight of the compound, implying that larger molecules are impeded by tissue structures more readily than smaller molecules. However, Lieberman *et al.* (1995) found no size dependence for molecule distribution in the rat brain. Thus, other parameters that may affect the distribution volume, such as concentration and infusion rate, need to be considered. Kroll *et al.* (1996) studied the effects of concentration and infusion rate on delivery of monocrystalline iron oxide nanocompounds (MIONs) in the brain. These authors demonstrated that high concentration and low flow rate might produce a greater distribution volume. They also noted that the infusion rate-dependence of the distribution volume was more significant at high concentrations. These relationships, nonetheless, were not corroborated by a later study by Chen *et al.* (1999), who found that the distribution volume of ^{14}C-albumin was independent of the concentration or the flow rate when the dose was diluted up to four times and the infusion rate was increased from 0.1 μl/min to 5 μl/min.

The conflicting results discussed above suggest that further studies are required for understanding mechanisms of convection. More specifically, it is important to investigate hydraulic conductivity, interstitial pressure, and retardation coefficient in different tumor tissues, and how these factors are coupled with infusion-induced tissue deformation.

Hydraulic conductivity

Hydraulic conductivity, K, is a measure of the fluid permeability of tissues. It is defined in Darcy's Law as a ratio of flow rate to pressure gradient. The value of K depends upon the viscosity of the fluid and structures of tissues. During intratumoral infusion, the viscosity can be experimentally controlled, but tissue structures may change with time and infusion conditions, presumably due to tissue deformation (Barry and Aldis, 1992; Dillehay, 1997; Lai and Mow, 1980; Zakaria *et al.*, 1997; Zhang *et al.*, 2000).

The hydraulic conductivity has been studied extensively in normal and tumor tissues (Baldwin and Wilson, 1993; Barry and Aldis, 1992; Boucher *et al.*, 1998; Daniels *et al.*, 1992; Guyton *et al.*, 1966; Huang *et al.*, 1997; Lai and Mow, 1980; Netti *et al.*, 2000; Swabb *et al.*, 1974; Tedgui and Lever, 1984; Zakaria *et al.*, 1997; Zhang *et al.*, 2000; Znati, 1995). However, quantification of K in all these studies involves interstitial perfusion. The perfusion will inevitably alter tissue structures through dehydration or edema (Fry *et al.*, 1986; Guyton *et al.*, 1966), volume compression or expansion (Barry and Aldis, 1992; Daniels *et al.*, 1992; Guyton, *et al.*, 1966; Huang *et al.*, 1997; Klaentschi *et al.*, 1998; Lai and Mow, 1980), and opening or closing of fluid channels in the tissue (Guyton *et al.*, 1966). Thus, only the apparent hydraulic conductivity (K_{app}), or the altered K, has been experimentally measured.

The value of K_{app} is tumor-dependent. It varies from $3.1 \times 10^{-8}\,cm^2/cmH_2O/sec$ in Morris hepatoma 5123 (Swabb *et al.*, 1974) to $1.8 \times 10^{-6}\,cm^2/cmH_2O/sec$ in a murine mammary carcinoma (MCaIV) (Netti *et al.*, 2000). The variation is likely due to the difference in tumor lines rather than experimental methods, because the same methods have also been used to quantify K_{app} in a human colon adenocarcinoma (LS174T) in three different studies and the data from these studies are nearly identical (Boucher *et al.*, 1998; Netti *et al.*, 2000; Znati, 1995).

In addition to tissue structures, K_{app} depends on perfusion conditions. In normal tissues Guyton *et al.* (1966) have demonstrated that K_{app} in a subcutaneous tissue of the abdominal wall is very sensitive to the perfusion pressure. When the pressure is changed from negative to positive values relative to the atmosphere, the value of K_{app} is increased by five orders of magnitude. The increase in K_{app} is presumably due to the opening of water channels within the tissue, which is induced by the pressure increase. Zakaria *et al.* (1997) studied K_{app} in the muscle of the abdominal wall. The value of K_{app} in an unconstrained muscle was increased from $0.9 \times 10^{-5}\,cm^2/min/mmHg$ to $4.7 \times 10^{-5}\,cm^2/min/mmHg$ when the hydrostatic pressure in the peritoneal cavity was increased from 1.5 to 8 mmHg. However, K_{app}, in the same muscle but mounted to a plexiglass, was decreased by one order of magnitude over the same range of pressure gradient. This study indicates that tissue deformation has a significant effect on K_{app}. In the unconstrained muscle, perfusion causes tissue stretching which may open water channels in the extracellular space and thus increase K_{app}. When the muscle is constrained by a plexiglass during perfusion, it is compressed. The compression may lead to closing of water channels and reduction in K_{app}. Effects of tissue deformation on K_{app} have also been found in the articular cartilage (Lai and Mow, 1980), although it is much less deformable than abdominal tissues.

The dependence of K_{app} on tissue deformation has a direct impact on intratumoral infusion of drugs and genes. During the infusion, tumor tissues are deformed due to the infusion induced interstitial pressure gradient. The pressure gradient may cause either compression or expansion of tumor tissues. The compressive strain can cause an exponential decrease in K_{app} in tumor tissues (Netti *et al.*, 2000). Zhang *et al.* (2000) have compared K_{app} in tumors under two different experimental conditions. In the first experiment, tumor slices are perfused in the direction normal to the surface, i.e., one-dimensional (1-D) perfusion. In the second experiment, tumor chunks are perfused through a needle inserted into the center of tumors. The perfusion is mainly in the radial direction, i.e., three-dimensional (3-D) perfusion. In both experiments, there exists a threshold pressure below which perfusion of tissues cannot be achieved. The existence of the threshold pressure suggests that the interstitial space may not be well connected prior to perfusion. Tissue perfusion can be achieved when the perfusion pressure is increased above the threshold level, presumably due to the formation of water channels in the interstitial space. Under this condition, K_{app} is greater than zero and depends on the perfusion pressure (Figure 20.2). During the 1-D perfusion, tumor tissues are compressed by the pressure difference across the slice and K_{app} decreases with the perfusion pressure (Figure 20.2). During the 3-D perfusion,

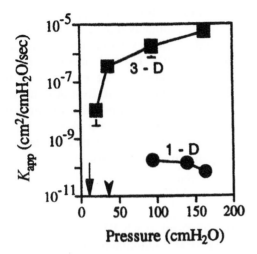

Figure 20.2 The apparent hydraulic conductivity (K_{app}) in fibrosarcomas at different perfusion pressures. The curve labeled with 1-D was obtained during one-dimensional perfusion of tumor slices. The curve labeled with 3-D was obtained during direct infusion into a tumor chunk via a 23G needle. The perfusion pressure varied between $20\,cmH_2O$ and $163\,cmH_2O$. The threshold pressures in 1-D and 3-D experiments are indicated by arrow-head and arrow, respectively. The symbols and error bars represent mean and SD, respectively. The number of tumors for each data point was six in 1-D experiments and three or four in 3-D experiments. Reprinted with permission (Zhang *et al.*, 2000).

tumor tissues are compressed radially and stretched longitudinally and latitudin-ally. Consequently, K_{app} is very sensitive to the perfusion pressure and the depen-dence of K_{app} on the perfusion pressure is always positive (Figure 20.2). When the values of K_{app} in both experiments are compared at the pressure of $163\,cmH_2O$, the difference is 80,260-fold (Figure 20.2). The large discrepancy is caused by the differences in tissue deformation.

Tissue deformation is dependent upon the mechanical properties of tissues, which are heterogeneous due to abnormal growth of tumors. At the macroscopic level, the heterogeneity is caused by necrotic regions and blood pockets in tumors (McGuire and Yuan, 2001). At the microscopic level, the heterogeneity is due to abnormal synthesis of extracellular matrix (Iozzo and Cohen, 1994; Netti *et al.*, 2000; Pucci-Minafra *et al.*, 1998). The heterogeneity may cause tissue rupture in weak locations during intratumoral infusion when the stress is greater than the strain energy release rate of local structures. The ruptures create low resistance pathways for infused molecules. Thus, distribution of molecules in tumors is likely to be irregular and unpredictable (Boucher *et al.*, 1998; Dillehay, 1997; McGuire and Yuan, 2001). Furthermore, the number of ruptured places may increase with tissue deformation or infusion pressure. Therefore, the unpredictability in the distribution of infused molecules may increase with the infusion pressure.

The dependence of the hydraulic conductivity on perfusion conditions has also been studied in polymeric gels (Johnson, 1996; Klaentschi *et al.*, 1998; Parker *et al.*,

1987). The relationship between K_{app} and perfusion pressure or gel compression is similar to that found in tissues, as discussed above. However, K_{app} in gels is less sensitive to volume change than that in tissues, presumably due to the lack of cells. Cells in tissues can be arranged in such a way that affects not only the size but also the connectedness of water channels (Yuan *et al.*, 2001). The lack of connectedness of water channels in tumor tissues has been indicated by the existence of the threshold pressure, as shown in Figure 20.2, for achieving intratumoral infusion of drugs. An increase in tissue deformation may enlarge both the size and the number of transport pathways, and thus cause a rapid increase in K_{app}. Taken together, the pressure-induced tissue deformation is an important consideration for improving the convection of drugs and genes in solid tumors.

Interstitial fluid pressure

IFP is elevated uniformly in solid tumors and can reach 94 mmHg in human cervical carcinomas (Jain, 1997). The elevated IFP eliminates the driving force for convective transport in the center of solid tumors. In addition, the elevated IFP has a significant impact on intratumoral infusion, since the driving force for infusion is the difference between the infusion pressure and the IFP. This driving force should be higher than a threshold level, as discussed above, in order to achieve the infusion.

Retardation coefficient

Interactions between solutes and tissue structures will retard the convective transport of solutes. Thus, the solute velocity is always smaller than the fluid velocity during convection. The ratio of the velocities is defined as the retardation coefficient (f) (Fry *et al.*, 1986; Levick, 1994), which is related to the reflection coefficient (σ) of solutes in transmembrane transport,

$$f = 1 - \sigma \tag{1}$$

Experimentally, f and σ have been poorly quantified (Levick, 1994; McGuire and Yuan, 2001; Parameswaran *et al.*, 1999). Retardation and reflection coefficients may depend on flow rate, solute and tissue properties.

Diffusion

Convection is driven by a pressure gradient, whereas diffusion relies on a concentration gradient. The ratio of convection versus diffusion is defined as the Péclet number. In normal tissues, the Péclet number is, in general, less than unity for small and hydrophilic molecules and larger than unity for macromolecules. Thus, interstitial transport is dominated by diffusion for small molecules and convection for large ones. In solid tumors, the pressure gradient is low due to the uniformly elevated IFP as discussed above. Thus, the Péclet number may also be smaller than unity for macromolecules. In this case, the transport of macromolecules relies on diffusion as well.

The rate of diffusion is proportional to the concentration gradient, and the proportionality constant is defined as the diffusion coefficient (D) in Fick's first law of diffusion. Experimental determination of D is commonly performed *ex vivo* due to the difficulty of measuring concentration gradients in the interstitium. *In vivo* measurement can be performed in specific tissues, using transparent chamber preparations in combination with the FRAP technique (Berk *et al.*, 1997; Jain *et al.*, 1997; Pluen *et al.*, 2001). However, the *in vivo* approach is limited only to fluorescent molecules or solutes whose D is not affected by labeling with fluorescent markers.

The diffusion coefficient depends on a number of factors, including the molecular properties of solutes; the structures of tissues, and; temperature. The temperature-dependence is less critical for drug delivery, since the temperature in tumors is stable and close to the body temperature. The dependence of D on tissue structures is significant (Netti *et al.*, 2000; Pluen *et al.*, 2001). It is mediated through the size and the volume fraction of pores, the tortuosity of diffusion pathways, and the connectedness of pores (Yuan *et al.*, 2001). Diffusion of macromolecules is faster in tissues with a lower collagen type I content (Pluen *et al.*, 2001) or tissues treated with collagenase (Netti *et al.*, 2000). However, there is no correlation between D and the concentration of total or sulfated glycosaminoglycans (Netti *et al.*, 2000).

The dependence of D on molecular properties of solutes is complicated and coupled with tissue structures. Empirically, effects of molecular weight (M_r) on D can be approximated by a power function,

$$D = a(M_r)^{-b}. \tag{2}$$

where a and b are functions of charge and configuration of solutes, as well as structures of tissues (Jain, 1987). Effects of tissue structures on D increase with the size of solutes. For example, the ratio of diffusion coefficients in tissue versus water is close to unity for oxygen (Bentley and Pittman, 1997), but reduced to 0.1–0.3 for albumin and IgG in tumor tissues (Berk *et al.*, 1997; Pluen *et al.*, 2001). This ratio will approach zero as the size of solutes is close to the cutoff size of pores in tissues.

The dependence of diffusion on molecular size has significant ramifications for nanoparticle delivery in tumors. For example, liposomes have been used as vehicles for systemic delivery of drugs and genes (Chesnoy and Huang, 2000; Drummond *et al.*, 2000; Kaneda, 2000; Kong and Dewhirst, 1999; Yuan *et al.*, 1994). Liposomes may improve delivery, reduce toxicity, and provide selectivity of therapeutic agents, because they preferentially extravasate in solid tumors through leaky vasculature (El-Kareh and Secomb, 1997; Hobbs *et al.*, 1998; Kong and Dewhirst, 1999; Yuan *et al.*, 1994). However, once the liposomes extravasate in tumors, they must rely on diffusion to move throughout the interstitial space. Due to the inverse relationship between particle size and D, most liposomes are trapped in perivascular regions. The maximum depth of interstitial penetration from the microvessel wall is ~30 μm over two days (Figure 20.3) (Yuan, 1998; Yuan *et al.*, 1994). The limited penetration may cause a large fraction of drugs released from liposomes to be carried away by the blood circulation, and thus reduce the efficacy of drugs. The penetration problem is an important concern in gene therapy, since genes cannot reach tumor cells located at several cell layers away from the microvessel

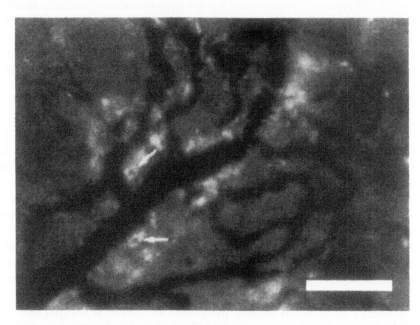

Figure 20.3 Heterogeneous distribution of liposomes in tumor tissues. Human colon adenocarcinoma cells (LS174T) were transplanted in dorsal skinfold chambers in severe combined immunodeficient mice. Fifteen to 32 days post tumor cell transplantation, fluorescently labeled liposomes were injected intravenously. The photos were taken at two days post injections. Liposomes accumulated only in perivascular regions in solid tumors. The arrows indicate liposomes internalized by cells. Bar = 100 μm. Reproduced with permission (Yuan *et al.*, 1994).

wall. Thus, damage to deeper tumor cells will rely on either diffusion of gene products secreted or released from transfected cells in perivascular regions or antiangiogenic strategies that reduce nutrient supply to deeper cells (Feldman and Libutti, 2000; Folkman, 1997; Kuo *et al.*, 2001).

Diffusion is also a dominant mechanism of transport for local drug delivery, using controlled release devices (Fung and Saltzman, 1997; Langer, 1995). The efficiency of local delivery is drug-dependent. For small drugs, diffusion is fast but the penetration distance is limited because of drug absorption by microvessels. To reduce the absorption, small drugs have been conjugated to larger carriers (Dang *et al.*, 1994). The size increase in drug conjugates not only improves interstitial penetration but also reduces the rate of diffusion. Therefore, effective delivery of drugs in the interstitial space will likely be achieved by conjugates with an intermediate size.

Available volume fraction

Diffusion in the interstitial space is closely related to the volume fraction of space that is available to fluid and solute transport in tissues. The volume fraction of tumor interstitial fluid space varies from 15% in human gliomas up to 60% in a rat fibrosarcoma 4956 (Jain, 1987). The available volume fraction (K_{AV}) of solutes is a measure of the steady state ratio of drug concentrations between tissues and the plasma (Krol *et al.*, 1999). Thus, drug and gene delivery can be significantly improved through increasing K_{AV}. In *ex vivo* experiments, K_{AV} determines the ratio of concentrations between tissues and external solutions at the equilibrium state. K_{AV} has been studied extensively in normal tissues but poorly in tumor tissues (Table 20.1) (Krol *et al.*, 1999). K_{AV} depends on the size of solutes and the dependence is determined by both the size and the connectedness of pores (Yuan *et al.*, 2001).

Binding

Binding to extravascular structures may improve selectivity and specificity of therapeutic agents but will also hinder interstitial transport. For example, specific antibodies delivered systemically accumulate only in perivascular regions with a very limited depth of interstitial penetration in solid tumors (Jain, 1997; Saga *et al.*, 1995). The binding-mediated retardation in interstitial transport has coined the phrase 'binding-site-barrier' (Juweid *et al.*, 1992). The barrier can be reduced through increasing the dose of antibodies, due to the saturation of available binding sites (Juweid *et al.*, 1992). However, the dose increase may reduce the advantage of the targeted delivery of antibodies. In addition to the dose, the binding-site-barrier depends on the binding strength, i.e., the avidity (Berk *et al.*, 1997; Kaufman and Jain, 1992). An increase in the avidity may increase the total accumulation of antibodies in tumors but may also enhance the barrier, resulting in a more heterogeneous distribution of antibodies in tumor tissues.

The avidity depends on binding valence and affinity. Kaufman and Jain (1992) have shown that the avidity can vary several orders of magnitude for the same pairs of IgG and antigen, depending on the ratio of IgG molecules that bind to the antigen with both binding paratopes (i.e., bivalent binding) versus that with a single paratope (i.e., monovalent binding). The ratio depends on the concentration of antigen or the distance between antigen molecules in tissues.

Binding to extravascular structures can also be non-specific, such as charge–charge interactions. Similar to antibody–antigen reactions, the strength of non-specific binding depends on the number of bonds formed between delivered molecules and fixed charges in tissues. This dependence has significant effects on DNA transport in tissues, because DNA molecules are highly negatively charged. The number of negatively charged groups is proportional to the length of DNA. Although the affinity between each pair of charge–charge interactions may be low compared with antibody–antigen binding, the avidity of DNA to tissues can be high. The high avidity may significantly reduce DNA transport via both diffusion and convection. Despite its importance in gene delivery, there are few quantitative studies on DNA transport in solid tumors (Nishikawa and Hashida, 1999; Nomura *et al.*, 1997). Most studies in the literature are focused on DNA transport in solutions or polymeric gels, which will be discussed later.

Effects of the microenvironment on interstitial transport in tumors

The microenvironment in solid tumors may significantly influence the interstitial transport of drugs and genes through various environmental factors. These factors

Table 20.1 Available volume fraction (K_{AV}) of macromolecules in various normal and tumor tissues

Tissue	Molecule	r^*	K_{AV}	References
Annulus Fibrosus	PEG	3.2	0.14	(Comper and Laurent, 1978)
Aorta	Albumin	3.6	0.11–0.20	(Fry, 1983)
	Albumin	3.6	0.16	(Thurn, 1982)
	PEG	3.2	0.20	(Comper and Laurent, 1978)
Cartilage	IGF-I	1.7	0.57	(Schneiderman *et al.*, 1995)
	Myoglobin	2.0	0.1	(Maroudas, 1976)
	Chymotrypsinogen	2.8	0.1	(Maroudas, 1976)
	Hemoglobin	2.8	0.01–0.03	(Maroudas, 1970)
	Ovalbumin	2.8	0.03	(Maroudas, 1976)
	Albumin	3.6	0.001–0.01	(Maroudas, 1976)
	Transferrin	3.7	0.001–0.01	(Maroudas, 1976)
	IgG	5.6	0.001–0.01	(Maroudas, 1976)
	PEG	3.2	0.02–0.09	(Comper and Laurent, 1978)
	Dextran	2.6	0.1–0.2	(Maroudas, 1970)
	Dextran	5.2	0.03–0.07	(Maroudas, 1970)
Cecum	Albumin	3.6	0.15	(Wiig *et al.*, 1992)
Colon	Albumin	3.6	0.12	(Wiig *et al.*, 1992)
Cornea	PEG	3.2	0.00	(Comper and Laurent, 1978)
Ileum	Albumin	3.6	0.10	(Wiig *et al.*, 1992)
Jejunum	Albumin	3.6	0.11	(Wiig *et al.*, 1992)
Nucleus Pulposus	PEG	3.2	0.00	(Comper and Laurent, 1978)
Muscle	Albumin	3.6	0.20	(Barr and Malvin, 1965)
	Albumin	3.6	0.04	(Wiig *et al.*, 1992)
Paw	Albumin	3.6	0.10	(Wiig *et al.*, 1992)
Skin	Albumin	3.6	0.14–0.22	(Bert *et al.*, 1986)
	Albumin	3.6	0.14–0.22	(Wiig *et al.*, 1992)
	PEG	3.2	0.6	(Comper and Laurent, 1978)
Subcutis	Albumin	3.6	0.16	(Reed and Lepsøe, 1989)
Tendon	Albumin	3.6	0.14	(Wiig *et al.*, 1992)
	PEG	3.2	0.46	(Comper and Laurent, 1978)
	Albumin	3.6	0.22	(Aukland, 1991)
Umbilical Cord	Myoglobin	2.0	0.68	(Meyer, 1983)
	Albumin	3.6	0.41	(Meyer, 1983)
	Thyroglobulin	3.8	0.44	(Meyer, 1983)
	Catalase	5.2	0.28	(Meyer, 1983)
	Transferrin	8.2	0.0	(Meyer, 1983)
	Dextran	8.0	0.62	(Meyer *et al.*, 1977)
	Dextran	11.7	0.55	(Meyer *et al.*, 1977)
	Dextran	16.0	0.42	(Meyer *et al.*, 1977)
Vitreous Body	PEG	3.2	0.00	(Comper and Laurent, 1978)
Fibrosarcoma	Albumin	3.6	0.13	(Krol *et al.*, 1999)
	Dextran	2.6	0.25	(Krol *et al.*, 1999)
	Dextran	3.7	0.33	(Krol *et al.*, 1999)
	Dextran	5.2	0.33	(Krol *et al.*, 1999)
	Dextran	6.9	0.14	(Krol *et al.*, 1999)
	Dextran	36.8	0.04	(Krol *et al.*, 1999)

Note

*r (nm) is the hydrodynamic radius of the molecules; it is either obtained from the literature or calculated based on the molecular weight of dextrans (Meyer *et al.*, 1977).

can, in general, be classified into four different categories: structural, physical, chemical, and biological. They are coupled together to form a complex micro-environment for interstitial transport in tumor tissues. The structural factors include the size and the connectedness of transport channels formed by cells and ECM. These channels directly determine the rate of drug and gene delivery, as well as the spatial and temporal distribution of therapeutic agents in tumor tissues. Furthermore, the network of transport channels is often dynamic and changes with time due to ECM remodeling and cell turnover.

The physical factors include mechanical stresses and temperature. As discussed above, IFP is uniformly elevated in solid tumors. It is likely that solid stresses are also increased due to rapid proliferation of tumor cells (Griffon-Etienne *et al.*, 1999; Helmlinger *et al.*, 1997; Yuan, 1997). The increase in IFP reduces convective transport, which is critical for delivery of macromolecules. The temperature effects on the interstitial transport of therapeutic agents are mediated by the viscosity of interstitial fluid, which directly affects the diffusion coefficient of solutes and the hydraulic conductivity of tumor tissues. The temperature in tumor tissues is stable and close to the body temperature under normal conditions, but it can be manipulated through either hypo- or hyper-thermia treatments, which are routine procedures in the clinic for cancer treatment.

The chemical environment may affect interstitial transport through various mechanisms. For example, the electric charge of drugs depends on local pH, which is low in solid tumors. The acidic environment can be exploited for improving the specificity of drug delivery to solid tumors (Drummond *et al.*, 2000; Gerweck, 1998; Kozin *et al.*, 2001; Kratz *et al.*, 1999; Prescott, *et al.*, 2000). The chemical environment can be modified for targeted drug delivery. One approach to the modification is the delivery of antibody–enzyme conjugates in the antibody directed enzyme prodrug therapy (ADEPT). The antibody is used to target tumor-associated antigens while the enzyme can locally convert a prodrug to drug in solid tumors. In this case, the interstitial transport of prodrugs and drugs are coupled with chemical reactions. ADEPT is just one example of two-step approaches to targeted drug delivery in solid tumors. The two-step approach can also be achieved through the DNA–DNA hybridization technique (Bos *et al.*, 1994). One of the major impacts of the chemical microenvironment on the interstitial transport is the clearance of drugs and nucleic acids from the interstitial space before reaching target cells. Pathways for chemical clearance include degradation, changes in molecular configuration, and binding to other molecules.

The chemical environment is often coupled with the biological environment. This is because cellular and ECM structures can be affected by chemicals while cells continuously release and clear chemicals in tissues. Effects of the biological environment on the interstitial transport can be either direct or indirect. Damage to cells and ECM will lead to an increase in the interstitial space for drug and gene transport. Drug and nucleic acid clearance discussed above can be achieved through internalization by cells. The indirect effects may involve changes in tissue structures induced by cytokines released from cells or proliferation of cells. Cell proliferation or death will also alter IFP and solid stresses in tumors. Changes in both tissue structures and mechanical stresses may have profound effects on interstitial transport, as discussed above.

TRANSPORT OF NUCLEIC ACIDS IN SOLUTIONS AND POLYMERIC GELS

Diffusion coefficients of nucleic acids in solutions and gels have been accurately measured with the development of advanced laboratory techniques, such as pulsed field-gradient NMR and FRAP (Lapham *et al.*, 1997; Pluen *et al.*, 1999; Politz *et al.*, 1998). These data may provide some semi-quantitative information applicable to interstitial transport of nucleic acids in tumor tissues.

Diffusion of nucleic acids in solutions

Nucleic acids are long, flexible macromolecules that exist in one of four configurations: linear, linear looped, circular and supercoiled. The configurations of RNA are either linear or linear looped. The linear looped configuration occurs spontaneously if the nucleic acid is long and there are at least two regions with complimentary bases. Single stranded DNA may exist with the first three configurations, whereas double stranded DNA is found to be either linear, circular, or supercoiled. Long nucleic acids with any configuration diffuse as randomly coiled globs in solutions. Thus, their diffusion coefficient in solutions is similar to that of globular proteins or solid spheres. It is related to the hydrodynamic radius (R_H) of nucleic acids through the Stokes-Einstein equation,

$$D_0 = \frac{K_B T}{6\pi\eta R_H} \tag{3}$$

where K_B is the Boltzmann constant, T is the solvent's absolute temperature, and η is the solvent viscosity. Nucleic acids, which are too short to form globs, diffuse as short and flexible chains. The diffusion coefficient of different nucleic acids in solutions has been quantified (Table 20.2). In dilute solutions of linear and double

Table 20.2 Diffusion coefficients of different nucleic acids in solutions

Nucleic acid	Diffusion coefficient (cm²/s)	References
12bp DNA fragment	1.23×10^{-6}	(Lapham *et al.*, 1997)
24bp DNA fragment	0.954×10^{-6}	(Lapham *et al.*, 1997)
5486bp DNA fragment	3.5×10^{-8}	(Pluen *et al.*, 1999)
9416bp DNA fragment	2×10^{-8}	(Pluen *et al.*, 1999)
23,130bp DNA fragment	1.5×10^{-8}	(Pluen *et al.*, 1999)
48,502bp DNA fragment	6.5×10^{-9}	(Pluen *et al.*, 1999)
164,000bp DNA fragment	2×10^{-9}	(Pluen *et al.*, 1999)
Yeast tRNA	7×10^{-7}	(Potts *et al.*, 1981)
14b RNA dimer	1.41×10^{-6}	(Lapham *et al.*, 1997)
14b RNA hairpin loop	0.918×10^{-6}	(Lapham *et al.*, 1997)
43mer oligonucleotide	5.7×10^{-6}	(Politz *et al.*, 1998)
T3 DNA	7.56×10^{-9}	(Lang and Coates, 1968)
Chi DNA	4.51×10^{-9}	(Lang and Coates, 1968)

stranded DNA, there exists a simple relationship between the diffusion coefficient and the number of base pairs (N_0) in the fragments (Doi and Edwards, 1986; Pluen *et al.*, 1999),

$$D_0 = \alpha N_0^{-0.50} \tag{4}$$

where α is a constant.

Diffusion of nucleic acids in polymeric gels

The behavior of long and flexible molecules in a gel depends on the ratio of R_g and a, which are the radius of gyration of nucleic acids and the pore radius in gels, respectively. R_g is a function of polymer length and rigidity (García Molina *et al.*, 1990),

$$R_g^2 = \frac{N_0 b_0 p}{3} \left[1 - 3 \cdot \frac{p}{N_0 b_0} + 6 \cdot \left(\frac{p}{N_0 b_0} \right)^2 - 6 \cdot \left(\frac{p}{N_0 b_0} \right)^3 \cdot \left(1 - \exp\left(-\frac{N_0 b_0}{p} \right) \right) \right] \tag{5}$$

where N_0 is the number of monomers or base-pairs, b_0 is the distance between bases (i.e., interbase spacing) and p is the persistence length of the molecule which is a measure of chain flexibility (García Molina *et al.*, 1990; Pluen *et al.*, 1999). For DNA, $p \approx 50$ nm and $b_0 \approx 0.34$ nm (Pluen *et al.*, 1999). Thus, Eq. 5 can be simplified to

$$R_g^2 = \frac{N_0 b_0 p}{3}, \tag{6}$$

if $N_0 >> p/b_0 \approx 150$. In this case, R_g^2 is proportional to the mean square end to end distance of DNA, $2N_0 b_0 p$. R_g is different from R_H. The ratio of R_g/R_H depends on configuration of molecules, excluded volume due to repulsive interactions of chain segments, and solvent quality (Doi and Edwards, 1986; Hiemenz, 1977; Pluen *et al.*, 1999).

When $R_g < a/2$ (i.e., the Rouse regime), the molecule, regardless of conformation, migrates as a glob and the diffusion coefficient, D_G, is described by the Zimm Model (Doi and Edwards, 1986).

$$D_G = \frac{0.196 \cdot k_B T}{\eta R_H} \approx \alpha N_0^{-0.5} \tag{7}$$

where α is a constant. When $R_g > a/2$, the molecule migrates by reptation, i.e., the snake-like movement of flexible polymers through porous media (Doi and Edwards, 1986). The diffusion coefficient for this regime can be approximated by

$$D_G = \frac{k_B a^2 T}{3 N_k^2 \zeta_k b^2} \tag{8}$$

where N_K is the number of Kuhn segments which can be approximated by the number of base-pairs (N_0), ζ_K is the friction coefficient of a Kuhn segment, and

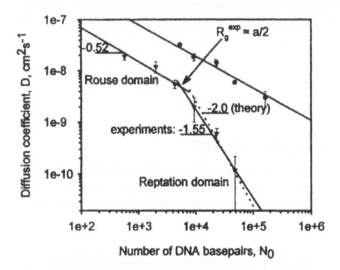

Figure 20.4 DNA diffusion coefficients, D_G, in 2% agarose gels (▼) and the DNA diffusion coefficients, D_0, in solutions (●) as a function of their base-pair number, N_0, in 0.1 M PBS at T = 25 °C. The slope indicated for the diffusion coefficients in gels corresponds to the scaling exponent −0.52, which is in good agreement with Zimm's predictions. The scaling exponent −2.0 is the theoretical scaling exponent given by the theory (Eq. 8), whereas the scaling exponent −1.55 is the result of experimental fit. The value of $R_g = a/2$ corresponds to the theoretical change regime between the Rouse regime and the reptation regime for the DNA in the gels. Reproduced with permission (Pluen *et al.*, 1999).

b is the Kuhn length ($b = 2p$) (de Gennes, 1979). Reptation applies mainly to nucleic acids in the linear configuration. Circular and supercoiled molecules are more rigid and less capable of reptation. Also, they frequently become impaled and trapped on gel fibers.

In 2% agarose gel, the diffusion coefficient of linear DNA is proportional to power functions of N_0 (Figure 20.4), as predicted by Eqs. 7 and 8. However, the experimental data are slightly different from theoretical predictions. The exponents of power functions are −0.52 and −1.55, rather than −0.5 and −2, in Rouse and reptation regimes, respectively (Pluen *et al.*, 1999).

Special considerations for improving interstitial transport of nucleic acids

One of the major concerns in nucleic acid delivery is its degradation in tissues. DNA can be degraded through depurination/β-elimination (Evans *et al.*, 2000; Lindahl, 1993), free radical oxidation (Evans *et al.*, 2000; Imlay and Linn, 1988), or enzymatic pathways (Barry *et al.*, 1999; De Smedt *et al.*, 2000; Mahato, *et al.*, 1997). A single cut in a strand of nucleic acid may cause it to lose its therapeutic effectiveness. A second concern is the heterogeneity and anisotropy of tumor tissue structures. As a result, both systemic and local deliveries of nucleic acids in tumors are likely to be anisotropic and heterogeneous. A third concern is the non-specific binding of highly negatively charged nucleic acids to positively charged extracellular matrix, which will reduce their transport in tissues as discussed above. The reduction is correlated with and sensitive to the length of nucleic acids. Finally, the pore size in tissues can be smaller than that in agarose gels. The average pore radius, a, in agarose gels depends on the concentration of agarose, ϕ, (Serwer and Hayes, 1986),

$$a \approx 118\phi^{-0.74} \tag{9}$$

When $\phi = 1\%$, $a = 118\,\text{nm}$, which is close to the size of plasmid DNA. In some tumor tissues, the interfiber distance of fibrillar collagen is only 20–42 nm for aligned fibrils and 75–130 nm for poorly organized fibrils (Pluen *et al.*, 2001). The space between collagen fibers is often occupied by cells and other extracellular matrix molecules (e.g., proteoglycans and glycosaminoglycans). Thus, the pore size in tissues can be much smaller than that in agarose gels, which makes both diffusion and convection sensitive to the size of pores, as discussed above. As a result, transport of nucleic acids in tissues is likely to be more difficult than that in gels. The transport problem may be reduced through treatments of tumor tissues with matrix enzymes, hyperosmotic solutions, and/or apoptotic agents that may temporarily increase the size and the connectedness of pores.

CONCLUDING REMARKS

Interstitial transport is a critical obstacle in nucleic acid-based therapies. The challenge is how to distribute nucleic acids uniformly and adequately within solid tumors. A complex set of mechanisms are involved in distributing large therapeutic agents in solid tumors. These mechanisms include convection, diffusion, and binding interactions, which are dependent on methods of administration, properties of therapeutic agents, and structures of tissues. Quantitative analyses of these mechanisms have been performed for many macromolecules and nanoparticles but not nucleic acids. Advanced imaging techniques, such as pulsed field-gradient NMR (Lapham *et al.*, 1997) and intravital microscopy techniques (Jain, 1997; Jain *et al.*, 1997), are now available for accurate measurement of transport parameters in tumor tissues. Once these data are obtained, interstitial transport of nucleic acids can be improved through developments of optimal administration methods, better nucleic acid carriers, and novel chemical and physical intervention techniques. Until this happens, nucleic acid-based therapies cannot reach their full potential.

ACKNOWLEDGMENTS

This work is supported in part by grants from the Whitaker Foundation and the National Science Foundation. S.M. is supported by a predoctoral fellowship from the Whitaker Foundation. D.Z. is supported by a predoctoral training grant from the National Institutes of Health.

REFERENCES

Aukland, K. (1991) Distribution volumes and macromolecular mobility in rat tail tendon interstitium. *Am. J. Physiol.*, **260**, H409–H419.

Baldwin, A.L. and Wilson, L.M. (1993) Endothelium increases medial hydraulic conductance of aorta, possibly by release of EDRF. *Am. J. Physiol.*, **264**, H26–H32.

Barr, L. and Malvin, R.L. (1965) Estimation of extracellular spaces of smooth muscle using different-sized molecules. *Am. J. Physiol.*, **208**, 1042–1045.

Barry, M.E., Pinto-Gonzalez, D., Orson, F.M., McKenzie, G.J., Petry, G.R. and Barry, M.A. (1999) Role of endogenous endonucleases and tissue site in transfection and CpG-mediated immune activation after naked DNA injection. *Hum. Gene Ther.*, **10**, 2461–2480.

Barry, S.I. and Aldis, G.K. (1992) Flow-induced deformation from pressurized cavities in absorbing porous tissues. *Bull. Math. Biol.*, **54**, 977–997.

Bentley, T.B. and Pittman, R.N. (1997) Influence of temperature on oxygen diffusion in hamster retractor muscle. *Am. J. Physiol.*, **272**, H1106–H1112.

Berk, D.A., Yuan, F., Leunig, M. and Jain, R.K. (1997) Direct *in vivo* measurement of targeted binding in a human tumor xenograft. *Proc. Natl. Acad. Sci. USA*, **94**, 1785–1790.

Bert, J.L., Pearce, R.H. and Mathieson, J.M. (1986) Concentration of plasma albumin in its accessible space in postmortem human dermis. *Microvasc. Res.*, **32**, 211–223.

Bobo, R.H., Laske, D.W., Akbasak, A., Morrison, P.F., Dedrick, R.L. and Oldfield, E.H. (1994) Convection-enhanced delivery of macromolecules in the brain. *Proc. Natl. Acad. Sci. USA*, **91**, 2076–2080.

Bos, E.S., Kuijpers, W.H., Meesters-Winters, M., Pham, D.T., de Haan, A.S., van Doornmalen, A.M. *et al.* (1994) *In vitro* evaluation of DNA–DNA hybridization as a two-step approach in radioimmunotherapy of cancer. *Cancer Res.*, **54**, 3479–3486.

Boucher, Y., Brekken, C., Netti, P.A., Baxter, L.T. and Jain, R.K. (1998) Intratumoral infusion of fluid: estimation of hydraulic conductivity and implications for the delivery of therapeutic agents. *Br. J. Cancer*, **78**, 1442–1448.

Butler, T.P., Grantham, F.H. and Gullino, P.M. (1975) Bulk transfer of fluid in the interstitial compartment of mammary tumors. *Cancer Res.*, **35**, 3085–3088.

Chary, S.R. and Jain, R.K. (1989) Direct measurement of interstitial convection and diffusion of albumin in normal and neoplastic tissues by fluorescence photobleaching. *Proc. Natl. Acad. Sci. USA*, **86**, 5385–5389.

Chen, M.Y., Lonser, R.R., Morrison, P.F., Governale, L.S. and Oldfield, E.H. (1999) Variables affecting convection-enhanced delivery to the striatum: a systematic examination of rate of infusion, cannula size, infusate concentration, and tissue-cannula sealing time. *J. Neurosurg.*, **90**, 315–320.

Chesnoy, S. and Huang, L. (2000) Structure and function of lipid–DNA complexes for gene delivery. *Ann. Rev. Biophys. Biomol. Struct.*, **29**, 27–47.

Comper, W.D. and Laurent, T.C. (1978) Physiological function of connective tissue polysaccharides. *Physiol. Rev.*, **58**, 255–315.

Dang, W., Colvin, O.M., Brem, H. and Saltzman, W.M. (1994) Covalent coupling of methotrexate to dextran enhances the penetration of cytotoxicity into a tissue-like matrix. *Cancer Res.*, **54**, 1729–1735.

Daniels, B.S., Hauser, E.B., Deen, W.M. and Hostetter, T.H. (1992) Glomerular basement membrane: *in vitro* studies of water and protein permeability. *Am. J. Physiol.*, **262**, F919–F926.

de Gennes, P.G. (1979) *Scaling Concepts in Polymer Physics*. Cornell University Press, Ithaca.

de Gennes, P.G. (1999) Passive entry of a DNA molecule into a small pore. *Proc. Nat. Acad. Sci. USA*, **96**, 7262–7264.

De Smedt, S.C., Demeester, J. and Hennink, W.E. (2000) Cationic polymer based gene delivery systems. *Pharm. Res.*, **17**, 113–126.

Dillehay, L.E. (1997) Decreasing resistance during fast infusion of a subcutaneous tumor. *Anticancer Res.*, **17**, 461–466.

Doi, M. and Edwards, S.F. (1986) *The Theory of Polymer Dynamics*. Oxford University Press, New York.

Drummond, D.C., Meyer, O., Hong, K., Kirpotin, D.B. and Papahadjopoulos, D. (1999) Optimizing liposomes for delivery of chemotherapeutic agents to solid tumors. *Pharmacol. Rev.*, **51**, 691–743.

El-Kareh, A.W. and Secomb, T.W. (1997) Theoretical models for drug delivery to solid tumors. *Crit. Rev. Biomed. Eng.*, **25**, 503–571.

Evans, R.K., Xu, Z., Bohannon, K.E., Wang, B., Bruner, M.W. and Volkin, D.B. (2000) Evaluation of degradation pathways for plasmid DNA in pharmaceutical formulations via accelerated stability studies. *J. Pharm. Sci.*, **89**, 76–87.

Feldman, A.L. and Libutti, S.K. (2000) Progress in antiangiogenic gene therapy of cancer. *Cancer*, **89**, 1181–1194.

Feuring-Buske, M., Buske, C., Unterhalt, M. and Hiddemann, W. (2000) Recent advances in antigen-targeted therapy in non-Hodgkin's lymphoma. *Ann. Hematol.*, **79**, 167–174.

Folkman, J. (1997) Angiogenesis and angiogenesis inhibition: an overview. *EXS*, **79**, 1–8.

Foon, K.A. (2000) Monoclonal antibody therapies for lymphomas. *Cancer J.*, **6**, 273–278.

Fry, D.L. (1983) Effect of pressure and stirring on *in vitro* aortic transmural ^{125}I-albumin transport. *Am. J. Physiol.*, **245**, H977–H991.

Fry, D.L., Cornhill, J.F., Sharma, H., Pap, J.M. and Mitschelen, J. (1986) Uptake of low density lipoprotein, albumin, and water by de-endothelialized *in vitro* minipig aorta. *Arteriosclerosis*, **6**, 475–490.

Fung, L.K. and Saltzman, W.M. (1997) Polymeric implants for cancer chemotherapy. *Adv. Drug Deliv. Rev.*, **26**, 209–230.

García Molina, J.J., López Martínez, M.C. and García de la Torre, J. (1990) Computer simulation of hydrodynamic properties of semiflexible macromolecules: Randomly broken chains, wormlike chains, and analysis of properties of DNA. *Biopolymers*, **29**, 883–900.

Gerweck, L.E. (1998) Tumor pH: implications for treatment and novel drug design. *Semin. Radiat. Oncol.*, **8**, 176–182.

Griffon-Etienne, G., Boucher, Y., Brekken, C., Suit, H.D. and Jain, R.K. (1999) Taxane-induced apoptosis decompresses blood vessels and lowers interstitial fluid pressure in solid tumors: clinical implications. *Cancer Res.*, **59**, 3776–3782.

Guyton, A.C., Scheel, K. and Murphree, D. (1966) Interstitial fluid pressure. 3. Its effect on resistance to tissue fluid mobility. *Circ. Res.*, **19**, 412–419.

Hall, F.L., Liu, L., Zhu, N.L., Stapfer, M., Anderson, W.F., Beart, R.W. *et al.* (2000) Molecular engineering of matrix-targeted retroviral vectors incorporating a surveillance function inherent in von Willebrand factor. *Hum. Gene Ther.*, **11**, 983–993.

Han, J., Turner, S.W. and Craighead, H.G. (1999) Entropic trapping and escape of long DNA molecules at submicron size constriction. *Phys. Rev. Lett.*, **83**, 1688–1691.

Helmlinger, G., Netti, P.A., Lichtenbeld, H.C., Melder, R.J. and Jain, R.K. (1997) Solid stress inhibits the growth of multicellular tumor spheroids. *Nat. Biotech.*, **15**, 778–783.

Hiemenz, P.C. (1977) *Principles of Colloid and Surface Chemistry*. Marcel Dekker, New York and Basel.

Hobbs, S.K., Monsky, W., Yuan, F., Roberts, W.G., Griffith, L., Torchillin, V.P. *et al.* (1998) Regulation of transport pathways in tumor vessels: Role of tumor type and microenvironment. *Proc. Nat. Acad. Sci. USA*, **95**, 4607–4612.

Huang, Y., Rumschitzki, D., Chien, S. and Weinbaum, S. (1997) A fiber matrix model for the filtration through fenestral pores in a compressible arterial intima. *Am. J. Physiol.*, **272**, H2023–H2039.

Imlay, J.A. and Linn, S. (1988) DNA damage and oxygen radical toxicity. *Science*, **240**, 1302–1308.

Iozzo, R.V. and Cohen, I. (1994) Altered proteoglycan gene expression and the tumor stroma. *EXS*, **70**, 199–214.

Jain, R.K. (1987) Transport of molecules in the tumor interstitium: a review. *Cancer Res.*, **47**, 3039–3051.

Jain, R.K. (1997) Delivery of molecular and cellular medicine to solid tumors. *Microcirculation*, **4**, 1–23.

Jain, R.K., Schlenger, K., Höckel, M. and Yuan, F. (1997) Quantitative angiogenesis assays: Progress and problems. *Nat. Med.*, **3**, 1203–1208.

Johnson, E.M. and Deen, W.M. (1996) Hydraulic permeability of agarose gels. *AIChE*, **42**, 1220–1224.

Juweid, M., Neumann, R., Paik, C., Perez-Bacete, M. J., Sato, J., van Osdol, W. *et al.* (1992) Micropharmacology of monoclonal antibodies in solid tumors: direct experimental evidence for a binding site barrier. *Cancer Res.*, **52**, 5144–5153.

Kaneda, Y. (2000) Virosomes: evolution of the liposome as a targeted drug delivery system. *Adv. Drug Deliv. Rev.*, **43**, 197–205.

Kaufman, E.N. and Jain, R.K. (1992) Effect of bivalent interaction upon apparent antibody affinity: experimental confirmation of theory using fluorescence photobleaching and implications for antibody binding assays. *Cancer Res.*, **52**, 4157–4167.

Klaentschi, K., Brown, J.A., Niblett, P.G., Shore, A.C. and Tooke, J.E. (1998) Pressure–permeability relationships in basement membrane: effects of static and dynamic pressures. *Am. J. Physiol.*, **274**, H1327–H1334.

Kong, G. and Dewhirst, M.W. (1999) Hyperthermia and liposomes. *Int. J. Hyperthermia*, **15**, 345–370.

Kozin, S.V., Shkarin, P. and Gerweck, L.E. (2001) The cell transmembrane pH gradient in tumors enhances cytotoxicity of specific weak acid chemotherapeutics. *Cancer Res.*, **61**, 4740–4743.

Kratz, F., Beyer, U. and Schutte, M.T. (1999) Drug-polymer conjugates containing acid-cleavable bonds. *Crit. Rev. Ther. Drug Carrier Syst.*, **16**, 245–288.

Kreitman, R.J., Wilson, W.H., White, J.D., Stetler-Stevenson, M., Jaffe, E.S., Giardina, S. *et al.* (2000) Phase I trial of recombinant immunotoxin anti-Tac(Fv)-PE38 (LMB-2) in patients with hematologic malignancies. *J. Clin. Oncol.*, **18**, 1622–1636.

Krol, A., Maresca, J., Dewhirst, M.W. and Yuan, F. (1999) Available volume fraction of macromolecules in a fibrosarcoma: Implications for drug delivery. *Cancer Res.*, **59**, 4136–4141.

Kroll, R.A., Pagel, M.A., Muldoon, L.L., Roman-Goldstein, S. and Neuwelt, E.A. (1996) Increasing volume of distribution to the brain with interstitial infusion: dose, rather than convection, might be the most important factor. *Neurosurgery*, **38**, 746–752.

Kuo, C.J., Farnebo, F., Yu, E.Y., Christofferson, R., Swearingen, R.A., Carter, R. *et al.* (2001) Comparative evaluation of the antitumor activity of antiangiogenic proteins delivered by gene transfer. *Proc. Nat. Acad. Sci. USA*, **98**, 4605–4610.

Lai, W.M. and Mow, V.C. (1980) Drag-induced compression of articular cartilage during a permeation experiment. *Biorheology*, **17**, 111–123.

Lang, D. and Coates, P. (1968) Diffusion coefficient of DNA in solution at 'zero' concentration as measured by electron microscopy. *J. Mol. Biol.*, **36**, 137–151.

Langer, R. (1995) 1994 Whitaker Lecture: polymers for drug delivery and tissue engineering. *Ann. Biomed. Eng.*, **23**, 101–111.

Lapham, J., Rife, J.P., Moore, P.B. and Crothers, D.M. (1997) Measurement of diffusion constants for nucleic acids by NMR. *J. Biomol. NMR*, **10**, 255–262.

Laske, D.W., Youle, R.J. and Oldfield, E.H. (1997) Tumor regression with regional distribution of the targeted toxin TF-CRM107 in patients with malignant brain tumors. *Nat. Med.*, **3**, 1362–1368.

Levick, J.R. (1994) An analysis of the interaction between interstitial plasma protein, interstitial flow, and fenestral filtration and its application to synovium. *Microvasc. Res.*, **47**, 90–125.

Lieberman, D.M., Laske, D.W., Morrison, P.F., Bankiewicz, K.S. and Oldfield, E.H. (1995) Convection-enhanced distribution of large molecules in gray matter during interstitial drug infusion. *J. Neurosurg.*, **82**, 1021–1029.

Lindahl, T. (1993) Instability and decay of the primary structure of DNA. *Nature*, **362**, 709–715.

Mahato, R.I., Rolland, A. and Tomlinson, E. (1997) Cationic lipid-based gene delivery systems: pharmaceutical perspectives. *Pharm. Res.*, **14**, 853–859.

Maroudas, A. (1970) Distribution and diffusion of solutes in articular cartilage. *Biophys. J.*, **10**, 365–379.

Maroudas, A. (1976) Transport of solutes through cartilage: permeability to large molecules. *J. Anat.*, **122**, 335–347.

McGuire, S. and Yuan, F. (2001) Quantitative analysis of intratumoral infusion of color molecules. *Am. J. Physiol.*, **281**, H715–H721.

Meyer, F.A. (1983) Macromolecular basis of globular protein exclusion and of swelling pressure in loose connective tissue (umbilical cord). *Biochim. Biophys. Acta.*, **755**, 388–399.

Meyer, F.A., Koblentz, M. and Silberberg, A. (1977) Structural investigation of loose connective tissue by using a series of dextran fractions as non-interacting macromolecular probes. *Biochem. J.*, **161**, 285–291.

Milenic, D.E., Yokota, T., Filpula, D.R., Finkelman, M.A., Dodd, S.W., Wood, J.F. *et al.* (1991) Construction, binding properties, metabolism, and tumor targeting of a single-chain Fv derived from the pancarcinoma monoclonal antibody CC49. *Cancer Res.*, **51**, 6363–6371.

Morrison, P.F., Laske, D.W., Bobo, H., Oldfield, E.H. and Dedrick, R.L. (1994) High-flow microinfusion: tissue penetration and pharmacodynamics. *Am. J. Physiol.*, **266**, R292–R305.

Netti, P.A., Berk, D.A., Swartz, M.A., Grodzinsky, A.J. and Jain, R.K. (2000) Role of extracellular matrix assembly in interstitial transport in solid tumors. *Cancer Res.*, **60**, 2497–2503.

Nishikawa, M. and Hashida, M. (1999) Pharmacokinetics of anticancer drugs, plasmid DNA, and their delivery systems in tissue-isolated perfused tumors. *Adv. Drug Deliv. Rev.*, **40**, 19–37.

Nomura, T., Nakajima, S., Kawabata, K., Yamashita, F., Takakura, Y. and Hashida, M. (1997) Intratumoral pharmacokinetics and *in vivo* gene expression of naked plasmid DNA and its cationic liposome complexes after direct gene transfer. *Cancer Res.*, **57**, 2681–2686.

Nomura, T., Yasuda, K., Yamada, T., Okamoto, S., Mahato, R.I., Watanabe, Y. *et al.* (1998) Gene expression and antitumor effects following direct interferon (IFN)-γ gene transfer with naked plasmid DNA and DC-chol liposome complexes in mice. *Gene Ther.*, **6**, 121–129.

Order, S.E., Siegel, J.A., Principato, R., Zeiger, L.E., Johnson, E., Lang, P. *et al.* (1996) Selective tumor irradiation by infusional brachytherapy in nonresectable pancreatic cancer: a phase I study. *Int. J. Radiat. Oncol. Biol. Phys.*, **36**, 1117–1126.

Parameswaran, S., Brown, L.V., Ibbott, G.S. and Lai-Fook, S.J. (1999) Hydraulic conductivity, albumin reflection and diffusion coefficients of pig mediastinal pleura. *Microvasc. Res.*, **58**, 114–127.

Parker, K.H., Mehta, R.V. and Caro, C.G. (1987) Steady flow in porous, elastically deformable materials. *J. Appl. Mech.*, **54**, 794–800.

Pluen, A., Boucher, Y., Ramanujan, S., McKee, T.D., Gohongi, T., di Tomaso, E. *et al.* (2001) Role of tumor–host interactions in interstitial diffusion of macromolecules: Cranial Verses subcutaneous tumors. *Proc. Natl. Acad. Sci. USA*, **98**, 4628–4633.

Pluen, A., Netti, P.A., Jain, R.K. and Berk, D.A. (1999) Diffusion of macromolecules in agarose gels: comparison of linear and globular configurations. *Biophys. J.*, **77**, 542–552.

Politz, J.C., Browne, E.S., Wolf, D.E. and Pederson, T. (1998) Intranuclear diffusion and hybridization state of oligonucleotides measured by fluorescence correlation spectroscopy in living cells. *Proc. Natl. Acad. Sci. USA*, **95**, 6043–6048.

Potts, R.O., Ford, Jr., N.C. and Fournier, M.J. (1981) Changes in the solution structure of yeast phenylalanine transfer ribonucleic acid associated with aminoacylation and magnesium binding. *Biochemistry*, **20**, 1653–1659.

Prescott, D.M., Charles, H.C., Poulson, J.M., Page, R.L., Thrall, D.E., Vujaskovic, Z. *et al.* (2000) The relationship between intracellular and extracellular pH in spontaneous canine tumors. *Clin. Cancer Res.*, **6**, 2501–2505.

Pucci-Minafra, I., Andriolo, M., Basirico, L., Alessandro, R., Luparello, C., Buccellato, C. *et al.* (1998) Absence of regular alpha2(I) collagen chains in colon carcinoma biopsy fragments. *Carcinogenesis*, **19**, 575–584.

Reed, R.K. and Lepsøe, S. (1989) Interstitial exclusion of albumin in rat dermis and subcutis in over- and dehydration. *Am. J. Physiol.*, **257**, H1819–H1827.

Saga, T., Neumann, R.D., Heya, T., Sato, J., Kinuya, S., Le, N., *et al.* (1995) Targeting cancer micrometastases with monoclonal antibodies: a binding-site barrier. *Proc. Nat. Acad. Sci. USA*, **92**, 8999–9003.

Schneiderman, R., Snir, E., Popper, O., Hiss, J., Stein, H. and Maroudas, A. (1995) Insulin-like growth factor-I and its complexes in normal human articular cartilage: studies of partition and diffusion. *Arch. Biochem. Biophys.*, **324**, 159–172.

Serwer, P. and Hayes, S.J. (1986) Exclusion of spheres by agarose gels during agarose gel electrophoresis: dependence on the sphere's radius and the gel's concentration. *Anal. Biochem.*, **158**, 72–78.

Shea, L.D., Smiley, E., Bonadio, J. and Mooney, D.J. (1999) DNA delivery from polymer matrices for tissue engineering. *Nat. Biotech.*, **17**, 551–554.

Swabb, E.A., Wei, J. and Gullino, P.M. (1974) Diffusion and convection in normal and neoplastic tissues. *Cancer Res.*, **34**, 2814–2822.

Tedgui, A. and Lever, M.J. (1984) Filtration through damaged and undamaged rabbit thoracic aorta. *Am. J. Physiol.*, **247**, H784–H791.

Thurn, A.L. (1982) Effects of endothelial injury on macromolecular transport in the arterial wall. *Ph.D. Thesis*. Columbia University, New York.

Weiner, L.M. (1999) An overview of monoclonal antibody therapy of cancer. *Semin. Oncol.*, **26**(Suppl. 12), 41–50.

Wiig, H., DeCarlo, M., Sibley, L. and Renkin, E.M. (1992) Interstitial exclusion of albumin in rat tissues measured by a continuous infusion method. *Am. J. Physiol.*, **263**, H1222–H1233.

Yuan, F. (1997) Stress is good and bad for tumors. *Nat. Biotech.*, **15**, 722–723.

Yuan, F. (1998) Transvascular drug delivery in solid tumors. *Semin. Rad. Oncol.*, **8**, 164–175.

Yuan, F., Krol, A. and Tong, S. (2001) Available space and extracellular transport of macromolecules: Effects of pore size and connectedness. *Ann. Biomed. Eng.*, **29**, 1150–1158.

Yuan, F., Leunig, M., Huang, S.K., Berk, D.A., Papahadjopoulos, D. and Jain, R.K. (1994) Microvascular permeability and interstitial penetration of sterically stabilized (Stealth) liposomes in a human tumor xenograft. *Cancer Res.*, **54**, 3352–3356.

Zakaria, E.R., Lofthouse, J. and Flessner, M.F. (1997) *In vivo* hydraulic conductivity of muscle: effects of hydrostatic pressure. *Am. J. Physiol.*, **273**, H2774–H2782.

Zhang, X.-Y., Luck, J., Dewhirst, M.W. and Yuan, F. (2000) Interstitial hydraulic conductivity in a fibrosarcoma. *Am. J. Physiol.*, **279**, H2726–H2734.

Znati, C.A. (1995) Transport phenomena in tumors: Effect of radiation. *Ph.D. Thesis*. Carnegie Mellon University, Pittsburgh.

21 Hepatic delivery of nucleic acids using hydrodynamics-based procedure

Dexi Liu and Guisheng Zhang

INTRODUCTION

Nucleic acids therapy using oligonucleotides (oligonucleotide therapy) or full coding sequence with regulatory elements for its expression (gene therapy) is a promising new modality in medical practice. This therapy intends to cure a disease through regulating the level of gene product(s), crucial for causing or maintaining a pathophysiological condition. In general, oligonucleotide therapy is designed to inhibit the synthesis of disease-related proteins, while gene therapy aims at correcting genetic defects by the import of a functional gene into target cells. As nucleic acid drugs are hydrophilic, large in molecular weight, and unable to cross the cell membrane freely, a delivery mechanism is often required for these genetic materials to reach their intracellular targets. Development of a safe and efficient method for nucleic acid delivery has been the focus of many studies in the past few years.

The most commonly used methods for nucleic acid delivery include the use of recombinant virus (Crystal, 1995) or synthetic compounds as a carrier (Felgner, 1990). As viral carriers (also called viral vectors) are often derived from disease causing viruses, there are persistent concerns about their safety, including the possibility of recombination with endogenous viruses, which could potentially mutate into a deleterious and infectious form (Boris-Lawrie and Temin, 1994; Cornetta *et al.*, 1991; Gunter *et al.*, 1993; Temin, 1990). In addition, viral vectors induce immune responses against the intrinsic viral antigen (Hugin *et al.*, 1993; Yang *et al.*, 1994, 1995) and cause side-effects.

Compared to viral vectors, the potential advantages of synthetic carriers (also called non-viral vectors) are apparent. Being synthetic, they could be made safe, non-immunogenic, easy to prepare and cost-effective. DNA delivered by these carriers may not be able to replicate or recombine into infectious forms. Among many reported non-viral carriers, including cationic polymers (Behr *et al.*, 1989; Kukowska-Latallo *et al.*, 1996; Wu and Wu, 1988) and cationic lipids (Felgner, 1990; Lee and Huang, 1997), the most frequently used form is cationic liposomes.

Cationic liposomes are lipid vesicles made of cationic lipids with or without additional neutral lipids. The first cationic lipid, N-2,3-dioleoyloxypropyl trimethyl ammonium chloride, was developed by Felgner and colleagues in 1987. Since then, many new cationic lipids have been synthesized and shown to be active in introducing DNA into target cells (for review see Huang *et al.*, 1999) when formulated into liposome (Felgner, 1990; Lee and Huang, 1997), emulsion or micellar form (Liu *et al.*, 1996a,b). When these lipid particles are mixed with plasmid DNA at an appropriate ratio, the resulting complexes show potent activity in transferring DNA molecules into cells. Although still controversial, the mechanism involved in non-viral carrier-mediated gene transfer into cells is likely through endocytosis (Zelpathi and Szoka, 1996; Plank *et al.*, 1994; Farhood *et al.*, 1995; Wrobel and Collins, 1995).

A broad success of liposome-based DNA delivery into cells *in vitro* has prompted many laboratories to develop a formulation that is effective *in vivo* for systemic DNA delivery. For the same reason, significant efforts have also been made in elucidating mechanisms under which the *in vivo* DNA transfer efficiency is regulated. These efforts have produced many important findings. First, it has been found that the optimal conditions for transfecting the established cell lines *in vitro* are not optimal for systemic transfection *in vivo* (Liu, 1997). Second, the type of cells transfected through a systemic administration of DNA/liposome complexes are largely limited to lung endothelial cells (Liu *et al.*, 1997; Song *et al.*, 1997). Furthermore, our work has shown that formation of DNA/liposome complexes is not essential for systemic DNA transfer into the lung endothelial cells. Sequential injection of free liposomes and plasmid DNA resulted in an identical level of gene expression to that of animals transfected with DNA/liposome complexes (Song *et al.*, 1998b). Our subsequent mechanistic studies revealed that the function of cationic liposomes in transfecting the lung endothelial cells via intravenous administration is to prolong the DNA retention time in the lung (Song *et al.*, 1998a,b; Liu, D. *et al.*, 1999).

The need for a safe and efficient method of DNA delivery has also encouraged pursuit of approaches where a carrier is not used. In contrast to DNA wrapped inside a virus or synthetic carrier, a more common name for the vectorless approaches is gene transfer with naked DNA. The first *in vivo* gene transfer using naked DNA was reported by Wolff and colleagues (1990), who demonstrated that a well detectable level of gene product could be achieved by the direct injection of a reporter gene into the muscle of a mouse. Following this study, similar results have been seen utilizing local regional administration of plasmid DNA into the liver (intrahepatic injection) (Hickman *et al.*, 1994; Budker *et al.*, 1996), melanomas in tumor bearing mice (intratumor injection) (Vile and Hart, 1993; Yang and Huang, 1996), heart (intramuscular injection) (Lin *et al.*, 1990), skin (intradermal injection) (Raz *et al.*, 1994) and thyroid gland (intraglandular injection) (Sikes *et al.*, 1994). Gene expression has also been reported in the lung after intratracheal instillation (Meyer *et al.*, 1995; Tsan *et al.*, 1995). However, these studies also showed that DNA transfer by the approach of intratissue injection is largely restricted to the injection site and has a relatively low efficiency.

To overcome these problems, ourselves (Liu *et al.*, 1999; Zhang *et al.*, 2000) and others (Zhang *et al.*, 1999) have worked on a different strategy with an emphasis on systemic DNA delivery. Under our consideration, DNA molecules are directly injected into the blood circulation, and thus have a better chance of reaching a large number of cells in different tissues. We are particularly interested in DNA delivery into liver cells due to their involvement in numerous metabolic and acquired diseases. The approach we took to ensure a successful DNA transfer into hepatocytes takes advantage of the anatomy of blood circulation, flow dynamics and the structural organization of liver cells. Our recent work (Liu *et al.*, 1999; Zhang *et al.*, 2000), and the work of others (Zhang *et al.*, 1999), has shown that this new technique called hydrodynamics-based DNA delivery (Liu *et al.*, 1999) is efficient for DNA delivery in mice. Results from these studies suggest that alteration of flow dynamics is a new and promising approach for nucleic acid delivery.

OVERCOMING CELLULAR AND BIOCHEMICAL BARRIERS FOR HEPATIC DNA DELIVERY USING HYDRODYNAMICS-BASED PROCEDURE

In animals, blood circulation is maintained by the regular contraction of the heart. Under ordinary conditions, arterial blood is carried by circulation to the capillary beds of different tissues, then merges into the veins and is finally brought back to the heart for a full cycle. Although blood is restrained in blood vessels, blood substances are able to reach parenchyma outside the blood vasculature through pores or fenestrial structures of the liver (Jones, 1982). Substance exchange between blood and hepatocytes takes place at the surface of plasma membrane. While it is known that hydrophobic substances are able to pass through cell membrane via defusion, charged molecules such as nucleic acids are prohibited from free entry into hepatocytes. Thus, the cell membrane has been considered a structural barrier for hepatic delivery of nucleic acids. The second barrier for systemic nucleic acid delivery is biochemical and involves serum nucleases. DNA molecules are readily degraded by various nucleases when intravenously injected. Therefore, cell membrane and nuclease-mediated DNA degradation serve as the major barriers for nucleic acid delivery to hepatocytes.

To overcome these structural and biochemical barriers, we have worked on a new method of DNA delivery based on the principle of hydrodynamics. This method uses a rapid intravenous injection of DNA solution in a volume equivalent to 8–12% of body weight. The rationale for our approach is as follows. Upon the tail vein injection of DNA solution into an animal, the large volume of DNA solution injected in a short period of time causes cardiac congestion, resulting in an accumulation of DNA solution in the inferior vena cava and consequently builds a higher pressure within this venous section. At the same time, DNA molecules injected were prevented from immediate mixing with nucleases in blood, as the large volume of injected DNA solution would push blood away from this venous section. As the liver has a large capillary bed, a more expandable structure and direct connection to inferior vena cava through the hepatic vein, the high pressure in inferior vena cava causes a reflux of DNA solution into the liver, building a hydrostatic pressure in the liver. Although such an increased pressure is not long-lasting, as the heart continues to pump the solution out of inferior vena cava, the extended exposure time of DNA to liver cells with a minimal presence of serum nucleases is sufficient for gene transfer to occur, and thus results in DNA transfer into liver cells.

EFFECT OF VOLUME AND INJECTION SPEED ON DNA DELIVERY TO HEPATOCYTES

The relationship between the efficiency of DNA transfer and injection volume was established in mice using plasmid DNA containing the luciferase gene (pCMV-Luc).

Table 21.1 Volume effect on the level of gene expression in liver*

Injection volume (ml/mouse)	Luciferase protein in liver (pg/mg)
0.5	2 (0.1)
1.0	12,210 (738)
1.3	180,348 (33,516)
1.6	356,706 (175,560)
2.0	327,180 (103,740)

Note
* Mice (18–20 g) were injected with 10 µg of pCMV-Luc plasmid DNA at various volumes of saline in approximately 3–5 seconds. Luciferase protein in the liver were analyzed eight hours post DNA injection according to method described in (Liu *et al.*, 1999). Data represent mean (SD), n=3.

Data summarized in Table 21.1 demonstrate that the level of luciferase gene expression increases with an increase in the volume of injected DNA solution. The maximal level of luciferase protein achieved was approximately 350 ng/mg of extracted protein from the liver. We also demonstrated in a previous study that the volume required for an optimal transfection varies with animal weight (Liu, F. *et al.*, 1999). The volume for a maximal level of gene expression was approximately 1.2 ml, 1.6 ml or 3.0 ml for animals with a body weight of 11–13 g, 18–20 g or 30–33 g, respectively. The estimated volume for an optimal activity in mice is approximately 8–12% of animal weight, which is higher than total blood, estimated to be 7.3% of the body weight in mice (Wu *et al.*, 1981).

Data in Table 21.2 show that gene expression level is dependent on injection speed. As DNA solution was injected through the tail vein, one would predict that a prolonged injection of the same volume of DNA solution into an animal would result in a lower level of transgene expression, because a high pressure is less likely to develop when DNA solution is injected slowly. Results summarized in Table 21.2 confirm such a prediction. Luciferase protein in the liver of animals receiving 1.6 ml DNA solution in five seconds was 130 ng/mg, compared to approximately 0.03 ng/mg when the same amount of plasmid DNA was injected into each mouse over 30 seconds, representing an approximately 4,000-fold decrease in the level of gene expression with about a six-fold increase in injection time.

Table 21.2 Effect of injection time on the level of gene expression*

Injection time (sec)	Luciferase protein in liver (pg/mg)
5	134,398 (25,301)
8	58,281 (56,995)
15	5,682 (7,731)
30	32 (20)

Note
* Mice (18–20 g) were intravenously injected with 10 µg of plasmid DNA in 1.6 ml saline. Mice were sacrificed eight hours after injection and luciferase protein in liver extracts was measured according to procedure in (Liu *et al.*, 1999). Data represent mean (SD), n=3.

TOXICITY EVALUATION ON HYDRODYNAMICS-BASED PROCEDURE

Serum biochemistry methods were used to evaluate the toxic effect of the procedure. The parameters evaluated include concentrations of major ions (Na^+, K^+, Cl^-); major proteins (albumin and total protein); liver-specific enzymes (alkaline phosphatase ALP); aspartate aminotransferase (AST), alanine aminotransferase (ALT) and total bilirubin. Both short- (one day) and long-term (seven days) effects of DNA administration on animal serum biochemistry were examined. With an exception of ALT value on day one, data presented in Table 21.3 show that all of these biochemical parameters were in normal range compared to those of an untreated animal. A transient increase of ALT value to 177 IU/L on day one was seen in animals injected with either saline or saline with DNA, compared to 45 IU/L in untreated animals. It was noted that ALT value fell into a normal range three days after injection. Animals injected with either saline or saline containing plasmid DNA gave an identical pattern of ALT change, suggesting that a transient increase of ALT value was procedure related, not caused by plasmid DNA or gene product. So far, we have performed this transfection procedure on over 500 mice and no procedure-related death has occurred. Different strains of mice tested including CD-1, Balb/c, C57BL/6, and nude mice showed the same level of transfection efficiency using this procedure.

EFFICIENCY OF HYDRODYNAMICS-BASED DNA DELIVERY

Three different types of plasmids containing either luciferase, β-galactosidase or the human α1-antitrypsin (hAAT) gene, were used to evaluate DNA transfer efficiency. Each animal received only one type of plasmid with one reporter gene. Data presented in Figure 21.1 show a significant level of luciferase gene expression in the liver when the amount of plasmid DNA injected was as low as 0.2 µg per mouse. Luciferase level increases by increasing the amounts of DNA injected and reaches the saturation level at approximately 5 µg per mouse. The amount of luciferase protein expressed at a dose of 5 µg per mouse is about 300 ng per mg of extracted protein from the liver, representing 45 µg of luciferase protein per gram of liver.

Table 21.3 Effect of hydrodynamics-based procedure on serum biochemistry

Time after injection (day)	Serum concentration*								
	Na^+ (mM)	K^+ (mM)	Cl^- (mM)	Alb (mg/L)	T.Prot (mg/L)	ALP (U/L)	AST (U/L)	ALT (U/L)	T.Bili (mg/L)
1	145 (1)	6.5 (0.2)	107 (2)	23 (2)	46 (3)	176 (39)	183 (17)	177 (56)	2 (1)
3	ND	ND	ND	ND	ND	ND	ND	58 (14)	ND
7	147 (2)	7.6 (0.4)	107 (1)	26 (2)	52 (3)	201 (32)	164 (29)	46 (9)	4 (1)
Normal mice	144 (1)	7.7 (0.8)	107 (1)	23 (3)	48 (4)	227 (40)	157 (43)	45 (3)	3 (2)

Notes
* Alb: albumin; T.Prot: total protein; ALP: alkaline phosphatase; AST: aspartate aminotrans-ferase; ALT: alanine aminotransferase; T.Bili: total bilirubin; ND: not determined. Data represent mean (SD), n = 5. Taken from (Liu *et al.*, 1999).

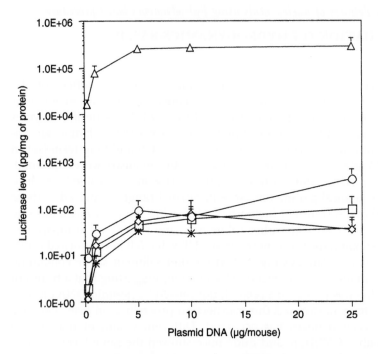

Figure 21.1 DNA dose-dependent gene expression. Various amounts of plasmid DNA (pCMV-Luc) were tail vein injected into mice (18–20 g). The level of luciferase gene expression in liver (△), kidney (○), spleen (▽), lung (□), and heart (*) was measured eight hours post injection. Error bar represents S.E.M. from three animals. Reproduced with permission from Liu *et al.* (1999).

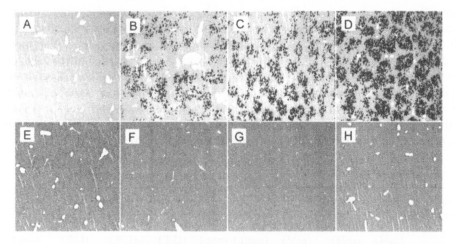

Figure 21.2 Histochemical analysis of β-galactosidase gene expression in liver. Mice were injected with 1.6 ml saline containing various amounts of pCMV-LacZ plasmid DNA. Animals were sacrificed eight hours post injection and liver sections were made using cryostat. Sections (A, B, C and D) were stained with X-gal solution followed by eosin for counter-stain. Sections (E, F, G and H) were stained by a standard hematoxylin/eosin staining method. Sections were made from animals each receiving 0 (A, E), 0.5 (B, F), 2.5 (C, G) and 25 µg (D, H) of pCMV-LacZ. (25x). (*see Color Plate 14*)

Transfection efficiency for mouse liver, with respect to the β-galactosidase gene, was examined using the histochemical method. Compared to control animals injected with saline only (Figure 21.2A), β-gal positive cells were easily seen in liver sections from animals injected with 0.5 µg of pCMV-LacZ plasmid DNA. The density of β-gal positive cells in liver sections increases with increasing doses of administered plasmid DNA. At a DNA dose of 25 µg per mouse, about 40% of cells expressed β-galactosidase (Figure 21.2D). Figures 21.2E, F, G and H are sections stained with hematoxylin/eosin (H&E) designed to identify potential liver damage. No β-gal positive cells were identifiable in other organs, including the lung, heart, kidney and spleen (Zhang *et al.*, 1999). Compared to a normal mouse without injection, no obvious physical damage to the liver at microscopic level was evident in animals injected with either saline (Figure 21.2E) or saline containing different amounts of pCMV-LacZ (Figures 21.2F, G and H).

The pattern of β-galactosidase gene expression was further examined at a higher magnification. Data in Figure 21.3 clearly show that β-gal positive cells are hepatocytes identifiable by their hexagonal shape. The transfected cells are

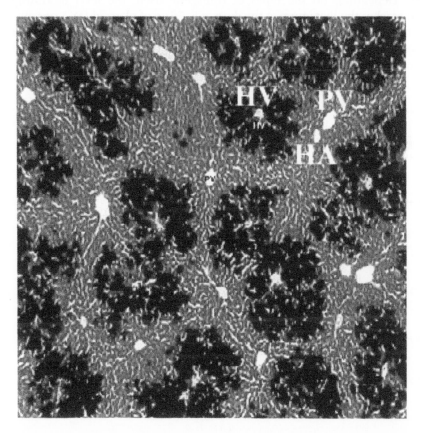

Figure 21.3 Histochemical analysis of β-galactosidase gene expression in liver. Ten µg of pCMV-LacZ plasmid DNA were injected into a mouse via the tail vein using the hydrodynamics-based procedure. β-galactosidase gene expression was assayed eight hours post injection. HV, hepatic vein; HA, hepatic artery; PV, portal vein (50x). (*see Color Plate 15*)

grouped around the hepatic vein and localize at the perivenular region in the cell plate.

Taking advantage of the unique function of the liver in synthesizing many types of proteins found in the circulation, we have also examined the efficiency of this transfection procedure in expressing secretory proteins using human α1-anti-trypsin (hAAT) as a model gene. Mice were injected with pCMV–hAAT plasmid at a dose of 0.05, 0.5, 5, 10, 25 and 50 µg per mouse, respectively, and human α1-antitrypsin concentration in serum was measured one day after the injection. Data presented in Figure 21.4 show that serum levels of human α1-antitrypsin increase with an increase of the amount of DNA injected. The highest level obtained was 200–800 µg/ml of serum in animals injected with 25–50 µg of pCMV–hAAT plasmid DNA. The detection limit of ELISA for hAAT under our experimental condition is 1 ng and the background for normal mouse serum is zero.

These results confirm that both types of genes, encoding either a cellular protein (e.g., luciferase and β-galactosidase) or a secretory protein (human α1-antitrypsin), can be efficiently introduced and expressed in mice by the hydrodynamics-based procedure. Depending on the types of transgene used, the level of transgene expression reaches the maximum at the dose of 5–50 µg of plasmid DNA per mouse. The level of transgene expression obtained by this new procedure is comparable to that of adenovirus at the maximal tolerant dose and is two- to eight-fold higher than that obtained using an adeno-associated virus through systemic administration.

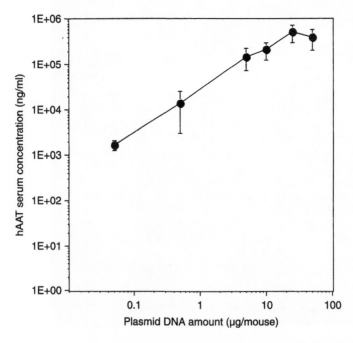

Figure 21.4 DNA dose dependent expression of human α1-antitrypsin gene in mice. Each mouse was transfected with various amounts of plasmid DNA (pCMV-hAAT). The serum concentration of human α1-antitrypsin in mice was determined 24 hours post injection using ELISA. Error bar represents S.E.M. from five mice.

INTRODUCTION AND EXPRESSION OF MULTIPLE GENES BY HYDRODYNAMICS-BASED PROCEDURE

The potential of the hydrodynamics-based procedure for introducing and expressing multiple genes was also examined. In this set of experiments, animals were injected with five different plasmids, each containing one gene encoding either luciferase (pCMV-Luc), β-galactosidase (pCMV-LacZ), mouse interleukin-12 (pCMV-mIL12), human α1 anti-trypsin (pCMV-hAAT) or human coagulation factor IX (pCMV-hFIX). Two of these five transgenes encode cellular protein (luciferase and LacZ) and others encode secretory proteins (hAAT, mIL-12, hFIX). Each animal was injected with 50 µg of plasmid DNA (10 µg for each type of plasmid). Twenty-four hours later, each animal was intravenously injected with 100 units of heparin to prevent coagulation two minutes before animals were killed. The level of gene expression for each reporter gene was analyzed using appropriate assays. Results summarized in Table 21.4 show that a sufficient level of gene product was obtained with respect to each transgene injected. While transgene encoding cellular protein (luciferase and LacZ) expressed in a similar level, the level of gene products from genes encoding secretory protein was significantly different with the highest seen with hAAT followed by IL-12. The lowest level was seen with human factor IX. While additional studies are needed to determine the cause of various product level among the transgenes used, the various protein levels from different transgenes are likely due to their difference in the half-life of their mRNA or/and protein. Additional experiments are ongoing to determine the maximal number of transgenes that one can express at the same time in the same animals.

PERSISTENCE OF GENE EXPRESSION

Time-dependent gene expression was determined for both the luciferase and human α1-antitrypsin gene. Animals were injected with 10 or 50 µg of either

Table 21.4 Level of gene expression by co-transfection of animals with multiple genes*

Plasmid	Reporter gene	Gene expression level
pCMV-Luc	luciferase	103 (18) (ng/mg extracted proteins in liver)
pCMV-LacZ	β-galactosidase	82 (25) (ng/mg extracted protein in liver)
pCMV-mIL12	mouse IL-12	108 (30) (µg/ml of blood)
pCMV-hFIX	human factor IX	23 (6) (µg/ml of blood)
pCMV-hAAT	human α1-antitrypsin	178 (20) (µg/ml of blood)

Notes

* A total of 50 µg of plasmid DNA (10 µg for each plasmid) was injected into each mouse (20–22 g) using the hydrodynamics-base procedure. Twenty-four hours later, animals were intravenously injected with 100 units of heparin/mouse to prevent coagulation two minutes before the animals were killed. Blood samples were collected by orbital puncture and liver was surgically removed from the sacrificed animal. Levels of luciferase and β-galactosidase proteins were analyzed using standard enzymatic luciferase and X-gal assay, respectively. Level of mouse IL-12 in the plasma was analyzed by ELISA using a kit from R&D System. hAAT level was also determined by ELISA (Zhang *et al.*, 2000). ELISA for hFIX was performed with commercially available antibodies. The level of each gene product in animals was calculated based on a standard curve established under the identical experimental conditions using commercially available pure proteins. Data represent mean (SD), n = 6.

pCMV-Luc or pCMV–hAAT plasmid DNA and the levels of transgene expression were measured at appropriate time points. For animals transfected with the luciferase gene, the luciferase level reached the maximum in approximately eight hours post injection and declined thereafter for about 30 days and then persisted at a lower level for more than six months (Figure 21.5A). A similar biphasic decline of gene product level was also observed in animals transfected with hAAT-containing plasmids. Serum level of human α1-antitrypsin dropped approximately 100-fold from day one to day 30 and persisted at a lower level for more than six months. Serum concentration of hAAT, six months post transfection, was approximately 10–50 µg/ml in animals, each of which were injected with 10 or 50 µg of pCMV–hAAT plasmid DNA (Figure 21.5B).

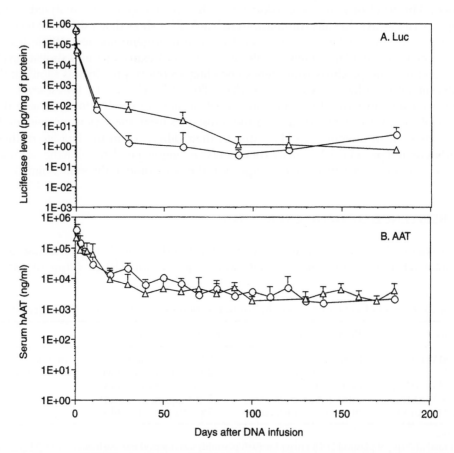

Figure 21.5 Persistence of transgene expression. Animals were injected with 1.6 ml saline containing 10 µg (△) or 50 µg (○) of either pCMV-Luc (A) or pCMV–hAAT (B) plasmid DNA. For luciferase gene expression, animals were sacrificed at various time intervals and luciferase activity in the liver was determined by standard luciferase assay. For human α1-antitrypsin gene expression, blood was collected at appropriate times and serum concentration of human α1-antitrypsin was determined by a standard ELISA. Error bars represent s.e.m. from three mice in A and five mice in B.

GENE FUNCTION ANALYSIS USING
HYDRODYNAMICS-BASED DNA DELIVERY

Considering the fact that the entire DNA sequence of human genome becomes available when the human genome project is completed, functional analysis of these DNA sequences, so called functional genomics, will become a center piece for biomedical research. Toward this end, one of the major applications for this hydrodynamics-based procedure would be for gene function analysis in the whole animal. To provide direct evidence in support of such a notion, we have tested the anti-tumor activity of the mouse interleukin 12 gene (mIL-12) in tumor-bearing mice. Antitumor activity of the mIL-12 gene has been previously demonstrated (Tahara and Lotze, 1995). In our experiments, C57BL6 mice were subcutaneously injected with 5×10^5 B16F1 cells per mouse. Animals were injected with $10\,\mu g$ of pCMV–mIL-12 plasmid DNA on days 7, 12, 19 and 25. Tumor growth was then monitored by the measurement of tumor size for 35 days. As evidenced in Figure 21.6, tumor growth was completely inhibited in treated groups compared to that of animals receiving reporter gene (pCMV-Luc). Four out of five treated animals were tumor free at the end of our experiments. These results validate the notion that hydrodynamics-based transfection is a viable tool for the rapid screening of large number of genes for antitumor activity. Based on the results from our multigene expression experiments described in a previous section, we postulate

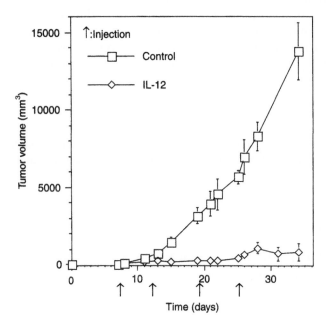

Figure 21.6 Antitumor effect of mouse IL-12 gene expression in tumor-bearing mice. B16F1 cells (5×10^5 cells/mouse) were subcutaneously injected in $100\,\mu l$ into C57BL6 mice. Animals were treated with $10\,\mu g$ of plasmid DNA containing mouse IL-12 (pCMV-mIL-12) or luciferase gene (pCMV-Luc, control) using hydrodynamics-based transfection at days 7, 12, 19 and 25. Tumor growth was monitored by measuring tumor size. Error bars represent S.E.M., n = 5.

that a large number of genes can be screened for anti-tumor activity in tumor bearing mice. For example, assuming that there are 100 genes to be tested, these 100 genes can be divided into 20 groups with five genes in each. The anti-tumor activity of each group of genes will be analyzed by monitoring the tumor growth after injecting gene constructs into tumor-bearing animals. The groups of genes that do not show anti-tumor activity will be identified and discarded. The group(s) of genes that show anti-tumor activity will then go to the second round of testing in the same animal model with fewer genes in each group. The testing cycle can be repeated until the effective gene is identified. The obvious advantage of this strategy is to allow researchers to discard the majority of genes that do not have anti-tumor activity and to identify the effective genes rather quickly. Evidently, a similar strategy can also be used to identify gene(s) or oligonucleotides for a particular biological activity should the functional end point be defined.

CONCLUDING REMARKS

A hydrodynamics-based method is the simplest, most convenient and efficient method developed so far for the hepatic delivery of nucleic acids. Its high efficiency, minimal toxicity, simplicity and ease of use make this technique a valuable tool for many studies that require the transfer of nucleic acids into hepatocytes in whole animals. As far as the transfection efficiency is concerned, the hydrodynamics-based procedure is as efficient as the adenovirus at the maximal tolerant dose in animals and better than that of adeno-associated virus. It is certainly the simplest method for introducing and expressing transgenes in mice. The potential of its application in gene function analysis in whole animals is extraordinary, considering the fact that the function of over 95% of estimated 30,000 genes revealed by the human genome project are yet to be defined. Furthermore, the high level of gene expression achieved by this new technique provides a powerful tool for protein production, which is critical for the success of proteomics and for protein structure studies. Its applications in pharmaceutical analysis of nucleic acids and the delivery of pharmaceutical agents into hepatocytes *in vivo* are also foreseeable.

ACKNOWLEDGMENTS

This work was supported in part by a grant from NIH (CA72925) and a research contract with Targeted Genetics Corporation.

REFERENCES

Behr, J.P., Demeneix, B., Loeffler, J.P. and Mutul, J.P. (1989) Efficient gene transfer into mammalian primary endocrine cells with lipopolyamine-coated DNA. *Proc. Natl. Acad. Sci. USA*, **86**, 6982–6986.
Boris-Lawrie, K. and Temin, H.M. (1994) The retroviral vector: replication cycle and safety considerations for retrovirus-mediated gene therapy. *Ann. N.Y. Acad. Sci.*, **716**, 59–70.

Budker, V., Zhang, G., Knechtle, S. and Wolff, J.A. (1996) Naked DNA delivered intra-portally expresses efficiently in hepatocytes. *Gene Ther.*, **3**, 593–598.

Cornetta, K., Morgan, R.A. and Anderson, W.F. (1991) Safety issues related to retroviral-mediated gene transfer in humans. *Hum. Gene Ther.*, **2**, 5–14.

Crystal, R.G. (1995) Transfer of genes to human: early lessons and obstacles to success. *Science*, **270**, 404–410.

Farhood, H., Serbina, N. and Huang, L. (1995) The role of dioleoylphosphatidylethanol-amine in cationic liposome mediated gene transfer. *Biochim. Biophys. Acta.*, **1235**, 289–295.

Felgner, P.L. (1990) Particulate systems and polymers for *in vitro* and *in vivo* delivery of polynucleotides. *Adv. Drug Deliv. Rev.*, **5**, 163–187.

Felgner, P.L., Gadek, T.R., Holm, M., Roman, R., Chan, H.W., Wenz, M., Northrop, J.P., Ringold, G.M. and Danielsen, M. (1987) Lipofectin: a highly efficient, lipid-mediated DNA-transfection procedure. *Proc. Natl. Acad. Sci. USA*, **84**, 7413–7417.

Gunter, K.C., Khan, A.S. and Noguchi, P.D. (1993) The safety of retroviral vectors. *Hum. Gene Ther.*, **4**, 643–645.

Hickman, M.A., Malone, R.W., Lehmann-Bruinsma, K., Sih, T.R., Knoell, D., Szoka, F.C. *et al.* (1994) Gene expression following direct injection of DNA into liver. *Hum. Gene Ther.*, **5**, 1477–1483.

Huang, L., Hung, M.C. and Wagner, E. (1999) *Nonviral Vectors for Gene Therapy*. Academic Press, New York.

Hugin, A.W., Flexner, C. and Moss, B. (1993) Clearance of recombinant vaccinia virus expressing IL-2: role of host immune response. *Cell. Immunol.*, **153**, 499–509.

Kukowska-Latallo, J.F., Bielinska, A.U., Johnson, J., Spindler, R., Tomalia, D.A. and Baker, Jr., J.R. (1996) Efficient transfer of genetic material into mammalian cells using Starburst polyamidoamine dendrimers. *Proc. Natl. Acad. Sci. USA*, **93**, 4897–4902.

Jones, A.L. (1982) Anatomy of normal liver. In: D. Zakim and T.D. Boyer (eds) *Hepatology: A Textbook of Liver Disease*. WB Sauders Company, Philadelphia, pp. 3–31.

Lee, R.J. and Huang, L. (1997) Lipid vector systems for gene transfer. *Crit. Rev. Ther. Drug Carrier Syst.*, **14**, 173–206.

Lin, H., Pharmacelc, M.S., Morle, G., Bolling, S. and Leiden, J.M. (1990) Expression of recombinant genes in myocardium *in vivo* after direct injection of DNA. *Circulation*, **82**, 2217–2221.

Liu, D. (1997) Cationic liposome-mediated gene delivery via systemic administration. *J. Liposome Res.*, **7**, 187–205.

Liu, D., Knapp, E.J. and Song, Y.K. (1999) Mechanisms of cationic liposome-mediated transfection of the lung endothelium. In: L. Huang, M.C. Hung and E. Wagner (eds) *Non-Viral Vectors for Gene Therapy*. Academic Press, New York, pp. 313–335.

Liu, F., Qi, H., Huang, L. and Liu, D. (1997) Factors controlling efficiency of cationic lipid-mediated transfection *in vivo* via intravenous administration. *Gene Ther.*, **4**, 517–523.

Liu, F., Song, Y.K. and Liu, D. (1999) Hydrodynamics-based transfection in animals by systemic administration of plasmid DNA. *Gene Ther.*, **6**, 1258–1266.

Liu, F., Yang, J.P., Huang, L. and Liu, D. (1996a) Effect of non-ionic surfactants on the formation of DNA/emulsion complexes and emulsion-mediated gene transfer. *Pharm. Res.*, **13**, 1642–1646.

Liu, F., Yang, J.P., Huang, L. and Liu, D. (1996b) New cationic lipid formulations for gene transfer. *Pharm. Res.*, **13**, 1856–1860.

Meyer, K.B., Thompson, M.M., Levy, M.Y., Barron, L.G. and Szoka, F.C. (1995) Intra-tracheal gene delivery to the mouse airway: characterization of plasmid DNA expression and pharmacokinetics. *Gene Ther.*, **2**, 450–460.

Plank, C., Oberhauser, B., Mechtler, K., Koch, C. and Wagner, E. (1994) The influence of endosome-disruptive peptide on gene transfer using synthetic virus-like gene transfer systems. *J. Biol. Chem.*, **269**, 12918–12924.

Raz, E., Carson, D.A., Parker, S.E., Parr, T.B., Abal, A.M., Aicjinger, G. *et al.* (1994) Intradermal gene immunization: the possible role of DNA uptake in the induction of cellular immunity to viruses. *Proc. Natl. Acad. Sci., USA*, **91**, 9519–9523.

Sikes, M.L., O'Malley, B.W., Finegold, M.J. and Ledley, F.D. (1994) *In vivo* gene transfer into rabbit thyroid follicular cells by direct DNA injection. *Hum. Gene Ther.*, **5**, 837–844.

Song, Y.K. and Liu, D. (1998a) Free liposomes enhance the transfection activity of DNA/lipid complexes *in vivo* by intravenous administration. *Biochim. Biophys. Acta.*, **1372**, 141–150.

Song, Y.K., Liu, F., Chu, S.Y. and Liu, D. (1997) Characterization of cationic liposome-mediated gene transfer *in vivo* by intravenous administration. *Hum. Gene Ther.*, **8**, 1585–1594.

Song, Y.K., Liu, F. and Liu, D. (1998b) Enhanced gene expression in mouse lung by prolonging the retention time of intravenously injected plasmid DNA. *Gene Ther.*, **5**, 1531–1537.

Tahara, H. and Lotze, M.T. (1995) Antitumor effects of interleukin-12 (IL-12): applications for the immunotherapy and gene therapy of cancer. *Gene Ther.*, **2**, 96–106.

Temin, H.M. (1990) Safety considerations in somatic gene therapy of human disease with retrovirus vectors. *Hum. Gene Ther.*, **1**, 111–123.

Tsan, M.F., White, J.E. and Shepard, B. (1995) Lung-specific and direct *in vivo* gene transfer with recombinant plasmid DNA. *Am. J. Physiol.*, **268**, L1052–L1056.

Vile, R.G. and Hart, I.R. (1993) Use of tissue-specific expression of the herpes simplex virus thymidine kinase gene to inhibit growth of established murine melanomas following direct intratumoral injection of DNA. *Cancer Res.*, **53**, 3860–3864.

Wolff, J.A., Malone, R.W., Williams, P., Chong, W., Acsadi, G., Jani, A. and Felgner, P.L. (1990) Direct gene transfer into mouse muscle *in vivo*. *Science*, **247**, 1465–1468.

Wrobel, I. and Collins, D. (1995) Fusion of cationic liposomes with mammalian cells occurs after endocytosis. *Biochim. Biophys. Acta.*, **1235**, 296–304.

Wu, M.S., Robbins, J.C., Bugianesi, R.L., Ponpipom, M.M. and Shen, T.Y. (1981) Modified *in vivo* behavior of liposomes containing synthetic glycolipids. *Biochim. Biophys. Acta.*, **674**, 19–26.

Wu, G.Y. and Wu, C.H. (1988) Receptor-mediated gene delivery and expression *in vivo*. *J. Biol. Chem.*, **263**, 14621–14624.

Yang, Y., Nunes, F.A., Berencsi, K., Furth, E.E., Gonczol, E. and Wilson, J.M. (1994) Cellular immunity to viral antigens limits E1-deleted adenoviruses for gene therapy. *Proc. Natl. Acad. Sci. USA*, **91**, 4407–4411.

Yang, Y., Li, Q., Ertl, H.C. and Wilson, J.M. (1995) Cellular and humoral immune responses to viral antigens create barriers to lung-directed gene therapy with recombinant adeno-viruses. *J. Virol.*, **69**, 2004–2015.

Yang, J.P. and Huang, L. (1996) Direct gene transfer to mouse melanoma by intratumor injection of free DNA. *Gene Ther.*, **3**, 542–548.

Zelphati, O. and Szoka, F.C. (1996) Intracellular distribution and mechanism of delivery of oligonucleotides mediated by cationic lipids. *Pharm. Res.*, **13**, 1367–1372.

Zhang, G., Budker, V. and Wolff, J.A. (1999) High levels of foreign gene expression in hepatocytes after tail vein injection of naked plasmid DNA. *Hum. Gene Ther.*, **10**, 1735–1737.

Zhang, G., Song, Y.K. and Liu, D. (2000) Long term expression of human alpha 1-anti-trypsin gene in mouse liver achieved by intravenous administration of plasmid DNA using hydrodynamics-based procedure. *Gene Ther.*, **7**, 1344–1349.

22 Role of CpG motifs in immunostimulation and gene expression

Paul J. Payette, Heather L. Davis and Arthur M. Krieg

INTRODUCTION

Discussions regarding the immune system typically focus on adaptive immune responses, namely the generation of pathogen specific B and T lymphocytes that help rid the body of pathogenic organisms and then protect against subsequent exposure to the same pathogen. These two qualities, antigenic specificity and immunological memory, highlight the evolution of the vertebrate immune system. However, in spite of its evolutionary complexity, the adaptive immune response is considered a second line of defense. The successful induction of adaptive immune responses ultimately relies on the recognition of invading dangers and the activation of innate immune responses. A better understanding of the innate immune system in recent years has revealed its paramount importance in the development of both innate and adaptive immune responses. The recognition of invading pathogens by the innate immune system is mediated in part by a family of receptors known as the pattern recognition receptors (PRRs). These receptors have evolved to recognize the pathogen-associated molecular patterns (PAMP) found in microbial products like lipopolysaccharide (LPS) and bacterial lipoproteins. Activation of these receptors generates signal transduction cascades and subsequent gene expression that leads to the activation of innate immune cells, such as professional antigen presenting cells, which in turn present antigenic information to the adaptive immune system, resulting in the induction of an adaptive immune response.

The first demonstration that bacterial DNA was in fact immunostimulatory came in 1984 when investigators discovered that the anti-tumor activity of the *Mycobacterium bovis* bacillus Calmette-Guerin (BCG) could be isolated to its deoxyribonucleic acid fraction (Tokunaga *et al.*, 1984). Subsequently, in 1991, investigators demonstrated that single stranded DNA (ssDNA) from *E. coli*, but not mammalian DNA, was capable of stimulating murine splenocytes *in vitro* in a dose dependent manner (Messina *et al.*, 1991). This stimulation was blocked following treatment with DNAse but was not affected when using cells from the endotoxin-resistant C3H/HeJ mouse, therefore ruling out a possible role for endotoxin contamination. Further, the elimination of T cell populations did not reduce the extent of splenocyte proliferation, suggesting that the predominant cell type induced to proliferate were B cells. In 1992 investigators discovered that the immunostimulatory properties of bacterial DNA could be reproduced using synthetically derived oligodeoxynucleotides (ODNs). The sequences of these ODNs contained palindromes (e.g., AACGTT) that were thought to be responsible for the immune stimulatory activity (Kataoka *et al.*, 1992; Tokunaga *et al.*, 1992; Yamamoto *et al.*, 1992).

In parallel to these initial descriptions, observations in the antisense field of study revealed that some antisense ODNs displayed sequence-specific immuno-stimulatory properties (Branda *et al.*, 1993; Krieg *et al.*, 1989, 1993; McIntyre *et al.*, 1993; Pisetsky and Reich 1994; Tanaka *et al.*, 1992). Exhaustive study revealed that immunostimulation by these ODNs could be attributed to the presence of CpG dinucleotides, in particular to base contexts (most importantly a hexamer) that were not restricted to a palindrome (Krieg *et al.*, 1995) (Figure 22.1). Further, methylation of the cytosine in the CpG dinucleotide completely abrogated any immunostimulatory properties, confirming that the immuno-stimulatory properties of these ODNs were dependent on the presence of the unmethylated CpG dinucleotides (Krieg *et al.*, 1995). Such immunostimulatory sequences based on unmethylated CpG dinucleotides are now known as CpG motifs.

In prokaryotic organisms, CpG dinucleotides are typically present at the expected random frequency of one in every sixteen pairs of bases along each single strand of DNA. In vertebrate DNA, CpG dinucleotides and CpG motifs are suppressed to one-third or one-quarter of the expected frequency (Bird, 1987). In addition, within mammalian DNA the cytosine residues in CpG dinucleotides are highly methylated (Bird, 1987) which eliminates any immuno-stimulatory properties (Klinman *et al.*, 1996; Krieg *et al.*, 1995). These differ-ences likely reflect an evolutionary divergence that has resulted in one of the many mechanisms by which vertebrates can recognize and respond to invading bacteria.

This chapter reviews the current understanding of how CpG motifs mediate the stimulation of the immune system and what their potential role in therapeutic based strategies might be.

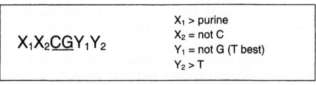

mouse motif GA<u>CG</u>TT, human motif GT<u>CG</u>TT

Figure 22.1 Optimal CpG motifs. The stimulatory effects of a particular sequence of DNA are determined by the base context in which the CpG dinucleotides appear. The most immune stimulatory CpG motifs are preceded by any base except a C, and followed by any base except a G. The positions of two bases further from the CpG are less important, although a purine on the *5'* side and pyrimidines on the *3'* side generally lead to a more immune stimulatory CpG motif. Although there is some cross-stimula-tion, the preferred human and mouse motifs are slightly different, as shown above.

IMMUNE RECOGNITION OF CpG MOTIFS

Cellular stimulation

Both bacterial DNA and synthetic oligodeoxynucleotides (ODNs) containing CpG motifs have been shown to induce or enhance the stimulation of a variety of immune cells (Figure 22.2). This stimulation includes:

(i)   the direct activation of murine and human B cells, resulting in immunoglobulin production, interleukin (IL)-6 and IL-10 secretion, major histocompatability complex (MHC) class II and B-7 upregulation, and resistance to apoptosis (Krieg *et al.*, 1995; Liang *et al.*, 1996; Wang *et al.*, 1997; Yi *et al.*, 1996a,b);

(ii) the direct activation of macrophages and dendritic cells, resulting in cluster designation (CD) 4 T cell independent maturation and subsequent release of chemokines and pro-inflammatory cytokines, including IL-12, upregulation of MHC class II, B7s expression and CD40 expression (Jakob *et al.*, 1998; Sparwasser *et al.*, 1997, 1998; Stacey *et al.*, 1996);

(iii) the activation of natural killer (NK) cells, resulting in the rapid induction of interferon gamma (IFNγ production and lytic capabilities) (Ballas *et al.*, 1996; Cowdery *et al.*, 1996; Yamamoto *et al.*, 1992). These effects appear to be

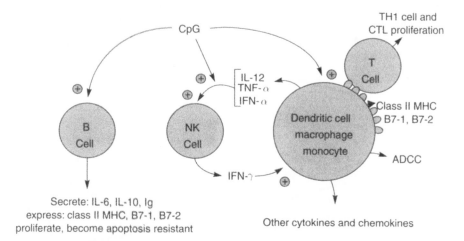

Figure 22.2 Cellular activation by CpG DNA. CpG DNA directly activates dendritic cells (DCs), monocytes and macrophages, to express increased levels of co-stimulatory molecules, to increase antigen presentation, and to secrete high levels of chemokines and cytokines, such as interleukin 12 (IL-12), interferon-α (IFN-α), and tumor necrosis factor-α (TNF-α), and monocytes and macrophages have increased antibody-dependent cellular cytotoxicity (ADCC) activity. NK cells are induced to express IFN-γ by these cytokines acting in concert with CpG, and have increased lytic activity. B cells rapidly produce IL-6 and IL-10 and express increased levels of co-stimulatory molecules. B cells rapidly enter the cell cycle and become resistant to some forms of activation-induced cell death. T cells are not directly activated by CpG, but because of the T helper 1 (Th1)-like cytokine environment, and the increased antigen presenting cell (APC) activity, antigen-specific Th1 cells and cytotoxic T lymphocytes (CTL) are generated.

indirectly mediated by the CpG DNA induced activation of antigen presenting cells (APCs) and the subsequent APC production of IL-12. However,
CpG DNA also has been reported to enhance NK cell IFN-γ production in
response to IL-12 alone (Iho *et al.*, 1999); and

(iv) the indirect influence on the activation of CD4+ and CD8+ T cells by the
CpG DNA mediated activation of APCs to produce cytokines such as type I
IFNs and IL-12, which lead to the development of a pro-Th1 immune
environment (Brunner *et al.*, 2000; Cho *et al.*, 2000; Kranzer *et al.*, 2000;
Lipford *et al.*, 2000; Sun *et al.*, 1998).

Signal transduction

The exact mechanism by which CpG DNA directly stimulates different cell populations is still being determined (Figure 22.3). Results from early investigations
supported a requirement for the internalization of the CpG DNA (Krieg *et al.*,
1995). CpG DNA mediated stimulation could be blocked by inhibitors of endosomal
acidification, suggesting that internalization involved the uptake of CpG DNA into
endosomes, which was subsequently subject to an acidification and maturation cycle
(Macfarlane and Manzel, 1998; Yi *et al.*, 1998; Hacker, 2000). In the absence of an
identifiable surface receptor it was thought that the CpG DNA might be translocated
from the endosomes to the cytoplasm, where it interacted with a putative CpG DNA
specific binding protein, which in turn mediated the intracellular signal cascade
(Krieg, 2000). However, a CpG specific receptor remained elusive.

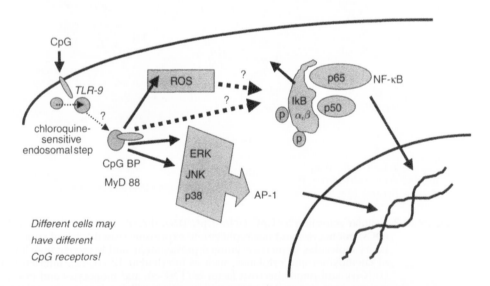

Figure 22.3 Signaling pathways activated by CpG DNA. CpG is thought to enter the
cell via a pH-dependent step that may be receptor mediated. There is a
possible role for the toll like receptor 9 (TLR-9). Once inside the cell, CpG
DNA appears to act, through a number of signal transduction pathways,
including the generation of reactive oxygen species (ROSs), the ubiquitination and degradation of IκB, and activation of the mitogen-activated
protein kinase (MAPK) pathways, which ultimately lead to the induction of
activating protein 1 (AP-1) and nuclear factor kappa B (NF-κB).

One of the earliest measurable events following stimulation with CpG DNA was the generation of reactive oxygen species (ROS) that was dependent upon endosomal acidification (Yi *et al.*, 1996c). It is thought that ROS may have an important role in the regulation of the redox balance in leukocytes. This role, in turn, influences the binding of transcription factors, such as the activation of protein 1 (AP-1), nuclear factor κB (NF-κB), p53 and SP-1, during cellular activation (Bogdan *et al.*, 2000; Krieg, 2000; Muller *et al.*, 1997).

How the signal-transduction cascade progressed from this point to the initiation of gene transcription was not known. At the transcriptional end of the cascade two of the major transcription factors induced by CpG DNA are NF-κB and AP-1 (Hacker, 2000). NF-κB is a key cellular transcription factor that is closely associated with the activation of immune cells of both the innate and acquired arms of the immune system (Ghosh *et al.*, 1998). The activation of the NF-κB is dependent on the phosphorylation, ubiquitination and subsequent degradation of the negative regulator of NF-κB, IκB. The signal transduction cascade induced by CpG DNA includes the activation of NF-κB (Stacey *et al.*, 1996), via the documented degradation of IκB (Yi and Krieg, 1998a).

The CpG induced degradation of IκB following phosphorylation supports the upstream activation of intracellular kinases. One such kinase that has been proposed to mediate this process is DNA dependent protein kinase (DNA-PK), which can phosphorylate p53, leading to increased transcriptional activation of genes involved in cell cycle arrest (Chu *et al.*, 2000). Animals lacking the catalytic subunit of this enzyme fail to respond to CpG DNA (Chu *et al.*, 2000), therefore it has been suggested that DNA-PK is involved in an upstream event that leads to the activation of IκB kinase (IKK) and the subsequent degradation of IκB (Chu *et al.*, 2000). However, DNA-PK activation cannot be solely responsible for mediating activation by CpG DNA, since studies in severe combined immunodeficient (SCID) mice, which lack the DNA-PK catalytic function, reveal highly effective immune stimulation by CpG DNA (Chace *et al.*, 1997).

The second major group of signal transduction pathways that has been identified as being influenced by CpG DNA is the mitogen-activated protein kinase (MAPK) pathways (Yi and Krieg, 1998b; Hacker, 2000). The MAPKs are a group of serine- and threonine-specific kinases that play an important role in mediating responses to extracellular signals (Robinson and Cobb, 1997). The three best-known pathways in this group, identified by the last kinase present in their respective cascades, are the extracellular signal-regulated (ERK)/MAPK pathway, the c-Jun N-terminal kinase (JNK)/stress-activated protein kinase (SAPK) pathway and the p38 pathway (Robinson and Cobb, 1997; Su and Karin, 1996). Each of these pathways has been reported to respond to CpG DNA and collectively lead to the generation and activation of the transcription factor AP-1 and, presumably, to other transcription factors (Hacker, 2000).

What has remained elusive, until recently, is the initiation event that leads to CpG DNA induced signal transduction cascades. Investigators have surmised that cellular activation by CpG DNA is similar to cellular activation following the recognition of PAMP present in other bacterial products, such as LPS and bacterial lipoproteins. Using mice deficient in either the myeloid differentiation marker 88 (MyD88) or the tumor necrosis factor receptor-associated factor 6 (TRAF6), investigators demonstrated that CpG DNA meditated activation was occurring via the Toll-like receptor (TLR)/interleukin 1 receptor (IL-1R) signaling pathway, much like with peptidoglycans and LPS specific activation mediated by TLR-2 and TLR-4, respectively (Hacker *et al.*, 2000; Schnare *et al.*, 2000; Takeuchi *et al.*, 1999).

The mammalian TLRs, so named for their striking homology to the toll receptors found in Drosophila (Medzhitov and Janeway, 2000), belong to the larger family of PRR that play an important role in innate immune activation following the recognition of PAMPs (Medzhitov and Janeway, 2000). Both MyD88 and TRAF6 have been identified as adapter molecules in the TLR/IL-1R pathways (Medzhitov and Janeway, 2000) and the deficiency of MyD88 has a negative effect on LPS mediated activation (Kawai *et al.*, 1999). Based on the documented similarities in signal transduction between CpG DNA and other bacterial products containing PAMPs, it was predicted that CpG DNA specific cell activation might be mediated in a similar fashion. However, knockout mice deficient in either TLR-2 or TLR-4 displayed normal responsiveness to CpG DNA specific activation (Hacker *et al.*, 2000; Schnare *et al.*, 2000). More recently it has been reported that TLR-9 deficient mice were completely unresponsive to CpG DNA, suggesting that TLR-9 may be the elusive CpG DNA specific receptor responsible for the upstream activation of the TLR/IL-1R signal transduction pathway (Hemmi *et al.*, 2000). However, although TLR-9 does possess a transmembrane region, direct associations are not generally observed between other TLRs and their ligands, suggesting that there potentially exists one or more co-factors for TLR-9 that remain to be identified.

It is important to note that the potential role for TLR-9 in immune activation by CpG DNA was elucidated using a single type of CpG motif in a synthetic ODN (Hemmi *et al.*, 2000). Since ODNs of different make-ups, with respect to backbones and sequence motifs, have generated different profiles and kinetics of immune activation (Ballas *et al.*, 1996; Kadowaki *et al.*, 2001; Sester *et al.*, 2000; Verthelyi *et al.*, 2001), TLR-9, like DNA-PK, may only be part of the story.

CpG ODNS AS PROPHYLACTIC AND THERAPEUTIC AGENTS

The immunostimulatory properties of CpG ODNs make them attractive candidates for the modulation of immune responses leading to the prevention and treatment of infectious diseases, atopic disease and malignancies.

Prophylactic vaccines

In a prophylactic setting, many studies have already highlighted the potential usefulness of CpG ODNs. As a vaccine adjuvant, CpG ODNs have been proven superior to other well-known adjuvants at inducing Th1 biased immune responses, including the gold standard, complete Freunds' adjuvant (CFA) (Chu *et al.*, 1997; Davis *et al.*, 1998; Kim *et al.*, 1999; Lipford *et al.*, 1997; Moldoveanu *et al.*, 1998; Roman *et al.*, 1997; Weeratna *et al.*, 2000; Weiner *et al.*, 1997). Interestingly, the immunostimulatory properties traditionally associated with CFA, which result in a Th1 biased response, have since been attributed to the presence of CpG-containing mycobacterial DNA (Chu *et al.*, 1997). Further, unlike other vaccine adjuvants that have worked well in mice but either do not work or are considered too toxic for human use, CpG ODNs have also proven highly effective in higher primates (Davis *et al.*, 2000; Hartmann and Krieg, 2000; Hartmann *et al.*, 2000; Jones *et al.*, 1999). More recently, early results from a phase I clinical trial in humans, where CpG ODN was combined with a hepatitis B virus vaccine, are suggestive that the ability of CpG ODNs to enhance antigen specific immune responses will be maintained in humans (Coley Pharmaceutical Group, unpublished data).

Synthetic CpG ODN has also proven effective as a stand alone agent in the protection from infectious disease. Pre-treatment of mice with CpG ODN alone was effective at inducing protection against subsequent challenge with pathogens such as *Plasmodium yoelli* and *Listeria monocytogenes* (Gramzinski *et al.*, 2001; Krieg *et al.*, 1998). In both of these models, protection was dependent on the CpG mediated induction of IL-12 and IFNγ. Therefore, in the absence of specific antigen, CpG can stimulate the innate immune response in a manner sufficient to mediate sterilizing immunity to the subsequent challenge with certain pathogens. This stimulation highlights tremendous possibilities for CpG ODNs in situations where no effective vaccine exists against pathogens that may be met, or where effective immunization with conventional vaccines is not possible, such as last minute travel, or during times of conflict when there is a threat of bio-warfare with unknown agents.

Therapeutic vaccines

Of course the corollary of preventing infectious disease is the treatment of chronic infection, and this may be where CpG ODN holds the most promise, with respect to infectious disease. There are populations throughout the world that are chronically infected with, and act as biological reservoirs for, intracellular pathogens, such as the hepatitis B and C viruses, the human immunodeficiency virus, *Mycobacterium leprae*, to name but a few. The existence of these populations represents a significant public health concern worldwide. In many cases, the basis for the development of chronic infection centers on the development of an inadequate pathogen specific cellular immune response that is required for the eradication of intracellular pathogens. Although direct evidence remains limited, observations made in the prophylactic setting suggest that the ability of CpG ODN to promote the development of Th1 biased immune response supports its potential as a therapy to overcome chronic infection. When CpG ODN was combined with a current HBV vaccine, the combination demonstrated the capability of overcoming hyporesponsiveness to HBV vaccine alone in at-risk orangutans (Davis *et al.*, 2000). This reaction demonstrates, in a prophylactic setting, that CpG ODN has the potential of altering immune phenotypes that may be predisposed for the development of chronic disease. This potential was further supported by observations made in a model of lethal murine *Leishmaniasis* (Zimmermann *et al.*, 1998). In this model, BALB/c mice succumb to infection by *Leishmania major* due to the generation of a Th2 biased immune response that, unlike a Th1 biased response, is incapable of controlling infection. It was shown that three consecutive doses of CpG ODN as late as 15 or 20 days post infection with *Leishmania major* lead to the control of infection in five of six animals (Zimmermann *et al.*, 1999). These results demonstrate the capability of CpG ODN to redirect immune activation in a situation of ongoing infection.

PREVENTION AND TREATMENT OF ATOPIC DISEASES

Atopy refers to the allergic sensitivity that certain individuals develop towards common and mostly innocuous environmental antigens such as dust mites, plant pollens and animal proteins. The condition of atopy generally manifests itself clinically in the form of asthma, hay fever, eczema or allergic rhinitis. The development of an atopic condition has been associated with the generation of predominately Th2 biased immune response to the particular allergen, and is thus often referred to as a Th2 based disease (Romagnani, 1994).

In recent decades, developed countries have experienced an alarming increase in the incidence of atopic diseases, in particular asthma, an increase that has not been paralleled in developing countries (Cookson and Moffatt, 1997; Seaton *et al.*, 1994). Although the exact reason for this discrepancy remains elusive, evidence suggests that this unparalleled increase in atopy may be related to the steady decline of infectious disease, particularly in early life, in the more developed parts of the world (Erb, 1999). In 1979, a measles epidemic occurred in Guinea-Bissau, West Africa, and children in this region were subsequently evaluated for the development of atopy. It was found that a history of measles infection was associated with a significant reduction in the risk of developing atopy (Shaheen *et al.*, 1996). Similarly, in a cohort of Japanese school children it was found that there was an inverse association between tuberculin responses and atopic disorders, with a positive response to a tuberculin test predicting a lower incidence of atopic disease. It is thought that the reduction in the development of childhood infections has resulted in populations that are more prone to developing atopy, possibly due to immune responses remaining skewed towards the Th2 bias of the immature immune system. If this is so, one would predict that the immunomodulating properties of CpG ODN that promote the development of Th1 biased immune responses may have a preventative and/or therapeutic influence on atopic disease. Indeed, such has been shown to be the case. Using different murine models of allergen-induced asthma, investigators have demonstrated that co-administration of CpG ODN with the allergen prevented the development of airway eosinophilia, Th2 cytokine induction, IgE production and bronchial hyperreactivity (Broide *et al.*, 1998; Kline *et al.*, 1998). These data suggest that combining CpG with potential allergens may serve as a protective vaccine against atopy in regions where the risk of developing atopy is deemed significant.

What of the people who have already been sensitized and are atopic? Could CpG technology benefit these individuals? Investigators have demonstrated, again using a murine model of allergic asthma, that treatment of a previously sensitized animal with CpG ODN combined with allergen, or CpG ODN alone, prevented the lung inflammation generally associated with re-exposure to allergen and that this protection lasted up to six weeks (Kline *et al.*, 1998; Sur *et al.*, 1999). Therefore, in combination with specific allergens or as a stand-alone agent, CpG ODN shows promise for the prophylaxis and therapy of atopic disease.

Cancer immunotherapy

The potential of bacterial infection and bacterial by-products to induce tumor regression was first evaluated in the 1890s by Dr. William Coley (Coley, 1893, 1894). His preparations, eventually referred to as Coley's toxins, did result in some tumor regression, but unfortunately they also remained quite toxic. More recently, a 17-year-old individual, suffering from metastatic Ewing's sarcoma, underwent a complete remission with the disappearance of his metastasized lesions following a postoperative bacterial infection. The individual had survived nine years tumor free (Mori *et al.*, 1997). The regression of the tumor following bacterial infection may be in part attributable to bacterial DNA. If so, then it would follow that synthetic CpG ODNs represent potential candidates for immunotherapeutic-based strategies for the treatment of malignancies. Indeed, with a better understanding of the immune system and the potential for immune-based anti-tumor strategies, CpG ODNs are being evaluated in a number of settings for their ability to either mediate tumor regression directly or to enhance other forms of anti-tumor immunotherapy.

CpG ODN as a stand-alone therapy

As a stand-alone therapy, CpG ODNs have the potential to activate a number of immune cells (discussed above) that could play an important role in mediating tumor regression. Direct injections into tumors would activate immune cells in the vicinity of the tumor and result in presentation of tumor antigens to the immune system by dendritic cells and destruction of the tumor by NK cells. Studies in a murine neuroblastoma model and a rat intracranial glioma model reveal that intralesional delivery of CpG ODN resulted in a dramatic decrease in tumor burden (Carpentier *et al.*, 1999, 2000). In both cases, the anti-tumor effect was attributable to immune activation by the CpG ODN. Systemic injection would lead to the activation of NK cells and result in enhanced antitumor activity. Investigations evaluating the effectiveness of antisense therapy to block the effect of the *c-myc* oncogene in a murine B-cell lymphoma transplant model, revealed that the inhibition of tumor growth was more likely the effect of the immunostimulatory properties associated with the ODN than the anti-sense activity (Smith and Wickstrom, 1998). Similar observations have been made for the prevention of tumor growth in a murine B16 melanoma model and a murine EL-4 T-cell lymphoma model following systemic delivery of CpG ODN (Ballas *et al.*, 2001). It is likely that NK cell activation plays a key role in the B16 model, since anti-tumor activity was maintained in SCID mice, which lack functional B and T cells. Therefore, these observations support the potential of CpG ODN in a non-tumor specific therapeutic regime that could stimulate the innate immune system efficiently enough to lead to tumor regression.

CpG ODN in combination with monoclonal antibodies

CpG ODN also holds great promise in combination-based therapies with other current anti-cancer technologies. One of the most exciting advances in the field of cancer therapy has been the development of humanized monoclonal antibodies (mAbs), which allow for the specific recognition of tumor cells by the immune system. The first two such mAbs approved by the FDA, Rituxan and Herceptin, have demonstrated significant clinical benefit and are now in use for the treatment of lymphoma and breast cancer (Maloney *et al.*, 1997; Pegram *et al.*, 1998). Directed towards specific proteins that are either unique to or primarily expressed by the tumor cells, the mAbs act either directly on the tumor cells through receptor modulation and inhibition of proliferation, or as signposts for the immune system mediating the destruction of tumor cells in part by antibody dependent cellular cytotoxicity (ADCC) by immune cells such as macrophage, neutrophils, and NK cells. Since CpG ODNs have demonstrated the ability to activate ADCC activity of immune cells, such as macrophage and NK cells, it follows that the addition of CpG ODNs to mAb therapy would potentiate any anti-tumor activity. In fact, a single dose of CpG ODN dramatically enhanced the anti-tumor response of a monoclonal antibody therapy in the 38C13 model of murine lymphoma (Wooldridge *et al.*, 1997). The potentiation effect of CpG ODN in this model was more dramatic than multiple doses of IL-2. Recently, it has been found that repeated doses of mAb and CpG ODN are capable of eliminating tumor loads 30 times greater than with antibody alone (Warren *et al.*, 2000). Based on these dramatic observations, the combination of CpG ODN with mAb therapy will shortly move into clinical trials.

CpG ODN in combination with chemotherapy and radiotherapy

Despite advances such as mAb therapy, traditional non-specific strategies such as chemotherapy and radiation therapy remain the mainstays of cancer therapy. Based on the immunostimulatory properties of CpG ODN it would be feasible to imagine that combining CpG ODN therapy with both of these traditional forms of cancer therapy would be beneficial. Following chemotherapy and radiation therapy there is usually substantial tumor cell death. Stimulating the immune system in a timely fashion following either chemotherapy or radiation therapy would result in the more efficient processing of potential tumor antigens for the presentation to effector immune cells, providing a situation where the immune system works in concert with the anti-cancer therapy in reducing tumor burden. In addition, the stress that is placed on tumor cells in response to therapy can increase MHC expression, effectively forcing them to reveal themselves on an antigenic level to the immune system, resulting in a more efficient disposal.

Cancer vaccines

As cancer research continues to evolve, more and more tumor antigens are being, and will continue to be, discovered that may have the potential in a vaccine-based strategy to fight cancer (Hodge *et al.*, 1995; Hsu *et al.*, 1997; Maeurer *et al.*, 1996; Pervin *et al.*, 1997). However, at this point the limitation is not necessarily due to the lack of a suitable antigen. Even once a potential antigen is identified, the hurdle becomes how to deliver it so as to induce an immune response that will include cellular immunity. It appears that for a cancer vaccine to be fully effective it must be able to induce both humoral and cellular immunity. Unfortunately, the only adjuvants licensed for human use in most countries at this point, derivatives of aluminum salts, induce a predominantly Th2-biased humoral immune response. This type of response will only be effective in situations where the tumor antigens are actually expressed as surface proteins, and even then, the cellular components necessary to recognize and kill the antibody-tagged cells may be inadequate. Novel experimental adjuvants that demonstrate the ability to induce cellular immune responses in mice are being evaluated, however their level of associated toxicity precludes their use in humans. CpG ODNs, on the other hand, have proven more effective than a variety of these novel adjuvants at inducing cellular immunity to exogenous antigen (Chu *et al.*, 1997; Davis *et al.*, 1998; Kim *et al.*, 1999; Lipford *et al.*, 1997; Moldoveanu *et al.*, 1998; Roman *et al.*, 1997; Weeratna *et al.*, 2000; Weiner *et al.*, 1997) and have demonstrated relatively little toxicity (Weeratna *et al.*, 2000). As for their potential in a cancer vaccine, studies employing an idiotypic mAb from the 38C13 murine lymphoma model as a target antigen revealed that CpG ODN was as effective as CFA at stimulating an antigen specific immune response that protected against a subsequent challenge with a tumor (Weiner *et al.*, 1997). In addition to the effectiveness of CpG ODN, there was less associated toxicity than with CFA. Similar protective effects have also been observed in a murine model of prostate cancer (Lubaroff *et al.*, unpublished data). Therefore, early observations support the effectiveness of CpG ODNs in the setting of cancer therapy and prevention. Based on these promising results, clinical trials have been initiated to evaluate whether the observed benefits of CpG ODN in animals will extend to humans.

Neutralizing CpG motifs and gene therapy

Much of the excitement about CpG DNA technology centers on the ability of CpG DNA to stimulate the immune system. However, another class of CpG motifs has been described which appears to be capable of neutralizing the effect of stimulatory CpG motifs. These neutralizing motifs were first discovered in adenoviral DNA (Krieg *et al.*, 1998). Among the many different serotypes of andenovirus, serotypes two and five are best known for their ability to establish persistent upper respiratory infections. It has been reported that most small DNA viruses and retro-viruses have evolved to suppress the occurrence of CpG dinucleotides in their genomes by 50–94% in an effort to evade immune activation following infection (Karlin *et al.*, 1994). The CpG content in the genomes of adenovirus serotypes two and five was evaluated to determine if there was any evidence of CpG suppression. However, CpG dinucleotide suppression did not appear to be present. What was noticeable was the occurrence of CpG dinucleotides in clusters of direct repeats, or flanked 5′ by a C or 3′ by a G, and which outnumbered stimulatory CpG motifs by 15- to 30-fold. Synthetic ODNs containing these types of motifs displayed the ability to neutralize immune activation by ODNs containing stimulatory CpG motifs *in vitro* and *in vivo*. The potential of neutralizing CpG motifs is highlighted by two closely related, but, in a sense, diametrically opposed fields of study, namely gene therapy and DNA-based immunization.

Gene therapy refers to the delivery of genetic material to cells for the correction or replacement of defective or absent endogenous genes. *In vitro* this is readily achievable using any number of mammalian expression vectors that can be found on the market. However, when the same delivery strategies are used *in vivo* the outcomes are not so promising. To date only limited success has been achieved in rare cases of genetic immune deficiencies (Cavazzana-Calvo *et al.*, 2000). In addition to the plethora of technical hurtles to overcome to ensure efficient gene expression, endogenous expression of foreign gene products ultimately leads to immune activation and eventual elimination of any cells expressing the transfected gene (Davis *et al.*, 1997). Indeed, it was these observations in the early history of gene therapy that spawned the field of DNA vaccines.

The field of DNA vaccines centers on the ability to deliver genetic material, coding, for desired protein antigens in the context of a mammalian expression vector (Donnelly *et al.*, 1997). It was realized that the immunostimulatory properties observed with DNA vaccines, namely the ability to induce a Th1 biased or cell mediated immune response, was attributable in part to the presence of CpG motifs within the plasmid DNA (Klinman *et al.*, 1997). In fact, it was demonstrated that the quality of immune activation by DNA vaccines could be influenced by the deliberate alteration of CpG content (Krieg *et al.*, 1998). Further, with the identification of neutralizing CpG motifs it became possible to remove any neutralizing influence from the DNA vaccine plasmids. The end result was the optimization of DNA vaccine plasmids, with respect to immune activation (Krieg *et al.*, 1998).

Unlike DNA vaccines, the ultimate goal of gene therapy is long-term endogenous expression of foreign proteins in the absence of immune induction. To achieve this expression, it will be necessary to eliminate the effect of stimulatory CpG motifs present in gene therapy vectors, either by removing or otherwise inactivating them, or by immune suppression for a period of time after gene transfer. Unfortunately, they cannot be inactivated simply through methylation of cytosine residues since this leads to a dramatic decrease in the level of gene expression due to the promoter shut down. Another strategy would be the deletion of all stimulatory CpG motifs from the gene therapy vector, however this is not possible since many of the motifs are located in essential portions of the vector that will not tolerate this degree of manipulation.

Since DNA vaccine vectors can be optimized for immune activation through the manipulation of both stimulatory and neutralizing CpG motifs, it follows that it should be possible to optimize gene therapy vectors with respect to minimizing or eliminating immune activation in the same fashion. The strategy would involve the removal of all stimulatory CpG sequences in non-essential parts of the expression vector and to add an optimized number of neutralizing CpG motifs to counteract the effect of any remaining stimulatory CpG motifs present in the essential parts of the expression vector. In summary, the use of neutralizing CpG motifs may show promise in a gene therapy setting by mimicking a natural strategy of minimizing immune activation following *in vivo* transfection of plasmid DNA. Studies to address this strategy are now underway.

CONCLUDING REMARKS

One can easily appreciate at the end of this review the phenomenal advances that have been made in the field of CpG DNA research in a short period of time. The ability to harness the power of the immune system for the prevention and treatment of human disease has been a priority of medical science since the concept of immunity was first identified. Along the way there have been exciting discoveries, such as the identification and reproduction of potent cytokines, and disappointing revelations, such as the limited effectiveness of these recombinant cytokines in the face of significantly toxic effects. CpG DNA offers an attractive alternative to medical science. Coming back to the natural stimulatory effect of bacterial DNA, CpG DNA offers the ability to stimulate the immune response to respond with a wide range of effector functions that work together in concert and lead to more effective and less toxic outcomes. From the point of gene therapy, the use of neutralizing CpG DNA to bypass immune activation following the delivery of gene therapy vectors might help overcome the inadvertent and undesirable immune activation caused by gene therapy vectors.

As outlined in this chapter, the prophylactic and therapeutic potential of CpG DNA has already been well established in a number of animal models. What remains to be confirmed is the extension of these observations in humans.

REFERENCES

Ballas, Z., Krieg, A., Warren, T., Rasmussen, W., Davis, H., Waldschmidt, M. and Weiner, G. (2001) CpG DNA in the treatment of murine malignancy (*submitted*).

Ballas, Z.K., Rasmussen, W.L. and Krieg, A.M. (1996) Induction of NK activity in murine and human cells by CpG motifs in oligodeoxynucleotides and bacterial DNA. *J. Immunol.*, **157**, 1840–1845.

Bird, A. (1987) CpG Islands as gene markers in the vertebrate nucleus. *Trends Genet.*, **3**, 342–347.

Bogdan, C., Rollinghoff, M. and Diefenbach, A. (2000) Reactive oxygen and reactive nitrogen intermediates in innate and specific immunity. *Curr. Opin. Immunol.*, **12**, 64–76.

Branda, R.F., Moore, A.L., Mathews, L., McCormack, J.J. and Zon, G. (1993) Immune stimulation by an antisense oligomer complementary to the rev gene of HIV-1. *Biochem. Pharmacol.*, **45**, 2037–2043.

Broide, D., Schwarze, J., Tighe, H., Gifford, T., Nguyen, M.D., Malek, S. *et al.* (1998) Immunostimulatory DNA sequences inhibit IL-5, eosinophilic inflammation, and airway hyperresponsiveness in mice. *J. Immunol.*, **161**, 7054–7062.

Brunner, C., Seiderer, J., Schlamp, A., Bidlingmaier, M., Eigler, A., Haimerl, W. *et al.* (2000) Enhanced dendritic cell maturation by TNF-alpha or cytidine-phosphate-guanosine DNA drives T cell activation *in vitro* and therapeutic anti-tumor immune responses *in vivo*. *J. Immunol.*, **165**, 6278–6286.

Carpentier, A.F., Chen, L., Maltonti, F. and Delattre, J.Y. (1999) Oligodeoxynucleotides containing CpG motifs can induce rejection of a neuroblastoma in mice. *Cancer Res.*, **59**, 5429–5432.

Carpentier, A.F., Xie, J., Mokhtari, K. and Delattre, J.Y. (2000) Successful treatment of intracranial gliomas in rat by oligodeoxynucleotides containing CpG motifs. *Clin. Cancer Res.*, **6**, 2469–2473.

Cavazzana-Calvo, M., Hacein-Bey, S., de Saint Basile, G., Gross, F., Yvon, E., Nusbaum, P. *et al.* (2000) Gene therapy of human severe combined immunodeficiency (SCID)-X1 disease. *Science*, **288**, 669–672.

Chace, J.H., Hooker, N.A., Mildenstein, K.L., Krieg, A.M. and Cowdery, J.S. (1997) Bacterial DNA-induced NK cell IFN-gamma production is dependent on macrophage secretion of IL-12. *Clin. Immunol. Immunopathol.*, **84**, 185–193.

Cho, H.J., Takabayashi, K., Cheng, P.M., Nguyen, M.D., Corr, M., Tuck, S. and Raz, E. (2000) Immunostimulatory DNA-based vaccines induce cytotoxic lymphocyte activity by a T-helper cell-independent mechanism. *Nat. Biotech.*, **18**, 509–514.

Chu, R.S., Targoni, O.S., Krieg, A.M., Lehmann, P.V. and Harding, C.V. (1997) CpG oligodeoxynucleotides act as adjuvants that switch on T helper 1 (Th1) immunity. *J. Exp. Med.*, **186**, 1623–1631.

Chu, W., Gong, X., Li, Z., Takabayashi, K., Ouyang, H., Chen, Y. *et al.* (2000) DNA-PKcs is required for activation of innate immunity by immunostimulatory DNA. *Cell*, **103**, 909–918.

Coley, W.B. (1893) The treatment of malignant tumors by repeated inoculations of *Erysipelas* with a report of ten original cases. *Am. J. Med. Sci.*, **105**, 487–511.

Coley, W.B. (1894) Treatment of inoperable malignant tumors with the toxins of *Erysipelas* and the bacillus. *Prodigious. Am. J. Med. Sci.*, **108**, 183–121.

Cookson, W.O. and Moffatt, M.F. (1997) Asthma: an epidemic in the absence of infection? *Science*, **275**(5296), 41–42.

Cowdery, J.S., Chace, J.H., Yi, A.K. and Krieg, A.M. (1996) Bacterial DNA induces NK cells to produce IFN-gamma *in vivo* and increases the toxicity of lipopolysaccharides. *J. Immunol.*, **156**, 4570–4575.

Davis, H.L., Millan, C.L. and Watkins, S.C. (1997) Immune-mediated destruction of transfected muscle fibers after direct gene transfer with antigen-expressing plasmid DNA. *Gene Ther.*, **4**, 181–188.

Davis, H.L., Suparto, II, Weeratna, R.R., Jumintarto, Iskandriati, D.D., Chamzah, S.S. *et al.* (2000) CpG DNA overcomes hyporesponsiveness to hepatitis B vaccine in orangutans. *Vaccine*, **18**, 1920–1924.

Davis, H.L., Weeranta, R., Waldschmidt, T.J., Tygrett, L., Schorr, J. and Krieg, A.M. (1998) CpG DNA is a potent enhancer of specific immunity in mice immunized with recombinant hepatitis B surface antigen. *J. Immunol.*, **160**, 870–876.

Donnelly, J.J., Ulmer, J.B., Shiver, J.W. and Liu, M.A. (1997) DNA vaccines. *Annu. Rev. Immunol.*, **15**, 617–648.

Erb, K.J. (1999) Atopic disorders: a default pathway in the absence of infection? *Immunol. Today*, **20**, 317–322.

Ghosh, S., May, M.J. and Kopp, E.B. (1998) NF-kappa B and Rel proteins: evolutionarily conserved mediators of immune responses. *Annu. Rev. Immunol.*, **16**, 225–260.

Gramzinski, R.A., Doolan, D.L., Sedegah, M., Davis, H.L., Krieg, A.M. and Hoffman, S.L. (2001) Interleukin-12- and gamma interferon-dependent protection against malaria conferred by CpG oligodeoxynucleotide in mice. *Infect. Immun.*, **69**, 1643–1649.

Hacker, H. (2000) Signal transduction pathways activated by CpG-DNA. *Curr. Top. Microbiol. Immunol.*, **247**, 77–92.

Hacker, H., Vabulas, R.M., Takeuchi, O., Hoshino, K., Akira, S. and Wagner, H. (2000) Immune cell activation by bacterial CpG-DNA through myeloid differentiation marker 88 and tumor necrosis factor receptor-associated factor (TRAF)6. *J. Exp. Med.*, **192**, 595–600.

Hartmann, G. and Krieg, A.M. (2000) Mechanism and function of a newly identified CpG DNA motif in human primary B cells. *J. Immunol.*, **164**, 944–953.

Hartmann, G., Weeratna, R.D., Ballas, Z.K., Payette, P., Blackwell, S., Suparto, I. *et al.* (2000) Delineation of a CpG phosphorothioate oligodeoxynucleotide for activating primate immune responses *in vitro* and *in vivo*. *J. Immunol.*, **164**, 1617–1624.

Hemmi, H., Takeuchi, O., Kawai, T., Kaisho, T., Sato, S., Sanjo, H. *et al.* (2000) A Toll-like receptor recognizes bacterial DNA. *Nature*, **408**, 740–745.

Hodge, J.W., Schlom, J., Donohue, S.J., Tomaszewski, J.E., Wheeler, C.W., Levine, B.S. *et al.* (1995) A recombinant vaccinia virus expressing human prostate-specific antigen (PSA): safety and immunogenicity in a non-human primate. *Int. J. Cancer*, **63**, 231–237.

Hsu, F.J., Caspar, C.B., Czerwinski, D., Kwak, L.W., Liles, T.M., Syrengelas, A. *et al.* (1997) Tumor-specific idiotype vaccines in the treatment of patients with B-cell lymphoma– long-term results of a clinical trial. *Blood*, **89**, 3129–3135.

Iho, S., Yamamoto, T., Takahashi, T. and Yamamoto, S. (1999) Oligodeoxynucleotides containing palindrome sequences with internal 5'-CpG-3' act directly on human NK and activated T cells to induce IFN-gamma production *in vitro*. *J. Immunol.*, **163**, 3642–3652.

Jakob, T., Walker, P.S., Krieg, A.M., Udey, M.C. and Vogel, J.C. (1998) Activation of cutaneous dendritic cells by CpG-containing oligodeoxynucleotides: a role for dendritic cells in the augmentation of Th1 responses by immunostimulatory DNA. *J. Immunol.*, **161**, 3042–3049.

Jones, T.R., Obaldia III, N., Gramzinski, R.A., Charoenvit, Y., Kolodny, N., Kitov, S. *et al.* (1999) Synthetic oligodeoxynucleotides containing CpG motifs enhance immunogenicity of a peptide malaria vaccine in Aotus monkeys. *Vaccine*, **17**, 3065–3071.

Kadowaki, N., Antonenko, S. and Liu, Y.J. (2001) Distinct CpG DNA and polyinosinic-poly-cytidylic acid double-stranded RNA, respectively, stimulate CD11c- type 2 dendritic cell precursors and CD11c+ dendritic cells to produce type I IFN. *J. Immunol.*, **166**, 2291–2295.

Karlin, S., Doerfler, W. and Cardon, L.R. (1994) Why is CpG suppressed in the genomes of virtually all small eukaryotic viruses but not in those of large eukaryotic viruses? *J. Virol.*, **68**, 2889–2897.

Kataoka, T., Yamamoto, S., Yamamoto, T., Kuramoto, E., Kimura, Y., Yano, O. and Tokunaga, T. (1992) Antitumor activity of synthetic oligonucleotides with sequences from cDNA encoding proteins of Mycobacterium bovis BCG. *Jpn. J. Cancer Res.*, **83**, 244–247.

Kawai, T., Adachi, O., Ogawa, T., Takeda, K. and Akira, S. (1999) Unresponsiveness of MyD88-deficient mice to endotoxin. *Immunity*, **11**, 115–122.

Kim, S.K., Ragupathi, G., Musselli, C., Choi, S.J., Park, Y.S. and Livingston, P.O. (1999) Comparison of the effect of different immunological adjuvants on the antibody and T-cell response to immunization with MUC1-KLH and GD3-KLH conjugate cancer vaccines. *Vaccine*, **18**, 597–603.

Kline, J.N., Waldschmidt, T.J., Businga, T.R., Lemish, J.E., Weinstock, J.V., Thorne, P.S. and Krieg, A.M. (1998) Modulation of airway inflammation by CpG oligodeoxynucleotides in a murine model of asthma. *J. Immunol.*, **160**, 2555–2559.

Klinman, D., Yamshchikov, G. and Ishigatsubo, Y. (1997) *Journal of Immunology*, **158**, 3635–3639

Klinman, D.M., Yi, A.K., Beaucage, S.L., Conover, J. and Krieg, A.M. (1996) CpG motifs present in bacteria DNA rapidly induce lymphocytes to secrete interleukin 6, interleukin 12, and interferon gamma. *Proc. Natl. Acad. Sci. USA*, **93**, 2879–2883.

Kranzer, K., Bauer, M., Lipford, G.B., Heeg, K., Wagner, H. and Lang, R. (2000) CpG-oligodeoxynucleotides enhance T-cell receptor-triggered interferon-gamma production and up-regulation of CD69 via induction of antigen-presenting cell-derived interferon type I and interleukin-12. *Immunology*, **99**, 170–178.

Krieg, A.M. (2000) Signal transduction induced by immunostimulatory CpG DNA. *Springer Semin. Immunopathol.*, **22**, 97–105.

Krieg, A.M., Gause, W.C., Gourley, M.F. and Steinberg, A.D. (1989) A role for endogenous retroviral sequences in the regulation of lymphocyte activation. *J. Immunol.*, **143**, 2448–2451.

Krieg, A.M., Love-Homan, L., Yi, A.K. and Harty, J.T. (1998) CpG DNA induces sustained IL-12 expression *in vivo* and resistance to Listeria monocytogenes challenge. *J. Immunol.*, **161**, 2428–2434.

Krieg, A.M., Tonkinson, J., Matson, S., Zhao, Q., Saxon, M., Zhang, L.M., Bhanja, U., Yakubov, L. and Stein, C.A. (1993) Modification of antisense phosphodiester oligodeoxynucleotides by a 5′ cholesteryl moiety increases cellular association and improves efficacy. *Proc. Natl. Acad. Sci. USA*, **90**, 1048–1052.

Krieg, A.M., Wu, T., Weeratna, R., Efler, S.M., Love-Homan, L., Yang, L., Yi, A.K. *et al.* (1998) Sequence motifs in adenoviral DNA block immune activation by stimulatory CpG motifs. *Proc. Natl. Acad. Sci. USA*, **95**, 12631–12636.

Krieg, A.M., Yi, A.K., Matson, S., Waldschmidt, T.J., Bishop, G.A., Teasdale, R. *et al.* (1995) CpG motifs in bacterial DNA trigger direct B-cell activation. *Nature*, **374**, 546–549.

Liang, H., Nishioka, Y., Reich, C.F., Pisetsky, D.S. and Lipsky, P.E. (1996) Activation of human B cells by phosphorothioate oligodeoxynucleotides. *J. Clin. Invest.*, **98**, 1119–1129.

Lipford, G.B., Bauer, M., Blank, C., Reiter, R., Wagner, H. and Heeg, K. (1997) CpG-containing synthetic oligonucleotides promote B and cytotoxic T cell responses to protein antigen: a new class of vaccine adjuvants. *Eur. J. Immunol.*, **27**, 2340–2344.

Lipford, G.B., Bendigs, S., Heeg, K. and Wagner, H. (2000) Poly-guanosine motifs costimulate antigen-reactive CD8 T cells while bacterial CpG-DNA affect T-cell activation via antigen-presenting cell-derived cytokines. *Immunology*, **101**, 46–52.

Macfarlane, D.E. and Manzel, L. (1998) Antagonism of immunostimulatory CpG-oligodeoxynucleotides by quinacrine, chloroquine, and structurally related compounds. *J. Immunol.*, **160**, 1122–1131.

Maeurer, M.J., Storkus, W.J., Kirkwood, J.M. and Lotze, M.T. (1996) New treatment options for patients with melanoma: review of melanoma-derived T-cell epitope-based peptide vaccines. *Melanoma Res.*, **6**, 11–24.

Maloney, D.G., Grillo-Lopez, A.J., White, C.A., Bodkin, D., Schilder, R.J., Neidhart, J.A. *et al.* (1997) IDEC-C2B8 (Rituximab) anti-CD20 monoclonal antibody therapy in patients with relapsed low-grade non-Hodgkin's lymphoma. *Blood*, **90**, 2188–2195.

McIntyre, K.W., Lombard-Gillooly, K., Perez, J.R., Kunsch, C., Sarmiento, U.M., Larigan, J.D. *et al.* (1993) A sense phosphorothioate oligonucleotide directed to the initiation codon of transcription factor NF-kappa B p65 causes sequence-specific immune stimulation. *Antisense Res. Dev.*, **3**, 309–322.

Medzhitov, R. and Janeway, C. (2000) The toll receptor family and microbial recognition. *Trends Microbiol.*, **8**, 452–456.

Messina, J.P., Gilkeson, G.S. and Pisetsky, D.S. (1991) Stimulation of *in vitro* murine lymphocyte proliferation by bacterial DNA. *J. Immunol.*, **147**, 1759–1764.

Moldoveanu, Z., Love-Homan, L., Huang, W.Q. and Krieg, A.M. (1998) CpG DNA, a novel immune enhancer for systemic and mucosal immunization with influenza virus. *Vaccine*, **16**, 1216–1224.

Mori, Y., Tsuchiya, H., Tsuchida, T., Asada, N., Nojima, T. and Tomita, K. (1997) Disappearance of Ewing's sarcoma following bacterial infection: a case report. *Anticancer Res.*, **17**, 1391–1397.

Muller, J.M., Rupec, R.A. and Baeuerle, P.A. (1997) Study of gene regulation by NF-kappa B and AP-1 in response to reactive oxygen intermediates. *Methods*, **11**, 301–312.

Pegram, M.D., Lipton, A., Hayes, D.F., Weber, B.L., Baselga, J.M., Tripathy, D. *et al.* (1998) Phase II study of receptor-enhanced chemosensitivity using recombinant humanized anti-p185HER2/neu monoclonal antibody plus cisplatin in patients with HER2/neu-overexpressing metastatic breast cancer refractory to chemotherapy treatment. *J. Clin. Oncol.*, **16**, 2659–2671.

Pervin, S., Chakraborty, M., Bhattacharya-Chatterjee, M., Zeytin, H., Foon, K.A. and Chatterjee, S.K. (1997) Induction of antitumor immunity by an anti-idiotype antibody mimicking carcinoembryonic antigen. *Cancer Res.*, **57**, 728–734.

Pisetsky, D.S. and Reich, C.F. (1994) Stimulation of murine lymphocyte proliferation by a phosphorothioate oligonucleotide with antisense activity for herpes simplex virus. *Life Sci.*, **54**, 101–107.

Robinson, M.J. and Cobb, M.H. (1997) Mitogen-activated protein kinase pathways. *Curr. Opin. Cell Biol.*, **9**, 180–186.

Romagnani, S. (1994) Lymphokine production by human T cells in disease states. *Annu. Rev. Immunol.*, **12**, 227–257.

Roman, M., Martin-Orozco, E., Goodman, J.S., Nguyen, M.D., Sato, Y., Ronaghy, A. *et al.* (1997) Immunostimulatory DNA sequences function as T helper-1-promoting adjuvants. *Nat. Med.*, **3**, 849–854.

Schnare, M., Holtdagger, A.C., Takeda, K., Akira, S. and Medzhitov, R. (2000) Recognition of CpG DNA is mediated by signaling pathways dependent on the adaptor protein MyD88. *Curr. Biol.*, **10**, 1139–1142.

Seaton, A., Godden, D.J. and Brown, K. (1994) Increase in asthma: a more toxic environment or a more susceptible population? *Thorax*, **49**, 171–174.

Sester, D.P., Naik, S., Beasley, S.J., Hume, D.A. and Stacey, K.J. (2000) Phosphorothioate backbone modification modulates macrophage activation by CpG DNA. *J. Immunol.*, **165**, 4165–4173.

Shaheen, S.O., Aaby, P., Hall, A.J., Barker, D.J., Heyes, C.B., Shiell, A.W. and Goudiaby, A. (1996) Measles and atopy in Guinea-Bissau. *Lancet*, **347**(9018), 1792–1796.

Smith, J.B. and Wickstrom, E. (1998) Antisense c-myc and immunostimulatory oligonucleotide inhibition of tumorigenesis in a murine B-cell lymphoma transplant model. *J. Natl. Cancer Inst.*, **90**, 1146–1154.

Sparwasser, T., Koch, E.S., Vabulas, R.M., Heeg, K., Lipford, G.B., Ellwart, J.W. and Wagner, H. (1998) Bacterial DNA and immunostimulatory CpG oligonucleotides trigger maturation and activation of murine dendritic cells. *Eur. J. Immunol.*, **28**, 2045–2054.

Sparwasser, T., Miethke, T., Lipford, G., Erdmann, A., Hacker, H., Heeg, K. and Wagner, H. (1997) Macrophages sense pathogens via DNA motifs: induction of tumor necrosis factor-alpha-mediated shock. *Eur. J. Immunol.*, **27**, 1671–1679.

Stacey, K.J., Sweet, M.J. and Hume, D.A. (1996) Macrophages ingest and are activated by bacterial DNA. *J. Immunol.*, **157**, 2116–2122.

Su, B. and Karin, M. (1996) Mitogen-activated protein kinase cascades and regulation of gene expression. *Curr. Opin. Immunol.*, **8**, 402–411.

Sun, S., Zhang, X., Tough, D.F. and Sprent, J. (1998) Type I interferon-mediated stimulation of T cells by CpG DNA. *J. Exp. Med.*, **188**, 2335–2342.

Sur, S., Wild, J.S., Choudhury, B.K., Sur, N., Alam, R. and Klinman, D.M. (1999) Long term prevention of allergic lung inflammation in a mouse model of asthma by CpG oligodeoxynucleotides. *J. Immunol.*, **162**, 6284–6293.

Takeuchi, O., Hoshino, K., Kawai, T., Sanjo, H., Takada, H., Ogawa, T., Takeda, K. and Akira, S. (1999) Differential roles of TLR2 and TLR4 in recognition of gram-negative and gram-positive bacterial cell wall components. *Immunity*, **11**, 443–451.

Tanaka, T., Chu, C.C. and Paul, W.E. (1992) An antisense oligonucleotide complementary to a sequence in I gamma 2b increases gamma 2b germline transcripts, stimulates B cell DNA synthesis, and inhibits immunoglobulin secretion. *J. Exp. Med.*, **175**, 597–607.

Tokunaga, T., Yamamoto, H., Shimada, S., Abe, H., Fukuda, T., Fujisawa, Y. *et al.* (1984) Antitumor activity of deoxyribonucleic acid fraction from Mycobacterium bovis BCG. I. Isolation, physicochemical characterization, and antitumor activity. *J. Natl. Cancer Inst.*, **72**, 955–962.

Tokunaga, T., Yano, O., Kuramoto, E., Kimura, Y., Yamamoto, T., Kataoka, T. and Yamamoto, S. (1992) Synthetic oligonucleotides with particular base sequences from the cDNA encoding proteins of Mycobacterium bovis BCG induce interferons and activate natural killer cells. *Microbiol. Immunol.*, **36**, 55–66.

Verthelyi, D., Ishii, K., Gursel, M., Takeshita, F. and Klinman, D. (2001) Human peripheral blood cells differentially recognize and respond to two distinct CPG motifs. *J. Immunol.*, **166**, 2372–2377.

Wang, Z., Karras, J.G., Colarusso, T.P., Foote, L.C. and Rothstein, T.L. (1997) Unmethylated CpG motifs protect murine B lymphocytes against Fas-mediated apoptosis. *Cell Immunol.*, **180**, 162–167.

Warren, T.L., Dahle, C.E. and Weiner, G.J. (2000) CpG Oligodeoxynucleotides enhance monoclonal antibody therapy of a murine lymphoma. *Clin. Lymphoma*, **1**, 58–61.

Weeratna, R.D., McCluskie, M.J., Xu, Y. and Davis, H.L. (2000) CpG DNA induces stronger immune responses with less toxicity than other adjuvants. *Vaccine*, **18**, 1755–1762.

Weiner, G.J., Liu, H.M., Wooldridge, J.E., Dahle, C.E. and Krieg, A.M. (1997) Immuno-stimulatory oligodeoxynucleotides containing the CpG motif are effective as immune adjuvants in tumor antigen immunization. *Proc. Natl. Acad. Sci. USA*, **94**, 10833–10837.

Wooldridge, J.E., Ballas, Z., Krieg, A.M. and Weiner, G.J. (1997) Immunostimulatory oligodeoxynucleotides containing CpG motifs enhance the efficacy of monoclonal antibody therapy of lymphoma. *Blood*, **89**, 2994–2998.

Yamamoto, S., Yamamoto, T., Kataoka, T., Kuramoto, E., Yano, O. and Tokunaga, T. (1992) Unique palindromic sequences in synthetic oligonucleotides are required to induce IFN and augment IFN-mediated natural killer activity. *J. Immunol.*, **148**, 4072–4076.

Yi, A.K., Chace, J.H., Cowdery, J.S. and Krieg, A.M. (1996a) IFN-gamma promotes IL-6 and IgM secretion in response to CpG motifs in bacterial DNA and oligodeoxynucleotides. *J. Immunol.*, **156**, 558–564.

Yi, A.K., Hornbeck, P., Lafrenz, D.E. and Krieg, A.M. (1996b) CpG DNA rescue of murine B lymphoma cells from anti-IgM-induced growth arrest and programmed cell death is associated with increased expression of c-myc and bcl-xL. *J. Immunol.*, **157**, 4918–4925.

Yi, A.K., Klinman, D.M., Martin, T.L., Matson, S. and Krieg, A.M. (1996c) Rapid immune activation by CpG motifs in bacterial DNA. Systemic induction of IL-6 transcription through an antioxidant-sensitive pathway. *J. Immunol.*, **157**, 5394–5402.

Yi, A.K. and Krieg, A.M. (1998a) CpG DNA rescue from anti-IgM-induced WEHI-231 B lymphoma apoptosis via modulation of I kappa B alpha and I kappa B beta and sustained activation of nuclear factor-kappa B/c-Rel. *J. Immunol.*, **160**, 1240–1245.

Yi, A.K. and Krieg, A.M. (1998b) Rapid induction of mitogen activated protein kinases by immune stimulatory CpG DNA. *J. Immunol.*, **161**, 4493–4497.

Yi, A.K., Tuetken, R., Redford, T., Waldschmidt, M., Kirsch, J. and Krieg, A.M. (1998) CpG motifs in bacterial DNA activate leukocytes through the pH-dependent generation of reactive oxygen species. *J. Immunol.*, **160**, 4755–4761.

Zimmermann, S., Egeter, O., Hausmann, S., Lipford, G.B., Rocken, M., Wagner, H. and Heeg, K. (1998) CpG oligodeoxynucleotides trigger protective and curative Th1 responses in lethal murine leishmaniasis. *J. Immunol.*, **160**, 3627–3630.

23 Local cardiovascular gene therapy

*Mikko P. Turunen, Mikko O. Hiltunen
and Seppo Ylä-Herttuala*

INTRODUCTION

The treatment of cardiovascular disease, such as atherosclerosis, postangioplasty restenosis, postbypass atherosclerosis, peripheral atherosclerotic vascular disease and graft failures is a major challenge in everyday clinical practice (Yla-Herttuala and Martin, 2000). New treatments, such as stenting, have provided new options for clinicians, but the outcome of these treatments still remains somewhat uncertain (Califf, 1995; Oesterle *et al.*, 1998; Yutani *et al.*, 1999). As the incidence of cardiovascular diseases is too high in western societies, new pharmaceutical approaches for the treatment of these disorders are constantly examined. The use of traditional drugs is often accompanied by unwanted side-effects in ectopic tissues. One of the main advantages of gene therapy over traditional pharmaceutical products is the possibility that a single administration of transgene could lead to a long-lasting therapeutic effect in the target tissue without inducing ectopic gene expression. Also, there is a good possibility of controlling gene expression to the target tissues or cells by use of tissue-specific promoters.

Blood vessels are good targets for gene therapy, since they are easily accessible with intravascular catheter-based methods, and gene transfer can be perfomed simultaneously with angioplasty operation or stenting (Isner *et al.*, 1996; Laitinen *et al.*, 2000; Yla-Herttuala and Martin, 2000). Current targets for cardiovascular gene therapy (see Table 23.1) include therapeutic angiogenesis in myocardium (Isner and Takayuki, 1998) and peripheral arteries (Laitinen *et al.*, 1998), prevention of postangioplasty and in-stent restenosis (Isner *et al.*, 1996; Rutanen *et al.*, 2001) and prevention of vein graft atherosclerosis and prosthesis failure (Mann, 1998; Mann *et al.*, 1995, 1997b, 1999).

The route of gene delivery largely determines the biodistribution profiles of vectors in the body (Hiltunen *et al.*, 2000; Mahato *et al.*, 1998; Thierry *et al.*, 1995; Zhu *et al.*, 1993). By optimal delivery methods the dosage of vector can be decreased while still achieving a maximal local effect. Therapeutic genes can be delivered to the target tissues via several routes. Direct injection in the target tissues has been utilized primarily in skeletal muscle and myocardium for gene delivery (Rosengart *et al.*, 1999; Safi *et al.*, 1999; Shyu *et al.*, 1998; Su *et al.*, 2000; Takeshita *et al.*, 1994; Tio *et al.*, 1999; Tsurumi *et al.*, 1996). Intravascular and extravascular delivery routes can also be used during surgical and catheter-mediated interventions (Nabel, 1992, 1995; Nabel *et al.*, 1990; Pakkanen *et al.*, 2000; Rekhter *et al.*, 1998). Figure 23.1 shows the gene delivery routes for treatment of myocardium and coronary heart diseases.

Table 23.1 Clinical gene therapy trials in cardiovascular disease

Disease	Delivery route	Treatment	Vector or protein	Investigator company	Location
Vein-graft stenosis, infrainguinal by-pass surgery	Pressure *ex vivo* delivery	E2F Decoy	Oligonucleotide	Mann, M.J., Dzau, V.J. *et al.*	Multicenter trial, USA
PAD, post PTA-DA restenosis	Hydrogel-coated balloon catheter after angioplasty	VEGF-A	Naked DNA	Isner, J.M. *et al.*	St. Elizabeth's Medical Center, Boston, MA, USA
PAD, post PTA restenosis	Infusion-perfusion catheter after abgioplasty	VEGF-A	Liposome/ Adenovirus	Mäkinen, K., Ylä-Herttuala, S. *et al.*	Kuopio University Central Hospital, Kuopio, Finland
PAD (Severe)	Adventitial delivery with biodegradable reservoir	VEGF-A	Plasmid/ Liposome	Eurogene Ltd	University Central Hospitals of Kuopio, Oulu and Tampere
PAD (Buerger's disease)	Intramuscular injection	VEGF-A	Naked DNA	Isner, J.M. *et al.*	St. Elizabeth's Medical Center, Boston, MA, USA
PAD	Intramuscular injection	VEGF-A	Naked DNA	Baumgartner, I., Isner, J.M. *et al.*	St. Elizabeth's Medical Center, Boston, MA, USA
PAD	Infusion-perfusion catheter after abgioplasty	LacZ	Adenovirus	Laitinen, M., Ylä-Herttuala, S. *et al.*	Kuopio University Central Hospital, Kuopio, Finland
PAD	Intramuscular injection	FGF-1	Plasmid (pCOR)	Aventis	Multicenter trial, USA
PAD	Intramuscular injection	VEGF-C	Naked plasmid	Isner, J.M. *et al.*	Multicenter trial, USA
PAD	Intramuscular injection	FGF-4	Adenovirus	Collateral therapeutics Inc/Schering	Multicenter trial, Europe
Myocardial ischaemia (Severe)	Intramyocardial injection	VEGF-C	Naked DNA	Isner, J.M. *et al.*/ Vascular Genetics Inc	St. Elizabeth's Medical Center, Boston, MA, USA
Myocardial ischaemia (Severe)	Catheter-based myocardial injection	VEGF-C	Naked DNA	Isner, J.M. *et al.*/ Vascular Genetics Inc	St. Elizabeth's Medical Center, Boston, MA, USA
End-stage ischaemic heart disease	Intramyocardial injection via thoracotomy	VEGF-A	Naked DNA	Sylven *et al.*	Huddinge Hospital, Karolinska Institute, Sweden
Coronary heart disease, post-PTCA restenosis	Infusion-perfusion catheter after angioplasty	LacZ/VEGF-A	Liposome/ adenovirus	Laitinen, M., Ylä-Herttuala, S. *et al.*	Kuopio University Central Hospital, Kuopio, Finland
Coronary heart disease (Severe)	Intramyocardial injection via thoracotomy	VEGF-A	Naked DNA	Symes, J.F., Isner, J.M. *et al.*	St. Elizabeth's Medical Center, Boston, MA, USA
Coronary heart disease	Intramyocardial injection during by-pass operation or minithoracotomy	VEGF-A$_{121}$	Adenovirus	Rosengart, T., Crystal, R.G. *et al.*/Gen Vec Inc	Cornell Medical Center, New York, USA

Coronary heart disease	Intracoronary injection	FGF-4	Adenovirus	Engler, R. *et al.*/ Collateral Therapeutics Inc/Berlex	Multicenter trial, USA

Notes
PAD = peripheral arterial disease; PTA = percutaneous transluminal angioplastry; PTCA = DA = directional atherectomy; PTCA = percutaneous transluminal coronary angioplasty.

INTRAVASCULAR DELIVERY

Intravascular gene transfer to arteries can be performed by using various types of catheters. A catheter is introduced into a target artery under fluoroscopical control after angioplasty operation. A basic principle in most catheters is that when the balloon is inflated, gene transfer solution can be infused through another port in the catheter and applied to the luminal surface of the target artery. Several types of commercially available catheters can be used for gene delivery. A double balloon catheter is made of two latex balloons, which, when inflated in a target arterial segment, isolate a transfection chamber of a varying length, into which gene transfer solution can be infused. This catheter was one of the first catheters used for *in vivo* gene transfer (Nabel *et al.*, 1990). Major limitations of this type of catheters are seized blood flow and a leakage through arterial side-branches.

A more advanced catheter is the Dispatch™ catheter, which is an infusion-perfusion balloon catheter that forms a separate compartment adjacent to target vessel wall when the catheter is inflated (Tahlil *et al.*, 1997). A prolonged vector infusion can be performed since blood flows through a central core of the catheter. This system has been successfully used to achieve efficient gene delivery into the endothelium and superficial medial layers of both normal and atherosclerotic rabbit and human arteries (Laitinen *et al.*, 1998). Porous and microporous catheters have also been used for arterial gene delivery. The channeled balloon catheter has 24 longitudinal channels, each containing 100 µm pores, that allows continuous blood flow into peripheral tissues (Hong *et al.*, 1993). Iontophoretic catheters use electroporation to facilitate the uptake of gene transfer solution into the arterial wall. New catheters are continuously being developed for intravascular injections. Among them are an infusasleeve, a transport catheter, a stented porous balloon catheter and a nipple infusion catheter (Bailey, 1997; Gonschior *et al.*, 1995; Marshall *et al.*, 2000; Willard *et al.*, 1994).

The advantage of these intravascular gene delivery methods is that gene transfer can be easily performed during angioplasty, stenting and other intravascular manipulations. Limitations of intravascular gene transfer are the presence of anatomical barriers, such as the internal elastic lamina and atherosclerotic lesions (Feldman *et al.*, 1995; Rome *et al.*, 1994) and the presence of a blood complement system which efficiently inactivates many gene transfer vectors (Plank *et al.*, 1996). Also, tissue damage induced by the gene delivery catheter is a problem that must be taken into account. Tissue injury (such as dissection, subintimal hemorrage, distortion of media) induced by the use of perforated balloon catheter for local gene delivery techniques has been reported (Willard *et al.*, 1994). Tissue injury and

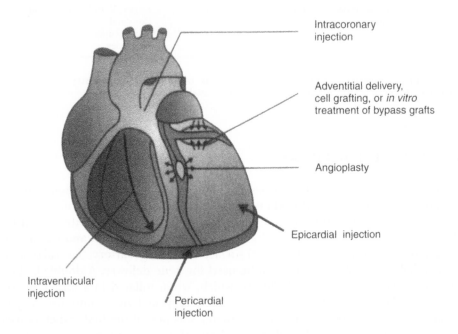

Intracoronary
injection

Adventitial delivery,
cell grafting, or *in vitro*
treatment of bypass grafts

Angioplasty

Epicardial injection

Intraventricular
injection

Pericardial
injection

Figure 23.1 Gene delivery routes for the treatment of myocardium and coronary heart
diseases.

cell loss after exposure to gene transfer solution may be related to lower levels of
transgene expression. Although intracoronary and intravenous delivery may be
preferred for their use to a large patient population, systemic re-circulation and
lack of sustained expression of these therapeutic agents may limit their usefulness
(Hiltunen *et al.*, 2000).

STENTS

Vascular stenting has become a common procedure during percutaneous transluminal angioplasty (PTA) and percutaneous transluminal coronary angioplasty
(PTCA) procedures because it has been found to reduce restenosis (Narins *et al.*,
1998). In both the STRESS (Stent Restenosis Study) and BENESTENT (Belgian
Netherlands Stent Study) trials, intracoronary stent placement reduced angio-
graphic restenosis rates to as low as 13% (Narins *et al.*, 1998; Serruys *et al.*, 1994).
However, local thrombosis and in-stent restenosis are continuing problems, as
long-term follow-up data of the stented patients has indicated (Bailey, 1997;
Caramori *et al.*, 1999). Polymer-coated stents impregnated with plasmid DNA
encoding therapeutic genes or stents covered with genetically engineered endothelial cells can be used for gene delivery (Dichek *et al.*, 1989). Stents can also be used
for local delivery of anticoagulant, thrombolytic or antiproliferative molecules
(Carter *et al.*, 1999; Hardhammar *et al.*, 1996; Serruys *et al.*, 1996). Vascular

endothelial growth factor (VEGF) has been shown to accelerate stent endothelialization, reducing stent thrombosis in rabbit models (Van Belle *et al.*, 1997).

PERIADVENTITIAL DELIVERY

Direct adventitial gene transfer can be used for vascular medicine. When gene transfer vector is administered on adventitial surface of the vessel wall it can stay in close contact with arterial cells for a long time (Laitinen *et al.*, 1997a; Laitinen and Ylä-Herttuala, 1998). Furthermore, with adventitial delivery the endothelium remains anatomically intact, which favours the rapid healing of the arteries after surgery. Also, an intact endothelium is advantegeous for gene delivery as the connective forces from the lumen are largely limited by the hydraulic resistance caused by the endothelium. Adventitial delivery can be used for gene delivery into the arterial wall during bypass operations, prosthesis and anastomosis surgery and endarterectomies. Adventitial gene delivery can be performed with silastic (Airenne *et al.*, 2000), or biodegradable collar (Pakkanen *et al.*, 2000), biodegradable gel (Stephan *et al.*, 1996), or direct injection into adventitia (Rios *et al.*, 1995). The limitation of this technique is that the gene transfer vector (or secreted/diffusible gene product) has to reach target cells, which, in the case of intimal cells, is difficult to accomplish (Laitinen *et al.*, 1997). The risk for systemic leakage of gene delivery vectors via the artery is much lower in the periadventitial than in the intravascular gene delivery. Moreover, positive biodistribution has been shown by PCR and X-gal stainings after both techniques (Hiltunen *et al.*, 2000). When using adventitial gene delivery, the leakage of vector to systemic circulation propably happens through extravascular capillaries, vasa vasorum and lymphatic vessels.

Cationic liposomes DOTMA/DOPE (Lipofectin™) have been used in adventitial gene delivery to rabbit carotid arteries by using silicone collar wrapped around the artery (Laitinen *et al.*, 1997). The gene transfer efficiency was very low (0.05% transfected cells in arterial segment). In pig carotid arteries DOTMA/DOPE liposomes/plasmid complexes have been shown to mediate transfection, but at a five- to seven-fold lower level than with adenoviruses (Pakkanen *et al.*, 2000). In that study, the marker gene expression was detected at seven days time point but was absent at 14 days timepoint. Cationic polymers, such as polyethylenimines and fractured dendrimers, have also been used for adventitial gene delivery to rabbit carotid arteries using silicone collar (Turunen *et al.*, 1999). With these systems the transfection efficiency, *in vitro* and *in vivo*, is largely dependent on the charge ratio of the polymer/plasmid complexes.

VEGFs AS THERAPEUTIC GENES

Vascular endothelial growth factors (VEGFs) are angiogenic growth factors that have significant roles in development, angiogenesis and cancer (Ferrara and Bunting, 1996). The VEGF family consists of several members: VEGFs A, B, C, D, E and placental growth factor. Some VEGFs stimulate endothelial cell proliferation, increase endothelial permeability, regulate vascular tone, act as an endothelial 'survival factor' in retinal vessels, and inhibit apoptosis in endothelial cells by inducing expression of anti-apoptotic genes (Gerber *et al.*, 1998a; Murohara *et al.*, 1998; Stephan and Brock, 1996). In addition to direct angiogenic effects, some VEGFs also induce the release of vasoactive molecules, such as nitric oxide and prostacyclin from vascular endothelium (Laitinen *et al.*, 1997b).

The VEGF-A gene is a distant relative of platelet-derived growth factor (PDGF) (Ferrara and Bunting, 1996). Five VEGF-A isoforms (VEGF121, VEGF145, VEGF165, VEGF189 and VEGF206) are generated through alternative splicing from a single gene that is mapped to 6p21, and they are distinguished by their heparan-sulfate binding properties (Ferrara and Bunting, 1996; Leung *et al.*, 1989; Poltorak *et al.*, 1997). All splice variants are glycosylated and expressed as dimeric proteins. They also possess a secretion signal sequence, but only VEGF121, VEGF145 and VEGF165 are secreted. In addition to mRNA splicing, expression of VEGF-A is regulated by proteolytic processing and hypoxia (Ferrara and Bunting, 1996; Risau, 1997; Plouet *et al.*, 1997). In response to hypoxia the levels of hypoxia-inducible factor-1 elevate and stimulate mRNA synthesis of VEGF-A. In addition, the stability of VEGF-A mRNA increases due to hypoxia. Most of these splice variants bind to two tyrosine-kinase receptors VEGFR-1 (flt-1) and VEGFR-2 (KDR/flk-1), which share 44% homology with each other and are expressed almost exclusively on the endothelial cells. The mitogenic effects of VEGF-A are mediated through VEGFR-2, but not VEGFR-1. Neuropilin-1 and Neuropilin-2 are tyrosine kinase receptors that also bind to VEGF165 (Neufeld *et al.*, 1999). VEGFR-2 mediates the mitogenic effect of VEGF-A by activating signaling pathways, like mitogen-activated protein kinase (MAPK) in endothelial cells. VEGFR-1 lacks this mitogenic capacity and its function in endothelial cells is mainly unknown, although the transduction pathway suggests that activation of VEGFR-1 induces endothelial cell migration. VEGF-A has also been shown to regulate apoptosis of endothelial cells (Gerber *et al.*, 1998b; Gupta *et al.*, 1999; Nor *et al.*, 1999).

Other members of the VEGF family have also been characterized. VEGFR-1 binds to VEGF-B, which share similar mitogenic characteristics as VEGF-A and is able to form heterodimers with VEGF-A (Olofsson *et al.*, 1996, 1998). VEGFR-2 and VEGFR-3 (flt-4) bind to VEGF-C and VEGF-D (Achen *et al.*, 1998). VEGFR-3 differs from other VEGF receptors by its characteristic expression and angiogenic effect in lymphatic vessels (Paavonen *et al.*, 2000). The newest member of the growing VEGF family is a secreted dimer VEGF-E, which has similar functional characteristics as VEGF165, but binds only to VEGFR-2 (Meyer *et al.*, 1999; Ogawa *et al.*, 1998).

A single dose of recombinant VEGF-A protein present in the blood stream or locally in the vessel wall has the capacity to accelerate reendothelization in balloon-injured rat carotid artery (Asahara *et al.*, 1995). Also, recombinant VEGF-C has the capacity to induce angiogenesis *in vivo* (Cao *et al.*, 1998). Injection of VEGF-A expression plasmid in ischemic rabbit hindlimbs and in the adventitial surface of rabbit carotid arteries has been shown to improve the status of the treated vessels (Laitinen *et al.*, 1997b; Tsurumi *et al.*, 1997). Preliminary results from beneficial effects of VEGF165 gene transfer in human peripheral arteries have also been reported (Baumgartner and Isner, 1998).

The effects of VEGFs are at least partially mediated by the enhanced production of NO and prostacyclin (Laitinen *et al.*, 1997b; Zachary, 1998). Furthermore, in addition to endothelial cell proliferation and inhibition of neointima formation, VEGF-A may also lead to neoangiogenesis in ischemic tissues (Baumgartner and Isner, 1998). This neoangiogenesis gives a potential advantage for VEGFs regarding gene therapy of ischemic atherosclerotic diseases.

Although it has been shown that angiogenesis inhibitors can reduce plaque area (Moulton *et al.*, 1999), no evidence of accelerated atherosclerosis has been observed after VEGF-A gene transfer to the vessel wall (Asahara *et al.*, 1996; Laitinen *et al.*, 1997b). In fact, it has been shown that local application of VEGF-A plasmid/liposome complexes in rabbit carotid arteries limits intimal thickening via a mechanism that is at least partially dependent on an increase in NO generation (Laitinen *et al.*, 1997b). Even though intravascular gene transfer efficiency in the artery wall is low, secreted products, such as VEGFs, can be used for therapeutic gene transfer trials. In addition to the ability to produce neovessels in ischemic tissues, VEGF-A can inhibit neointimal proliferation induced by angioplasty. This inhibitory property makes VEGF-A an optimal candidate for gene therapy studies aimed at the prevention of postangioplasty restenosis in ischemic coronary heart disease.

VEGF-A, however, has certain characteristics that may not be protective in the vessel wall. For example, it increases vascular permeability putatively via formation of capillary fenestrations or by opening the trans-cellular gaps. This change in permeability leads to leakage of plasma coagulation factors and other plasma proteins into both the vessel wall and the adventitial compartment. VEGF-A also induces expression of tissue factor, which is a coagulation factor. Together with other proteins in the vessel wall, this tissue factor may provide a scaffold for migrating cells, in addition to its putative mitogenic effect on SMCs (Carmeliet *et al.*, 1996). By inducing the expression of VCAM-1 and ICAM-1 in endothelial cells, VEGF-A may enhance leukocyte adhesion to the endothelium (Melder *et al.*, 1996). It has also been shown that VEGFs are expressed in tumors promoting tumor angiogenesis and that tumor growth can be inhibited with anti-VEGF-A antibodies (Nicosia, 1998; Ferrara and Bunting, 1996). Thus, it is possible that VEGF-A, if released to systemic circulation during gene transfer, may promote tumor growth elsewhere in the body.

CARDIOVASCULAR GENE THERAPY CLINICAL TRIALS

Both viral and non-viral vectors are used in current clinical gene therapy trials (Table 23.1). Succesful gene transfer, shown by marker gene expression, to human atherosclerotic arteries after intravascular catheter-mediated technique using adenovirus has been demonstrated (Laitinen *et al.*, 1998). These patients, who had been programmed for lower limb amputation, volunteered for the phase I clinical trial. This trial was followed by phase II clinical trials with intravascular catheter-mediated gene transfer to patients suffering from chronic leg ischemia and/or coronary heart disease. VEGF has also been shown to cause beneficial clinical effects after high dose intramuscular gene transfer of naked DNA to patients (Baumgartner and Isner, 1998). In spite of the promising results aimed to prevent neointimal hyperplasia with gene therapy in animal experiments, there are still a limited number of published clinical trials that have a beneficial clinical outcome.

CONCLUDING REMARKS

Gene therapy offers new possibilities for the treatment of cardiovascular diseases. This area of research has focused mainly on the treatment of postangioplasty restenosis, in-stent restenosis, and vein graft thickening. First clinical trials have shown that vascular gene transfer to humans is generally safe and well tolerated. Even though the feasibility of current gene transfer vectors to deliver therapeutic genes *in vitro* and *in vivo* has been shown in various cell types and tissues, more efficient and safer gene transfer methods should still be developed.

ACKNOWLEDGMENTS

This study was supported by grants from the Finnish Foundation for Cardiovascular Research, Finnish Academy, Kuopio University Hospital (EVO grant 5130), and the Sigrid Juselius Foundation.

REFERENCES

Achen, M.G., Jeltsch, M., Kukk, E., Makinen, T., Vitali, A., Wilks, A.F. *et al.* (1998) Vascular endothelial growth factor D (VEGF-D) is a ligand for the tyrosine kinases VEGF receptor 2 (Flk1) and VEGF receptor 3 (Flt4). *Proc. Natl. Acad. Sci., USA*, **95**, 548–553.

Airenne, K.J., Hiltunen, M.O., Turunen, M.P., Turunen, A.M., Laitinen, O.H., Kulomaa, M.S. *et al.* (2000) Baculovirus-mediated periadventitial gene transfer to rabbit carotid artery. *Gene Ther.*, **7**, 1499–1504.

Asahara, T., Bauters, C., Zheng, L.P., Takeshita, S., Bunting, S., Ferrara, N. *et al.* (1995) Synergistic effect of vascular endothelial growth factor and basic fibroblast growth factor on angiogenesis *in vivo*. *Circulation*, **92**, II365–II371.

Asahara, T., Chen, D., Tsurumi, Y., Kearney, M., Rossow, S., Passeri, J. *et al.* (1996) Accelerated restitution of endothelial integrity and endothelium-dependent function after phVEGF165 gene transfer. *Circulation*, **94**, 3291–3302.

Bailey, S.R. (1997) Local drug delivery: current applications. *Prog. Cardiovasc. Dis.*, **40**, 183–204.

Baumgartner, I. and Isner, J.M. (1998) Stimulation of peripheral angiogenesis by vascular endothelial growth factor (VEGF). *Vasa.*, **27**, 201–206.

Califf, R.M. (1995) Restenosis: the cost to society. *Am. Heart J.*, **130**, 680–684.

Cao, Y., Linden, P., Farnebo, J., Cao, R., Eriksson, A., Kumar, V. *et al.* (1998) Vascular endothelial growth factor C induces angiogenesis *in vivo*. *Proc. Natl. Acad. Sci. USA*, **95**, 14389–14394.

Caramori, P.R., Lima, V.C., Seidelin, P.H., Newton, G.E., Parker, J.D. and Adelman, A.G. (1999) Long-term endothelial dysfunction after coronary artery stenting. *J. Am. Coll. Cardiol.*, **34**, 1675–1679.

Carmeliet, P., Ferreira, V., Breier, G., Pollefeyt, S., Kieckens, L., Gertsenstein, M. *et al.* (1996) Abnormal blood vessel development and lethality in embryos lacking a single VEGF allele. *Nature*, **380**, 435–439.

Carter, A.J., Scott, D., Bailey, L., Hoopes, T., Jones, R. and Virmani, R. (1999) Dose-response effects of ^{32}P radioactive stents in an atherosclerotic porcine coronary model. *Circulation*, **100**, 1548–1554.

Dichek, D.A., Neville, R.F., Zwiebel, J.A., Freeman, S.M., Leon, M.B. and Anderson, W.F. (1989) Seeding of intravascular stents with genetically engineered endothelial cells. *Circulation*, **80**, 1347–1353.

Feldman, L.J., Steg, P.G., Zheng, L.P., Chen, D., Kearney, M., McGarr, S.E. *et al.* (1995) Low-efficiency of percutaneous adenovirus-mediated arterial gene transfer in the athero-sclerotic rabbit. *J. Clin. Invest.*, **95**, 2662–2671.

Ferrara, N. and Bunting, S. (1996) Vascular endothelial growth factor, a specific regulator of angiogenesis. *Curr. Opin. Nephrol. Hypertens.*, **5**, 35–44.

Gerber, H.P., Dixit, V. and Ferrara, N. (1998a) Vascular endothelial growth factor induces expression of the antiapoptotic proteins Bcl-2 and A1 in vascular endothelial cells. *J. Biol. Chem.*, **273**, 13313–13316.

Gerber, H.P., McMurtrey, A., Kowalski, J., Yan, M., Keyt, B.A., Dixit, V. *et al.* (1998b) Vascular endothelial growth factor regulates endothelial cell survival through the phosphatidylinositol 3'-kinase/Akt signal transduction pathway. Requirement for Flk-1/KDR activation. *J. Biol. Chem.*, **273**, 30336–30343.

Gonschior, P., Pahl, C., Huehns, T.Y., Gerheuser, F., Erdemci, A., Larisch, K. *et al.* (1995) Comparison of local intravascular drug-delivery catheter systems. *Am. Heart J.*, **130**, 1174–1181.

Gupta, K., Kshirsagar, S., Li, W., Gui, L., Ramakrishnan, S., Gupta, P. *et al.* (1999) VEGF prevents apoptosis of human microvascular endothelial cells via opposing effects on MAPK/ERK and SAPK/JNK signaling. *Exp. Cell Res.*, **247**, 495–504.

Hardhammar, P.A., van Beusekom, H.M., Emanuelsson, H.U., Hofma, S.H., Albertsson, P.A., Verdouw, P.D. *et al.* (1996) Reduction in thrombotic events with heparin-coated Palmaz-Schatz stents in normal porcine coronary arteries. *Circulation*, **93**, 423–430.

Hiltunen, M.O., Turunen, M.P., Turunen, A.M., Rissanen, T.T., Laitinen, M., Kosma, V.M. *et al.* (2000) Biodistribution of adenoviral vector to non-target tissues after local *in vivo* gene transfer to arterial wall using intravascular and periadventitial gene delivery methods. *FASEB J.*, **14**, 2230–2236.

Hong, M.K., Wong, S.C., Farb, A., Mehlman, M.D., Virmani, R., Barry, J.J. *et al.* (1993) Feasibility and drug delivery efficiency of a new balloon angioplasty catheter capable of performing simultaneous local drug delivery. *Coron. Artery. Dis.*, **4**, 1023–1027.

Isner, J.M., Pieczek, A., Schainfeld, R., Blair, R., Haley, L., Asahara, T. *et al.* (1996) Clinical evidence of angiogenesis after arterial gene transfer of phVEGF165 in patient with ischaemic limb. *Lancet*, **348**, 370–374.

Isner, J.M. and Takayuki, A. (1998) Therapeutic angiogenesis. *Front. Biosci.*, **3**, e49–e69.

Isner, J.M., Walsh, K., Rosenfield, K., Schainfeld, R., Asahara, T., Hogan, K. *et al.* (1996) Arterial gene therapy for restenosis. *Hum. Gene Ther.*, **7**, 989–1011.

Laitinen, M., Hartikainen, J., Hiltunen, M.O., Eränen, J., Kiviniemi, M., Närvänen, O. *et al.* (2000) Catheter-mediated vascular endothelial growth factor gene transfer to human coronary arteries after angioplasty. *Hum. Gene Ther.*, **11**, 263–270.

Laitinen, M., Mäkinen, K., Manninen, H., Matsi, P., Kossila, M., Agrawal, R.S. *et al.* (1998) Adenovirus-mediated gene transfer to lower limb artery of patients with chronic critical leg ischemia. *Hum. Gene Ther.*, **9**, 1481–1486.

Laitinen, M., Pakkanen, T., Donetti, E., Baetta, R., Luoma, J., Lehtolainen, P. *et al.* (1997a) Gene transfer into the carotid artery using an adventitial collar: comparison of the effectiveness of the plasmid–liposome complexes, retroviruses, pseudotyped retroviruses, and adenoviruses. *Hum. Gene Ther.*, **8**, 1645–1650.

Laitinen, M. and Ylä-Herttuala, S. (1998) Adventitial gene transfer to arterial wall. *Pharmacol. Res.*, **37**, 251–254.

Laitinen, M., Zachary, I., Breier, G., Pakkanen, T., Häkkinen, T., Luoma, J. *et al.* (1997b) Vegf gene transfer reduces intimal thickening via increased production of nitric oxide in carotid arteries. *Hum. Gene Ther.*, **8**, 1737–1744.

Leung, D.W., Cachianes, G., Kuang, W.J., Goeddel, D.V. and Ferrara, N. (1989) Vascular endothelial growth factor is a secreted angiogenic mitogen. *Science*, **246**, 1306–1309.

Mahato, R.I., Anwer, K., Tagliaferri, F., Meaney, G., Leonard, P., Wadhwa, M.S. *et al.* (1998) Biodistribution and gene expression of lipid/plasmid complexes after systemic administration. *Hum. Gene Ther.*, **9**, 2083–2099.

Mann, M.J. (1998) E2F decoy oligonucleotide for genetic engineering of vascular bypass grafts. *Antisense Nucleic Acids Drug Dev.*, **8**, 171–176.

Mann, M.J., Gibbons, G.H., Kernoff, R.S., Diet, F.P., Tsao, P.S., Cooke, J.P. *et al.* (1995) Genetic engineering of vein grafts resistant to atherosclerosis. *Proc. Natl. Acad. Sci. USA*, **92**, 4502–4506.

Mann, M.J., Gibbons, G.H., Tsao, P.S., von der Leyen, H.E., Cooke, J.P., Buitrago, R. *et al.* (1997) Cell cycle inhibition preserves endothelial function in genetically engineered rabbit vein grafts. *J. Clin. Invest.*, **99**, 1295–1301.

Mann, M.J., Whittemore, A.D., Donaldson, M.C., Belkin, M., Conte, M.S., Polak, J.F. *et al.* (1999) *Ex-vivo* gene therapy of human vascular bypass grafts with E2F decoy: the PREVENT single-centre, randomized, controlled trial. *Lancet*, **354**, 1493–1498.

Marshall, D.J., Palasis, M., Lepore, J.J. and Leiden, J.M. (2000) Biocompatibility of cardiovascular gene delivery catheters with adenovirus vectors: An important determinant of the efficiency of cardiovascular gene transfer. *Mol. Ther.*, **1**, 423–429.

Melder, R.J., Koenig, G.C., Witwer, B.P., Safabakhsh, N., Munn, L.L. and Jain, R.K. (1996) During angiogenesis, vascular endothelial growth factor and basic fibroblast growth factor regulate natural killer cell adhesion to tumor endothelium. *Nat. Med.*, **2**, 992–997.

Meyer, M., Clauss, M., Lepple-Wienhues, A., Waltenberger, J., Augustin, H.G., Ziche, M. *et al.* (1999) A novel vascular endothelial growth factor encoded by orf virus, VEGF-E, mediates angiogenesis via signalling through VEGFR-2 (KDR) but not VEGFR-1 (Flt-1) receptor tyrosine kinases. *EMBO J.*, **18**, 363–374.

Moulton, K.S., Heller, E., Konerding, M.A., Flynn, E., Palinski, W. and Folkman, J. (1999) Angiogenesis inhibitors endostatin or TNP-470 reduce intimal neovascularization and plaque growth in apolipoprotein E-deficient mice. *Circulation*, **99**, 1726–1732.

Murohara, T., Horowitz, J.R., Silver, M., Tsurumi, Y., Chen, D., Sullivan, A. *et al.* (1998) Vascular endothelial growth factor/vascular permeability factor enhances vascular permeability via nitric oxide and prostacyclin. *Circulation*, **97**, 99–107.

Nabel, E.G. (1992) Direct gene transfer into the arterial wall. *J. Vasc. Surg.*, **15**, 931–932.

Nabel, E.G. (1995) Gene therapy for vascular diseases. *Atherosclerosis*, **118** (Suppl.), S51–S56.

Nabel, E.G., Plautz, G. and Nabel, G.J. (1990) Site-specific gene expression *in vivo* by direct gene transfer into the arterial wall. *Science*, **249**, 1285–1288.

Narins, C.R., Holmes, D.R.J. and Topol, E.J. (1998) A call for provisional stenting: the balloon is back! *Circulation*, **97**, 1298–1305.

Neufeld, G., Cohen, T., Gengrinovitch, S. and Poltorak, Z. (1999) Vascular endothelial growth factor (VEGF) and its receptors. *FASEB J.* **13**, 9–22.

Nicosia, R.F. (1998) What is the role of vascular endothelial growth factor-related molecules in tumor angiogenesis? *Am. J. Pathol.* **153**, 11–16.

Nor, J.E., Christensen, J., Mooney, D.J. and Polverini, P.J. (1999) Vascular endothelial growth factor (VEGF)-mediated angiogenesis is associated with enhanced endothelial cell survival and induction of Bcl-2 expression. *Am. J. Pathol.*, **154**, 375–384.

Oesterle, S.N., Whitbourn, R., Fitzgerald, P.J., Yeung, A.C., Stertzer, S.H., Dake, M.D., Yock, P.G. and Virmani, R. (1998) The stent decade: 1987 to 1997. Stanford Stent Summit faculty. *Am. Heart J.*, **136**, 578–599.

Ogawa, S., Oku, A., Sawano, A., Yamaguchi, S., Yazaki, Y. and Shibuya, M. (1998) A novel type of vascular endothelial growth factor, VEGF-E (NZ-7 VEGF), preferentially utilizes KDR/Flk-1 receptor and carries a potent mitotic activity without heparin-binding domain. *J. Biol. Chem.*, **273**, 31273–31282.

Olofsson, B., Korpelainen, E., Pepper, M.S., Mandriota, S.J., Aase, K., Kumar, V., Gunji, Y., Jeltsch, M.M., Shibuya, M., Alitalo, K. and Eriksson, U. (1998) Vascular endothelial growth factor B (VEGF-B) binds to VEGF receptor-1 and regulates plasminogen activator activity in endothelial cells. *Proc. Natl. Acad. Sci. USA*, **95**, 11709–11714.

Olofsson, B., Pajusola, K., Kaipainen, A., von Euler, G., Joukov, V., Saksela, O., Orpana, A., Pettersson, R.F., Alitalo, K. and Eriksson, U. (1996) Vascular endothelial growth factor B, a novel growth factor for endothelial cells. *Proc. Natl. Acad. Sci. USA*, **93**, 2576–2581.

Paavonen, K., Puolakkainen, P., Jussila, L., Jahkola, T. and Alitalo, K. (2000) Vascular endothelial growth factor receptor-3 in lymphangiogenesis in wound healing. *Am. J. Pathol.*, **156**, 1499–1504.

Pakkanen, T.M., Laitinen, M., Hippeläinen, M., Hiltunen, M.O., Alhava, E. and Ylä-Herttuala, S. (2000) Periadventitial lacZ gene transfer to pig carotid arteries using a biodegradable collagen collar or a wrap of collagen sheet with adenoviruses and plasmid–liposome complexes. *J. Gene Med.* **2**, 52–60.

Plank, C., Mechtler, K., Szoka-FC, J. and Wagner, E. (1996) Activation of the complement system by synthetic DNA complexes: a potential barrier for intravenous gene delivery. *Hum. Gene Ther.*, **7**, 1437–1446.

Plouet, J., Moro, F., Bertagnolli, S., Coldeboeuf, N., Mazarguil, H., Clamens, S. and Bayard, F. (1997) Extracellular cleavage of the vascular endothelial growth factor 189-amino acid form by urokinase is required for its mitogenic effect. *J. Biol. Chem.*, **272**, 13390–13396.

Poltorak, Z., Cohen, T., Sivan, R., Kandelis, Y., Spira, G., Vlodavsky, I., Keshet, E. and Neufeld, G. (1997) VEGF145, a secreted vascular endothelial growth factor isoform that binds to extracellular matrix. *J. Biol. Chem.*, **272**, 7151–7158.

Rekhter, M.D., Simari, R.D., Work, C.W., Nabel, G.J., Nabel, E.G. and Gordon, D. (1998) Gene transfer into normal and atherosclerotic human blood vessels. *Circ. Res.* **82**, 1243–1252.

Rios, C.D., Ooboshi, H., Piegors, D., Davidson, B.L. and Heistad, D.D. (1995) Adeno-virus-mediated gene transfer to normal and atherosclerotic arteries. A novel approach. *Arterioscler. Thromb. Vasc. Biol.*, **15**, 2241–2245.

Risau, W. (1997) Mechanisms of angiogenesis. *Nature*, **386**, 671–674.

Rome, J.J., Shayani, V., Flugelman, M.Y., Newman, K.D., Farb, A., Virmani, R. and Dichek, D.A. (1994) Anatomic barriers influence the distribution of *in vivo* gene transfer into the arterial wall. Modeling with microscopic tracer particles and verification with a recombinant adenoviral vector. *Arterioscler. Thromb.*, **14**, 148–161.

Rosengart, T.K., Lee, L.Y., Patel, S.R., Sanborn, T.A., Parikh, M., Bergman, G.W., Hachamovitch, R., Szulc, M., Kligfield, P.D., Okin, P.M., Hahn, R.T., Devereux, R.B., Post, M.R., Hackett, N.R., Foster, T., Grasso, T.M., Lesser, M.L., Isom, O.W. and Crystal, R.G. (1999) Angiogenesis gene therapy: phase I assessment of direct intramyocardial administration of an adenovirus vector expressing VEGF121 cDNA to individuals with clinically significant severe coronary artery disease. *Circulation*, **100**, 468–474.

Rutanen, J., Rissanen, T.T., Kivela, A., Vajanto, I. and Ylä-Herttuala, S. (2001) Clinical applications of vascular gene therapy. *Curr. Cardiol. Rep.*, **3**, 29–36.

Safi, J.J., DiPaula, A.F.J., Riccioni, T., Kajstura, J., Ambrosio, G., Becker, L.C. *et al.* (1999) Adenovirus-mediated acidic fibroblast growth factor gene transfer induces angiogenesis in the nonischemic rabbit heart. *Microvasc. Res.*, **58**, 238–249.

Serruys, P.W., de Jaegere, P., Kiemeneij, F., Macaya, C., Rutsch, W., Heyndrickx, G. *et al.* (1994) A comparison of balloon-expandable-stent implantation with balloon angioplasty in patients with coronary artery disease. Benestent Study Group. *N. Engl. J. Med.*, **331**, 489–495.

Serruys, P.W., Emanuelsson, H., van der Giessen, W., Lunn, A.C., Kiemeney, F., Macaya, C. *et al.* (1996) Heparin-coated Palmaz-Schatz stents in human coronary arteries. Early outcome of the Benestent-II Pilot Study. *Circulation*, **93**, 412–422.

Shyu, K.G., Manor, O., Magner, M., Yancopoulos, G.D. and Isner, J.M. (1998) Direct intramuscular injection of plasmid DNA encoding angiopoietin-1 but not angiopoietin-2 augments revascularization in the rabbit ischemic hindlimb. *Circulation*, **98**, 2081–2087.

Stephan, C.C. and Brock, T.A. (1996) Vascular endothelial growth factor, a multifunctional polypeptide. *P.R. Health Sci. J.*, **15**, 169–178.

Stephan, D.J., Yang, Z.Y., San, H., Simari, R.D., Wheeler, C.J., Felgner, P.L. *et al.* (1996) A new cationic liposome/DNA complex enhances the efficiency of arterial gene transfer *in vivo. Hum. Gene Ther.*, **7**, 1803–1812.

Su, H., Lu, R. and Kan, Y.W. (2000) Adeno-associated viral vector-mediated vascular endothelial growth factor gene transfer induces neovascular formation in ischemic heart. *Proc. Natl. Acad. Sci. USA*, **97**, 13801–13806.

Tahlil, O., Brami, M., Feldman, L.J., Branellec, D. and Steg, P.G. (1997) The dispatch(tm) catheter as a delivery tool for arterial gene transfer. *Cardiovasc. Res.*, **33**, 181–187.

Takeshita, S., Pu, L.Q., Stein, L.A., Sniderman, A.D., Bunting, S., Ferrara, N. *et al.* (1994) Intramuscular administration of vascular endothelial growth factor induces dose-dependent collateral artery augmentation in a rabbit model of chronic limb ischemia. *Circulation*, **90**, II228–II234.

Thierry, A.R., Lunardi-Iskandar, Y., Bryant, J.L., Rabinovich, P., Gallo, R.C. and Mahan, L.C. (1995) Systemic gene therapy: biodistribution and long-term expression of a transgene in mice. *Proc. Natl. Acad. Sci. USA*, **92**, 9742–9746.

Tio, R.A., Tkebuchava, T., Scheuermann, T.H., Lebherz, C., Magner, M., Kearny, M. *et al.* (1999) Intramyocardial gene therapy with naked DNA encoding vascular endothelial growth factor improves collateral flow to ischemic myocardium. *Hum. Gene Ther.*, **10**, 2953–2960.

Tsurumi, Y., Kearney, M., Chen, D.F., Silver, M., Takeshita, S., Yang, J.H. *et al.* (1997) Treatment of acute limb ischemia by intramuscular injection of vascular endothelial growth factor gene. *Circulation*, **96**, 382–388.

Tsurumi, Y., Takeshita, S., Chen, D., Kearney, M., Rossow, S.T., Passeri, J. *et al.* (1996) Direct intramuscular gene transfer of naked DNA encoding vascular endothelial growth factor augments collateral development and tissue perfusion. *Circulation*, **94**, 3281–3290.

Turunen, M.P., Hiltunen, M.O., Ruponen, M., Virkamäki, L., Szoka, F.C.J., Urtti, A. *et al.* (1999) Efficient adventitial gene delivery to rabbit carotid artery with cationic polymer-plasmid complexes. *Gene Ther.*, **6**, 6–11.

Van Belle, E., Tio, F.O., Couffinhal, T., Maillard, L., Passeri, J. and Isner, J.M. (1997) Stent endothelialization: time course, impact of local catheter delivery, feasibility of recombinant protein administration, and response to cytokine expedition. *Circulation*, **95**, 438–448.

Willard, J.E., Landau, C., Glamann, D.B., Burns, D., Jessen, M.E., Pirwitz, M.J. *et al.* (1994) Genetic modification of the vessel wall. Comparison of surgical and catheter-based techniques for delivery of recombinant adenovirus. *Circulation*, **89**, 2190–2197.

Ylä-Herttuala, S. and Martin, J.F (2000) Cardiovascular gene therapy. *Lancet*, **355**, 213–222.

Yutani, C., Imakita, M., Ishibashi-Ueda, H., Tsukamoto, Y., Nishida, N. and Ikeda, Y. (1999) Coronary atherosclerosis and interventions: pathological sequences and restenosis. *Pathol. Int.*, **49**, 273–290.

Zachary, I. (1998) Vascular endothelial growth factor. *Int. J. Biochem. Cell Biol.*, **30**, 1169–1174.

Zhu, N., Liggitt, D., Liu, Y. and Debs, R. (1993) Systemic gene expression after intravenous DNA delivery into adult mice. *Science*, **261**, 209–211.

24 Gene therapy for cardiovascular disease

David A. Bull, Stephen H. Bailey, Lei Yu,
David G. Affleck and Sung Wan Kim

INTRODUCTION

Ischemic heart disease is the leading cause of death in the United States today (American Heart Association, 2001). In 1998, over 450,000 deaths were attributable to ischemic heart disease. This year over 1.1 million citizens will have a new or recurrent myocardial infarction. One of the consequences of non-fatal myocardial infarction is congestive heart failure (CHF), afflicting 22% of men and 46% of women surviving heart attacks over the subsequent five years. Currently, there are over 4.7 million Americans living with CHF, and these patients have a five year mortality of 50%. The mainstay of therapy for ischemic heart disease is revascularization. Nearly 2,000,000 cardiac catheterizations and 553,000 coronary artery bypass surgical procedures are performed annually (American Heart Association, 2001).

The development of these technologies has led to an improved survival and quality of life for patients with ischemic heart disease. Growing evidence suggests, however, that revascularization alone is insufficient for the longer-term management of many of these patients. A significant number will develop CHF each year following ischemic events to the myocardium, despite undergoing revascularization. Revascularization of ischemic myocardium can also result in reperfusion injury, which is associated with a cascade of events promoting additional myocyte loss and detrimental ventricular remodeling. To address these issues, innovative therapies that can complement and extend the benefits of revascularization are required. Fortunately, developments in genetics and molecular biology have led to a better understanding of the pathophysiology of ischemic heart disease, CHF and a number of other cardiovascular diseases. The emergence of gene therapy offers the potential for innovative prophylactic and treatment strategies for cardiovascular disease.

GENE THERAPY CLINICAL TRIALS

Trials of gene therapy for cardiovascular disease are already a clinical reality. To date, these clinical trials have focused primarily on the treatment of patients with end-stage ischemic heart disease (Rosengart *et al.*, 1999a,b; Losordo *et al.*, 1998; Symes *et al.*, 1999). Other cardiovascular diseases to which gene therapy may be applied include congestive heart failure (Maurice *et al.*, 1999; Del Monte *et al.*,

1999), cardiomyopathies and congenital disease. If gene therapy for cardiovascular disease is to become a clinical reality, however, many questions remain to be answered. Among these questions are: (1) What are the appropriate genes to be used to treat a particular disease state within the cardiovascular system? (2) What is the appropriate carrier vehicle for these genes? (3) Should gene therapy within the cardiovascular system be focused on maximum initial transfection efficiency, or is less efficient but chronic gene transfer more appropriate? (4) What is the optimal route of administration of gene medicines? (5) What are the potential complications of genetic transfection of the myocardium? (6) Should gene expression within the myocardium be inducible relative to the disease being treated to minimize complications related to over-expression of the transgene? Initial studies provide partial answers to some of these questions. A review of these studies can provide important clues as to the future direction of gene therapy for the treatment of cardiovascular disease.

ISCHEMIC HEART DISEASE (IHD)

Ischemic heart disease (IHD) is a disease of the coronary arterial wall manifesting as a progressive narrowing of the coronary artery lumen. The progressive luminal narrowing can restrict blood flow to the myocardium, resulting in an imbalance between the oxygen requirements of the myocardium and the oxygen delivery through the coronary arteries. This imbalance between oxygen demand and delivery can result in chest pain, or angina pectoris, and when severe and prolonged can result in heart attack or myocardial infarction.

The growth of collateral coronary vessels occurs naturally in the setting of native coronary artery stenoses and can dramatically change the natural history of coronary disease. Adequate collateralization can overcome severe stenoses, relieving ischemia, provided that the narrowing of the native artery does not progress too quickly. With well established collateral vessels, even acute obstruction of a coronary artery may not lead to myocardial infarction. In most patients, however, the stenoses within the coronary arteries progress more rapidly than the compensatory development of collateral vessels, resulting in one or more regions of the myocardium being acutely or chronically ischemic.

The current therapy for ischemic heart disease is revascularization with angioplasty, stent placement or coronary artery bypass surgery. The development of these techniques has led to an improved survival and quality of life for patients with ischemic heart disease. Despite these advances, there remains a large number of patients who suffer from symptomatic myocardial ischemia who are not candidates for conventional revascularization procedures. Over the past ten years, our knowledge of the molecular processes that affect angiogenesis and collateralization has significantly increased. The description of growth factors that promote new blood vessel growth, i.e., angiogenesis, offers the possibility of a 'biologic bypass' for these patients. Gene therapy for end-stage ischemic heart disease attempts to introduce genes directly into the heart to induce angiogenesis within the myocardium of affected patients (Rosengart *et al.*, 1999a,b; Losordo *et al.*, 1998; Symes *et al.*, 1999). While nearly 2,000,000 cardiac catheterizations and 553,000 coronary artery bypass procedures are performed annually, it has been estimated that at least

200,000 patients annually would be candidates for therapeutic angiogenesis (American Heart Association, 2001).

Gene therapy to promote therapeutic angiogenesis within the myocardium has already been reported in several clinical trials (Rosengart *et al.*, 1999a,b; Losordo *et al.*, 1998; Symes *et al.*, 1999). The two genes, that have primarily been used in these trials are Vascular Endothelial Growth Factor (VEGF) (Rosengart *et al.*, 1999a,b; Losordo *et al.*, 1998; Symes *et al.*, 1999) and basic Fibroblast Growth Factor (bFGF) (Giordano *et al.*, 1996; Carmeliet, 2000). The protein products of these genes have also been used in clinical trials, either as sole therapy or in combination with gene therapy (Post *et al.*, 2001). The initial results of these trials suggest a benefit for gene therapy in these patients, and manifest typically as a reduction in symptoms of disabling angina (Rosengart *et al.*, 1999a,b; Losordo *et al.*, 1998; Symes *et al.*, 1999). These are important findings as patients in these trials have typically exhausted all other forms of conventional therapy (Rosengart *et al.*, 1999a,b; Losordo *et al.*, 1998; Symes *et al.*, 1999). Gene therapy, therefore, may be an effective form of treatment in these patients who at the present time have no other options.

CONGESTIVE HEART FAILURE (CHF)

Gene therapy has also been proposed as a potential treatment for congestive heart failure (CHF), which is an important clinical problem in the United States today, with an estimated 5,000,000 Americans affected. While medical therapy can help patients in the early stages of the disease, once they progress to stage III or stage IV congestive heart failure, their prognosis is poor. Cardiac transplantation is an effective therapy for younger patients with congestive heart failure, but this modality is limited to just several thousand patients per year because of a shortage of donor organs. Among the mechanisms contributing to the development of congestive heart failure is a decrease in sarcoplasmic reticulum Ca^{2+}-ATPase (SERCA2a) pump activity, resulting in alterations in calcium fluxes and calcium levels within the myocardium (Del Monte *et al.*, 1999). Restoration of contractile function in isolated cardiomyocytes from failing human hearts has been demonstrated by gene transfer of SERCA2a (Del Monte *et al.*, 1999). Another potential therapy is the genetic transfer of the beta-adrenergic signaling components to treat CHF (Maurice *et al.*, 1999). Enhancement of the cardiac function has been demonstrated after adeno-viral-mediated *in vivo* intracoronary β_2-adrenergic receptor (BARK) gene delivery (Maurice *et al.*, 1999). Both the SERCA2a gene and the BARK gene, then, show promise as potential therapies in animal models of CHF. Hopefully, future studies will show efficacy in humans.

CARDIAC TRANSPLANTATION

Patients undergoing cardiac transplantation represent another potential group of patients who might benefit from gene therapy. Early and mid-term survival following cardiac transplantation is good, often exceeding 70% at many centers. Five years following transplantation, however, many of these patients manifest accelerated coronary vasculopathy, which is the leading cause of death following cardiac transplantation. This vasculopathy targets the coronary arteries of the transplanted heart, resulting in progressive stenoses of the major coronary arteries and more particularly, of their small distal branches. The etiology has been proposed to be an immune-mediated chronic rejection directed toward the endothelium of the transplanted heart. Gene therapy, which could alter the immune response to the endothelium of the transplanted heart, might slow or even prevent the development of graft vasculopathy (Jayakumar *et al.*, 2000; Iwata *et al.*, 2000).

HYPERTROPHIC CARDIOMYOPATHY

Hypertrophic cardiomyopathy is another cardiovascular disease which may benefit from gene therapy. This is a spectrum of inherited conditions which affect various elements controlling functions of the sarcomere. Many of the specific genetic changes responsible for the development of hypertrophic cardiomyopathy have been delineated. Interestingly, the specific genetic changes differ in their pathogenicity, with some lesions known to be lethal at an early age and other lesions which are clinically silent and do not appreciably alter the life span of the individual. For potentially lethal lesions, gene transfer to the myocardium may represent a means to reverse the inherited disorder (Bowles *et al.*, 2000).

GENE DELIVERY SYSTEMS

As important as determining which gene to use to treat a particular condition is the vector in which the gene will be packaged to facilitate transfection. At the present time, the vectors used for genetic transfection of the myocardium include attenuated adenovirus (AV) (Rosengart *et al.*, 1999a,b), adeno-associated virus (AAV) (Alexander *et al.*, 1999; Kaplitt *et al.*, 1996; Lee *et al.*, 1996), plasmid-based polyplexes and lipoplexes. Each of these gene delivery systems has particular advantages and disadvantages.

Adenoviral vectors allow initial high transfection efficiency, but are limited by the development of an immune response to the viruses themselves (Alexander *et al.*, 1999). This limitation reduces transfection efficiency on repeated dosing, a concern in settings where subsequent dosing is required to achieve an optimal level of the transgene, or where later dosing may be desired to repeat a therapeutic effect (Alexander *et al.*, 1999). Also of concern is the possibility of inducing a systemic inflammatory response with the use of an adenoviral vector (Alexander *et al.*, 1999), a safety issue which has led to poor clinical outcomes for gene therapies used in other clinical settings. Other drawbacks of the attenuated adenovirus include the limited size of therapeutic DNA which can be incorporated into the virion, the potential for systemic spread of the virus and its widespread tropism. The concerns regarding repeated dosing and induction of an immune response has led researchers to propose using an adeno-associated virus in which the transfection efficiency of the adenovirus is maintained while the immunogenicity of the virus itself has been modified (Alexander *et al.*, 1999). These vectors do appear to offer superior transfection efficiency. The adeno-associated virus, however, can only accommodate small transgenes (<4.5 kb), is low titer and is difficult to prepare. Furthermore, the possibility of a systemic host response still exists with the adeno-associated virus despite its immunologic modification. Finally, both the adenovirus and the adeno-asssociated virus have the potential for regeneration of wild-type, replication-competent strains.

The limitations of viral vector systems have promoted interest in non-viral vectors. Polymers are macromolecules that provide opportunities for the design of novel systems for gene delivery. The major drawback of a polymeric gene carrier is low transfection efficiency. The introduction of lipid components into polymeric carriers dramatically enhances gene transfer efficiency both *in vitro* and *in vivo*. The advantages of using polyplexes and lipoplexes for gene delivery to the myocardium are their non-toxicity, capability for repeated dosing and the potential for cell-specific targeting. The use of low density lipoprotein (LDL) moieties with the carrier vehicle allows targeting of the LDL receptor and the potential for directed gene therapy within the myocardium. Utilizing these principles, we have recently described the use of a novel gene delivery system for the myocardium: TerplexDNA (Affleck *et al.*, 2001). The Terplex gene delivery system significantly augments myocardial transfection, compared to naked plasmid DNA (Affleck *et al.*, 2001). The efficacy of TerplexDNA suggests that it is possible for gene delivery systems within the myocardium to be tailored to the site, as dictated by the disease state and the proposed therapy. Such targeted gene therapy may ultimately prove to be more useful than approaches that rely on more efficient but less specific transfection of host cells.

ROUTE OF ADMINISTRATION

Another important issue, with regard to genetic transfection of the myocardium, is the route of administration. Among the possible routes are intra-coronary arterial delivery (Rosengart *et al.*, 1999; Miao *et al.*, 2000), retrograde coronary sinus delivery (Boekstegers *et al.*, 2000; Boekstegers, 2001), direct myocardial injection (Rosengart *et al.*, 1999; Losordo *et al.*, 1998) and intra-pericardial instillation (Fromes *et al.*, 1999). Each of these routes has potential advantages and disadvantages. Gene delivery via the coronary arteries offers the potential for catheter-based delivery. Unfortunately, studies examining the therapeutic efficacy of growth factor gene and protein therapy using this route for induction of angiogenesis within the myocardium have yielded conflicting results. While some studies have shown the induction of angiogenesis with delivery via the coronary arteries (Laitinen *et al.*, 2000), other studies have found no induction of angiogenesis compared to controls.

Intra-coronary arterial delivery may result in significant distribution of the gene to unaffected areas of the myocardium, resulting in a decrease in gene delivery to the desired site of action. This decrease is of concern when trying to induce angiogenesis within a particular region of the myocardium. Further, coronary arterial gene delivery to induce angiogenesis in the setting of ischemic heart disease in humans may be limited by the inability to deliver the gene at therapeutic levels beyond high-grade coronary artery stenoses or occlusions. Intra-coronary arterial delivery of gene medicines may be more applicable in the setting of inherited cardiomyopathies, where the coronary arteries are often widely patent and the myocardium is diffusely affected. The need for alternate routes to reach the myocardium via the vascular system has led to studies examining the feasibility of gene delivery via the coronary sinus venous system. Initial studies examining this route suggest that there is the potential for effective transfection of the myocardium, perhaps potentiated by the administration of the genes into a low-pressure vascular bed (Boekstegers *et al.*, 2000; Boekstegers, 2001). This route may ultimately prove to be desirable in patients with significant stenoses from coronary artery disease, where effective delivery of genes via the arterial route may not be possible for the reasons discussed above (Boekstegers *et al.*, 2000; Boekstegers, 2001).

Delivery for intra-myocardial gene therapy is typically performed with the aid of a needle and syringe based assembly. Using this technique, genes can be delivered to the targeted area with strictly controlled dosing. Several studies have demonstrated efficacy of this technique in animals and humans (Rosengart *et al.*, 1999a,b). With targeted delivery, re-distribution of the gene outside of the myocardium is less of a concern than it is with other delivery techniques. A disadvantage of injection of genes directly into the myocardium is the potential for fibrosis at the site of injection. At present, direct intra-myocardial injection requires a surgical procedure (Rosengart *et al.*, 1999a,b; Losordo *et al.*, 1998; Symes *et al.*, 1999). While this technique allows concomitant administration of gene therapy at the time of surgical therapies, dependence on opening of the thoracic cavity for gene delivery may limit its wider applicability. The development of less invasive means of targeted intra-myocardial delivery would help solve this problem and is presently underway (Kornowski *et al.*, 2000).

Intra-pericardial delivery has been proposed as an alternative means by which to accomplish genetic transfection of the myocardium. With this technique, a catheter is inserted via a sub-xyphoid approach and the gene is delivered into the pericardial space (Fromes *et al.*, 1999). While this technique might seem to result in dilution of the delivered gene, reasonable transfection of the epicardial surface of the myocardium has been reported with intra-pericardial delivery (Fromes *et al.*, 1999). A review of these different routes for gene delivery suggests that the route of delivery will likely have to be tailored to the anatomy and physiology of the myocardium being treated as well as the required level of transgene expression.

SAFETY CONSIDERATIONS

Paramount in any consideration of gene therapy for cardiovascular disease is the safety of the proposed therapy, both short-term and long-term. The potential benefit to the patient must be weighed against the potential risks of the therapy. Recent clinical experience has demonstrated that fatalities can occur with gene therapy and so careful consideration must be given to the disease state being treated and the potential for complications (Senior, 2000). Gene therapy to induce angiogenesis for inoperable coronary artery disease has received the most clinical attention to date. The concerns raised by gene therapy for this condition are whether unregulated expression of the transgene within the myocardium may lead to complications. Over-expression of vascular endothelial growth factor

(VEGF) can lead to several important problems, including the formation of vasculartumors, or angiomas. This formation is of particular concern within the heart as angiomas constitute space-occupying lesions, which can lead to heart failure and death (Lee *et al.*, 2000). Over-expression of VEGF may also accelerate atherosclerotic plaque formation and rupture in animals (Celleti *et al.*, 2001).

These studies suggest that while gene therapy can be beneficial, it will be important to develop gene constructs whose expression is inducible, so that the gene is expressed only when required, preventing complications related to unregulated expression. In addition, careful attention must be paid to the construction and delivery of carrier vehicles such that expression is limited to the target area of interest within the myocardium. With genes that promote angiogenesis, re-distribution of the gene into the systemic circulation raises concerns regarding promotion of occult tumor angiogenesis or undesired angiogenesis in other organ systems. Studies examining the effects of gene therapy on the myocardium also need to assess the potential for the unanticipated consequences of the gene therapy outside of the cardiovascular system.

CONCLUDING REMARKS

Gene therapy is a promising new approach to treat a variety of acquired and congenital diseases. Many problems need to be solved, however, before gene therapy can be broadly applicable to treat cardiovascular disease. It will be important to develop carrier vehicles for gene delivery that allow for efficient transfection, tissue specific targeting, minimal toxicity and a negligible immunologic or inflamatory response. As the above review indicates, the gene therapy will need to be tailored to the particular disease being treated. It will also be essential that therapeutic gene expression within the cardiovascular system is regulated to avoid complications of unregulated gene expression. Therapeutic gene expression should be limited to the targeted cells and tissues to avoid systemic spread where gene expression within other organ systems may be deleterious. Solving these problems will require extensive animal and human studies to determine the optimal role of gene therapy for the treatment of cardiovascular disease. Cardiovascular gene therapy should be a productive area of study for many years to come.

REFERENCES

Affleck, D.G., Yu, L., Bull, D.A., Bailey, S.H. and Kim, S.W. (2001) Augmentation of myocardial transfection using TerplexDNA: a novel gene delivery system. *Gene Ther.*, 8, 349–353.

Alexander, M.Y., Webster, K.A., McDonald, P.H. and Prentice, H.M. (1999) Gene transfer and models of gene therapy for the myocardium. *Clin. Exp. Pharmacol. Physiol.*, 26, 661–668.

American Heart Association 2001 Heart and Stroke Statistical Update. Dallas, Texas. American Heart Association, 2001.

Boekstegers, P. (2001) Perspectives on selective retroinfusion of coronary veins as an alternative approach for myocardial gene transfer and angiogenesis. *J. Inv. Cardiol.*, 13, 339–342.

Boekstegers, P., Von Degenfeld, G., Giehrl, W., Kupatt, C., Franz, W. and Steinbeck, G. (2000) Selective pressure-regulated retroinfusion of coronary veins as an alternative access of ischemic myocardium: Implications for myocardial protection, myocardial gene transfer and angiogenesis. *Z Kardiol. 89 Suppl.*, **9**, IX/109–112.

Bowles, N.E., Bowles, K. and Towbin, J.A. (2000) Prospects for gene therapy for inherited cardiomyopathies. *Prog. Pediatr. Cardiol.*, **12**, 133–145.

Carmeliet, P. (2000) Fibroblast growth factor-1 stimulates branching and survival of myocardial arteries. *Circ. Res.*, **87**, 176–183.

Celletti, F.L., Waugh, J.M., Amabile, P.G., Brendolan, A., Hilfiker, P.R. and Drake, M.D. (2001) Vascular endothelial growth factor enhances atherosclerotic plaque progression. *Nat. Med.*, **7**, 425–429.

Del Monte, F., Harding, S.E., Schmidt, U., Matsui, T., Kang, Z.B., Dec, G.W. *et al.* (1999) Restoration of contractile function in isolated cardiomyocytes from failing human hearts by gene transfer of SERCA2a. *Circulation*, **100**, 2308–2311.

Fromes, Y., Salmon, A., Wang, X., Collin, H., Rouche, A., Hagege, A. *et al.* (1999) Gene delivery to the myocardium by intrapericardial injection. *Gene Ther.*, **6**, 683–688.

Giordano, F.J., Ping, P., McKirnan, M.D., Nozaki, S., DeMaria, A.N., Dillman, W.H. *et al.* (1996) Intracoronary gene transfer of fibroblast growth factor-5 increases blood flow and contractile function in an ischemic region of the heart. *Nat. Med.*, **2**, 534–539.

Iwata, A., Sai, S., Moore, M., Nyhuis, J., de Fries-Hallstrand, R., Quetingco, G.C. *et al.* (2000) Gene therapy of transplant arteriopathy by liposome-mediated transfection of endothelial nitric oxide synthase. *J. Heart Lung Transplant*, **19**, 1017–1028.

Jayakumar, J., Suzuki, K., Khan, M., Smolenski, R.T., Farrell, A., Latif, N. *et al.* (2000) Gene therapy for myocardial protection: Transfection of donor hearts with heat shock protein 70 gene protects cardiac function against ischemia-reperfusion injury. *Circulation*, **102** (19 Suppl. 3), III302–306.

Kaplitt, M.G., Xiao, X., Samulski, R.J., Li, J., Ojamaa, K., Klein, I.L. *et al.* (1996) Long-term gene transfer in porcine myocardium after coronary infusion of an adeno-associated virus vector. *Ann. Thorac. Surg.*, **62**, 1669–1676.

Kornowski, R., Fuchs, S., Epstein, S.E., Branellec, D. and Schwartz, B. (2000) Catheter-based plasmid-mediated transfer of genes into ischemic myocardium using the pCOR plasmid. *Coron. Art. Dis.*, **11**, 615–619.

Laitinen, M., Hartikainen, J., Hiltunen, M.O., Eranen, J., Kiviniemi, M., Narvanen, O. *et al.* (2000) Catheter-mediated vascular endothelial growth factor gene transfer to human coronary arteries after angioplasty. *Hum. Gene Ther.*, **11**, 263–270.

Lee, L.Y., Zhou, X., Polce, D.R., El-Sawy, T., Patel, S.R., Thakker, G.D. *et al.* (1996) Exogenous control of cardiac gene therapy: Evidence of regulated myocardial transgene expression after adenovirus and adeno-associated virus transfer of expression cassettes containing corticosteroid response element promoters. *J. Thorac. Cardiovasc. Surg.*, **118**, 26–35.

Lee, R.J., Springer, M.L., Blanco-Bose, W.E., Shaw, R., Ursell, P.C. and Blau, H.M. (2000) VEGF gene delivery tomyocardium: Deleterious effects of unregulated expression. *Circulation*, **102**, 898–901.

Losordo, D.W., Vale, P.R., Symes, J.F., Dunnigton, C.H., Esakof, D.D., Maysky, M. *et al.* (1998) Gene therapy for myocardial angiogenesis: Initial clinical results with direct myocardial injection of phVEGF$_{165}$ as sole therapy for myocardial ischemia. *Circulation*, **98**, 2800–2804.

Maurice, J.P., Hata, J.A., Shah, A.S., White, D.C., McDonald, P.H., Dolber, P.C. *et al.* (1999) Enhancement of cardiac function after adenoviral-mediated *in vivo* intracoronary β_2-adrenergic receptor gene delivery. *J. Clin. Invest.*, **104**, 21–29.

Miao, W., Luo, Z., Kitsis, R. and Walsh, K. (2000) Intracoronary, adenovirus-mediated Akt gene transfer in heart limits infarct size following ischemia-reperfusion injury *in vivo*. *J. Mol. Cell. Cardiol.*, **32**, 2397–2402.

Post, M.J., Laham, R., Sellke, F.W. and Simons, M. (2001) Therapeutic angiogenesis in cardiology using protein formulations. *Cardiovasc. Res.*, **49**, 522–531.

Rosengart, T.K., Lee, L.Y., Patel, S.R., Sanburn, T.A., Parikh, M., Bergman, G.W. *et al.* (1999a) Phase I assessment of direct intramyocardial administration of an adenovirus vector expressing VEGF121 cDNA to individuals with clinically significant severe coronary artery disease. *Circulation*, **100**, 468–474.

Rosengart, T.J., Lee, L.Y., Patel, S.R., Kligfield, P.D., Okin, P.M., Hackett, N.R. *et al.* (1999b) Six-month assessment of a phase I trial of angiogenic gene therapy for the treatment of coronary artery disease using direct intramyocardial administration of an adenovirus vector expressing the VEGF121 cDNA. *Ann. Surg.*, **230**, 466–472.

Senior, K. (2000) Gene therapy: A rocky start to the new millennium. *Mol. Med. Today*, **6**, 93.

Symes, J.F., Losordo, D.W., Vale, P.R., Lathi, K.G., Esakof, D.D., Mayskiy, M. *et al.* (1999) Gene therapy with vascular endothelial growth factor for inoperable coronary artery disease. *Ann. Thorac. Surg.*, **68**, 830–837.

25 Gene therapy for the prevention of autoimmune diabetes

Kyung Soo Ko, Minhyung Lee and
Sung Wan Kim

INTRODUCTION

The advent of new techniques in gene therapy gives hope to many patients suffering from diseases that are difficult to cure. Until now, the scope of gene therapy has been limited to a refractory disease because of safety issues, effectiveness, and long-term adverse effects. Although a small number of patients benefit from gene therapy, the recent revelation of pathogenesis, the development of new technology and tools, and a huge research activity will enable us to treat genetic and acquired diseases with gene therapy.

Current clinical trials mostly focus on the malignancy, cardiovascular and hematologic diseases. However, autoimmune disease is a good candidate for gene therapy for several reasons. Autoimmune disease originates from the loss of self-tolerance, and its prevalence increases along with industrialization. The chronic course of autoimmune disease, prolongation of life expectancy, and the development of treatment modality result in the loss of labor and exponential increase of economic burden. Recent gene therapy research activities for the prevention and treatment of autoimmune diseases are quite promising.

There are several reasons why autoimmune disease is a good candidate for gene therapy. First, most autoimmune disease stems form a similar abnormality of the immune system. Therefore, it can be a good candidate for immune intervention. Second, the slow progressive nature of immune destruction enables us to predict the onset of disease by using genetic, immunologic, and metabolic markers. So, it is realistic to prevent the autoimmune disease at the pre-clinical stage. Current experimental immune intervention modality can be replaced with gene therapy, which may overcome several drawbacks of protein delivery. In this chapter, we describe the current trends and future prospects of gene therapy for autoimmune diabetes.

PATHOGENESIS OF AUTOIMMUNE DIABETES

The current concept of autoimmune diabetes is that pancreas islet β cells are destroyed by an autoimmune response mediated by T lymphocytes that react specifically to one or more β cell proteins (Bach, 1994). Figure 25.1 shows the pathogenesis of type 1 diabetes. This concept gave rise to the idea that auto-immune diabetes can be prevented by the manipulation of autoreactive T cells or

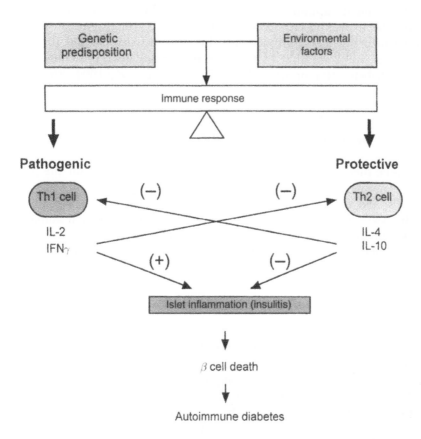

Figure 25.1 Pathogenesis of type 1 diabetes.

autoantigen, such as transgenic mice (Mueller *et al.*, 1996), administration of cyto-kine (Pennline *et al.*, 1994), injection of autoantigen to induce immune tolerance (Tisch *et al.*, 1993) and administration of autoantibody (Menard *et al.*, 1999).

The complete destruction of β cells due to autoimmune mechanism results in absolute insulin deficiency, which requires life-long insulin supplementation for survival. This autoimmune response afflicts patients who have a specific susceptible major histocommpatibility complex (MHC) allele or who lack protective allele. Certain environmental factors, including microbial, chemical, and dietary factors are known to trigger the immune system to attack self-organs. Also, some environmental factors suppress the autoimmune response. Therefore, the clinical expression of autoimmune diabetes is determined by the net sum of promotional (or suppressional) genetic (or environmental) factors. The use of non-specific immuno-suppressant showed only temporary effect, but serious side-effects, such as infection and organ toxicity, were seen. Current immune prevention of autoimmune diabetes is mainly based on the suppression of immune reaction to specific autoantigen.

Autoimmune diabetes is a Th1-mediated disease and β cell destruction is also mediated by the subset of CD4 and CD8 positive T lymphocytes secreting IFN-γ, thus favoring cellular immunity (Rabinovitch and Skyler, 1998). Th1 activities are downregulated by Th2 cells secreting IL-4 and IL-10. In animal models of autoimmune diabetes, any approach favoring Th2 activity has led to diabetes prevention. The administration of these immuno-regulatory cytokines reduces autoimmune diabetes (Rapoport *et al.*, 1993; Pennline *et al.*, 1994; Zheng *et al.*, 1997).

PREVENTION OF AUTOIMMUNE DIABETES

Two main gene therapy strategies have been intensively studied for the prevention of autoimmune diabetes. One is to suppress the expression of autoantigen in islet β-cells, and the other is to use immune suppression cytokines. Glutamic acid decarboxylase (GAD) has been shown to be the most important autoantigen and thus suppression of the GAD expression can treat diabetes (Yoon *et al.*, 1999). For cytokine gene therapy, IL-4 and IL-10 have been the most widely explored.

Autoantigen-related gene therapy for the prevention of autoimmune diabetes

Autoimmunity develops from a failure in self-nonself discrimination. Therefore, many animal studies have been conducted to interfere with the recognition of autoantigen by autoreactive T cells. Among several candidate autoantigens, which induce the autoimmune destruction of pancreas β cells, GAD is the most important one. GAD is a rate-limiting enzyme in the synthesis of a major inhibitory neurotransmitter, γ-aminobutyric acid (GABA), and is distributed in neural system and pancreas islets. Although the function of GAD in the pancreas remains unknown, the presence of both GAD and GABA within islet β cells, and the presence of GABA receptors on these cells, suggests that GABA is involved in paracrine signaling in the islet.

Oral (Pleau *et al.*, 1995), nasal (Tian *et al.*, 1996), or intrathymic (Tisch *et al.*, 1993) administrations of GAD have been shown to accomplish immune regulation or immune tolerance, and the development of autoimmune diabetes was prevented by GAD challenge. The mechanism of prevention was thought to be the enhancement of Th2 cell function. Immunization using antigenic determinant peptide of GAD was also successful. These prevention trials confirmed that the GAD antibody does not play a role in destruction of β cells. Menard *et al.* (1999) suggested that the anti-GAD antibody binds to the GAD antigen, or perhaps binds to the epitope presented in association with the antigen presenting cell (APC)-MHC and prevents T cell recognition, thereby delaying disease onset.

The GAD-related gene therapy trial was β cell specific and induced suppression of GAD expression in antisense GAD transgenic mice (Yoon *et al.*, 1999). In this report, antisense GAD RNA expression was driven by rat insulin promoter for specific expression in the pancreas. The complete suppression of β cell GAD expression blocked the generation of diabetogenic T cells and prevented the development of autoimmune diabetes. These findings indicate that β cell GAD expression is a requirement for the development of autoimmune diabetes in NOD mice. GAD expression in the brain was detected equally in the brain tissue of transgene-negative NOD mice and antisense GAD transgenic NOD mice, suggesting that the suppression of GAD by antisense GAD RNA may not have any effect on normal expression of GAD in other organs. Also, the pancreatic insulin content and plasma insulin concentration of antisense GAD transgenic mice were indistinguishable from that of transgene negative NOD mice. It suggests that suppression of GAD expression does not have any side effect on the normal function of the pancreas. The possibility of somatic antisense GAD gene therapy was proved by delivery of antisense GAD plasmid *in vitro* and *in vivo* (Lee *et al.*, 2001b). In this study, antisense GAD plasmid complexed with PEG-*g*-PLL was transfected to mouse insulinoma 6 (MIN6) cells. The results showed that GAD expression can be suppressed by antisense GAD RNA. Since the antisense GAD RNA was driven by rat insulin promoter, the antisense GAD RNA was expressed in pancreas in mice. However, the development of a more efficient and β cell specific transfection is indispensable. For β cell specific delivery, several kinds of new gene carriers have been designed. These gene carriers include the conjugation of β cell specific ligands such as anti-GAD antibody and sulfonyl urea. However, further study is needed to verify the clinical applicability of this approach.

Although a GAD directed prevention trial is an attractive option, some animal experiments, which showed oral antigen challenge, can induce or accelerate an autoimmune disease (Blanas *et al.*, 1996; McFarland, 1996). The nature of autoantigen, the route of administration, and the concentration of the autoantigen are likely to influence whether immune response leads to tolerance or attack. Moreover, GAD autoimmunity is also associated with a neurological disease, Stiff-Man syndrome (though the epitopes are different from autoimmune diabetes). So particular caution should be exercised in modulating the immune response to GAD, lest the consequence of preventing autoimmune diabetes is to induce Stiff-Man syndrome (Butler *et al.*, 1993; Daw *et al.*, 1996). The other trial of GAD gene therapy is the potential for the treatment of drug-resistant epilepsy because GAD is a synthesizing enzyme of GABA, which is a major neuro-inhibitory transmitter (Robert *et al.*, 1997).

CYTOKINES IN AUTOIMMUNE DIABETES

Autoimmune diabetes favors the concept that β cells are destroyed by an autoimmune response directed against certain β cell constituents (autoantigen). There are several lines of evidence to support the concept that autoimmune diabetes is a T cell-mediated autoimmune disease, including the transfer of disease into non-diabetic recipients of bone marrow transplantation who are human leukocyte antigen (HLA)-compatible siblings (Lampeter, 1993) and recurrence of auto-immune diabetes after pancreas transplantation (Sibley *et al.*, 1985). These findings suggest that normal islet β cells can be the targets of an autoimmune response.

The nonobese diabetic mouse (NOD), as well as the biobreeding (BB) rats are the two rodent models whose diabetes-related immunopathology is considered to be quite similar to that in humans. Studies in these animal models have revealed that autoreactive T cells that mediate islet β cell destruction belong to the Th1 subset of T cells (produce IL-2 and IFN-γ), whereas regulatory T cells are of the Th2 type (produce IL-4 and IL-10). Because Th1 and Th2 cells are mutually inhibitory, there have been many trials using IL-4 and/or IL-10 for the prevention of autoimmune disease, like autoimmune diabetes, rheumatoid arthritis (Evans *et al.*, 1996; Boyle *et al.*, 1999), and inflammatory bowel disease (Rogy *et al.*, 2000).

A variety of cytokines implicated in the pathogenesis of autoimmune diabetes have been found to express at the gene or protein level, or both, in the insulitis lesion of animal models and diabetic patients. Studies involving the systemic administration of cytokines to diabetes-prone NOD mice and BB rats have revealed that several cytokines can prevent the development of autoimmune diabetes. These include IL-1 (Wilson *et al.*, 1990), IL-2 (Zielasek *et al.*, 1990), IL-4 (Rapoport *et al.*, 1993), IL-10 (Pennline *et al.*, 1994), TNF-α (Jacob *et al.*, 1990), and TNF-β (Seino *et al.*, 1993). Systemically administered IL-4 or IL-10 have been shown to prevent diabetes. A combination of IL-4 and IL-10 exerts a synergistic effect on the suppression of cell-mediated immunity *in vivo* (Powrie *et al.*, 1993; Faust *et al.*, 1996). Although the underlying mechanism is not yet known, both data establish IL-4 and IL-10 as potent inhibitors of the Th1 effector function *in vivo* and suggest their utility in controlling deleterious Th1-mediated inflammatory response that occur in some infectious and autoimmune disease.

For cytokine gene therapy of autoimmune diabetes, several kinds of cytokine expression plasmids have been designed and constructed. In general, the mammalian expression plasmids are composed of promoter, intron, cDNA, and polyadenylation sequences. Transgene expression is regulated by promoter and enhancers motifs, which is usually located at the 5' end of a gene. To date, several promoters and enhancers have been employed to regulate cytokine gene expression.

Systemic delivery of cytokine expression plasmids

Promoters from cytomegalovirus (CMV) or simian virus 40 (SV40) have been widely used because they are known to be strong promoters (Qin *et al.*, 1997). When we evaluated mouse interleukin-4 (IL-4) and interleukin-10 (IL-10) expression plasmids, pCMV-mIL-4 and pCMV-mIL-10, respectively, we found a high expression level of IL-4 or IL-10 *in vitro* and *in vivo* Koh *et al.* (2001). However, CMV promoter appears to show a decrease in activity when administered *in vivo*. The duration of gene expression by CMV promoter is short compared with cellular promoters such as β-actin promoter. Also, CMV promoter shows lower activity than chicken β-actin promoter in the liver (Xu *et al.*, 2001).

Nitta *et al.* (1998) reported that intramuscular injection of pCAGGS-mIL-10, which contains the chicken β-actin promoter, prevented the development of autoimmune diabetes in NOD mice. The intravenous injection of pCAGGS-mIL-10 complexed with biodegradable polymeric carrier, poly[α-(4-aminobutyl)-L-glycolic acid] (PAGA) in NOD mice showed significant expression levels of IL-10 in the liver, leading to the prevention of autoimmune insulitis (Koh *et al.*, 2000). PAGA is a biodegradable gene carrier and can stabilize the plasmid in the blood stream, leading to increased availability of the plasmid for gene expression. The efficiency of PAGA in systemic administration of cytokine plasmids was also proved in gene therapy with another immune suppression cytokine, IL-4. pCAGGS-mIL10/PAGA complex was intravenously injected to NOD mice (Lee *et al.*, 2001a). IL-4 was expressed mainly in the liver. Autoimmune insulitis also prevented the expression of IL-4. The most impressive results were obtained from the combined administration of pCAGGS-mIL-4 and pCAGGS-mIL-10 (Ko *et al.*, 2001). We found that the co-administration of IL-4 and IL-10 plasmid complexed with PAGA exerted long lasting and augmented immune regulatory effects. Insulitis and diabetes were prevented by a single injection of IL-4 and IL-10 plasmids, because the cell source of IL-4 and IL-10 is a little different. In the case of cytokine combination, we can obtain the maximum effect by optimizing the timing and sequencing of injection, and the therapeutic dose of plasmid.

To further enhance the expression of IL-4 and IL-10, a chimeric expression plasmid was constructed, in which the expression of IL-4 and IL-10 was under the control of two independent CMV promoters and enhancers (Figure 25.2). The expressions of two genes in a plasmid can also be achieved by using the internal ribosome entry site (IRES) under the control of one promoter or two independent promoter units. However, it is well known that IRES has drawbacks and that the second gene expression is lower than the first gene expression. Mahato *et al.* (2001) showed that two promoter plasmid was much more efficient than IRES plasmid in gene expression. Also, by constructing this kind of chimeric plasmid, we can regulate the specific therapeutic gene and cell-targeting process; the process will be more simplified by the incorporation of the on-off system or by tissue-specific promoter for each gene.

TGF-β1 was also evaluated with NOD mice for the prevention of autoimmune diabetes, since it down-regulates many immune responses (Piccirillo *et al.*, 1998). In TGF-β1 expression plasmid, pCMV-TGF-β1, the mTGF-β1 cDNA is under the

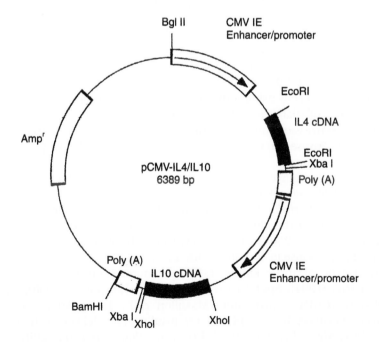

Figure 25.2 The map of chimeric plasmid, pCMV-IL4/IL10.

transcriptional control of a CMV promoter/enhancer. Intramuscular injection of the plasmid showed TGF-β1 mRNA expression in skeletal muscle cells, as well as an increased level of TGF-β1 in the plasma of treated mice. Administration of pCMV-TGF-β1 was effective in protecting NOD mice from insulitis and diabetes. In addition, there was a decreased expression of IL-12 and IFNγ mRNA in the pancreas of protected mice.

Delivery of tissue-specific or glucose responsive expression plasmid

To minimize the adverse effects of systemic expression, targeted organ-specific expression is one of the goals in designing gene therapy strategy. The unique characteristics of diabetes (high glucose concentration) can be either a hurdle or an advantage. The insulin promoter is pancreas specific in gene expression (Sharma and Stein, 1994). In addition, elevations in extraceullular glucose concentration activate the insulin promoter (German *et al.*, 1990; Efrat *et al.*, 1991; Goodison *et al.*, 1992; Redmon *et al.*, 1994; Odagiri *et al.*, 1996; Kennedy *et al.*, 1999). Therefore, the insulin promoter has been used for pancreas targeting and glucose responsive expression of a gene (Mueller *et al.*, 1996; Khachatryan *et al.*, 1997; Yang and Kotin, 2000). A previous report showed that autoimmune diabetes was completely prevented in the transgenic NOD mice, in which IL-4 was expressed in the pancreas by human insulin promoter (Mueller *et al.*, 1996). This approach was effective in that it expressed IL-4 pancreas specifically, without any side-effects from the systemic expression of IL-4. These results also indicated that autoimmune diabetes in NOD mice is not a systemic disease, and it can be modulated from the islet compartment. Therefore, for somatic gene therapy, the rat insulin promoter was inserted upstream of the IL-4 cDNA (Lee *et al.*, 2001a). This plasmid, pRIP-mIL-4 was complexed with water soluble lipopolymer and transfected *in vitro*. The results indicated that pRIP-mIL-4 expressed IL-4 cell-type specifically.

Another application of insulin promoter was the repression of GAD autoantigen in the pancreas. Yoon *et al.* (1999) reported that silencing of the expression of GAD65 and GAD67 in the β cells using antisense techniques completely protected against the development of diabetes in the transgenic NOD mice. For pancreas specific antisense RNA expression, insulin promoter was incorporated upstream of antisense GAD cDNAs. Antisense GAD RNA was expressed exclusively in the pancreas of the transgenic mice.

Elevations in extracellular glucose concentration activate the insulin promoter (German *et al.*, 1990; Efrat *et al.*, 1991; Goodison *et al.*, 1992; Redmon *et al.*, 1994; Odagiri *et al.*, 1996; Kennedy *et al.*, 1999). pRIP-mIL-4 expressed IL-4 *in vitro* in a glucose-responsive manner, as the glucose concentration increases the level of IL-4 expression elevated (Lee *et al.*, 2001). In the liver, some glycolytic genes are transcriptionally induced in response to carbohydrates. Liver specific glucose responsive promoters include L-type pyruvate kinase (L-PK) promoter (Lefrancois-Martinez *et al.*, 1994; Doiron *et al.*, 1994), Spot 14 (S14) promoter (Jump *et al.*, 1990), and glucose-6-phosphatase (G6Pase) promoter (Massillon *et al.*, 1996; Argaud *et al.*, 1997). These promoters have been explored for insulin gene delivery (Lu *et al.*, 1998; Gros *et al.*, 1997; Mitanchez *et al.*, 1997; Lee *et al.*, 2000; Chen *et al.*, 2001). It is clear that they are applicable to glucose responsive cytokine expression plasmids.

OTHER TRIALS FOR AUTOIMMUNE DIABETES

Recently, the broad concept of gene therapy for autoimmune diabetes has extended the applicability and includes preventive trial, insulin supplementation, and manipulation of many kinds of cells. For the prevention of autoimmune diabetes, besides the antigen challenge and cytokine administration, over-expression of the anti-apoptotic gene (Liu *et al.*, 1996; Rabinovitch *et al.*, 1999) or the radical scavenging enzyme, manganese superoxide dismutase (MnSOD), resulted in increased cell resistance to cytokines (Hohmeier *et al.*, 1998). Anti-apoptotic gene, Bcl-2 is a cellular protein that regulates apoptosis and over-expression of the Bcl-2 can prevent apoptosis (Kroemer, 1997). Transfection of the Bcl-2 gene into human pancreatic islets protects β-cells from cytokine-induced destruction (Rabinovitch *et al.*, 1999).

Gene therapy for the insulin delivery requires a precise regulation of insulin expression in terms of plasma glucose concentration because of the risk of hypoglycemic shock. There is a time lag between the decrease in glucose concentration and the cessation of the effect of expressed insulin. However, Lee *et al.* (2000) reported that the risk of hypoglycemia was very low when they used single chain insulin analog. The development of more sensitive glucose-responsive promoter will be beneficial to avoid this potential side effect.

Genetic modification of the islet transplant *in vitro* prior to transplantation could improve its survival, function, and safety following transplantation. The shortage of transplantable β cells can be overcome by the generation of β-cell lines. In addition to providing an abundant source of β cells, cell lines represent a more reproducible source, compared with islets, with respect to functional properties. Another advantage of cell lines is the ability to modify the cells by gene transfer in culture to improve their properties.

Pancreatic islets consist predominantly of extremely slow-dividing α-, β-, and δ-cells. This aspect of the islet cells demands the use of gene transfer vehicles that can deliver genes into quiescent cells. One of the gene therapy methods to address this point is to use islet-specific Th1 lymphocytes. Islet-specific Th1 clones was used as a vehicle to deliver IL-10 to pancreatic islets (Moritani *et al.*, 1996). Islet-specific Th1 lymphocytes were transduced with the IL-10 gene and transferred into NOD mice. IL-10-transduced Th1 cells could deliver IL-10 to islets according to their T-cell antigen receptor specificity, and they could prevent insulitis and destruction of islet β-cell in NOD mice. Similarly, another way to deliver the cytokine gene to pancreatic β-cells is at the level of activation and function of the antigen presenting cells (APC) in the islets. These APCs will take up antigen at the damage sites and produce pro-inflammatory molecules. Thus, the APCs of the islets of Langerhans, inducing macrophages and dendritic cells (DC), are possible targets for gene therapy.

FUTURE PROSPECTS

Although the history of gene therapy for autoimmune diabetes is rather short, the current accumulated data are quite encouraging. A thorough understanding of the underlying pathogenesis will help us design several treatment options. The development of molecular biology and chemistry makes it possible to construct a pancreas-specific plasmid or modify gene carrier directed to the pancreas. To prevent autoimmune diabetes without any side-effects, pancreas targeting gene carriers as well as β cell targeting plasmid should be developed.

An accurate prediction of the clinical onset in the human diabetic patient is necessary for gene therapy to be successful. We need to investigate the therapeutic dose of gene expression plasmid for the treatment of insulitis. Since insulin gene delivery should be closely coupled to the plasma glucose concentration, the knowledge of glucose responsive elements will enable us to deliver therapeutic plasmid more efficiently to β-cells. Finally, for the human trial we need to develop a more efficient and safer gene carrier, which should be applicable to repeated injections.

REFERENCES

Argaud, D., Kirby, T.L., Newgard, C.B. and Lange, A.J. (1997) Stimulation of glucose-6-phosphatase gene expression by glucose and fructose-2, 6-bisphosphate. *J. Biol. Chem.*, **272**, 12854–12861.

Bach, J.F. (1994) Insulin-dependent diabetes mellitus as an autoimmune disease. *Endocr. Rev.*, **15**, 516–542.

Blanas, E., Carbone, F.R., Allismi, J., Miller, J.F. and Heath, W.R. (1996) Induction of autoimmune diabetes by oral administration of autoantigen. *Science*, **274**, 1707–1709.

Boyle, D.L., Nguyen, K.H., Zhuang, S., Shi, Y., McCormack, J.E., Chada, S. *et al.* (1999) Intra-articular IL-4 gene therapy in arthritis: anti-inflammatory effect and enhanced Th2 activity. *Gene Ther.*, **6**, 1911–1918.

Butler, M.H., Solimena, M., Dirkz, R.J., Hayday, A. and DeCamilli, P. (1993) Identification of a dominant epitope of glutamic acid decarboxylase (GAD65) recognized by autoantibodies in stiff man syndrome. *J. Exp. Med.*, **178**, 2097–2106.

Chen, R., Meseck, M.L. and Woo, S.L.C. (2001) Auto-regulated hepatic insulin gene expression in type 1 diabetic rats. *Mol. Ther.*, **3**, 584–590.

Daw, K., Ujihara, N., Atkinson, M.A. and Powers, A.C. (1996) Glutamic acid decarboxylase autoantibodies in stiff man syndrome and insulin-dependent diabetes mellitus exhibit similarities and differences in epitope recognition. *J. Immunol.*, **156**, 818–825.

Doiron, B., Cuif, M.H., Kahn, A. and Diaz-Guerra, M.J. (1994) Respective roles of glucose, fructose, and insulin in the regulation of the liver-specific pyruvate kinase gene promoter. *J. Biol. Chem.*, **269**, 10213–10216.

Efrat, S., Surana, M. and Fleischer, N. (1991) Glucose induces insulin gene transcription in a murine pancreatic β-cell line. *J. Biol. Chem.*, **266**, 11141–11143.

Evans, C.H., Robbins, P.D., Ghivizzani, S.C., Herdon, J.H., Kang, R., Bahnson, A.B. *et al.* (1996) Clinical trial to assess the safety, feasibility, and efficacy of transferring a potentially anti-arthritic cytokine gene to human joints with rheumatoid arthritis. *Hum. Gene Ther.*, **7**, 1261–1280.

Faust, A., Rothe, H., Schade, U., Lampeter, E. and Kolb, H. (1996) Primary nonfunction of islet grafts in autoimmune diabetic nonobese diabetic mice is prevented by treatment with interleukin-4 and interleukin-10. *Transplantation*, **62**, 648–652.

German, M.S., Moss, L.G. and Rutter, W.J. (1990) Regulation of insulin gene expression by glucose and calcium in transfected primary islet cultures. *J. Biol. Chem.*, **265**, 22063–22066.

Goodison, S., Kenna, S. and Ashcroft, S.J.H. (1992) Control of insulin gene expression by glucose. *Biochem. J.*, **285**, 563–568.

Gros, L., Montoliu, L., Riu, E., Lebrigand, L. and Bosch, F. (1997) Regulated production of mature insulin by non-beta-cells. *Hum. Gene Ther.*, **8**, 2249–2259.

Hohmeier, H.E., Thigpen, A., Tran, V.V., Davis, R. and Newgard, C.B. (1998) Stable expression of manganese superoxide dismutase (MnSOD) in insulinoma cells prevents IL-1 beta-induced cytotoxicity and reduces nitric oxide production. *J. Clin. Invest.*, **101**, 1811–1820.

Jacob, C.O., Asiso, S., Michie, S.A., McDevitt, H.O. and Acha-Orbea, H. (1990) Prevention of diabetes in nonobese diabetic mice by tumor necrosis factor (TNF): similarities between TNF-α and interleukin 1. *Proc. Natl. Acad. Sci. USA*, **87**, 968–972.

Jump, D.B., Bell, A. and Santiago, V. (1990) Thyroid hormone and dietary carbohydrate interact to regulate rat liver S14 gene transcription and chromatin structure. *J. Biol. Chem.*, **265**, 3474–3478.

Khachatryan, A., Guerder, S., Palluault, F., Cote, G., Solimena, M., Valentijn, K. *et al.* (1997) Targeted expression of the neuropeptide calcitonin gene-related peptide to β cells prevents diabetes in NOD mice. *J. Immunol.*, **158**, 1409–1416.

Kennedy, H.J., Rafiq, I., Pouli, A.E. and Rutter, G.A. (1999) Glucose enhances insulin promoter activity in MIN6 β-cells independently of changes in intracellular Ca^{2+} concentration and insulin secretion. *Biochem. J.*, **342**, 275–280.

Ko, K.S., Lee, M., Koh, J.J. and Kim, S.W. (2001) Combined administration of IL-4 and IL-10 plasmids to prevent the development of autoimmune diabetes in NOD mice. *Mol. Ther.* (*in press*).

Koh, J.J., Ko, K.S., Lee, M., Han, S., Park, J.S. and Kim, S.W. (2000) Degradable polymeric carrier for the delivery of IL-10 plasmid DNA to prevent autoimmune insulitis of NOD mice. *Gene Ther.*, **7**, 2099–2105.

Kroemer, G. (1997) The proto-oncogene Bcl-2 and its role in regulating apoptosis. *Nat. Med.*, **3**, 614–620.

Lee, H.C., Kim, S.J., Kim, K.S., Shin, H.C. and Yoon, J.W. (2000) Remission in models of type 1 diabetes by gene therapy using a single-chain insulin analogue. *Nature*, **408**, 483–488.

Lee, M., Han, S., Ko, K.S. and Kim, S.W. (2001a) Cell type specific and glucose responsive expression of interleukin-4 by using insulin promoter and water soluble lipopolymer. *J. Control. Rel.*, **75**, 421–429.

Lee, M., Han, S., Ko, K.S., Koh, J.J., Park, J.S., Yoon, J.-W. *et al.* (2001b) Repression of GAD autoantigen in pancreas β cell by delivery of antisense plasmid/PEG-*g*-PLL complex. *Mol. Ther.*, **4**, 339–346.

Lefrancois-Martinez, A.M., Diaz-Guerra, M.J., Vallet, V., Kahn, A. and Antoine, B. (1994) Glucose-dependent regulation of the L-pyruvate kinase gene in a hepatoma cell line is independent of insulin and cyclic AMP. *FASEB. J.*, **8**, 89–96.

Lampeter, E.B. (1993) Discussion remark to session 24: BMT in autoimmune disease. *Exp. Hematol.*, **21**, 1155.

Liu, Y., Rabinovitch, A., Suarez-Pinzon, W., Muhkerjee, B., Brownlee, M., Edelstein, D. *et al.* (1996) Expression of the bcl-2 gene from a defective HSV-1 amplicon vector protects pancreatic beta-cells from apoptosis. *Hum. Gene Ther.*, **7**, 1719–1726.

Lu, D., Tamemoto, H., Shibata, H., Saito, I. and Takeuchi, T. (1998) Regulatable production of insulin from primary-cultured hepatocytes: Insulin production is up-regulated by glucagon and cAMP and down-regulated by insulin. *Gene Ther.*, **5**, 888–895.

Mahato, R.I., Lee, M., Han, S., Maheshwari, A. and Kim, S.W. (2001) Intratumoral delivery of p2CMVmIL-12 using water-soluble lipopolymers. *Mol. Ther.*, **4**, 130–138.

Massillon, D., Barzilai, N., Chen, W., Hu, M. and Rossetti, L. (1996) Glucose regulates *in vivo* glucose-6-phosphatase gene expression in the liver of diabetic rats. *J. Biol. Chem.*, **271**, 9871–9874.

McFarland, H.F. (1996) Complexities in the treatment of autoimmune disease. *Science*, **274**, 2037–2038.

518   *Kyung Soo Ko, Minhyung Lee and Sung Wan Kim*

Menard, V., Jacobs, H., Jun, H.-S., Yoon, J.-W. and Kim, S.W. (1999) Anti-GAD monoclonal antibody delays the onset of diabetes mellitus in NOD mice. *Pharm. Res.*, **16**, 1059–1066.

Mitanchez, D., Chen, R., Massias, J.F., Proteu, A., Mignon, A., Bertagna, X. and Kahn, A. (1997) Regulated expression of mature human insulin in the liver of transgenic mice. *FEBS lett.*, **421**, 285–289.

Moritani, M., Yoshimoto, K., Ii, S., Kondo, M., Iwahana, H., Yamaoka, T. *et al.* (1996) Prevention of adoptively transferred diabetes in nonobese diabetic mice with IL-10-transduced islet-specific Th1 lymphocytes. *J. Clin. Invest.*, **98**, 1851–1859.

Mueller, R., Krahl, T. and Sarvetnick, N. (1996) Pancreatic expression of interleukin-4 abrogates insulitis and autoimmune diabetes in nonobese diabetic (NOD) mice. *J. Exp. Med.*, **184**, 1093–1099.

Nitta, Y., Tashiro, F., Tokui, M., Shimada, A., Takei, I., Tabayashi, K. *et al.* (1998) Systemic delivery of interleukin 10 by intramuscular injection of expression plasmid DNA prevents autoimmune diabetes in nonobese diabetic mice. *Hum. Gene Ther.*, **9**, 1701–1707.

Odagiri, H., Wang, J. and German, M.S. (1996) Function of the human insulin promoter in primary cultured islet cells. *J. Biol. Chem.*, **271**, 1909–1915.

Pennline, K.J., Roque-Gaffney, E. and Monahan, M. (1994) Recombinant human IL-10 prevents the onset of diabetes in the nonobese diabetic mouse. *Clin. Immunol. Immuno-pathol.*, **71**, 169–175.

Piccirillo, C.A., Chang, Y. and Prud'homme, G.J. (1998) TGF-β1 somatic gene therapy prevents autoimmune disease in nonobese diabetic mice. *J. Immunol.*, **161**, 3950–3956.

Pleau, J.M., Fernandez-Saravia, F., Esling, A., Homo-Delarche, F. and Dardenne, M. (1995) Prevention of autoimmune diabetes in non-obese diabetic female mice by treatment with recombinant glutamic acid decarboxylase (GAD65). *Clin. Immunol. Immunopathol.*, **751**, 90–95.

Powrie, F., Menon, S. and Coffman, R.L. (1993) Interleukin-4 and interleukin-10 synergize to inhibit cell-mediated immunity *in vivo. Eur. J. Immunol.*, **23**, 2223–2229.

Qin, L., Ding, Y., Pahud, D.R., Chang, E., Imeriale, M.J. and Bromberg, J.S. (1997) Promoter attenuation in gene therapy: Interferon-γ and tumor necrosis factor-α inhibit transgene expression. *Hum. Gene Ther.*, **8**, 2019–2029.

Rabinovitch, A. and Skyler, J.S. (1998) Prevention of type 1 diabetes. *Med. Clin. North Am.*, **82**, 739–755.

Rabinovitch, A., Suarez-Pinzon, W., Stryanadka, K., Ju, Q., Edelstein, D., Brownlee, M. *et al.* (1999) Transfection of human pancreatic islets with an anti-apoptotic gene (bcl-2) protects b-cells from cytokine-induced destruction. *Diabetes*, **48**, 1223–1229.

Rapoport, M.J., Jaramillo, A., Zipris, D., Lazarus, A.H., Serreze, D.V., Leiter, E.H. *et al.* (1993) Interleukin 4 reverse T cell proliferative unresponsiveness and prevents the onset of diabetes in nonobese diabetic mice. *J. Exp. Med.*, **178**, 87–99.

Redmon, J.B., Towle, H.C. and Robertson, R.P. (1994) Regulation of human insulin gene transcription by glucose, epinephrine, and somatostatin. *Diabetes*, **43**, 546–551.

Robert, J.J., Bouilleret, V., Ridoux, V., Valin, A., Geoffroy, M.C., Mallet, J. *et al.* (1997) Adenovirus-mediated transfer of a functional GAD gene into nerve cells: potential for the treatment of neurological diseases. *Gene Ther.*, **4**, 1237–1245.

Rogy, M.A., Beinhauer, B.G., Reinisch, W., Huang, L. and Pokieser, P. (2000) Transfer of interleukin-4 and inleukin-10 in patients with severe inflammatory bowel disease of the rectum. *Hum. Gene Ther.*, **11**, 1731–1741.

Seino, H., Takahashi, K., Satoh, J., Zhu, X.P., Sagara, M., Masuda, T. *et al.* (1993) Prevention of autoimmune diabetes with lymphotoxin in NOD mice. *Diabetes*, **42**, 398–404.

Sharma, A. and Stein, R. (1994) Glucose-induced transcription of the insulin gene is mediated by factors required for β-cell-type specific expression. *Mol. Cell. Biol.*, **14**, 871–879.

Sibley, R.K., Sutherland, D.E.R., Goetz, F. and Michael, A.F. (1985) Recurrent diabetes mellitus in the pancreas iso- and allograft. *Lab. Invest.*, **53**, 132–144.

Tian, J., Atkinson, M., Clare-Salzler, M., Herschenfeld, A., Forsthuber, T., Lehmann, P. *et al.* (1996) Nasal administration of glutamic decarboxylase peptides induces Th2 responses and prevents murine insulin-dependent diabetes. *J. Exp. Med.*, **183**, 1561–1567.

Tisch, R., Yang, X.D., Singer, S., Liblau, R.S., Fugger, L. and McDevitt, H.O. (1993) Immune response to glutamic acid decarboxylase correlates with insulitis in non-obese diabetic mice. *Nature*, **366**, 72–75.

Wilson, C.A., Jacobs, C., Baker, P., Baskin, D.G., Dower, S., Lernmark, A. *et al.* (1990) IL-1 beta modulation of spontaneous autoimmune diabetes and thyroiditis in the BB rat. *J. Immunol.*, **144**, 3784–3788.

Xu, L., Daly, T., Gao, C., Flotte, T.R., Song, S., Byrne, B.J. *et al.* (2001) CMV-β-actin promoter directs higher expression from an adeno-associated viral vector in the liver than the cytomegalovirus or elongation factor 1α promoter and results in therapeutic levels of human factor X in mice. *Hum. Gene Ther.*, **12**, 563–573.

Yang, Y.-W. and Kotin, R.M. (2000) Glucose-responsive gene delivery in pancreatic islet cells via recombinant adeno-associated viral vectors. *Pharm. Res.*, **17**, 1056–1060.

Yoon, J.-W., Yoon, C.-S., Lim, H-W., Huang, Q.Q., Kang, Y., Pyun, K.H. *et al.* (1999) Control of autoimmune diabetes in NOD mice by GAD expression or suppression in β cells. *Science*, **284**, 1183–1187.

Zheng, X.X., Steele, A.W., Hancock, W.W., Stevens, A.C., Nickerson, P.W., Roy-Chaudhury, P., Tian, Y. and Strom, T.B. (1997) A noncytolytic IL-10/Fc fusion protein prevents diabetes, blocks autoimmunity, and promotes suppressor phenomena in NOD mice. *J. Immunol.*, **158**, 4507–4513.

Zielasek, J., Burkart, V., Naylor, P., Goldstein, A., Kiesel, U. and Kolb, H. (1990) Interleukin-2-dependent control of disease development in spontaneously diabetic BB rats. *Immunology*, **69**, 209–214.

Index

Printed and bound by CPI Group (UK) Ltd, Croydon, CR0 4YY

23/10/2024

01778226-0009